AF694149

Medical Radiology

Radiation Oncology

Series Editors

Luther W. Brady
Hans-Peter Heilmann
Michael Molls
Carsten Nieder

For further volumes:
http://www.springer.com/series/4353

Associate Editors

Zeljko Vujaskovic, Ph.D., Professor of Radiation Oncology, Department of Radiation Oncology, Duke University Medical Center, Box 3085, Durham, NC, 27710, USA

Kishan J. Pandya, MD, Professor Emeritus, School of Medicine and Dentistry, University of Rochester, 601 Elmwood Ave, Box HH67, Rochester, NY, 14620, USA

Advisory Editors

Yuhchyau Chen, MD, Ph.D., Department Chair and Richard Bell Professor, Director of Clinical Investigation, Department of Radiation Oncology, Professor in Oncology, James P. Wilmot Cancer Center, 601 Elmwood Ave, Box 647, Rochester, NY, 14642, USA

Luis Felipe Fajardo, L-G, MD, Emeritus Professor of Pathology, Stanford University School of Medicine, 4190 Cherry Oaks Place, Palo Alto, CA, 94306, USA

John Hansen, Ph.D., Professor of Neurobiology and Anatomy, and Associate Dean, School of Medicine and Dentistry, University of Rochester, Rochester, NY, USA

Managing Editor

Sisi Lisa Chen, Executive Coordinator of the Survivorship Advisory Committee, Editorial Assistant, University of Rochester Medical Center, 601 Elmwood Ave, Box 647, Rochester, NY, 14642, USA

Co-Managing Editor

Liyi Xie, MD, Department of Radiation Oncology, University of North Carolina, Chapel Hill, NC, USA; Department of Radiation Oncology, Fudan University of Shanghai Cancer Center, Shanghai, China

Assistant Managing Editor

Callise Wiley, Editorial Assistant to Dr. Philip Rubin, Oncoideas, Inc

Philip Rubin • Louis S. Constine
Lawrence B. Marks
Editors

ALERT – Adverse Late Effects of Cancer Treatment

Volume 1: General Concepts and Specific Precepts

Springer

Editors
Philip Rubin MD
Professor and Chair Emeritus
Department of Radiation Oncology
Former Associate Director of the James.
P. Wilmot Cancer Center, University
of Rochester Medical Center
Rochester, NY
USA

Louis S. Constine MD, FASTRO
The Philip Rubin Professor of Radiation
Oncology and Pediatrics, Vice Chair
Department of Radiation Oncology, James P.
Wilmot Cancer Center
University of Rochester Medical Center
Rochester, NY
USA

Lawrence B. Marks MD, FASTRO
Dr. Sidney K. Simon Distinguished Professor
of Oncology Research, Professor and Chairman
Department of Radiation Oncology
University of North Carolina and Lineberger,
Comprehensive Cancer Center
Chapel Hill, NC
USA

ISSN 0942-5373
ISBN 978-3-662-50134-4 ISBN 978-3-540-72314-1 (eBook)
DOI 10.1007/978-3-540-72314-1
Springer Heidelberg New York Dordrecht London

© Springer-Verlag Berlin Heidelberg 2014
Softcover reprint of the hardcover 1st edition 2014
This work is subject to copyright. All rights are reserved by the Publisher, whether the whole or part of the material is concerned, specifically the rights of translation, reprinting, reuse of illustrations, recitation, broadcasting, reproduction on microfilms or in any other physical way, and transmission or information storage and retrieval, electronic adaptation, computer software, or by similar or dissimilar methodology now known or hereafter developed. Exempted from this legal reservation are brief excerpts in connection with reviews or scholarly analysis or material supplied specifically for the purpose of being entered and executed on a computer system, for exclusive use by the purchaser of the work. Duplication of this publication or parts thereof is permitted only under the provisions of the Copyright Law of the Publisher's location, in its current version, and permission for use must always be obtained from Springer. Permissions for use may be obtained through RightsLink at the Copyright Clearance Center. Violations are liable to prosecution under the respective Copyright Law.
The use of general descriptive names, registered names, trademarks, service marks, etc. in this publication does not imply, even in the absence of a specific statement, that such names are exempt from the relevant protective laws and regulations and therefore free for general use.

While the advice and information in this book are believed to be true and accurate at the date of publication, neither the authors nor the editors nor the publisher can accept any legal responsibility for any errors or omissions that may be made. The publisher makes no warranty, express or implied, with respect to the material contained herein.

Printed on acid-free paper

Springer is part of Springer Science+Business Media (www.springer.com)

This volume recognizes our patients…
Cancer Survivors who have benefited from the treatment and lived with its consequences
To save one life is to save the whole world
I dedicate this book to my long-time friend Mayer Mitchell (Bubba), who recently succumbed to cancer and the late effects of cancer therapy. Mayer's life epitomized the challenges of a cancer survivor. He had stage IV Hodgkin's disease, Breast cancer, Prostate cancer, Urinary Bladder cancer, and Rectal cancer. Each cured cancer was followed by a radiation/chemotherapy-associated complication. Nevertheless, he endured and, with his brother Abe, built thousands of homes, shopping centers in five southern states over five decades.

Philip Rubin

I dedicate this book to my many teachers and mentors. My parents were both teachers in the NYC public schools and I grew up with a strong sense of respect for teachers. As I have always been drawn to the physical sciences, I have particularly fond feelings towards many instructors in math, chemistry, physics and engineering. At the completion of my third year of medical school at the University of Rochester (in New York), I could not envision practicing in any one of the core clinical specialties; I missed the quantitative aspects of the physical sciences. While I was contemplating a career change to become a math teacher, my then girl friend (now wife) Caryn, who was also a medical student at Rochester, said to me, "I heard a talk today from someone who is a radiation oncologist, you should go talk to them, I think you might like that field." Serendipity. And she was right!

My subsequent visit to the radiation oncology department started my >30 year relationship with Dr. Rubin. As a student at Rochester, I have fond memories of shadowing Dr. Rubin on Wednesday afternoons. As I remember it, he used to see all of the patients under treatment in his department each week. So, the patients all had two "weekly checks"; one with their primary treating radiation oncologist, and a second with Dr. Rubin. He used to take great pride in explaining the rationale for the radiation treatment, and always emphasized the need to understand the risks of the radiation treatment when choosing fields and doses.

Over the next three decades, Dr. Rubin proved to be a great mentor, role model, and friend. He has supported and nurtured my interests in radiation-induced normal tissue injury; e.g. getting me involved with his LENT-SOMA initiatives and helping me to formulate ideas and projects. Helping to write a book with Dr. Rubin, who has helped our field understand so much about the effects of radiation, has been and honor. Thank you Phil. Thanks also to Sandy Constine- a long-time friend and colleague. Sandy has made tremendous contributions to better understand the effects of radiation, particularly in children. Your dedication to ameliorating pediatric late effects is inspiring. I am glad that we were able to help Phil with this book- published approximately 35 years after Phil's landmark contribution Clinical Radiation Pathology (published with George Casarett). This book proved to be a labor of love for us all.

I am thankful to all who contributed to this book; the authors, editors, administrative assistants, and our publisher. Your efforts and expertise are much appreciated. Thank you to my many excellent teachers and mentors throughout school, including college (Cooper Union), medical school (University of Rochester), internship (Sinai Hospital of Baltimore) and residency (Mass General). Thanks also to my many colleagues at UNC and Duke for providing a fertile and productive environment, and for serving as teachers and mentors. Special thanks to Drs. Leonard R. Prosnitz, Edward C. Halperin and Gustavo S. Montana for their mentorship and guidance.

Thank you to my family for their support: to my

parents (Hyman and Helen Marks), to my wife Caryn-whose love, caring and encouragement are ongoing sources of strength, and to our three children (Noah, Samuel and Benjamin).

Lawrence B. Marks

"For the person fighting cancer, each day is precious and must be faced with courage. For the physician, each patient is an inspiration. For the survivor of cancer, the world is full and each day is a celebration." I wrote these words many years ago, and continue to reflect on the many sources of inspiration that grace my life. I feel tremendous gratitude for my good fortune to work in a field and live a life that refreshes my spirit on a daily basis. This book honors the memory of our patients who did not survive cancer, but also those who have faced mortality but found a way to embrace all that life offers. A friend of mine once said: "That is the essence of surviving cancer—making your life a passionate statement instead of just marking time."

I am surrounded by individuals who have helped me understand the wonder of my life, and afforded me the opportunity to contribute what I can. Philip Rubin, a giant in our field, towers above all others in my professional life. On a snowy night in Rochester 32 years ago he persuaded me to join his faculty by clearly outlining my future…one in which he would work with me to fulfill whatever personal destiny I might have. He defined the trait that I value above all others, curiosity. He combined that with enthusiasm and creativity, and a drive to benefit others. I have strived to emulate this great man. I have been fortunate to have other mentors who also demonstrated these qualities, notably John Felstiner who was my English teacher at Stanford, Leigh Thompson who was a professor at The Johns Hopkins medical school, Archie Bleyer during my fellowship in Pediatric Oncology at the University of Washington, Sarah Donaldson during my residency in radiation oncology at Stanford, and Edward Halperin and Larry Marks who have been friends and colleagues during many of these years. However, I am also appreciative of the many young physicians, nurses, social workers, and others who are focused on improving the lives of cancer patients and enable me to do my job.

My personal life has been graced by the lady who I met 42 years ago, and then married 41 years ago. Sally has a spirit of giving to others that cannot be extinguished, and on a daily basis rekindles my flame. The joy that we both receive from our remarkable children, Alysia and Josh, fills us and affirms the relevance of our lives. For me, they demonstrate the gifts that life affords, and foster my dedication to provide my patients with the opportunity to live their lives as fully as possible.

Louis S. Constine

Foreword

The publication in 1968 of the book by Rubin and Casarett entitled *Clinical Radiation Pathology*, in Volumes I and II, represented a hallmark statement regarding the late effects related to radiation therapy. Since that time, there has been no significant comprehensive publication dealing with early and late effects in normal tissues from all forms of cancer treatment.

The new text by Rubin and his co-workers comprehensively documents contemporary understanding of the adverse late effects of cancer treatment in a coherent, multidisciplinary approach related to the care of cancer survivors. All major organs are affected by the treatment program, whether it be radiation, chemotherapy, or surgical treatment, and these impacts must be taken into consideration in any discussion on what might be the most appropriate treatment in cancer management. Modern cancer treatment is clearly based on safe intensification of radiation therapy, chemotherapy, and biologic modifiers. Not only has this resulted in a significant general increase in survivorship from cancer to 64 % overall, but the survival rate is considerably higher for selected malignancies, such as 87 % for breast cancer and 80 % for childhood cancers. Malignancies resistant to therapy have necessitated the utilization of aggressive treatment approaches associated with improvement in survivorship but also with increased risk of normal tissue complications. Late effects can occur years after the cessation of the treatment regimen, tending to arise earlier with radiation therapy than with chemotherapy. The present text, reflecting more recent publications, offers landmark statements with regard to the potential for such effects, the general concepts and principles relating to their development, and the dynamic interplay among molecular cytologic and histopathologic events. There is now much greater awareness that modern cancer treatment leads to not only physiologic and metabolic abnormalities, but also clinical manifestations that dictate the need for innovative new aggressive programs of management.

Without question the present text represents a dramatic step forward from the original Rubin/Casarett text, with more emphasis on the contemporary situations that each oncologist faces in their practice on a day-to-day basis. The efforts on the part of Rubin and his colleagues have borne fruit. This new book provides readers with significant information about late effects and how they might be managed. It is recommended for inclusion on the shelf of every oncologist and should be at the forefront of practitioners' minds when considering the various treatment regimens.

Luther W. Brady, MD
Hans-Peter Heilmann, MD
Michael Molls, MD
Carsten Nieder, MD

Preface

Concept of the Biocontinuum

"The past is the beginning of the beginning"

H. G Wells

In 1968, Casarett and Rubin proposed a paradigm to formally link acute and late effects as a biophysiopathologic and clinical continuum. Over the past four decades, numerous laboratory and clinical studies have provided additional insights to refine this paradigm. The first section of this book reviews the general concepts that frame the initial paradigm, and a series of paradigm shifts. These introductory chapters provide the foundation to the Organ/Site-specific chapters that form the core of this book.

The introductory section:

- "Prologue: Surviving Cancer: SEER Statistics": Biocontinuum of the radiation-induced pathophysiology was conceptualized as a course of events beginning with acute injury, followed by recovery, and then arteriocapillary fibrosis that leads to cell senescence (Casarett paradigm). These concepts of the waxing and waning clinical expressions of organ damage were based on observations from the beginning of the supervoltage era that are translated into greater depth doses and increased organ injury. The natural history of this organ damage was carefully traced, and mechanisms were postulated. (Rubin paradigm).
- "Biocontinuum of the Pathophysiology Paradigm": The importance of the microvasculature and the vascular endothelial cells as the most radiosensitive cell among the various elements of the mesenchyme was carefully studied in the laboratory and in pathologic specimens. For many organs, the late effects appeared to be mediated through injury of the microcirculation reinforcing Casarett's observations (Fajardo Paradigm shift). The importance of the interaction of various organs to both radiation and chemotherapy during a prolonged course of multimodal treatment is embodied in the multiorgan domino effect and host effects. (Sutherland and Seimann Paradigm Shift).
- "Biophysiopathology of the Microvasculature and Microcirculation": A series of in vivo/in vitro experiments demonstrated a perpetual cytokine cascade following radiation that fortified Casarett's "there is latent period histologically" after radiation or other cytotoxic treatment. The release of proinflammatory chemokines and cytokines (ILI, IL6, and TNF) simultaneously with profibrotic cytokines (TGFb and RDGF) indicated that the biocontinuum, once initiated, continues over time. The incremental persistence and interrelationships of these families of cytokines after chemotherapy and surgical wound healing provides a commonality to explain increased toxicity. (Finklestein and Williams Paradigm Shift).

- "Molecular Mechanisms of Radiation Induced Injury": An improved understanding of the biological processes that underlie the evolving clinical events affords the opportunity to target specific mediators of these processes in order to mitigate (i.e., reduce or prevent) subsequent late effects.
- "Biodetection and Biointervention: Cytokine Pathways as a Rationale for Anti-cytokine Interventions Post-Radiation": Advances in Imaging (e.g., CT, SPECT, MRI, and MRS) were exploited as a powerful means to objectively characterize *regional* organ injury in a variety of tissues (e.g., lung, heart, liver, brain, and parotid). By relating regional dose to the degree of regional injury, dose–response relationships for regional injury can be defined. These dose–response relationships are largely volume independent, and thus might be taken as an objective measure of inherent radiation sensitivity. For a parallel organ, the sum of regional injuries might be expected to be related to the degree of global injury (Marks paradigm). The available data for the lung does suggest such a relationship, albeit weak.
- "Quantitative/Objective Analyses of RT-Induced Late Normal Tissue Injury Using Functional Imaging": Many systems have evolved for grading the adverse effects of cancer treatment. In 1995 Rubin, Constine, and colleagues developed the SOMA-LENT scoring system. This approach systematically and objectively distinguished the subjective, objective, management-based, and analytical-based components of scoring treatment-related organ injury. A new common toxicity criteria sponsored by all cancer disciplines and the NCI evolved into a single uniform system merging acute and late effects. It applied to all modalities a grading dictionary of common terms to measure toxicity, i.e., CTC version 3.0. (Rubin and Trotti Paradigm Shift).
- "Biograding of Normal Tissue TNM Toxicity Taxonomy: Scoring the Adverse Effects of Cancer Treatment": The link between radiation exposure to a particular organ and the clinical manifestation of injury may be complex. It depends on several obvious factors such as the inherent sensitivity of the target cells and the volume of the organ irradiated (e.g., parameters from the DVH). Less obvious, but equally important, factors include the architecture of the organ (series vs. parallel), the "size/structure" of the organ's functional subunits, and the distribution of function within the organ (homogeneous vs. heterogeneous). Further, some clinical endpoints reflect focal injury to an organ; while others reflect global organ injury, and some endpoints may be affected by injury to several organs (i.e., endpoints may not be specific to a particular organ). Milano, Rubin, and Marks review the impact of these various factors, and how they interact with each other, on one's ability to relate DVHs to clinical outcomes. They also review and compare prior attempts to summarize the relationship between dose/volume and clinical outcomes. (Byfield and Marks Paradigm Shift)
- "Understanding and Predicting Radiation-Associated Normal Tissue Injury: A Global and Historical Perspective": A variety of chemotherapeutic agents, and newer biological agents, may both directly affect target organs, and also influence the impact of radiation on many organs. This is meticulously explored by Kishan and Fung.
- "Biotoxicity of Chemotherapy": Patients treated with cytotoxic therapy are at risk for a multiplicity of long-term side effects. Systematic strategies for post-treatment surveillance are often available for survivors of pediatric cancer, but are largely lacking for adult survivors. Ng and Hudson review the surveillance strategies that have been suggested, and make some recommendations where well-accepted follow-up recommendations do not exist.

- "BioSurveillance and Longitudinal Lifelong Guidelines": Children appear to be at particular risk for treatment-related late effects. This heightened sensitivity appears to be related to their relatively rapid cellular kinetics (i.e., more mitotic activity than in adults). Interorgan variations in sensitivity might be related to variations in the cellular kinetics between the different organs. Organ "growth" might reflect hypertrophy, proliferation, and/or stromal accumulation. In children, therapies might also reduce their mitotic potential thereby leading to late effects. (Constine Paradigm Shift). The concept of aging/senescence is portrayed as the loss of "mitotic potential" over time. Numerous radiation studies have verified this concept and the loss of cell renewal capacity after chemotherapy (established by exposing mice to busulfan and uncovering a loss in bone marrow renewal capacity). (Botnik and Hellman Paradigm Shift)
- "BioPediatric Complexities of Growth and Development": Genetic and epigenetic factors that might influence the sensitivity to cytotoxic therapies are reviewed. This is an area of increasingly active investigation.

The Organ/Site-specific section

- This section comprises 26 chapters. Each of these is organized in a relatively uniform manner. Where practical, the site-specific chapters share common figures and tables, and include the following sections:
- *Literature Landmarks and Milestones* that have contributed to understanding adverse acute/late effects. There will be more numerous citations in the bibliography
- *Anatomy* section illustrations are based on "Tillman's Anatomy Atlas" (Springer) and each organ's macrostructure is described as parallel (often solid) or serial (often hollow) structures, and provide a basis for defining the anatomic/physiologic functional subunits.
- *Histology* section defines the normal tissue's microarchitecture often illustrated utilizing "Zhang's Histology Atlas" (Springer); the parenchymal cell's mitotic potential will be notated with Casarett, Cowdry Schema and Relate to cell's radiosensitivity to insult by radiation.
- *Physiology* section enhances the understanding of the functional subunit and provides parameters and metrics to assess toxicity.
- *Biology* section describes the molecular events within the normal tissue's cells (e.g., parenchymal, endothelial, macrophageal/lymphocyte, and interstitial stromal fibroblasts), and the associated cytokine cascade induced by therapies.
- *Pathophysiology* section includes histopathologic illustrations of acute/late effects in the normal tissue.
- *Clinical Syndromes* section provides an overview of clinical issues including items such as means of detection, differential diagnoses, risk factors, comorbidities, and management. Tables from CTC V3.0 and LENT-SOMA will tabulate symptoms and signs and the grading of treatment toxicity.
- *Imaging* section will provide illustrations of acute/late events as seen on diagnostic images (e.g., CT, SPECT, or MRI).
- *Endoscopy and Laboratory* tests of function are discussed and correlated with treatment-related injury as well.
- *Radiation tolerance* sections summarize the dose/volume/outcome data and highlight typical Dose/Time and Dose/Volume limits commonly used clinically. The predictive ability of measurements such as Mean Dose, V20, and V40 or equivalents is discussed.

- *Chemotherapy* agents are tabulated, along with their associated toxicity, and specific anatomic/physiologic features. The interactions between Radiation and Chemotherapy (and surgery where applicable) in causing toxicity are reviewed.
- *Mitigators*, preventive agents, and Interventions are described.
- *Future Directions and Special Topics* section addresses unique aspects for the specific site being addressed with prospects for future clinical investigational studies and laboratory research.
- *Literature Landmarks and Milestones* that have contributed to understanding adverse acute/late effects.
- *Bibliography* provides a selected list of recommended reading (*).

This book represents the most-recent attempt of the authors to summarize/categorize/understand LENT (late effects of normal tissues) over the last several decades:

1. Rubin & Casarett: Clinical Radiation Pathology, 1968
2. Rubin & Bartelink et al: LENT SOMA IJROBP, 1995
3. Trotti & Rubin et al: NCI common toxicity criteria, CTC version 3, incorporated adverse late effects, and subsequent updates
4. QUANTEC, 2010
5. Rubin, Constine, Marks: ALERT, 2013

Dr. Marks is supported by NCI Grant CA69579

Philip Rubin
Louis S. Constine
Lawrence B. Marks

Acknowledgements

The editors are grateful for the tremendous effort of Lisa Chen, our managing editor. She indeed was the glue that held all the pieces of this effort together. She nurtured the elements through their gestation and now its birth.

Global Acknowledgement

The editors sought to create a comprehensive book covering a wide array of information. As such, we relied heavily on prior works addressing similar topics, including many works that we helped to create. Portions of this book were adopted, with permission, from the following sources:

Special Issue of the Int J Radiat Oncol Biol and Phys from March 30, 1995 dedicated to the SOMA (subjective, objective, management, analytic) system to assess Late Effects of Normal Tissues (LENT). This initiative aimed to better standardize the manner in which normal tissue effects are quantitatively scored.

Special Issue of the Int J Radiat Oncol Biol and Phys from March 1, 2010 dedicated to QUANTEC (quantitative Analysis of normal tissue effects in the clinic). This initiative aimed to summarize the available dose/volume/outcome data for normal tissue effects.

Rubin and Casarett's textbook, Radiation Pathology, from 1968. This book offered a comprehensive summary of the effects of radiation on normal tissues.

Cindy L. Schwartz (Editor), Wendy L. Hobbie (Editor), Louis S. Constine (Editor), & Kathleen S. Ruccione (Editor). Survivors of Childhood and Adolescent Cancer: A Multidisciplinary Approach (Pediatric Oncology) 2nd ed. Springer-Verlag Berlin Heidelberg New York: 2005.

Luis Fajardo's textbook, Radiation Pathology, from 2001. Fajardo, L, Berthrong M, Anderson R (2001). Radiation Pathology. Oxford University Press, New York.

Tillman, B.N., & Elbermani, W, ed. Atlas of Human Anatomy, Clinical Edition. 1st ed. New York: Mud Puddle Books Inc.; 2007.

Zhang, Shu-Xin. An Atlas of Histology. New York: Springer-Verlag Inc.; 1999.

Updated and Supplemental information

Interested readers are encouraged to view additional information from other sources including:

Common Terminology Criteria for Adverse Events (CTCAE) from the U.S. Department Of Health And Human Services (National Institutes of Health and National Cancer Institute). This report provides a grading system for the common toxicities. It is updated periodically with the last update, version 4.03, published June 14, 2010. Available at http://evs.nci.nih.gov/ftp1/CTCAE/About.html.

Contents

Contributors

Mitchell S. Anscher Department of Radiation Oncology, Virginia Commonwealth University School of Medicine, Richmond, VA, USA

David J. Brenner Center for Radiological Research, Columbia University Medical Center, New York, NY, USA

George Casarett Department of Radiation Oncology, University of Rochester School of Medicine and Dentistry, Rochester, NY, USA

C. Norman Coleman Department of Health and Human Services (HHS), Office of the Assistant Secretary for Preparedness and Response (ASPR), Washington, USA

Louis S. Constine The Philip Rubin Professor of Radiation Oncology and Pediatrics, Vice Chair Director, the Judy DiMarzo Cancer Survivorship Program Department of Radiation Oncology, University of Rochester Medical Center, Rochester, NY, USA

Tom V. Darling Department of Kinesiology and Physical Education, Valdosta State University, Valdosta, GA, USA

Sughosh Dhakal Radiation Oncology, Department of Radiation Oncology, University of Rochester School of Medicine and Dentistry, Rochester, NY, USA

Craig C. Earle Department of Medical Oncology, Dana-Farber Cancer Institute, Boston, MA, USA

Michael W. Epperly Department of Radiation Oncology, University of Pittsburgh Cancer Institute, Pittsburgh, PA, USA

Luis Fajardo Stanford Medical School, Palo Alto, CA, USA

Chunkit Fung James P Wilmot Cancer Center, University of Rochester Medical Center, Rochester, USA

Paul R. Graves Department of Radiation Oncology, New York Methodist Hospital, Brooklyn, NY, USA

Joel S. Greenberger Department of Radiation Oncology, University of Pittsburgh Cancer Institute, Pittsburgh, PA, USA

Caroline Hadley Baylor University School of Medicine, Houston, Texas, USA

Philip Rubin Professor and Chair Emeritus Department of Radiation Oncology, University of Rochester School of Medicine and Dentistry, Rochester, NY, USA

Nathaniel Hafer National Institutes of Health (NIH), National Institute of Allergy and Infectious Diseases (NIAID), Bethesda, USA; The American Association for the Advancement of Science (AAAS) Science and Technology Policy Fellow, Washington, USA

David C. Hodgson Department of Radiation Oncology, Princess Margaret Hospital, University of Toronto, Toronto, ON, Canada

Melissa M. Hudson Cancer Survivorship Division, St. Jude Children's Research Hospital, Memphis, TN, USA

Isabel L. Jackson Department of Radiation Oncology, University of Maryland Medical Center, Greenbaum Cancer Center, Baltimore, MD, USA

Pascal Jean-Pierre Department of Psychology, University of Notre Dame, Notre Dame, IN, USA

Andre Konski Department of Radiation Oncology, Wayne State University School of Medicine Barbara Ann Karmanos Cancer Center, Detroit, Michigan, USA

Bert Maidment National Institutes of Health (NIH), National Institute of Allergy and Infectious Diseases (NIAID), Bethesda, USA

Ronald Manning ASPR, Biomedical Advanced Research and Development Authority (BARDA), Washington, USA

Lawrence B. Marks Department of Radiation Oncology, Lineberger Cancer Center, University of North Carolina, Chapel Hill, NC, USA

Ross Mikkelsen Department of Radiation Oncology, Virginia Commonwealth University School of Medicine, Richmond, VA, USA

Michael T. Milano Department of Radiation Oncology, University of Rochester School of Medicine and Dentistry, Rochester, NY, USA

Supriya G. Mohile Department of Medical Hematology/Oncology, Rochester, NY, USA

Gary R. Morrow Departments of Radiation Oncology & Psychiatry, Director University of Rochester Cancer Center Community Clinical Oncology Program Research Base, Rochester, NY, USA

Karen Mustian Departments of Radiation Oncology and Community and Preventive Medicine, University of Rochester Medical Center, Rochester, NY, USA

Jiho Nam Department of Radiation Oncology, University of North Carolina at Chapel Hill Campus, Chapel Hill, NC, USA; Department of Radiation Oncology, Pusan National University, Yangsan, South Korea

Andrea K. Ng Department of Radiation Oncology, Harvard Medical School, Brigham and Women's Hospital, Dana-Farber Cancer Institute, Boston, MA, USA

Paul Okunieff Department of Radiation Oncology, University of Florida Shands Cancer Center, Gainesville, USA

Oxana Palesh Department of Psychiatry & Behavioral Sciences, Stanford School of Medicine, Stanford, CA, USA

Kishan J. Pandya Department of Radiation Oncology, Former Associate Director of the James. P. Wilmot Cancer Center, University of Rochester Medical Center, Rochester, NY, USA

Arnold C. Paulino Department of Radiation Oncology, The Methodist Hospital, Houston, TX, USA

Luke J. Peppone Department of Kinesiology and Physical Education, Valdosta State University, Valdosta, GA, USA

Pat Prasanna Division of Cancer Treatment and Diagnosis (DCTD)/Radiation Research Program (RRP), National Cancer Institute (NCI), Bethesda, USA

Jason Q. Purnell The Brown School/Institute for Public Health, Washington University in St. Louis, St. Louis, MO, USA

Mike E. Robbins Department of Radiation Oncology, Wake Forest School of Medicine, Brain Tumor Center of Excellence, Winston-Salem, NC, USA

Barry S. Rosenstein Radiation Oncology, Dermatology and Community and Preventive Medicine, Mount Sinai School of Medicine, NYU School of Medicine, New York, NY, USA

Madelyn Rubin Yale University School of Nursing, New Haven, CT, USA

Rainer K. Sachs Departments of Mathematics and Physics, University of California, Berkeley, CA, USA

Sheila Judge Santacroce Yale University School of Nursing, New Haven, CT, USA

Igor Shuryak Center for Radiological Research, Columbia University Medical Center, New York, NY, USA

Lois B. Travis Department of Radiation Oncology, University of Rochester, James P. Wilmot Cancer Center, Rochester, NY, USA

Andy M. Trotti H. Lee Moffit Cancer Center Research Institute, Tampa, FL, USA

Zeljko Vujaskovic Department of Radiation Oncology, University of Maryland Medical Center, Greenbaum Cancer Center, Baltimore, MD, USA

Introduction

Our country formally declared war on cancer four decades ago. While many skirmishes have been won, the battle rages on. Far too many patients still succumb to cancer. Nevertheless, an increasing number of patients are successfully treated, and the population of cancer survivors is increasing. An estimated 13.7 million Americans (almost 4 % of the United States population) were living with a history of cancer on January 1, 2012. By January 1, 2022 that number is expected to increase to nearly 18 million (Siegel et al. 2012). Overall, approximately 65 % of adults will survive their malignancy, and this is much higher for selected cancers such as breast and the lymphomas.

Living beyond cancer should be cause for celebration. However, cancer survivors are vulnerable to the late effects of their therapy. They have complicated needs including physical problems, financial obstacles, and mountains of emotions that must be addressed. All of these hurdles can compromise the quality of life of cancer survivors and their family.

The modern era of cancer therapy is predicated on the safe intensification of surgery, radiation, chemotherapy, and biologic adjuvants. Malignancies resistant to therapy have demanded an aggressive treatment approach that often resides on the edge of normal tissue tolerance, or even exceeds tolerance to some "acceptable" degree. Clearly, the potential to ameliorate or prevent such normal tissue damage, or to manage and rehabilitate affected patients, requires an understanding of tissue tolerance to therapy. Because "late effects" can manifest months or years after cessation of treatment, therapeutic decisions intended to obviate such effects can be based only on the probability, not the certainty, that such effects will develop. In making such decisions, the balance between efficacy and potential for toxicity should be considered and may be influenced by host-, disease-, and treatment-related risk factors. The determination of the frequency and pathogenesis of late effects is difficult for several reasons: (a) patients must survive long enough for damage to develop, (b) the number of patients both affected and unaffected by therapy must be known, and (c) the latent period to the manifestation of damage compromises discernment of the responsible component of multimodality therapy. Further complicating our understanding of organ tolerance to therapy is that tumor and host factors interact with therapy in the causation of late effects.

This book represents a monumental effort by numerous experts on the adverse consequences of radiation and chemotherapy. It was inspired by our patients, both those fortunate enough to have survived, but also those who did not. For our survivors, it is our responsibility to understand, mitigate, treat, and prevent their "late effects." However, this book was also inspired by our mentor, Philip Rubin. With George Casarett (Rubin and Casarett 1968), he pioneered the field of radiation-associated normal tissue damage. At a time when many radiation oncologists were satisfied to be effectively combating cancer, Phil Rubin recognized that the *quality* of survival after cancer was paramount. He was driven to teach his colleagues and emerging oncologists the critical need to appreciate normal tissue toxicity and the pathophysiology by which it evolved. At the University of Rochester, he successfully obtained a succession of program project grants to study normal tissue toxicity. It has been his lifelong goal to educate future generations of oncologists about the power and also the consequences of cancer therapy. His motto was always: "there is no free lunch."

Finally, he encouraged numerous protégé to follow in his footsteps. His inspiration to oncologists, pathologists, and biologists throughout the world has allowed for the safe treatment of an uncountable number of patients.

Louis S. Constine, MD, FASTRO
Lawrence B. Marks, MD, FASTRO

References

Siegel R, DeSantis C, Virgo K et al (2012) Cancer treatment and survivorship statistics. CA Cancer J Clin 62:220–231

Rubin P, Casarett G (1968) Clinical radiation pathology, vol 1 and 2. WB Saunders, Philadelphia

Prologue: Surviving Cancer: SEER Statistics

Craig C. Earle, Lois B. Travis, and Louis S. Constine

Contents

Abstract

- The number of cancer survivors is increasing rapidly because of a combination of demographic forces, public health success, and improving medical treatments.
- Projections are that the oncology workforce will be unable to meet the demand for cancer care in coming decades.
- Survivorship care planning can improve the quality of care and open up the possibility for survivorship care to be delivered by an array of health care providers.

1 Introduction

There are numerous definitions of the term cancer survivor. Doctors have traditionally thought of survivors as those patients whose cancers have been cured. A commonly used generic milestone is being cancer-free for 5 years, although the reality is that oncologists use different time frames for various cancers and even for similar situations within a given cancer type. The advocacy community, on the other hand, has commonly used a more expanded definition to assert that "from the time of its discovery and for the balance of life, an individual diagnosed with cancer is a survivor" (National Coalition of Cancer Survivorship charter), a definition which includes situations in which the cancer is incurable. Family and friends affected by the patient's cancer are sometimes also called survivors (considered 'secondary survivors' by the National Cancer Institute's (NCI) Office of Cancer Survivorship (OCS)). More recently, in the 2005 report *From Cancer Patient to Cancer Survivor: Lost in Transition* (Institute of Medicine 2005), the Institute of Medicine (IOM) put forth the pragmatic definition of cancer survivors as those patients in the period after the completion of primary cancer treatment until the time of recurrence or death.

C. C. Earle (✉)
Department of Medical Oncology, Dana-Farber Cancer Institute, Boston, MA, USA
e-mail: craig_earle@dfci.harvard.edu

L. B. Travis
Division of Cancer Epidemiology and Genetics, National Cancer Institute, National Institutes of Health, DHHS, Bethesda, MD 20892, USA

L. S. Constine
Department of Radiation Oncology, James P. Wilmot Cancer Center, University of Rochester Medical Center, 647Rochester, NY 14642, USA

P. Rubin et al. (eds.), *ALERT – Adverse Late Effects of Cancer Treatment*, Medical Radiology. Radiation Oncology,
DOI: 10.1007/978-3-540-72314-1_1, © Springer-Verlag Berlin Heidelberg 2014

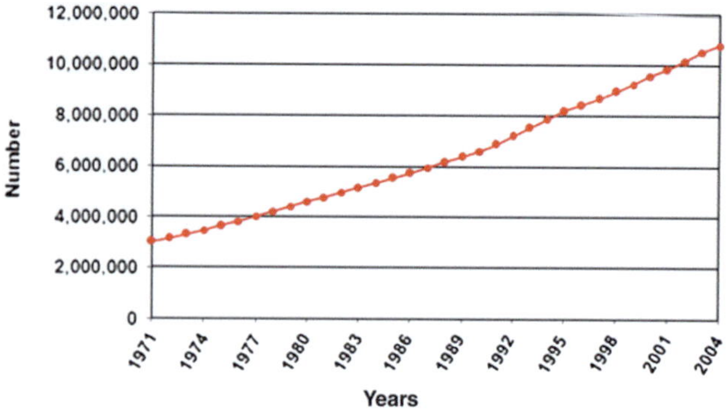

Fig. 1 Estimated number of cancer survivors in the United States from 1971 to 2004. Based on November 2006 SEER data submission

2 Statistics

Cancer is now the leading cause of mortality for adults in the United States. It will directly afflict one in three persons, and most of us are affected by cancer in some way. The NCI estimated that as of January 1st, 2005 there were 10.8 million Americans with a personal history of cancer (Fig. 1), approximately 3.7 % of the population (http://dccps.nci.nih.gov/ocs/prevalence). This number has been steadily increasing such that it may be greater than 12 million in 2008. Worldwide, the number of cancer survivors was over 25 million in 2002 (Parkin et al. 2005). There are several reasons for this growth in numbers, but demographics are likely a major contributor. Cancer is, in general, a disease of the elderly (Fig. 2), and the baby-boom generation is now entering the years during which cancer incidence rates increase. Consequently, there are more cancer patients, and as a result more survivors.

Demographics, however, do not alone account for the increasing number of cancer survivors. Other factors, including public health successes and medical advances, have also contributed to the rising numbers. As Fig. 3 demonstrates, between 1993 and 2005 the annual age-adjusted cancer death rates have fallen by an average of 1.1 % per year. These statistics reflect incidence rates that have finally plateaued and started to decrease (Fig. 4) due to factors such as lower smoking rates, combined with the growing proportion of patients cured of cancer. Figure 5 shows that in 1975, the 5 year relative survival rate for all cancer patients considered together was about 50 %. By 2000, the 5 year relative survival rate had increased to about 66 %. Effective screening tests which detect cancer at earlier stages are responsible for much of this improvement in survival, but increasingly successful primary and adjuvant treatments also contribute to these increases.

The estimated number of cancer survivors by time since initial diagnosis and gender is shown in Fig. 6, with 14 % of all patients having survived for 20 or more years. Breast is

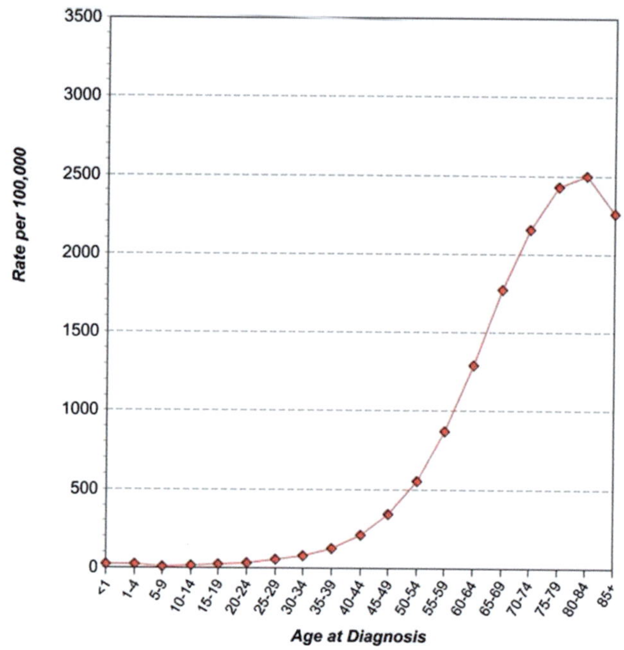

Fig. 2 Age-specific crude SEER cancer incidence rates. For all cancer sites, all ages, all races, both sexes 2000–2005

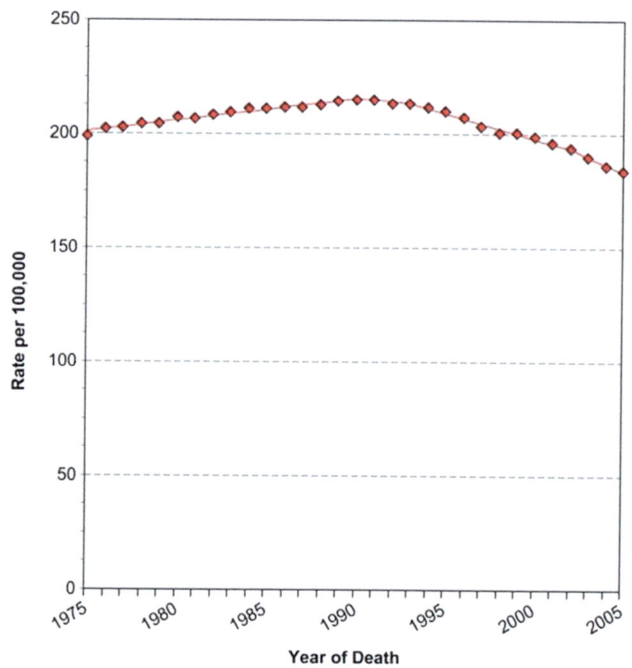

Fig. 3 Age-adjusted U.S. cancer mortality rates. For all cancer sites, all ages, all races, both sexes 1975–2005. Mortality source: U.S. mortality files, National Center for Health Statistics, CDC. Rates are age-adjusted to the 2000 U.S. standard population (19 age groups – Census P25–1130). Regression lines are calculated using the join point regression program version 3.3, April 2008, National Cancer Institute

the most common primary site (22 %), followed by prostate (19 %), colorectal (10 %), and gynecological malignancies (9 %, Fig. 7); these cancers have relatively high incidence

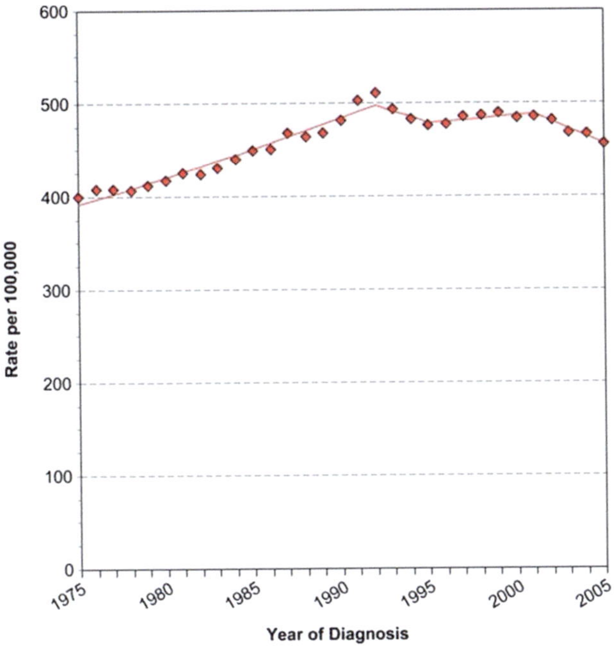

Fig. 4 Age-adjusted SEER cancer incidence rates. For all cancer sites, all ages, all races, both sexes 1975–2005. Incidence source: SEER 9 areas (San Francisco, Connecticut, Detroit, Hawaii, Iowa, New Mexico, Seattle, Utah, and Atlanta). Rates are age-adjusted to the 2000 U.S. standard population (19 age groups – Census P25–1130). Regression lines are calculated using the join point regression program version 3.3, April 2008, National Cancer Institute

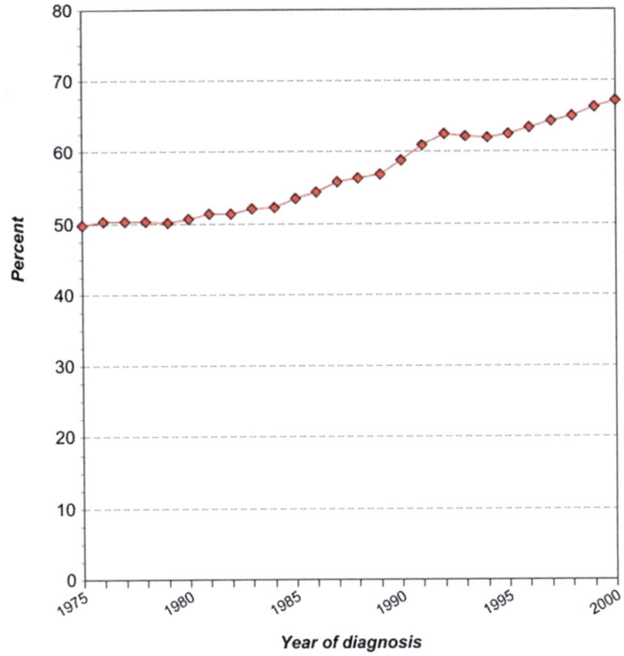

Fig. 5 5 year relative cancer survival rate by year of diagnosis. For all cancer sites, all ages, all races, both sexes 1975–2000. Survival source: SEER 9 areas (San Francisco, Connecticut, Detroit, Hawaii, Iowa, New Mexico, Seattle, Utah, and Atlanta). Survival rates are relative rates expressed as percents. The 5 year estimates are calculated using monthly intervals

rates and depending on stage, are generally curable. Lung cancer, on the other hand, despite being the most common cancer overall, accounts for only 3 % of survivors because of its generally poor outcomes. Conversely, the proportion of cancer survivors under age 19 is only 1 %, given the rarity of childhood cancers, although these tumors are typically accompanied by high cure rates. The estimated proportion of cancer survivors by current age is shown in Fig. 8, with 60 % of patients over age 65.

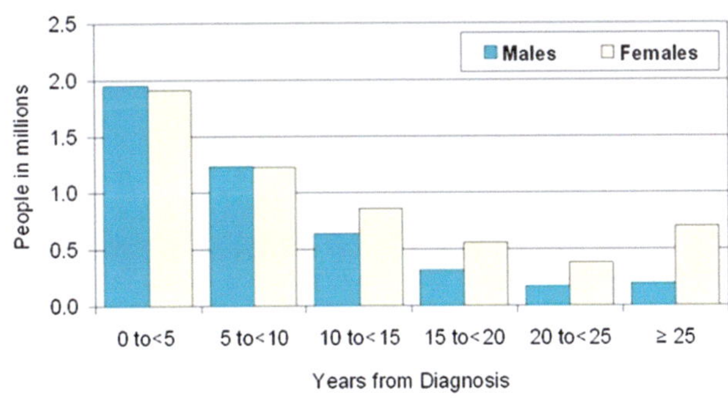

Fig. 6 Estimated number of cancer survivors by time from diagnosis and gender. Estimate for January 1, 2004 based on November 2006 SEER data submission. Invasive/first primary cases only; n = 10.8 million survivors

3 The Oncology Workforce

As the number of cancer survivors has grown, so has the recognition that the care of the patient requires attention to issues that go well beyond treatment of the cancer itself. The first recommendation in the IOM report was that cancer survivorship should be recognized "as a distinct phase of cancer care." This viewpoint represented a remarkable shift in thinking. Previously, patients had been viewed as survivors of a specific cancer, sometimes with a narrow spectrum of lasting effects related only to that cancer and/or its treatment. The IOM articulated a view that there are important cross-cutting issues with which all cancer survivors must contend. These include concerns about the following issues: appropriate surveillance for relapse; effects of treatment such as organ damage, mobility, fatigue, fertility, and sexual dysfunction; and the possibility of second cancers either due to shared genetic or environmental exposures that caused the index tumor or that are related to treatment. Other shared issues relate to the following factors: the effect of a cancer history on the ability to obtain health, life, or disability insurance, and related concerns of how insurability might affect employability and finances; and a host of psychosocial effects including fear,

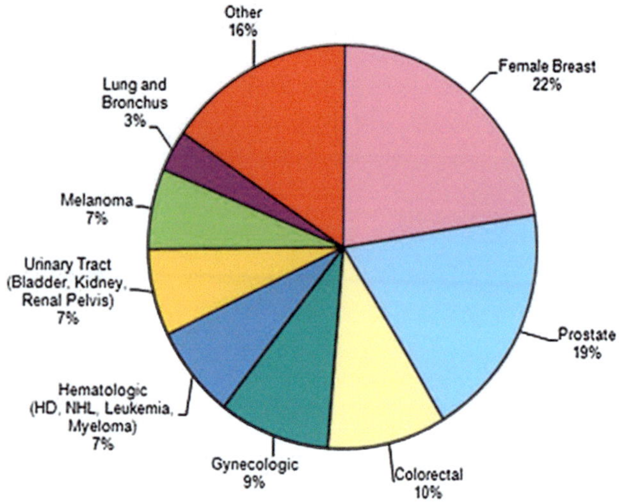

Fig. 7 Estimated proportion of cancer survivors in the U.S. by site. Based on November 2006 SEER data submission

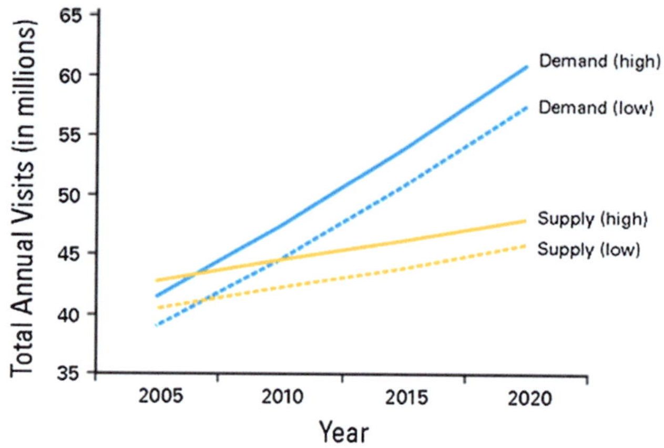

Fig. 9 Baseline projected supply of and demand for oncologist visits, 2005–2020. Reprinted with permission. ©2008 American Society of Clinical Oncology. All rights reserved. Erikson C et al.: J Oncol Practice Vol. 3 (2), 2007:79–86

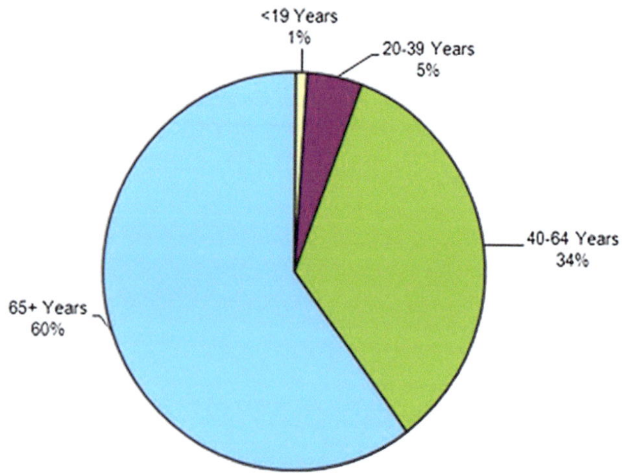

Fig. 8 Estimated proportion of cancer survivors by current age. Based on November 2006 SEER data submission

altered interpersonal relationships, cosmesis, and cognitive effects (e.g., 'chemo brain') stemming from cancer treatment. These domains of concern depend less on the particular type of cancer, and more on therapeutic exposures and individual reactions to them. Moreover, the end of primary treatment for cancer has been called a 'teachable moment'(Ganz 2005) in recognition that patients may be more receptive to recommendations to change risk behaviors related to diet, exercise, smoking, etc., and messages about general health maintenance (e.g., immunizations, other screenings) around the time of a major health crisis, such as a cancer diagnosis.

This more holistic view of caring for cancer survivors promises to provide them great benefit, but raises questions about how such care can practically be delivered. The demographic trends, which were mentioned previously, predict increasing numbers of cancer patients and survivors who will require ongoing care and monitoring. These statistics prompted the American Society of Clinical Oncology (ASCO) to create in 2005 a Workforce in Oncology Taskforce to study the equilibrium of supply and demand. By gathering information through professional databases and surveys on the demographics and career plans of the current oncology workforce as well as those in training, ASCO was able to project that demand for cancer care is expected to rise 48 % between 2005 and 2020, while the supply of oncologists will grow by only about 14 % (Fig. 9). This is due to a combination of an aging oncology workforce and a limited number of oncology fellowship positions. The Workforce Taskforce concluded that the health care system will likely have major shortages in its capacity to meet future demand for oncology services and that no single action (such as training more oncologists or engaging primary care physicians (PCPs) and physician-extenders in cancer care) will fill the gap between supply and demand. Instead, policymakers will need to employ a multifaceted strategy in meeting this challenge.

It is important to note that the assumptions in the Workforce Taskforce analysis included no change in current oncology practices. This is a very conservative assumption given that oncologists generally have increasingly more management options and treatments to offer patients with each passing year. Even those cancer patients who may not be cured are living longer and requiring care for extended periods of time. Further, this model specifically does not take into account the changing standards and trends in survivorship care discussed herein.

4 Survivorship Care Planning

It is important to recognize that there is no single optimal strategy by which survivorship care can be provided. Follow-up care can be carried out by specialists, generalists, physician assistants, or nurse practitioners, combinations of these providers in a 'shared care' model, or in a specialized survivorship clinic. The mechanism(s) by which care are delivered, however, are less important than ensuring communication and coordination of care among all involved health personnel.

The IOM had as its second recommendation that 'patients completing treatment should be provided with a comprehensive care summary and follow-up plan…(the) "Survivorship Care Plan". The intent of this recommendation was to create an actionable document that is specific to each individual patient so that the patient and all providers would have a guide as to what treatments were rendered and what procedures should be performed in the future. In this way, communication and coordination could be enhanced. As most elements of survivorship care are not technically demanding, the specifics of which provider is responsible for the different components of care can be customized to best suit each patient's situation, depending on resource availability and preferences.

High-quality data exist on which these new care models are based. For example, randomized trials have shown that primary care providers (PCPs) who have been given a brief survivorship care plan with explicit directions for follow-up can achieve the same outcomes as specialists (Grunfeld et al. 1995a, b, 1996a, 1999a, 2006). In breast cancer, the time to diagnosis of recurrence is unchanged when follow up is randomized between PCPs and specialists (Grunfeld et al. 1996a) and there is no excess of serious clinical events such as pathological fractures or spinal cord compression from an unrecognized recurrence (Grunfeld et al. 2006). In addition, physical quality of life and mental health (including anxiety and depression) do not differ, though satisfaction with care actually favors non-specialist providers (Grunfeld et al. 1999). Randomized trials that examine the follow-up of patients with both breast or colorectal cancer have shown that care is delivered at lower cost both to the health care system (fewer, less expensive tests), as well as to the patient (out of pocket costs related to travel) when delivered by non-specialist providers (Grunfeld et al. 1996a, 1999b; Wattchow et al. 2006). Moreover, PCPs are generally willing to take on the role of follow-up care (Grunfeld et al. 1995) and patients may prefer it, (Grunfeld et al. 1996) while surveys have shown that most oncologists would like to focus on delivering cancer treatment (American Society of Clinical Oncology 1996). Consequently, shared-care models appear to be safe and feasible. These models may be particularly attractive for managing breast cancer survivors, where the evidence is strongest and the manpower concerns are greatest (Ganz and Hahn 2008). Still, there are also workforce issues facing many other physician specialties, including primary care providers, (Bodenheimer 2006) and there are currently insufficient allied providers to completely solve the human resource problem (Erikson et al. 2007). Consequently, creative solutions will be needed to address the above issues.

The care *summary* envisioned by the IOM should include the following (adapted from the IOM Report: 'From Cancer Patient to Cancer Survivor: Lost in Transition, Box 3-16, pp. 152–153, which can be found at www.iom.edu and which was adapted from the President's Cancer Panel (2004):

(1) Diagnostic tests performed and results.
(2) Tumor characteristics (e.g., site(s), stage and grade, hormone receptor status, marker information).
(3) Dates of treatment initiation and completion.
(4) Surgery, chemotherapy, radiotherapy, transplant, hormonal therapy, or gene or other therapies provided, including agents used, treatment regimen, total dosage, identifying number and title of clinical trials (if any), indicators of treatment response, and toxicities experienced during treatment.
(5) Psychosocial, nutritional, and other supportive services provided.
(6) Full contact information on treating institutions and key individual providers.
(7) Identification of a key point of contact and coordinator of continuing care.

The care *plan*, on the other hand, would provide recommendations regarding both cancer and non-cancer care. It is not reasonable to expect non-specialist providers to remain up to date on surveillance recommendations and the potential side effects of new cancer treatments, but they are well-able to act on specific information for a particular patient and implement a care plan. Recommendations for surveillance of cancer are available from several sources. The American Society of Clinical Oncology (ASCO) has *evidence-based* surveillance guidelines for breast and colorectal cancer that can be found at: www.asco.org under the Quality Care & Guidelines tab. *Consensus* guidelines for surveillance for recurrence of other cancers after treatment are incorporated into the National Comprehensive Cancer Network (NCCN) guidelines, found at:

www.nccn.org. In Europe, the European Society for Medical Oncology also publishes consensus guidelines at www.esmo.org/resources/clinicalguidelines.

Long-term effects are those that first occur during cancer treatment and persist after completion of primary therapy, such as peripheral neuropathy from oxaliplatin. *Late effects*, on the other hand, are those signs/symptoms that were not apparent during primary treatment, but become evident at some later time, such as bone loss and increased risk of hip fracture from pelvic radiation (Baxter et al. 2005). Unfortunately, there are no comprehensive guidelines for monitoring or managing long-term and late effects of cancer therapy for survivors of adult cancer, however, the major issues can be extrapolated from the *consensus* guidelines of the Children's Oncology Group, found at www.survivorshipguidelines.org.

According to the IOM, the care plan should include:

(1) The likely course of recovery from acute treatment toxicities, as well as the need for ongoing health maintenance or adjuvant therapy.
(2) A description of recommended cancer screening and other periodic testing and examinations, and the schedule on which they should be performed (and who should provide them).
(3) Information on possible late and long-term effects of treatment and symptoms of such effects.
(4) Information on possible signs of recurrence and second tumors.
(5) Information on the possible effects of cancer on marital/partner relationship, sexual functioning, work, and parenting, and the potential future need for psychosocial support.
(6) Information on the potential insurance, employment, and financial consequences of cancer and, as necessary, referral to counseling, legal aid, and financial assistance.
(7) Specific recommendations for healthy behaviors (e.g., diet, exercise, healthy weight, sunscreen use, immunizations, smoking cessation, osteoporosis prevention). When appropriate, recommendations that first-degree relatives be informed about their increased risk and the need for cancer screening (e.g., breast cancer, colorectal cancer, prostate cancer).
(8) As appropriate, information on genetic counseling and testing to identify high-risk individuals who could benefit from more comprehensive cancer surveillance, chemoprevention, or risk-reducing surgery.
(9) As appropriate, information on known effective chemoprevention and behavioral strategies for secondary prevention (e.g., tamoxifen in women at high risk for breast cancer; smoking cessation after lung cancer) and monitoring of adherence to these recommendations.
(10) Referrals to specific follow-up care providers (e.g., rehabilitation, fertility, psychology), support groups, and/or the patient's primary care provider.
(11) A listing of cancer-related resources and information (e.g., Internet-based sources and telephone listings for major cancer support organizations).

5 Conclusion

The data reviewed in this chapter show that demographic trends in both the general population and the oncology workforce, combined with the results of our success in the war against cancer, have now presented us with a major health service delivery challenge for cancer survivors. Multifaceted enhancements to the workforce and many coexisting models of care delivery will be needed in the future. Careful survivorship care planning has the potential to improve the quality of care for cancer survivors, enhance patient satisfaction through empowerment, and possibly contribute to solutions to the looming concerns with regard to the oncology workforce (Erikson et al. 2007).

References

American Society of Clinical Oncology (1996): Status of the medical oncology workforce. J Clin Oncol 14:2612–2621

Baxter NN, Habermann EB, Tepper JE et al (2005) Risk of pelvic fractures in older women following pelvic irradiation. JAMA 294:2587–2593

Bodenheimer T (2006) Primary care–will it survive? N Engl J Med 355:861–864

Erikson C, Salsberg E, Forte G et al (2007) Future supply and demand for oncologists: challenges to assuring access to oncology services. J Oncol Pract 3:79–86

Ganz PA (2005) A teachable moment for oncologists: cancer survivors, 10 million strong and growing! J Clin Oncol 23:5458–5460

Ganz PA, Hahn EE (2008) Implementing a survivorship care plan for patients with breast cancer. J Clin Oncol 26:759–767

Grunfeld E, Yudkin P, Adewuyl-Dalton R, et al (1995a) Follow up in breast cancer: Quality of life unaffected by general practice follow up. BMJ 311:54

Grunfeld E, Mant D, Vessey MP et al (1995b) Evaluating primary care follow-up of breast cancer: methods and preliminary results of three studies. Ann Oncol 6(Suppl 2):47–52

Grunfeld E, Mant D, Vessey MP et al (1995c) Specialist and general practice views on routine follow-up of breast cancer patients in general practice. Fam Pract 12:60–65

Grunfeld E, Mant D, Yudkin P et al (1996a) Routine follow up of breast cancer in primary care: randomised trial. BMJ 313:665–669

Grunfeld E, Mant D, Yudkin P et al (1996b) Routine follow-up of breast cancer in primary care: randomised trial. BMJ 313:665–669

Grunfeld E, Fitzpatrick R, Mant D et al (1999a) Comparison of breast cancer patient satisfaction with follow-up in primary care versus specialist care: results from a randomized controlled trial. Br J Gen Pract 49:705–710

Grunfeld E, Gray A, Mant D et al (1999b) Follow-up of breast cancer in primary care vs specialist care: results of an economic evaluation. Br J Cancer 79:1227–1233

Grunfeld E, Levine MN, Julian JA et al (2006) Randomized trial of long-term follow-up for early-stage breast cancer: a comparison of family physician versus specialist care. J Clin Oncol 24: 848–855

Institute of Medicine (2005) From cancer patient to cancer survivor: lost in transition. National Academies Press, Washington

Parkin DM, Bray F, Ferlay J et al (2005) Global cancer statistics, 2002. CA Cancer J Clin 55:74–108

Wattchow DA, Weller DP, Esterman A et al (2006) General practice vs surgical-based follow-up for patients with colon cancer: randomised controlled trial. Br J Cancer 94:1116–1121

Biocontinuum of the Pathophysiology Paradigm

Biocontinuum of Radiation Pathogenesis of Normal Tissue: The Past is the Prologue to the Future

Philip Rubin and George Casarett

Contents

Abstract

Under the various conditions of radiation therapy, the period of time from irradiation to the end of life may be characterized by continuous complications of clinical significance arising from irradiation of normal organs, alternating with clinical complication with clinically "silent" periods of the absence of such clinically significant complications. However, *there is at no time a "silent" histopathologic period*, i.e., absence of radiation-induced changes in the irradiated organs, although their degree of rate of progression may vary considerably. Furthermore, the addition of further stress of insult, e.g., from trauma or infection, to the organs that have sustained residual radiation damage (e.g. deterioration of the vasculature) may precipitate clinically significant complications during otherwise clinically "silent" periods. The histopathologic sequence of events after a brief radiation exposure is divided into four general phases (see Fig. 5): *Casarett Hypothesis*. The Biocontinuum diagram illustrates generally, with respect to clinical periods, the waxing and waning (vertically), or organ damage with time and persistence or progression of residual damage. The upper lines depict radiation damage of different degrees. The bottom line indicates the accumulation of organ damage with time of "aging", may be additive to radiation damage in effect. The rising arrows indicate the precipitation of damage from subclinical or clinical levels to clinically significant or even lethal levels, as a result of complications such as trauma or infection or as a result of deterioration of vasculature and failure of the blood circulation. No precise values of relationships are intended for the slopes or shapes of the graph lines: *Rubin Paradigm*.

In memory of George Casarett.

P. Rubin (✉) · G. Casarett
Department of Radiation Oncology, University of Rochester School of Medicine and Dentistry, 601 Elmwood Ave, Box 647 Rochester, NY 14642, USA
e-mail: oncophilip@earthlink.net

P. Rubin et al. (eds.), *ALERT – Adverse Late Effects of Cancer Treatment*, Medical Radiology. Radiation Oncology, DOI: 10.1007/978-3-540-72314-1_2, © Springer-Verlag Berlin Heidelberg 2014

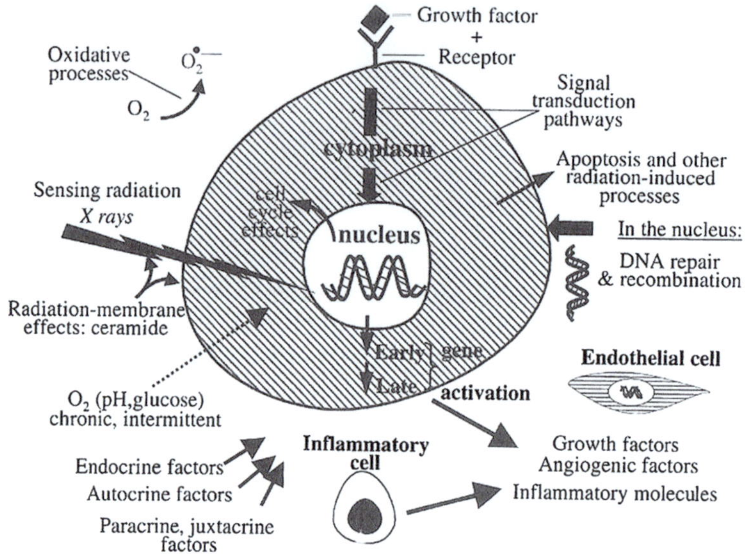

Fig. 1 Potential radiation biologic targets for translational research. For each of the pathways detailed molecular and cellular knowledge is continuously becoming available that explains cellular phenotype and provides novel therapeutic targets (Modified from Coleman CN. Harris JR: Current Scientific issues related to clinical radiation oncology. Radiat Res 1998:150:125.)

1 Introduction: Historical Annotation

In the 1960s, the "Manhattan Project", code for the "Atomic Bomb" was declassified and thereby allowed for access to numerous radiation biologic and pathologic research theses. George Casarett was the senior biopathologist and in collaboration the two-volume work entitled "Clinical Radiation Pathology" was published in 1968. The paradigm we developed was the "Biocontinuum" in which we postulated that once normal tissues are irradiated a sequence of cellular responses continues for a lifetime ranging from acute-subacute-late, and chronic clinical manifestations over decades. Recent molecular biology studies of a 'Perpetual Cytokine Cascade' induced immediately after tissues are exposed to radiation, which confirms his observations, "*there is at no time a 'silent' histopathologic latent period*" prior to the clinical expression of radiation reactions.

2 Prologue I

2.1 Normal Cell and Potential Targets for Radiation

A knowledge of the normal cell, its structure, and its function is essential to an understanding of the complexities of radiation cytopathology, which is, in turn, essential to the understanding of radiation biopathology and its clinical manifestations. Once initiated, these normal tissue responses result in sequence of acute to chronic late effects. This "Biocontinuum" of longitudinal alterations is expressed differently over the patients' lifetime. Paradoxically, radiation can save an individual's life and may ultimately lead to his demise decades later.

The potential radiation biologic targets for translational research are illustrated in Fig. 1 and Table 1. For each of the pathways, detailed molecular and cellular knowledge is continually becoming available to explain different cellular phenotypes and may provide novel therapeutic targets. Many of the concepts of the induction of chronic oxidative stress and the inflammatory process followed by fibrogenesis inherent to radiation-induced pathogenesis have parallels in chemotherapy and biologics, which includes a similar cytohistologic toxicity. The surgical wound healing has a parallel sequence of inflammation, then fibrosis in its histologic appearance.

2.2 Cell Types According to Mitotic Frequency

In his classification of body cells on the basis of the kinds of individual lives they lead, Cowdry (1950) named four general classes: vegetative intermitotic, differentiating intermitotic, reverting postmitotic, and fixed postmitotic (Fig. 2a, b). Table 2 outlines the properties of these classes of cells and gives examples.

2.2.1 Vegetative Intermitotic Cells

These cells divide relatively frequently, have relatively short individual lives between divisions, differentiate little or not at all during their individual lives between divisions, show minimal aging changes, and function chiefly as producers of cells to replace themselves and the more differentiated cells of relatively short life span which die or are regularly lost from the body. The division of cells of this type produces daughter cells, some of which differentiate and others of which remain vegetative intermitotic cells.

Table 1 Application of molecular biologic concepts to radiation therapy

Process	Potential manipulation	Examples of therapy[a]
DNA damage	Increase damage in tumor cells	Hypoxic-cell sensitizers, thymidine analogues
DNA repair	Decrease repair in tumor cells	Fluoropyrimidines, hydroxyurea, cisplatin
Signal transduction	Inhibit protective signalling cascades in tumor cells	Protein kinase C inhibitors (?) phosphotyrosine kinase inhibitors(?)
Radiation-induced gene expression	Use gene therapy	Tumour necrosis factor linked to radiation responsive promotor(?)
Growth factor expression	Administer or increase expression of protective factors	Interleukin-1, granulocyte colony-stimulating factor granulocyte—macrophage colony-stimulating factor, basic fibroblast growth factor (?)
	Block expression of factors producing long-term toxicity	Antibodies or antisense RNA against epidermal growth factor, transforming growth factor β (?)
Apoptosis	Force tumor cells to undergo apoptosis	Transfection of wild-type TP53(?)
Cell cycle	Synchronize tumor cells in sensitive phase of cycle (early S or M phase)	Antimetabolites (early S phase), paclitaxel phase (M), cyclin inhibitors(G, to S phase)
	Prevent G_2 arrest in tumor cells	Cyclin inhibitors(G_2 to M phase)(?)

[a] A question mark indicates potential therapy

From Licter As, Lawrence TS; Recent advances in radiation oncology, N Engl J Med 1995; 332:371, permission. Copyright © 1995 Massachusetts Medical Society. All rights reserved

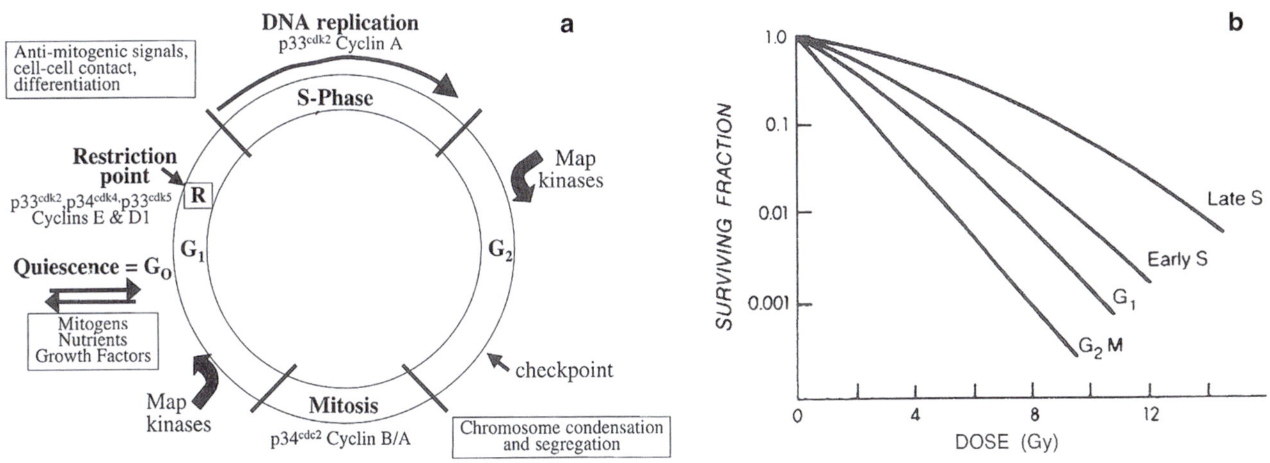

Fig. 2 **a** Cell cycle progression, with the major regulatory kinases indicated. Once a cell passes the restriction point (R), it is committed to progress through S-phase, even in the absence of mitogenic signals checkpoints (indicated in G_2) have also been identified in G_1, S_1 and mitosis. **b** Patterns of radiosensitivity change through the cell cycle. This change is known as the "age function," and varies widely among different cell types. Cells in mitosis are almost always sensitive, followed by cells at the G_1/S boundary, whereas the period of greatest resistance is at late S. *G* gaps; G_1 first gap before DNA synthesis; G_2M Second gap before mitosis; *S* DNA synthesis phase (Adapted from Sinclair WK: Cyclic X-ray responses in mammalian cells in vitro. Radiat Res 1968; 33:620, with permission. Copyright © 1967 OPA (Overseas Publishers Association) N.V.)

2.2.2 Differentiating Intermitotic Cells

These cells also divide relatively frequently; have relatively short individual lives between divisions and show only slight aging changes. However, they undergo steps in the process of differentiation between divisions. Each individual differentiation intermitotic cell becomes increasingly more differentiated between divisions until it becomes fully capable of performing its specialized function, at which time it becomes either a reverting or a fixed postmitotic cell. The number of successive divisions in a line of differentiating intermitotic cells before the completion of differentiation varies with the type of specialized cell in question. For the sake of simplicity, only one row of differentiating intermitotic cells is represented in the diagram. Actually there may be several divisions, as in the production of mature blood cells in bone marrow, or there may be omission of this stage in other tissues, as in thin epidermis.

2.2.3 Reverting Postmitotic Cells

Reverting postmitotic cells are highly differentiated, functionally mature cells with relatively long individual lives

Table 2 Kinds of cell lives

	Vegetative intermitotics	Differentiating intermitotics	Reverting postmitotics	Fixed postmitotics
Life span	Begins at mitosis Ends at mitosis Duration short	Same. Duration short, perhaps even shorter	Begins at mitosis Ordinarily ends at death. When demand for more cells is great, ends at mitosis. Duration longer	Begins at mitosis Ends at death. Duration still longer; for nerve cells very long, very short for neutrophilic leucocytes
Differentiation	Least. Constitutes reservoir of cells. Aging minimal	More as steps in acquisition of specific functions. Aging slight	Still more. Functionally mature. Aging marked	Most. Functionally mature. Aging greatest, ending in death
Service	As cell producers	As cells learning how to work	As cell specialists	As cell specialists even after death. Erythrocytes, epidermal cells, corneal cells, and ganoblasts
Examples	Basal epidermal cells, spermatogonia of testicle, hemocytoblasts of bone marrow	Spinous cells of epidermis, spermatocytes, erythroblasts, myelocytes.	Renal epithelial cells, smooth muscle cells, hepatic epithelial cells.	Nerve cells. Neutrophilic leucocytes
Principal locations	In stratified epithelia nearer to arterial bloodstream.	Sometimes farther away as in spinous layer of epidermis	In liver and adrenals nearest the arterial bloodstream	Almost anywhere needed
Malignant transformation	Occasional	Occasional	Rare	After youth, never

which show marked aging changes and may die without producing daughter cells. These cells do not normally undergo regular or frequent divisions, but when the demand for more cells of their kind is great, e.g., after pathologic destruction, some of them may "revert" for a time to an intermitotic state, in that they divide exuberantly to replace cells lost.

2.2.4 Fixed Postmitotic Cells

Fixed postmitotic cells are very highly differentiated, functionally mature cells which have lost completely their ability to divide, regardless of functional demand. They show marked aging changes ending in death. Some cell types of this class, such as neurons, have long lives and die without replacement, whereas others, such as neutrophilic leukocytes, are relatively short-lived but are replaced by a supply of precursors produced by the divisions of vegetative and differentiating intermitotic cells and sometimes by the division of reverting postmitotic cells.

2.3 Classification of Cells According to Relative Radiosensitivity

The relative radiosensitivity of cells according to the kinds of lives they lead is illustrated in Fig. 3. This classification is given in the order of decreasing relative radiosensitivity and is based upon the criterion of cell death.

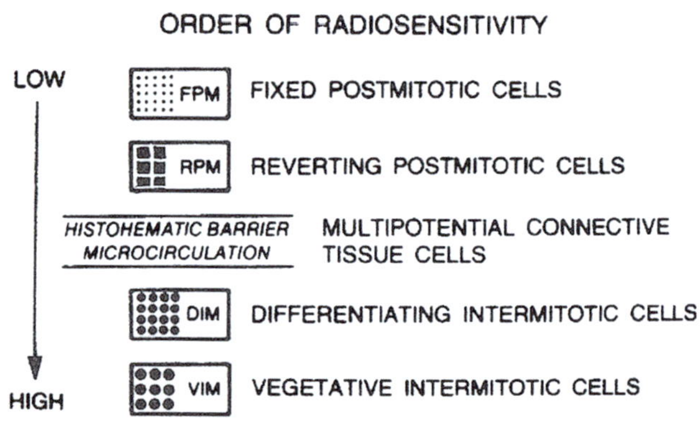

Fig. 3 Relative cell radiosensitivity. (From Rubin P, Casarett GW: Clinical Radiation Pathology. Philadelphia, W.B. Saunders, 1968, with permission.)

Radiation acts at molecular and cellular levels, and tissue effects represent a summation of those effects. Because the key target cells for the survival of a complex organ depends on the organization of all its tissues, cellular damage in one key cell population may result in death of the whole tissue. For example, small blood vessels are fairly sensitive to irradiation, so the effects on a tissue from disruption of its blood supply may be greater than those from the irradiation of the parenchymal cells themselves.

A relative cell radiosensitivity is illustrated in Fig. 3, which is based on the classification schema related to cellular division and differentiation by Cowdry. The uncommitted

Table 3 Classification of cells according to relative radiosensitivity

Tissues	Relative radiosensitivity	Chief mechanisms of hypoplasia
Lymphoid, hemopoietic (marrow), spermatogenic epithelium, ovarian follicular epithelium, intestinal epithelium	High	Destruction of vegetative or differentiating tissue cells of high mitotic frequency
Oropharyngeal stratified epithelium, epidermal epithelium, hair follicle epithelium, sebaceous gland epithelium, urinary bladder epithelium, esophageal epithelium, optic lens epithelium, gastric gland epithelium, ureteral epithelium	Fairly high	Destruction of vegetative or differentiating tissue cells of fairly high mitotic frequency
Ordinary interstitial connective tissue, neurological tissue (connective tissue of nervous system), finely vasculature, growing cartilage, or bone tissue	Medium	Damage or destruction of connective tissue cells of moderate mitotic frequency and damage to the fine vasculature
Mature cartilage or bone tissue, mucous or serous gland epithelium, salivary gland epithelium, sweat gland epithelium, nasopharyngeal simple epithelium, renal epithelium, pulmonary epithelium, renal epithelium, hepatic epithelium, pancreatic epithelium, pituitary epithelium, thyroid epithelium, adrenal epithelium	Fairly low	Hypoplasia secondary to damage to associated fine vasculature and connective tissue elements, with relatively less contribution by the direct effects on parenchymal cells, which normally divide infrequently
Neuronal tissue, muscle tissue	Low	Hypoplasia secondary to damage to associated fine vasculature and connective tissue elements, with little contribution by the direct effects on the parenchymal cells, which do not normally divide

stem cell is a vegetative intermitotic cell; the committed stem cell is a differentiating intermitotic cell. Reverting postmitotic cells have the ability to divide when conditioned or challenged, such as hepatocytes after liver resection. The organization of tissues and organs by these cell types determines their radiosensitivity, which is based on their most radiosensitive cells. Table 3 reviews cell and tissue radiosensitivity.

2.3.1 Class 1: Vegetative Intermitotic Cells

These are generally the most radiation sensitive of cells. They are short-lived as individual cells, they are primitive, and they normally divide regularly to produce daughter cells, some of which will enter into a process of differentiation and others of which will not differentiate, but remain vegetative intermitotic cells. This class includes cells such as free stem cells of the hematopoietic tissues, e.g., hemocytoblasts, primitive lymphoblasts, primitive erythroblasts, and primitive myeloblasts; the dividing of cells deep in the intestinal glands (crypts of Lieberkuhn); the primitive Type A spermatogonia in the seminiferous epithelium; granulosa cells of developing and mature ovarian follicles; basal germinal cells of the epidermis and germinal cells of the gastric glands and of holocrine glands such as the sebaceous glands. Large and medium-sized lymphocytes also belong to this class. Small lymphocytes are also highly radiosensitive, but they do not divide as small lymphocytes. They have been observed on occasion to divide after first increasing in size. Nevertheless, they are exceptional in this class, although they are among the most radiosensitive cell types.

2.3.2 Class 2: Differentiating Intermitotic Cells

These cells are relatively radiosensitive, but are generally somewhat less sensitive to radiation than vegetative intermitotic cells. They are also relatively short-lived as individuals and are produced by divisions of vegetative intermitotic cells. They normally divide from time to time for a limited number of divisions, and they differentiate to some degree between divisions. The more differentiated they become, the less sensitive to radiation they become. This class includes cells such as dividing differentiating cells of the hematopoietic series in the intermediate stages of differentiation in both granulocytic and erythrocytic series in bone marrow, the more differentiated spermatogonia (intermediate and Type B), and the spermatocytes in the seminiferous epithelium and ovocytes.

2.3.3 Class 3: Multipotential Connective Tissue Cells and Endothelial Cells

This class of cells is intermediate in position between relatively radiosensitive cells in classes 1 and 2 and the relatively radioresistant cells in classes 4 and 5. These cells may divide irregularly or sporadically in time and in response to a variety of special stimuli, and they are generally capable of undergoing transitions from one to another morphologic and functional form under the influence of various stimuli. Their life span as individuals with respect to one form of function may be highly variable, but under normal conditions it is on average longer than that of cells in classes 1 and 2. This class includes such cells as endothelial cells, especially those of the smaller vessels, which distinction

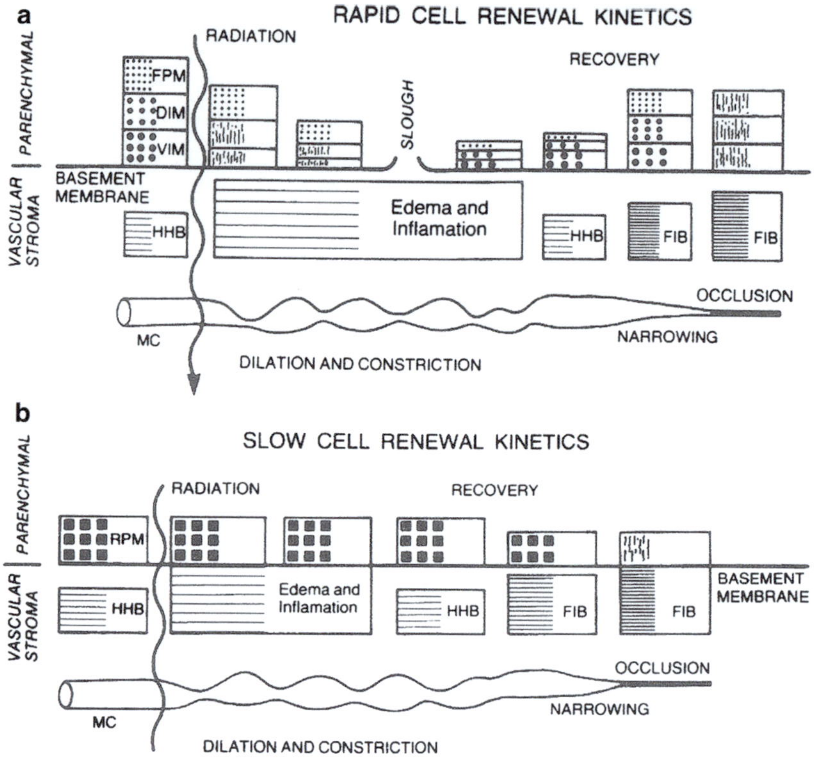

Fig. 4 **a** Rapid renewal system illustrating radiation effects on both parenchyma and micro vasculature compartments. *VIM* vegetative intermitotic cells; *DIM* differentiating intermitotic cells; *FPM* fixed postmitotic cells; *HHB* histo-hernatic barrier; *FIB* increased fibrosis; *MC* microcirculation (From Rubin P. Casarett GW: Clinical Radiation Pathology. Philadelphia, W.B. Saunders, 1968, with permission). **b** Slow renewal system illustrating effects on the vascular compartment, which leads to a late effect in the parenchymal cells as the capillary sclerosis and fibrosis increases. *RPM* reverting postmitotic cells (From Rubin P. Casarett GW: Clinical Radiation Pathology. Philadelphia, W.B. Saunders, 1968, with permission.)

would imply the existence of some indirect mechanisms as yet unknown, and fibroblasts and mesenchymal cells.

2.3.4 Class 4: Reverting Postmitotic Cells

In general this class of cells is relatively radiation resistant. These cells experience relatively long lives as individuals, do not normally undergo regular or periodic division in the adult and generally do not divide except under abnormal conditions presenting special stimuli. Under an appropriate stimulus, usually involving damage, destruction, or loss of considerable numbers of cells of their kind or of cells which they are capable of producing, they can revert to a condition in which they divide to produce more cells of their kind or they undergo heterotypic transformations to produce cells of certain other kinds.

Some of the cell types of this class are highly specialized in function, while others are not. Some are epithelial and some are connective tissue elements. This class includes cells such as the epithelial parenchymal cells and the duct cells in the salivary glands, liver, kidney, and pancreas; basal and parenchymal cells of merocrine glands such as the sweat glands and of endocrine glands such as the adrenal, thyroid, parathyroid, and pituitary glands; cells of interstitial gland tissue of the gonads; cells of corpora lutea; Sertoli cells; septal cells of the lung; fixed stem cells of various tissues, such as the reticulum cells in hematopoietic tissues and perhaps some smooth muscle cells. The cells in this class may show considerable aging changes, but on division their daughter cells show a relative rejuvenation, with the disappearance of aging changes.

2.3.5 Class 5: Fixed Postmitotic Cells

The cells in this class are generally the most radiation resistant of cells. They normally do not divide or have lost completely the ability to divide under any circumstances and are highly differentiated morphologically and highly specialized in function. Some of them have very long lives and others have relatively short lives, but all undergo progressive aging changes until death, If not killed prematurely. The short-lived fixed postmitotic cells, when lost, are replaced by the action of vegetative and/or differentiating intermitotic precursor cells. If the loss of precursor cells is also reverting postmitotic primitive fixed stem cells. This class includes cells such as the long-lived neurons and perhaps some muscle cells, which are not replaceable, and the short-lived polymorphonuclear granulocytes, erythrocytes, spermatids, spermatozoa, superficial epithelial cells of the alimentary tract and epithelial cells of the sebaceous glands, all of which are replaceable.

2.4 Normal Tissues and Their Relative Radiosensitivity

The histopathologic manifestations of radiation cellular death are pyknosis and karyolysis, swollen vacuolated cells with loss of staining capacity, and altered permeability, with eventual degeneration and phagocytosis. The events following exposure to radiation doses are determined, in part, by the radiosensitivity of the cells in the parenchymal compartment as well as related to the radiosensitivity of vascular stroma and its turnover rate. A rapid renewal system, illustrated in Fig. 4a, consists of vegetative intermitotic cells, differentiating intermitotic cells, and fixed postmitotic cells as found in the skin or the mucous membrane of the alimentary tract in the testes. The initial fractional doses of irradiation destroy the stem cell compartments (vegetative intermitotic cells and differentiating intermitotic cells) and reduce the production of cells that normally flow into the postmitotic compartment. The lining or mucous membrane thins and, as the dose increases, the connective tissue becomes edematous. With large doses, the parenchymal compartment may be lifted or sloughed as a result of the edema. The ability of the tissue to regenerate depends on the survival of stem cells (vegetative intermitotic cells), which gradually increase in number, differentiate, and rebuild the postmitotic compartment. The compartments eventually stabilize, but they might be relatively reduced as a result of increased fibrosis and an increased histo-hematic barrier. If large doses have been given, the microcirculation might become occluded at a later time, leading to frank delayed necrosis. With lesser degrees of fibrosis, the parenchymal compartment might atrophy, and when stressed, as by infection, might show its limited stem cell reserve capacity or mitotic potential to respond.

The sequence of events differs in a slow renewal system or nonrenewal system (Fig. 4b). The parenchymal compartment consists of reverting postmitotic cells or fixed postmitotic cells. Little or no change occurs in the parenchymal compartment with the fractional dose schemes used clinically. The vascular stromal compartment more often determines the course of events, although there are effects that can be attributed to a direct effect on parenchymal cells. The late expression of injury of these cells is caused by their slow renewal, hence the slow expression of injury.

2.4.1 Concept and Criteria of Radiosensitivity of Tissues

As in the case of the cell, the radiosensitivity or radioresistance of tissues, relates to differences in degree of response to similar doses to differences in doses required to produce similar responses. These terms are relative designations and depend upon the criterion or effect used as a basis for classification. The criterion of relative radiosensitivity of tissue types used here is the relatively direct loss (hypoplasia) of the parenchymal (definitive) cells of the tissue, with resulting tissue atrophy. The term "relatively direct" is defined as the result of mechanisms entirely contained within the tissue specified.

2.4.2 Range and Basis of Radiosensitivity of Tissue Types

The mechanisms of relatively direct radiation-induced hypoplasia and atrophy of rapidly and continually self-repopulating tissues, i.e., tissues which contain the frequently dividing intermitotic cells, may chiefly include temporary or permanent inhibition of mitosis, normal and precocious maturation and loss of cells without replacement for a time, and much mitosis-linked death of cells. Since these tissues are self-repopulating from vegetative and/or differentiating intermitotic cells, they are highly radiosensitive during mitosis. These cellular effects require relatively small doses, such tissues being highly radiosensitive.

In the case of in frequently or slowly repopulating tissues, i.e., those in which the only source of repopulation are the rarely dividing, long-lived reverting postmitotic cells, the chief and almost the only mechanism of relatively direct radiation-induced hypoplasia and atrophy is interphase death, which requires large doses. Therefore such tissues are relatively radioresistant.

In the case of tissues which cannot repopulate their parenchymal cells, i.e., tissues containing irreplaceable, long-lived fixed postmitotic cells, the only mechanism of relatively direct radiation-induced hypoplasia and atrophy is interphase death, and therefore such tissues are extremely radioresistant.

As the dose is gradually increased in the irradiation of an organ, more and more indirect effects at the intertissue level are brought to bear on the irradiated tissues, reducing the degree of selectivity that is associated with relatively direct effects on the tissue. In the case of the relatively resistant, slowly repopulating tissues or nonrepopulating tissues, the hypoplasia and atrophy which may be caused by large doses is often due in large measure to relatively indirect (intertissue) mechanisms, prominent among which are effects mediated through damage reactions of the cellular elements of interstitial connective tissue and the fine vasculature. The microvasculature has a relative radiosensitivity which is intermediate between dividing intermitotic cells on the one hand and reverting or fixed postmitotic cells. Similarly, in the irradiation of organs or segments of the body, more remote indirect (interorgan or systemic) mechanisms may contribute to the total effect on tissues being irradiated.

The *relative radiosensitivity* of a tissue is determined largely by the relative radiosensitivity of its parenchymal cells. Therefore, the essential radiosensitivity of the fine vasculature and connective tissue cells is modified by the radiosensitivity of the different tissue types in which it is embedded. The radiation sensitivity of the fine vasculature and interstitial connective tissue is generally less than that of tissues containing vegetative and/or differentiating intermitotic parenchymal cells, but is generally greater than that of tissues composed only of reverting or fixed

Table 4 Normal tissues and their relative radiosensitivity

Organs	Relative radiosensitivity	Chief mechanisms of parenchymal hypoplasia
Lymphoid organs, bone marrow (and blood), testes, ovaries, intestines	High	Destruction of parenchymal cells, especially the vegetative or differentiating intermitotic cells that are precursors of the mature parenchymal cells
Skin and other organs with epidermoid linings (cornea, oral cavity, esophagus, rectum, vagina, uterine cervix, urinary bladder, ureters, etc.)	Fairly high	Destruction of vegetative and differentiating intermitotic cells of stratified epithelium
Optic lens, stomach	Fairly high	Destruction of proliferating epithelial cells
Growing cartilage	Medium	Destruction of proliferating chondroblasts, plus some damage to the fine vasculature and connective tissue elements
Fine vasculature	Medium	Damage to the endothelium, plus some inflammatory reaction to the destruction of associated, dependent, sensitive parenchymal cells
Growing bone	Medium	Destruction of connective tissue cells and chondroblasts or osteoblasts, plus some damage to the fine vasculature
Mature cartilage or bone, salivary glands, respiratory organs, kidneys, liver, pancreas, thyroid, adrenal, pituitary	Fairly low	Hypoplasia secondary to damage to the fine vasculature and connective tissue elements with relatively less contribution by the direct effects on parenchymal tissues
Muscle, brain, spinal cord	Low	Hypoplasia secondary to damage to the fine vasculature and connective tissue elements, with little contribution by the direct effects on parenchymal tissues

postmitotic parenchymal cells. Consequently, in tissues of the former type (containing sensitive parenchymal cells), radiation can cause early or acute lesions (hypoplasia, atrophy) largely through relatively direct mechanisms at the tissue level, with relatively little mediation of the effect through damage to the fine vasculature and interstitial connective tissue. On the other hand, in tissues of the latter type (containing resistant parenchymal cells), the production of early or acute lesions requires larger doses and is usually associated with more marked mediation of the effect through damage to the fine vasculature and/or connective tissue elements and a relatively lesser contribution to the lesion from relatively direct mechanisms of tissue effect.

The radiation damage changes in the fine vasculature and interstitial connective tissue play a very important role in the production of chronic or delayed lesions in tissues of all kinds. The chronic and delayed radiation lesions are associated with nutritional and metabolic disturbances of the tissues.

2.4.3 Classification of Tissues

In keeping with the above considerations, various types of *tissues* are listed in Table 3 in the order of decreasing radiosensitivity, on the basis of the relatively direct radiation effect (hypoplasia) on the tissues specified; the chief mechanisms of the tissue effect are indicated. Similarly, in Table 4 are listed various *organs* in the order of decreasing radiosensitivity, on the basis of the relatively direct radiation effect (parenchymal hypoplasia), which would include effects due to inter tissue mechanisms within the organs, such as effects on parenchymal tissues mediated through damage to the local fine vasculature and connective tissue; here, too, the chief mechanisms of the organ effect are indicated.

2.4.4 Organs According to Relative Radiosensitivity

The order of relative radiosensitivity is given in terms of high, fairly high, medium, fairly low, and low. Tissue or organ parenchymal hypoplasia secondary to damage to the vasculature and interstitial connective tissue varies according to the progressive nature of the damage to these supporting tissues. A moderate radiation dose may result in the development over a long period of time of a degree of parenchymal hypoplasia similar to that which may be caused by a large dose in a short period of time. Therefore the order of relative radiosensitivity of the tissues and organs listed in Tables 3 and 4 is based arbitrarily on the maximal degree of hypoplasia observed within two months, a period of time sufficient to observe most of the relatively direct destructive actions of radiation in tissues.

2.5 Biocontinuum of Histologic Sequence of Events

The development of the cellular and histopathologic effects of radiation in various organs, from the subclinical levels to the levels of clinical importance in radiotherapy, is also greatly dependent on (1) organ radiosensitivity, (2) dose,

(3) time, and (4) volume of organ. But beyond this, such development is dependent upon additional factors, including (5) the structural nature of the organ as related to its function, (6) the reserve functional capacity of the organ, and therefore (7) the fraction of the organ irradiated, (8) the relative functional importance of the organ to the body, and (9) the clinical detectability of the related functional changes.

The acuteness or chronicity of the histopathologic changes underlying the first appearance of clinical complications depends to a considerable extent on the relative radiosensitivity of the parenchyma of the organ in relation to the relative sensitivity of the fine vasculature and supporting tissue. Under a given set of conditions, the first appearance of clinical effects in organs containing parenchymal tissue that is relatively highly sensitive to the cytocidal action of radiation is more likely to be associated with the histopathologic development of acute degeneration of the parenchyma, whereas in organs containing relatively radioresistant parenchyma the underlying histopathologic change is more likely to involve a predominance of chronic deterioration of the fine vasculature and secondary degeneration of the parenchyma.

Consequently, under the various conditions of radiation therapy, the period of time from irradiation to the end of life may be characterized by continuous complications of clinical significance arising from irradiation of normal organs, by alternation of periods of such clinical complication with clinically "silent" periods of the absence of such clinically significant complications. However, *there is at no time a "silent" histopathologic period,* i.e., absence of radiation induced changes in the irradiated organs, although their degree or rate of progression may vary considerably. Furthermore, the addition of further stress or insult, e.g., from trauma or infection, to organs that have sustained residual radiation damage may precipitate clinically significant complications during otherwise clinically "silent" periods. The histopathologic sequence of events after a brief radiation exposure is divided into four general phases: *Casarett Hypothesis*.

2.5.1 Phase I

This phase is characterized chiefly by the development of *acute damage* to cells and tissues that are sufficiently sensitive to the dose administered, although recovery processes begin during this phase also. In highly radiosensitive tissues there may be conspicuous inhibition of mitosis and destruction of parenchymal cells, leading to hypoplasia and atrophy of the tissues. Lesser degrees of such changes are seen in this phase in the more radio-resistant tissues. There may also be damage to small blood vessels and connective tissues in this phase, partly as a result of the relatively direct effects of radiation on these structures and partly as a result of the secondary effects of parenchymal cell destruction and the resulting inflammatory processes.

2.5.2 Phase II

This phase is characterized chiefly by *processes of recovery from acute damage,* although there may be some evidence of cell necrosis or tissue hypoplasia still persisting and there may be evidence of the beginning of chronic or permanent tissue damage. In the tissues that can repopulate themselves with parenchymal cells to replace those lost, regenerative replacement is prominent during this phase. If cell regeneration is very slow or inadequate owing to marked damage, repair by secondary intention (replacement fibrosis) may become relatively prominent. Subtle evidence of continuing spotty degeneration of the fine vasculature may persist in this phase, as well as evidence of both typical repair of the endothelium in some regions and atypical repair of the fine vasculature in the form of spotty fibroblastic activity and early fibrosis in and around the walls of these vessels and interstitially. These early atypical repair processes represent the beginning of increases in arteriolocapillary fibrosis and the histo-hematic connective tissue barrier described earlier.

The severe damage to the fine vasculature caused by large radiation doses results in poor support for continuing viability or regeneration of any kind of dependent cell, radiosensitive or radioresistant. Under these conditions this recovery phase is usually characterized by marked lesions in which repair by secondary intention (fibrosis) may be the most prominent repair process.

2.5.3 Phase III

This phase is an intermediate phase of *little or no change in parenchymal cellularity* after the irradiated tissue has regenerated parenchymal cells to the extent of its capability. The duration of this phase, before the beginning of the later phase of parenchymal tissue hypoplasia or premature involution or necrosis, varies widely and inversely with the dose. If the dose is very large, this intermediate phase may be virtually nonexistent, with failure of parenchymal regeneration and with continued or progressive deterioration of the parenchyma cells and fine vasculature. On the other hand, after small or moderate doses that permit parenchymal cell regeneration to normal or near normal levels of cellularity, this intermediate phase may be relatively long in duration. Even under these conditions, however, the degenerative changes in fine vasculature and the interstitial fibrosis, once initiated, progress in degree or may be added to other similar changes that develop with time or increasing age.

2.5.4 Phase IV

This phase is characterized by *delayed or late parenchymal degeneration,* either in the form of gradual premature involution of tissues, with hypoplasia, atrophy and replacement fibrosis, as in premature aging, or in the form of a more rapid breakdown or necrosis of tissues. The possibility that unrepaired intracellular damage such as chromosomal damage

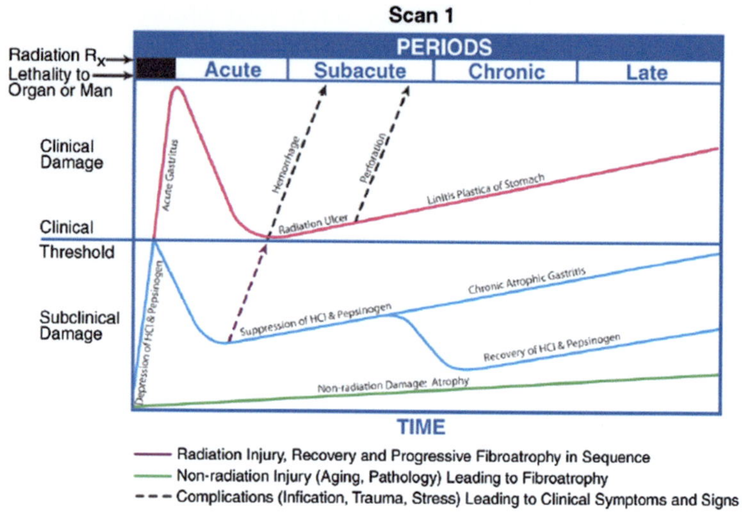

Fig. 5 Clinical expression events of the biocontinuum

may contribute to such delayed effects is not precluded. However, at the histologic level, both these types of delayed effects seem to be sequentially secondary to the progressively increasing degrees of degeneration of the fine vasculature and increasing density of quantity of fibrous connective tissue. In general, the larger the dose, the earlier and more rapidly these late effects develop.

2.6 Clinical Expression Events of the Biocontinuum

The sequence of clinical events after the initiation of radiation therapy will be considered in terms of four successive periods of time of arbitrary length, as follows: acute clinical period (first 6 months), subacute clinical period (second 6 months), chronic clinical period (second through fifth years), and late clinical period (after 5 years): *Rubin Hypothesis* (Fig. 5).

The diagram illustrates generally, with respect to these clinical periods, the waxing and waning (vertically) or organ damage with time and persistence or progression of residual damage. The upper lines depict radiation damage of different degrees. The bottom line indicates the accumulation of organ damage with time or "aging," may be additive to radiation damage in effect. The rising arrows indicate the precipitation of damage from subclinical or clinical levels to clinically significant or even lethal levels, as a result of complications such as trauma or infection or as a result of deterioration of the vasculature and failure of the blood circulation. No precise values or relationships are intended for the slopes or shapes of the graph lines.

2.6.1 Acute Clinical Periods (First 6 Months)

The accumulation of acute organ damage (histopathologic phase I) during the first part of this period, i.e., during the course of the fractionated radiation treatment, is depicted on the graph by the sharp initial rise in the radiation damage. Although recovery processes are operating between radiation exposures, the destructive processes predominate during the course of radiotherapy. The steepness of the radiation damage curve depends upon the relative radiosensitivity of the organ, the dose, and the schedule of fractionation. The recovery from acute organ damage (histopathologic phase II) after the cessation of the course of radiotherapy is depicted by the gradual decline in the radiation damage after the peak of acute damage. The steepness of the recovery curve is usually greater with lesser degrees of acute radiation damage and complicating factors.

Whether or not the radiation damage of an organ is sufficient to reach levels of clinical significance or to exceed tolerance limits and cause death in the acute clinical periods depends upon the relative radiosensitivity of the organ, the dose, the schedule of fractionation, and the occurrence or absence of complicating factors. In the case of some organs, with certain schedules of radiotherapy, the first part of the acute clinical period or even the whole of this period may be clinically silent, with clinically significant changes appearing for the first time, if at all, in later clinical periods as a result of deterioration of the vasculature and the occurrence of complications.

2.6.2 Subacute Clinical Period (Second 6 Months)

In the radiation damage graph in Fig. 5, the leveling of the slope or the plateau of the recovery portions of the curves above the threshold or "aging" damage levels during the subacute clinical period depicts the end of recovery from acute damage (end of histopathologic phase II) or the persistence or early progression of permanent residual damage (histopathologic phase III).

2.6.3 Chronic Clinical Period (Second Through Fifth Years)

In the radiation damage graphs in Fig. 5, the gradually rising lines depict an increase in degree of chronic organ damage, in terms of the progression of permanent residual radiation damage and/or the addition of aging damage (histopathologic phases III and IV). The clinically significant problems arising during this clinical period are usually the result of chronic deterioration of the organ's vasculature and circulation, an increase in the histo-hematic connective tissue barrier, degeneration of dependent parenchyma, and a reduction in resistance to complicating factors such as infection, trauma, or functional stress.

2.6.4 Late Clinical Period (After the Fifth Year)

The histopathologic and clinical developments during this clinical period are essentially similar to those described for the chronic clinical period, except for the slower progression of permanent residual radiation damage and a greater dependence upon the addition of the damage of aging. Radiation carcinogenesis can be manifested during this period and is usually preceded by some manifestation of chronic radiation damage.

3 Prologue II: Concept of Radiation Tolerance Dose

3.1 Introduction: Historical Annotation

The Tolerance Dose is an important concept first generated in collaboration with radiation oncology colleagues in national cooperative oncology groups. In the decades as radiation therapy was separating from radiologic diagnosis (1960–1970), NCI supported radiation research symposia during which controversial concepts were addressed. "The Biology of dose Limiting Tissues: Time and Dose Relationships in Radiation Biology as applied to Radiotherapy". Mendlesohn indicated how "Dose Response Data/Curves" were generated in the laboratory but clinical prudence limited the ability to create valid data since clinicians avoided producing severe radiation complications. In response, Rubin (Vice Chairman of RTOG and Chairman of Late Effects Committee) reviewed the available literature, consulted with colleagues (Ted Phillips), and generated the following definitions 3.

3.2 Tolerance Dose Effect

The Tolerance Dose is an attempt to express the minimal and maximal injurious dose acceptable to the clinician. This requires the assignment of an arbitrary but useful percentage for the risk of complications.

- The minimal tolerance dose is defined as $TD_{5/5}$, i.e., the dose to which a given population of patients is exposed under a standard set of treatment conditions resulting in no more than a 5 % severe complication rate within 5 years after treatment.
- The maximal tolerance dose is defined as $TD_{50/5}$ i.e., the dose to which a given population of patients is exposed under a standard set of treatment conditions resulting in a 50 % severe complication rate at 5 years after treatment.

The "dose limiting tissues or organs" in radiation therapy are based upon our inability to define an optimum tumor dose (many biological factors are unknown clinically) so that the radiation oncologist is often required to treat to tolerance. These dose limiting tissues have been defined into three categories or classes:

The concept was based on utilizing standard radiation regimes as supervoltage radiation became available, i.e., 60–70 Gy, in 6–7 weeks, 10 Gy a week, 5 days each week, daily dose of 1.8–2.0 cGy. Normal Tissues/Organs were divided into 3 classes:

- Class I—Organs in which radiation lesions are fatal or result in severe morbidity.
  - Vital Organs (Table 5).
- Class II—Organs in which radiation lesions result in moderate to mild morbidity and in exceptional circumstances a fatality, but generally late effects are compatible with survival.
  - Essential Organs (Table 6).
- Class III—Organs in which radiation lesions result in mild, transient, reversible effects or in no morbidity.
  - Tolerant Organs (Table 7).

3.3 Tolerance Volume Effect

The "Volume Effect" was based on whether the whole organ or partial organ was irradiated based on field size and length according to the available literature. The concept of tolerance volume needs to be defined in the same fashion as tolerance dose. The volume frequently proves to be more critical to complications outcome and also serves as a clinical guide because it is possible to obliterate or lose a certain volume of a vital organ with large doses; exceeding the TD_{50-100} is akin to surgical resection (stereotactic radiation surgery). Loss of some volume generally does not affect organ survival because the organ can often compensate for volume loss, up to a threshold volume, through regeneration or hypertrophy and remain, although impaired,

Table 5 Tolerance dose effect

Class I organs	Injury	$TD_{5/5}$	$TD_{50/5}$	Whole or partial organ (Field size or length)	Reference[a]
Bone marrow	Aplasia, pancytopenia	250 3,000	450 4,000	Whole Segmental	Bond et al. Rubin et al.
Liver	Acute and chronic hepatitis	2,500 1,500	4,000 2,000	Whole Whole strip	Ingold et al. Kraut et al.
Stomach	Perforation, ulcer hemorrhage	4,500	5,500	100 cm^2	Friedman
Intestine	Ulcer, perforation, hemorrhage	4,500 5,000	5,500 6,500	400 cm^2 100 cm^2	Friedman Roswit et al. Palmer
Brain	Infraction, necrosis	6,000 7,000	7,000 8,000	Whole 25 %	Kramer et al. Lindgren
Spinal Cord	Infraction, necrosis	4,500	5,500	10 cm	Phillips and Buschke Wara et al.
Heart	Pericarditis and pancarditis	4,500	5,500	60 %	Newton Stewart and Fajardo
Lung	Acute and chronic pneumonitis	3,000 1,500	3,500 2,500	100 cm^2 Whole	Gish et al. Lokick et al. Wara et al.
Kidney	Acute and chronic nephrosclerosis	1,500 2,000	2,000 2,500	Whole (strip) Whole	Kraut et al., Tefft Kunkler et al.
Fetus	Death	200	400	Whole	Rugh

Table 6 Tolerance dose effect

Class II organs	Injury	$TD_{5/5}$	$TD_{50/5}$	Whole or partial organ (Field size or length)
Oral cavity/pharynx Skin	Ulceration, mucositis acute and chronic dermatitis	6,000 5,500	7,500 7,000	50 cm^2 100 cm^2
Esophagus	Esophagitis, ulceration	6,000	7,500	75 cm^2
Rectum	Ulcer, stricture	6,000	8,000	100 cm^2
Salivary glands	Xerostomia	5,000	7,000	50 cm^2
Urinary bladder	Contracture	6,000	8,000	Whole
Ureters	Stricture	7,500	10,000	5–10 cm
Testes Ovaries	Sterilization Sterilization	100 200–300	200 625–1200	Whole whole
Growing cartilage, Growing bone (Child) Pure cartilage, Mature bone (Adult)	Growth arrest, Dwarfting Necrosis, Fracture, sclerosis	1,000 1,000 6,000 6,000	3,000 3,000 10,000 10,000	Whole 10 cm^2 Whole 10 cm^2
Eye retina		5,500	7,000	Whole
Cornea		5,000	6,000	Whole
Lens		500	1,200	Whole or part
Endocrine glands Thyroid Adrenal Pituitary	Hypothyroidism Hypoadrenalism Hypopituitarism	4,500 >6,000 4,500	15,000 – 20,000–30,000	Whole Whole Whole
Peripheral nerves	Neuritis	6,000	10,000	10 cm
Ear middle Ear inner vestibular	Serous otitis Meniere's syndrome	5,000 6,000	7,000 7,000	Whole Whole

Table 7 Tolerance dose effect

Class III organs	Injury	$TD_{5/5}$	$TD_{50/5}$	Whole or partial organ (field size or length)
Muscle (Child) Muscle (Adult)	Atrophy Fibrosis	2,000–3,000 6,000	4,000–5,000 8,000	Whole Whole
Lymph nodes and Lymphatics	Atrophy Sclerosis	5,000	>7,000	Whole node
Large arteries/veins	Sclerosis	>8,000	>10,000	10 cm^2
Articular cartilage Uterus	None Necrosis, Perforation	>50,000 >10,000	>500,000 >20,000	Joint surface (mm^2) Whole
Vagina	Ulcer, fistula	9,000	>10,000	Whole
Breast (Child)	No development	1,000	1,500	Whole
Breast (Adult)	Atrophy, Necrosis	>5,000	>10,000	Whole

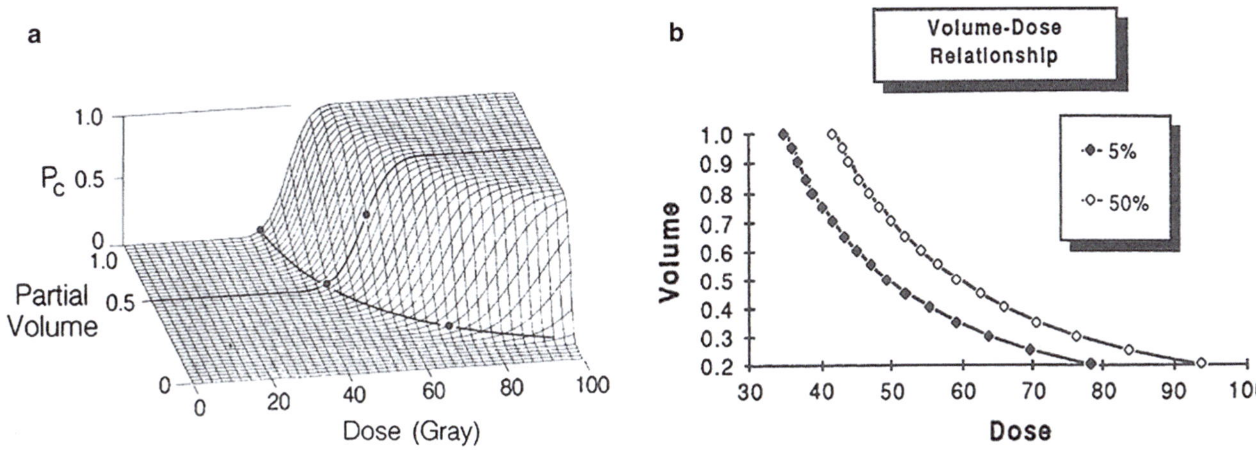

Fig. 6 Volume effect: **a** The dose–response curve is not an absolute or fixed effect but varies as a function of volume. This important concept allows the radiation oncologist to give much larger doses to partial volumes. (From Lyman JT, Wolbarst AB: Optimization of radiation therapy. III: a method of assessing complication probabilities from dose–volume histograms. Inst J Radiat Oncol Biol Phys 1987; 13:103, with permission from Elsevier Science). **b** for TD_5 and TD_{50}, the dose increases as the volume decreases. Note that the slope changes as more than 50 % of the whole organ is included. Small increments in dose, that is 10–20 %, can prove to be lethal

within functional tolerance for survival. Different organs demonstrate a range of tolerance volume (TV) parameters:

1. TV_{5-25}: 5–25 % of the organ volume irradiated can result in a life-threatening or lethal complication.
2. TV_{50-90}: 50–90 % of the organ volume irradiated can result in a life-threatening or lethal complication.

There are generally two levels of critical volume for dose-limiting or vital organs. Only the gastrointestinal tract and the central nervous system (CNS) can have disastrous outcomes after small volumes (TV 5–10 %) are exposed to doses exceeding TD_{5-50}. However, it is important to note that necrotic bowel and, on occasion, CNS necrotic foci can be resected successfully. For the majority of organs considered dose limiting, such as bone marrow, lung, kidney, and, in all probability, heart and liver, high doses can be tolerated to smaller volumes. Such organs may decompensate when more than 50 % of the total volume (as applied to paired organs) is exceeded and threatens survival.

The time when organ decompensation begins clearly depends on the compensatory regenerative mechanisms that come into play when significant organ volume loss occurs. The dose–response curve is not an absolute or fixed effect but varies as a function of volume. This is an important concept because it allows the radiation oncologist to give much larger doses to partial volumes. For TD_5 and TD_{50}, the dose increases as the volume decreases. Note that the slope changes as more than 50 % of the whole organ is included and is steeper. Small increments in dose, that is, 10–20 % of the total dose, can be lethal. The dose–volume histogram is being adopted by numerous investigators to predict unfavorable outcomes as a result of volume loss in a critical structure.

An important and insightful concept was developed by Lyman, in which the dose response curve is not an absolute

Table 8 Parameters of therapy: tolerance doses ($TD_{5/5}$–$TD_{50/5}$)

Single dose (Gy)		Fractionated dose (Gy)	
Lymphoid	2–20	Testes	1–2
Bone marrow	2–10	Ovary	6–10
Ovary	2–6	Eye (lens)	6–12
Testes	2–10	Kidney	20–30
Eye (lens)	2–10	Thyroid	20–40
Mucosa	5–20	Lung	23–28
Lung	7–10	Skin	30–40
GI	5–10	Liver	35–40
Colorectal	10–20	Bone Marrow	40–50
Kidney	10–20	Heart	43–50
Heart	18–20	GI	50–55
Vasculo connective tissue	10–20	Vasculo connective tissue	50–60
Liver	15–20	Spinal cord	50–60
Skin	15–20	Brain	55–70
Peripheral nerve	15–20	Peripheral nerve	65–77
Spinal cord	15–20	Mucosa	65–77
Brain	15–25	Bone and cartilage	>70
Bone and cartilage	>30	Muscle	>70
Muscle	>70		

or fixed effect but varies as a function of organ volume. A 3-D construct allowed for a method of assessing complication probabilities from dose–volume histograms (Fig. 6a) this concept provided the radiation oncologist with a guide as to varying the dose depending on volume (Fig. 6b). This concept applied to organ tolerance doses, arbitrarily choosing 1/3 and 2/3 organ volumes was then published with Enami et al.

3.4 Tolerance of Organs

3.4.1 Dose–Time–Volume Factors

Dose-limiting organs and tissues in radiation oncology have been defined according to their tolerance doses (Table 8). The minimal tolerance dose ($TD_{5/5}$) and the maximal tissue tolerance dose ($TD_{50/5}$) refer to severe to life-threatening complications occurring in 5 and 50 % of patients within 5 years of therapeutic radiation treatment. However, in this era of multimodality, there are many factors that affect our concepts of radiosensitivity. The rapid advances of radiation oncology and the related sciences of radiation biology and radiation physics and accumulating information about interactions with other therapeutic modalities (e.g., chemotherapy or biologic response modifiers) impact our understanding of normal tissue toxicities. Thus, although previously defined radiation tolerance doses (TD_5 and TD_{50}) remain as valuable guides, their applicability has changed. Radiation doses customarily deemed to be safe may no longer be so. When combined with another therapy, such doses can lead to severe late effects with regard to different vital organs. Factors relevant to defining tolerance doses include those from therapy, the host, and the tumor.

3.4.2 General Therapy Modifying Factors

- *Dose*: There is no absolute or fixed dose that ablates a normal tissue because the $TD_{5/5}$ and $TD_{50/5}$ are dependent on dose, time, and volume factors.
- *Fractionation*: The radiation fraction dose, the interval between fractions, and the overall duration of therapy are major determinants of both early and late effects. The time to expression of the effect is related to the cell kinetics of different subpopulations within a tissue organ. With alternate fractionation regimens under investigation, the $TD_{5/5}$ and $TD_{50/5}$ will shift for different organs. Hyper fractionation, accelerated fractionation, and hypo fractionation have different effects on tolerance doses.
- *Volume*: A major factor in determining a tolerance dose is whether the whole or part of an organ is exposed to radiation. With more widespread use of large fields, for example, total body irradiation (TBI) and hemibody irradiation (HBI), compared with very defined or small fields, for example, intraoperative radiation therapy and stereotactic radiosurgery, single or brief radiation exposures with various dose rates to different volumes, will create a new set of normal tissue toxicities.
- *Chemotherapy*: Of the various modalities, the addition of chemotherapy and the timing of its delivery relative to irradiation have a major impact on organ sensitivity. The use of an agent may dramatically affect either the same cells or different cell subpopulations, leading to lower threshold doses for organ injury. The widespread use of drugs is the most common factor altering the tolerance dose concepts of normal tissues.
- *Innovations*: The new modalities, radiosensitizers and radioprotectors, and immunologic and biologic response modifiers, including gene therapy, may each or all alter late effects.

The concept of an optimal radiation dose that provides maximal curability and minimal toxicity is the basis of varying fractionation schedules. Strandqvist lines or isoeffect plots based on varying dose-time regimens suggest that an optimal zone can be found, yielding a favorable therapeutic ratio. Although these lines were originally drawn with parallel slopes, it became apparent to many investigators that tumors respond differently to normal tissues, and a divergence in isoeffect slopes occurs. The importance of the volume of normal tissue in the field and dose-time factors needs

Table 9 Parameters of therapy: tolerance dose $TD_{5/5}$–$TD_{50/5}$

Target cell	Complication end point	Dose range (Gy)[a] $TD_{5/5}$–$TD_{50/5}$
Range: 2–10 Gy		
Testes/spermatogonia	Sterility	1–2
Lymphoid tissue/lymphocytes	Lymphopenia	2–10
Diseased bone marrow	Severe leukopenia and thrombocytopenia	3–5
(CLL or multiple myeloma)		6–10
Ovary/oocytes		
Range: 10–20 Gy		
Lens	Cataract	6–12
Bone marrow stem cells	Acute aplasia	15–20
Range: 20–30 Gy		
Lung-type II cells, vasculo connective tissue	Pneumonitis/fibrosis	20–30
Kidney-glomeruli	Arterionephrosclerosis	23–28
Range: 30–40 Gy		25–35
Bone marrow	Hypoplasia	35–40
Liver-central veins	Radiation hepatitis	
Range: 40–50 Gy		43–50
Heart (whole)	Pericarditis and pancarditis	45–50
Bone marrow microenvironments, sinuses	Permanent aplasia	
Range: 50–60 Gy		50–55
GI organ	Infarction necrosis	50–60
Spinal cord	Myelopathy	50–60
Brain	Encephalopathy	55–65
Heart (partial)	Cardiomyopathy	
Range: >60–70 Gy		65–75
Mucosa	Ulcer	65–75
Rectum	Ulcer	65–75
Bladder	Ulcer	65–75
Mature bones	Fracture	

CCL Chronic lymphocytic leukemia
[a] Doses are given as the total fractionated dose to whole or partial organs
From Rubin P: Law and order of radiation sensitivity. Absolutely versus relative. In: Vaeth JM, Meyer JL (eds): Frontiers of Radiation Therapy and Oncology, 23rd edn, p7. Basel, Karger, 1989, with permission

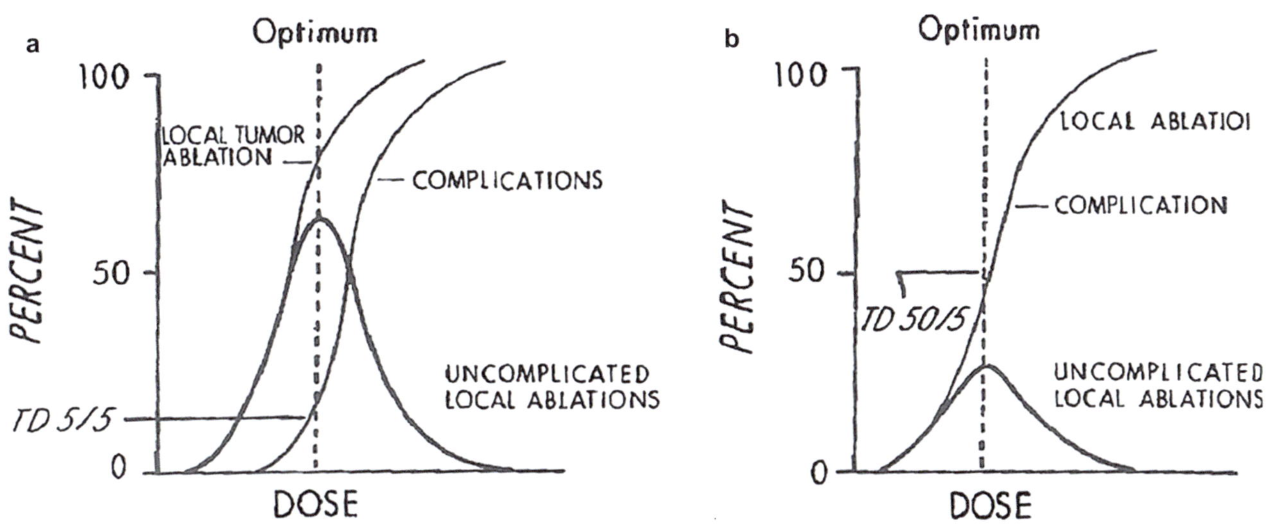

Fig. 7 **a** The modification of this figure is the line indicating the $TD_{5/5}$ proposed. In favorable circumstances, the radiation therapist would not be willing to exceed the numerical rate of complication. Modified from Mendelsohn (9). **b** The modification of this figure is the line indicating the $TD_{50/5}$. In unfavorable circumstances, the radiation therapist is often unwilling to exceed the maximal rate since the dose–response curve rises sharply. Modified from Mendelsohn (9)

to be stressed when considering tolerance of normal tissue or organs (Rf: Von Essen). In re-examining and revising the tolerance doses for different vital dose-limiting tissues and organs, the volume factor is even more relevant today in view of the increasing use of TBI and HBI, in which whole organ systems are exposed. More time concentrated schedules are in use, varying from single exposures to short, intense hypo fractionation schedules of stereotactic radiosurgery. Another modality—intraoperative radiation therapy—has led to the use of large, single doses to large tissue volumes and has provided new insights into tolerance doses.

At present, the prescribed tolerance dose is, at best, a calculated estimate of the TD_5 and TD_{50} based on recorded human and animal data. The complication probability of either 5 (TD_5) or 50 % (TD_{50}) assumes uniform irradiation of all or part of an organ, conventional fractionation schedules (1.8–2.0 Gy per fraction and five fractions per week), relatively normal organ function as a baseline, no adjuvant drugs or surgical manipulations, and age ranges that exclude children and the elderly (Table 9). In ordering the organ radiosensitivity according to dose level, a variety of factors are considered, including the end point chosen (late rather than acute effects), the use of single or fractionated regimens, and the volume of the organs. Because the literature is not always complete or precise, extrapolation is inevitably involved when using either clinical or experimental animal data. The dose levels are rounded off rather than recorded precisely to one or two decimals, as is occasionally reported. Such accuracy can be as misleading as the general estimates of tolerance doses offered.

3.4.3 Specific Organ Tolerances: Dose-Limiting Tissues

Most organ systems are composed of many cell subpopulations (20–40 or more), each performing an important activity. Therefore, organ tolerance is determined by the radiosensitivity or relevant stem cell subpopulations that may not always be proliferating or dividing; the most radiosensitive, vital cell population determines organ tolerance and organ failure. Just as the degree of importance held by an irradiated organ determines the survival of an organism, the functional capacity of cells is often distinct from their regenerative capacity, permitting organ physiology to be preserved in the face of injury and allowing for recovery or repair from the insult.

Late Effects of Normal Tissue (LENT) syndromes at each organ site are not random events but are specific entities that occur at certain times and are expressed in a recognizable fashion and often can be ameliorated. A LENT paradigm is presented in diagrammatic form for each organ site (Fig. 7a and b). Additional detailed information regarding specific organ tolerances are summarized in Chap. 8 (Understanding and Predicting Radiation-Associated Normal Tissue Injury: A Global and Historical Perspective), as well as in the site-specific chapters throughout the book.

4 Prologue III: The Concept of Pediatric Radiation Sensitivity

4.1 Introduction: Historical Annotation

"Pediatric Radiation Tolerance Doses" were graduated as a function of age in Children Oncology Cooperative groups for most normal tissues. Discovering the postnatal pediatric growth curves, radiation tolerance doses were redefined as a function of normal tissues evolution from infant to child to adolescence. Uncovering the seminal research thesis and basis which we published in the 1920s is acknowledged to SCAMMON for the first time (not Tanner or Harris). His remarkable thesis is presented to illustrate the importance of identifying the original reference; counter to emphasizing the most recent publications to be current. In 1980, a "new hypothesis" of relating pediatric normal tissue/organ tolerance to the classic "Growth curves of different normal tissues/organs" was developed with Sandy Constine.

4.2 Concept of Mitotic Potential Versus Mitotic Activity

The child, like the embryo, is a mosaic of numerous tissues and organs which are undergoing continual growth and maturation. These tissues and organs have cells that are in various stages of development: totipotential, multipotential, and eventually unipotential which are either resting or in active proliferation without or with differentiation into specialized tissues or organs. Just as the fetus in its development is continually changing in its tissue and cellular kinetics, so in turn is its radiosensitivity with critical points in time of exquisite vulnerability to irradiation for specific organs. Similarly, the infant and child consist of an array of tissues and organ that vary in radiosensitivity at different times according to their developmental stage.

The hypothesis advanced for understanding the changing radiosensitivity and radioresistance of pediatric tissues is in comprehending their periods of active proliferation and differentiation and eventual maturation. Growth of an organ varies from infancy, childhood, and puberty and is not constant. Correction factors applied for radiation dose are modified by age but do not recognize that various organs indeed develop and mature at different rates (Table 9). No one formula can be applied universally to all tissues.

Adjusted doses for age assumes that growth occurs at a constant rate. The growth rate and maturation of each tissue or organ is the major determinant of its radiosensitivity. A model for pediatric radiosensitivity of normal tissues and organs is developed in an analogous fashion to fetal organ radiosensitivity.

4.3 The Fetal Model of Radiosensitivity: Prenatal Organogenesis

The susceptibility of the fetus to radiation and the resultant dramatic occurrence of congenital abnormalities has been the subject of intense study. Analogies have been drawn between experimental studies in mammalian fetal radiobiology and abnormalities observed in human circumstances. It is possible to extrapolate from these laboratory studies to man.

The principle events in the development of an embryo include implantation, placentation, organogenesis, and the differentiation of the various organs. The sequence of events tends to be the same in different mammalian species with only the timescale differing (11, 16, 36). Both in the experimental model and in clinical experience, moderate doses of ionizing radiation have been shown to produce catastrophic effects in the fetus which include growth retardation, fetal death, or gross congenital malformations (36). In the mouse, a dose of 200 rad will lead to prenatal deaths in the preimplantation phases, abnormalities, or neonatal deaths during the organogenesis (38). Neural tissues are interestingly the most exquisitely sensitive and most rapidly dividing in early fetal development. An exposure of 100–500 rad during the course of embryogenesis suffices to produce neural malformations, mainly an overall reduction of brain size as micro-opthalmy or micro-cephaly (16). In comparison, 2 weeks after birth, doses greater than 1,000 rad are necessary to produce neurologic abnormalities in rats (9, 52). Information available from Japanese survivors of the A bomb attacks show an increase in fetal deaths, infant deaths, and neurologic abnormalities (24). Doses lower than 250 rad delivered between the 4th and 20th weeks of gestation may lead to severe abnormalities.

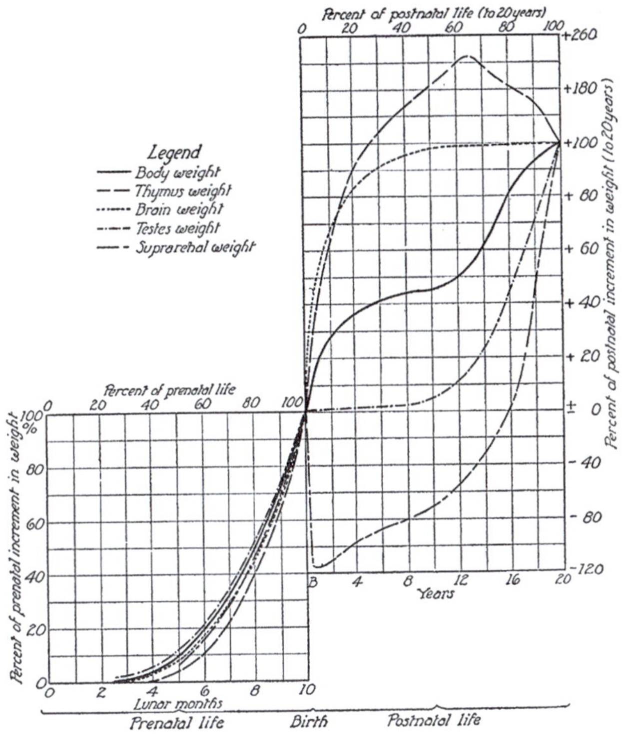

Fig. 8 The pediatric model of radiosensitivity: postnatal growth spurts

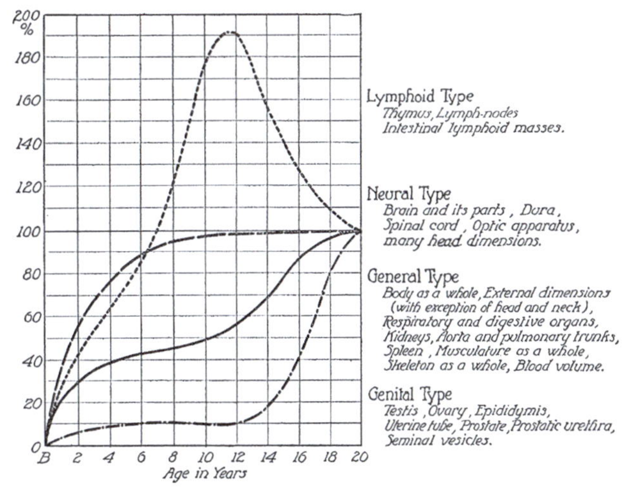

Fig. 9 The pediatric model of radiosensitivity: postnatal growth spurts

4.4 The Pediatric Model of Radiosensitivity: Postnatal Growth Spurts

Instead of critical moments, days or weeks for fetal organ induction and rapid development, in the child there are longer periods of months of rapid proliferation when the entire parenchyma of an organ is in a phase of active mitosis. At some point the collection of tissues or cells becomes mature and differentiates into a specialized system. Some systems have rapid proliferation or cell cycle kinetic characteristics whereas others behave as slow renewal systems and only become active again if challenged or stimulated. 'When does a pediatric tissue or organ become similar to an adult tissue or organ?' is a question that needs to be answered. Postnatal development has been studied much less than prenatal development and information about variation in growth characteristics is less well known.

In the child, there are two major periods of rapid rate of growth development: the postnatal period and puberty. The growth of the different organs follows four general patterns (14, 42–44). The first is a general skeletal pattern which has the two peak periods aforementioned. The organs of circulation and digestion follow the pattern of the body as a whole (postnatal and pubertal activity). The neural type is characterized by a rapid postnatal growth which slows in late infancy and ceases in adolescence. The respiratory and renal organs tend to follow this pattern according to their maturation. The genital type shows little change during early life but rapid development just before the coincident with puberty. This is particularly true of breast tissue and applies to testis and ovarian tissue. The lymphoid type is characterized by a gradual evolution and involution to the time of puberty.

The number of different organs will be reviewed regarding their growth maturation and radiosensitivity for the different stages of proliferation and differentiation. Organ weight and size may be helpful guides, but it is essential to determine when an organ is through or is entering its phase of rapid proliferation. It is important to distinguish hyperplasia from hypertrophy as to the mechanism of organ growth. To fully understand an organ's radiosensitivity it is necessary first to comprehend its biology.

The following tenets were offered as guidelines to pediatric organ radiosensitivity:

(1) The stage of organogenesis, during fetal development when an organ is being formed, is the most highly radiosensitive phase.
(2) Specific phases of tissue proliferation during infancy and childhood when rapid growth spurts occur determine the organ's radiosensitivity. Radiosensitivity of a tissue/organ is highest prior to and at the time of onset of proliferative activity in each organ system.
(3) Maturation occurs at different ages for each tissue/organ and its identification allows for recognition when the radiosensitivity in children is similar to adults.
(4) Growth of an organ due to increase in cell size is less vulnerable to irradiation than when due to an increase in cell number, i.e., hypertrophy versus hyperplasia.
(5) Radiation therapy and chemotherapy can be additive even when safe schedules are given and can lead to late effects despite intervals up to months or years between time of administration of these modes.
(6) Correction factors applied for radiation dose must take into account the maturation of each organ irradiated and not the child as a unit. The doses recommended for several organs appears to be in the same range as for adults: heart, kidney, lung, liver. Data available in the current literature suggest two periods of increased sensitivity: the first years of life and the puberty growth spurt. This latter applies for the genital organs, bone, and muscle.

The origin of the "post-natal pediatric curves" (PNPC) are most often attributed to Tanner (1962); however, the PNPC are referenced to Harris 1927. Obtaining this 100-year-old book, upon inspection was an assemblage of four research PhD theses, entitled: "The Measurement of Man". The most remarkable work was by *Scammon: The Measurement of The Body in Childhood.* It is truly an outstanding research project based on autopsy specimens and radiographs involving thousands of children and adolescents, some followed longitudinally for two decades (1–20 years). Two graphs are presented (Figs. 8 and 9).

At birth, all of these structures are growing at a rate of between 5–10 % per month of their attained magnitudes and all undergo a very marked reduction in these relative rates of growth in infancy and early childhood. But thereafter the trends of this measure of increment become different. The relative growth of the body as a whole (general type) as exemplified by body weight, falls to a minimum at about 7 years. This shows a distinct para puberal rise to about 12 years and a decline thereafter. The genital organs (the general type), as exemplified by the testis show an even more pronounced reduction in relative growth rate but a tremendous prepubertal rise, which like the rise in relative growth of the body as a whole, reaches its peak at puberty and declines thereafter. The nervous system (the neural type) as represented by the brain, shows no rise in relative rate of growth in later childhood or adolescence. On the contrary, there is a steady but slow decline in this measure from childhood to maturity. And the lymphoid organs (lymphoid type) as illustrated by the thymus show not only a decline, in relative velocity, but in actual negative velocity (indicating a loss of weight) in the years following puberty. Thus, measures of rates, as well as the amounts of growth, illustrate the essential similarities of prenatal growth at a remarkable diversity of post natal growth of various parts of the human body.—SCAMMON 1910–1930.

Biophysiopathology of the Microvasculature and Microcirculation

Philip Rubin and Luis Fajardo

Contents

Abstract

The microvasculature and microcirculation are the largest single organ in the human body. The essential radiosensitivity of the fine vasculature and connective tissue cells associated with various types of dependent tissue seems to vary much less on the basis of the relatively direct effects rather, than the relative radiosensitivity of various dependent tissue types themselves. The radiation sensitivity of the fine vasculature and interstitial connective tissue is generally less than that of the radiosensitive tissues containing more mitotically active parenchymal cells. Generally the greater that the tissues are composed of sensitive parenchymal cells, radiation can cause early or acute lesions. The tissues that contain resistant parenchymal cells, the production of early or acute lesions require large doses and is usually associated with more marked mediation of the effect through damage to the fine vasculature and or connective tissue elements. The radiation damage and subsequent progressive changes in fine vasculature and interstitial connective tissue play a very important role in the production of chronic delayed lesions in a large variety of tissues. The discussion of microvasculature injury varies with the cell kinetics of the different tissues and parenchymal cells that constitute the various organs and viscera in the body.

1 Introduction

The largest normal tissue structure in the human body is the microvasculature. It is generally estimated that there are 50,000 miles of capillaries with a surface area of approximately 1000 square miles. The ubiquitous distribution and presence of the microvasculature is essential for survival of all normal tissue/organs; the microcirculation supplies oxygen and nutrients and removes wastes. The fine

P. Rubin (✉)
Professor and Chair Emeritus, Department of Radiation Oncology, University of Rochester School of Medicine and Dentistry, 601 Elmwood Ave, Box 647, Rochester, NY 14642, USA
e-mail: oncophilip@earthlink.net

L. Fajardo
Stanford Medical School, 3801 Miranda Ave, Palo Alto, CA 94304, USA

P. Rubin et al. (eds.), *ALERT – Adverse Late Effects of Cancer Treatment*, Medical Radiology. Radiation Oncology, DOI: 10.1007/978-3-540-72314-1_3, © Springer-Verlag Berlin Heidelberg 2014

vasculature is widespread, occurs as a component of most other organs (including larger vessels), and responds to irradiation in a more sensitive fashion than large vessels and is directly, intimately, and critically involved in the radiation responses of tissues dependent upon it for metabolic support.

2 Anatomy

A metarteriole gives rise to capillaries. The precapillary sphincters of the arteriole and metarteriole control the entry of blood into capillaries. The distal segment of the thoroughfare channel receives capillaries from the microcirculatory bed, but no sphincters are present where the afferent capillaries enter the thoroughfare channels. Blind-ending lymphatic vessels are shown in association with the capillary bed. Note the presence of anchoring filaments and the valve system within the lymphatic capillaries (Fig. 1) (Ross et al. 2003). Most arterioles can dilate 60–100 % from their resting diameters and can maintain constriction for a long time.

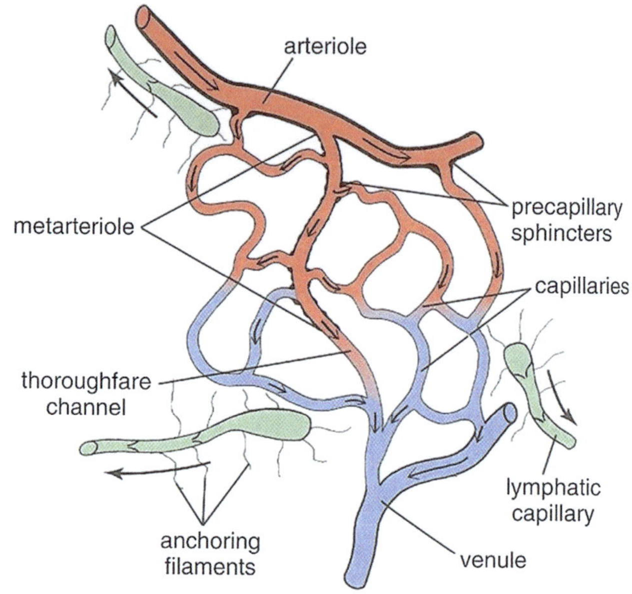

Fig. 1 Diagram of microvasculature (with permission from Ross et al. 2003)

3 Histology of Microvasculature

- Capillaries: structurally the fundamental vascular units are simple endothelial tubes connecting terminal arterioles or precapillaries and venules. There is usually a semi fluid intercellular cement between the endothelial cells of the capillary, and only a delicate reticular network surrounds the endothelial tube. Outside their walls may be found fixed macrophages and fibroblasts. The average diameter of normal blood capillaries is about 8 microns; thus erythrocytes are permitted to pass in single file. The largest normal capillary has a diameter of about 12 microns. Capillaries form networks which may be flattened or spongy and vary in shape, conforming to the character of the region they supply. The closeness of the mesh generally varies directly with the intensity of the tissue metabolism in the region supplied. Lymphatic capillaries are somewhat broader than blood capillaries and not as uniform in caliber, showing dilatations and constrictions. Their walls are composed of endothelium alone, embedded in connective tissue. These capillaries form dense networks roughly paralleling networks of blood capillaries, and they are often close neighbors of blood capillaries. They are found in nearly all parts of the body. Near surfaces, such as the skin and internal membranes, they often begin as loops or as blind swollen tubules. There are certain other small blood channels resembling capillaries in some respects, but which can be distinguished from them. Prominent examples are sinusoids and the rete mirabile.
- Sinusoids are special channels between larger vessels. Some of them connect arterioles with venules, as in the spleen, adrenal cortex, and bone marrow. Others connect venule with venule, as in the liver and in the anterior lobe of the pituitary gland. There are also lymphatic sinusoids which interconnect lymphatic vessels, as in the lymph nodes. Sinusoids are relatively wide, up to 30 microns, and are not uniform in caliber. They are lined by an incomplete layer of scattered fixed microphages that project into the lumen, by flat cells that are apparently potential macrophages and by cells in every transition between these two forms. These lining cells are separated from the surrounding parenchyma only by a network of reticular fibrils.
- The rete mirabile is a capillary-like plexus inserted in the course of an arteriole or venule, with an afferent arteriole or venule carrying blood to it and efferent arteriole or venule draining it. An example is the renal glomerulus, and similar structures are the sinusoids of the anterior pituitary (venule-sinusoid-venule) and of the lymph nodes (lymphatic-sinusoid-lymphatic).
- Precapillaries are vessels intermediate between capillaries and arterioles or venules. They are larger than capillaries but have incomplete accessory coats as compared

with arterioles and venules. Arterial precapillaries are less than 40 microns in diameter. The smallest of them consist of an endothelial tube surrounded by scattered smooth muscle fibers; the largest are, in addition, surrounded discontinuously by connective tissue cells and fibers. Venous precapillaries are less than 200 microns in diameter; the smallest consist of endothelium surrounded by scattered connective tissue elements, and the larger ones are, in addition, surrounded discontinuously by smooth muscle fibers. With the smooth muscle in the precapillaries to act as sphincters, the control of vessel size and blood flow through the capillary beds becomes possible.

- Arterioles: All blood vessels larger than precapillaries exhibit a common generally structural organization. However, each specific type of vessel shows characteristic adaptive variations in which certain features of the general plan may be emphasized, minimized, or omitted, or certain new features may be added. Every typical blood vessel larger than a precapillary is composed of three concentric coats of tunics, namely, the tunica intima or interna, the tunica media, and the tunica adventitia or externa. The *tunica intima* consists of an endothelium (simple squamous epithelium) bounding the lumen, a subendothelial coat of delicate fibroelastic tissue and a fenestrated internal elastic membrane, which is the outermost component of the intima. The *tunica media* consists primarily of smooth muscle circularly arranged, with variable amounts of elastic fibers, or circular elastic networks, or concentric elastic tubes in certain large vessels. The *tunica adventitia,* the outer coat, usually contains a concentration of elastic tissue as an elastic layer, and close to the tunica media there may be a definite external elastic membrane. The remainder of this coat consists of moderately compact fibroelastic tissue which merges gradually with areolar connective tissue. Blood vessels most than 1 mm in diameter contain nutrient vessels called *vasa vasorum*. In arteries these are usually limited to the tunica adventitia, but in veins they may extend through the tunica media. Lymphatic vessels are also present in the walls of the larger blood vessels. The arteries include *arterioles,* the smallest arteries (40–300 microns in diameter), which are predominantly muscular; small to *medium-sized arteries,* which are predominantly muscular; and large arteries, which are predominantly elastic. The transition from muscular to elastic composition is usually gradual, and there are intermediate mixed types. The size and composition of arteries are not always typically correlated. The arterioles have relatively thick walls and narrow lumens, the walls being thicker relative to the caliber of the lumen than in any other type of blood vessel. As compared with arterioles, venules have a large diameter (between 200 and 100 microns) but a relatively thin wall and broad lumen. The tunica intima consists only of an endothelial layer, the thin tunica media is almost exclusively smooth muscle, and the tunica adventitia is a relatively thick component of the very thin wall. An arterial lumen is always smaller than that of its companion vein of the combined lumens of its companion veins, and the arterial wall is thicker, more rigid, and more resistant to collapse.

4 Physiology of Microcirculation

The microcirculatory apparatus is of special importance in any consideration of damage and recovery of organs because of its intimate and vital supportive relationship to the metabolism of tissues and tissue components. The fine blood vessels, and usually the fine lymphatic vessels also, enter into the composition of most organs. The one-way microcirculatory flow carries nutrients, oxygen, hormones, and blood cells to all parts of the body, and collects metabolic wastes from the tissues and transports them to the kidneys or, in the case of carbon dioxide, to the lungs.

Capillaries are the most important of all vessels functionally, since they are in a close relationship with the various tissue elements at the site of cellular metabolism, where they deliver nutrients and oxygen and receive wastes, their thin walls and slow blood flow favor diffusive interchanges. Capillary blood flow varies in amount and extent with tissue activity, being intermittent in resting or relatively inactive tissues and voluminous and extensive in active tissues. Although capillaries are closed tubes they are normally semi permeable. Water, gases, salts, and nutrients in simple form are among those substances which pass through their walls, but most colloids and all microscopically visible particles do not normally pass through. However, the degree of permeability of capillary walls varies regionally and also with local changes in condition. Leukocytes occasionally pass through the endothelium under normal conditions, and when the endothelium is altered, as in inflammatory conditions, the passage of leukocytes may be greatly increased; even erythrocytes may escape from the blood through the altered endothelium. True endothelial cells are not normally phagocytic, as are the cells lining the sinusoids.

The muscular arteries can regulate the blood flow to any part of the body according to its changing needs by means of nervous control of the muscular layer of the vessels. The arterioles, with their relatively thick walls and narrow lumens, are the chief controllers of systemic blood pressure and local blood flow. Most of the decline in blood pressure in the mascular system occurs within the arterioles, so that the delicate capillaries normally receive blood gently in a slow stream.

Endothelial cells normally divide from time to time with moderate frequency to replace those cells that die and are lost. They are capable of much more rapid proliferation under pathologic conditions, e.g., during recovery from local injuries to the vasculature and during neovascular formation in the healing of wounds or lesions. In neovascular formation, the endothelium from capillaries forms solid sprouts which enter injured and regenerating areas. The sprouts become hollow, fibroblasts are at hand, myoblasts soon differentiate, and accessory coats are formed around the endothelial tubes as needed.

The aging arteries seem to be a physiologic process that passes gradually into arteriosclerosis. Each type of artery normally shows a characteristic pattern and schedule of change with increasing time.

5 Pathogenesis

A discussion of the radiation effects on endothelial cells should be preceded by some review of the complex physiology of the endothelium. Aside from those activities common to all cells, certain specialized functions are characteristic of Endothelial cells (EC):

- EC are the most radiosensitive among the fixed elements of the mesenchyme. Depending on dose, ionizing radiation can produce lethal or sublethal injury to EC. The latter may alter considerably the complex physiology of the endothelium. Some functions are inhibited or abolished: fibronolysis, synthesis of various enzymes and cytokines, attachment of EC to the basal lamina, angiogenesis, etc. Other functions are enhanced, including permeability, soluble coagulation, platelet adhesion, and aggregation. There is also upregulation of adhesion molecules for leukocytes. Endothelial cells are heterogeneous; accordingly, radiation effects vary in quality and severity from one site to another, and from one animal species to another.
- Coagulation: EC participate in the soluble coagulation system by producing both procoagulants (e.g., tissue factor and Factor V) and anticoagulants (e.g., plasminogen activators and thrombomodulin.). In addition, EC regulate the adhesion and aggregation of platelets through von Willebrand Factor (vWill F), nitric oxide, etc.
- Permeability: transport of certain molecules across the EC cytoplasm.
- Inflammation and immune response: EC express multiple antigens, including MHCs I and II, and ABO. Several cytokines are produced in EC, such as IL1 and GM-CSF. Depending on activation state, lymphocytes, granulocytes, and macrophages adhere to specific EC receptors.
- Synthesis of stromal components: EC produce their own basement membrane (mainly collagens IV, V, and laminin), as well as various collagens for the surrounding tissue matrix.
- Vascular tone regulation: through angiotensin converting enzyme and endothelin, EC contract smooth muscle while nitric oxide relaxes it.
- Angiogenesis: this, the formation of microvessels in the fully developed vertebrate, is the most dynamic function of the endothelium; it occurs in response to a large number of agonists and antagonists. It is either physiologic (e.g., in wound healing and cyclical endometrial growth) or pathologic (e.g., in neoplasia and many inflammatory disease).

The above, and other endothelial cell functions, are regulated by numerous genes, many of which have been characterized. EC vary greatly from tissue to tissue and from one animal species to another. This heterogeneity is evident morphologically, functionally, and in response to injury. Figure 2 outlines diagrammatically the most important of the functions characteristic of EC (compare with Fig. 3) (Fig. 2) (Fajardo 1989).

The impact of ionizing radiation on the endothelium has been studied in vivo and in vitro, the latter using various EC lines, including human umbilical vein cells (HUVEC), bovine aortic cells (BAEC), or capillary EC (e.g., HDMEC). The doses varied between < 1 Gy and as much as 60 Gy, with various fractionation schemes. For the in vitro studies, the doses were often 5 Gy or less. From a review of various in vitro experiments (too many to list here), it appears that radiation becomes lethal to endothelial cells when it reaches Do values of the order of 100–200 cGy in the clonogenic survival curves (higher values are required in vivo).

EC may undergo mitotic death or apoptosis, the latter through a pathway that probably involves the formation of ceramide.

Sublethal doses of radiation affect the morphology and various functions of EC.

Common morphologic changes include hypertrophy of EC associated with reorganization of F-actin filaments, and detachments from the basement membrane. The in vivo changes include vascular constrictions, thromboses, and rupture of microvascular walls with resulting hypoperfusion. Most studies show an increase in permeability for various molecules (however, serotonin transport is decreased). There is hypercoagulation, and platelet aggregation due to enhanced release of vWill F, causing an increased tendency to thrombosis. In addition, ineffective fibrinolysis results from a decrease in plasminogen activators. The eicosanoid metabolism is altered, with early decrease and late increase in PGI-2. There is enhanced chemoattraction for leukocytes and upregulation of adhesion molecules (e.g., ELAM-1). EC show decrease in endothelial enzyme activity (e.g., angiotensin converting

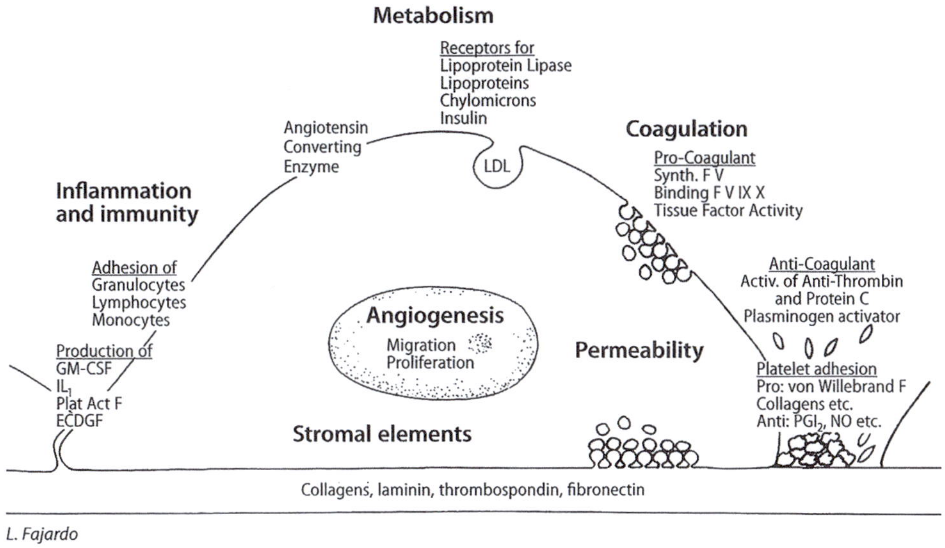

Fig. 2 Physiology of normal endothelial cell a normal endothelial cell attached to its basal lamina (*bottom*), which is partially denuded on the *right*. The main functions described here are indicated in *bold uppercase letters*, with examples in *lowercase*. *ABO*, blood antigens; *ACE*, angiotensin converting enzyme; *GM-CSF*, granulocyte–monocyte colony stimulating factor; *LDL*, low density lipoproteins; *MHC I & II*, major histocompatibility complexes; *NO*, nitric oxide; PGI_2,prostacyclin (Reproduced , with permission, from (Fajardo 1989))

Fig. 3 Radiation effects of radiation on endothelial = F3.2 P21 CURED I LENT; general effects of radiation on endothelial cells. This is a diagrammatical summary of the most important , lethal, and sublethal effects of ionizing radiation on endothelial cells. It combines in vitro and in vivo data and is based on multiple sources of information (Reproduced, with permission, from (Fajardo 1998))

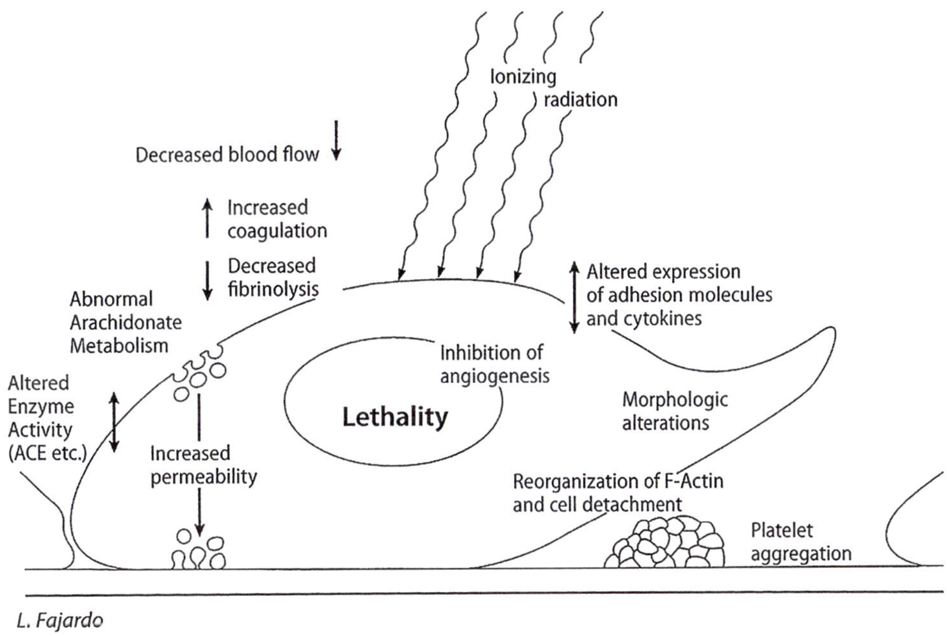

enzyme, alkaline phosphatase). Radiation inhibits angiogenesis: the magnitude of this effect depends in part on the sequence of angiogenic stimulus versus radiation. Various data suggest that the inhibition of angiogenesis is greater when the radiation exposure occurs prior to the angiogenic stimulus instead of following it. This information may be important when designing the sequence of radiation therapy versus surgery (the angiogenic stimulus, and depends on the timing of radiation with regard to the time interval for surgery.

Like other normal cells, EC have some innate protection from ionizing radiation. For instance, glutathione and superoxide dismutase provide some defense of EC from reactive oxygen species (e.g., hydroxyl radical and superoxide respectively). Nevertheless, it appears that endothelial cells are the most radiosensitive elements in the vessel wall. They may even be the most sensitive among the fixed cells of the mesenchyme. Many of the studies suggest that EC are more radioresponsive in vitro than in vivo. Sublethal endothelial radiation injury not only contributes to the very early, acute effects, but also accounts for many of the delayed effects, such as stromal fibrinous exudate and ischemia.

Several of the above described deleterious effects of radiation on the EC can be ameliorated or even abrogated by pharmacologic modifiers. However, as far as we know, there is no single compound that prevents all of these effects in the endothelium (Fig. 3) (Fajardo 1998).

6 Capillaries and Arterioles

There are differences in radiation response between small and large vessels. The endothelial tissue of the small blood vessels seems to be moderately sensitive to ionizing radiation. Its radiosensitivity seems to be intermediate between the highly radiosensitive parenchymal tissues containing vegetative and differentiating intermitotic cells of high mitotic frequency and the radioresistant tissues composed of reverting and fixed postmitotic cells. However, the endothelium of large blood vessels does not seem to be quite as responsive to radiation as that of smaller blood vessels. This difference in itself suggests either an enhanced conditional sensitivity of endothelium of small vessels or an influence of indirect mechanisms of alteration at the intertissue level, or perhaps even more remote indirect mechanisms contributing to the total radiation effect observed in the fine vasculature after moderate doses of radiation.

The reasons for this difference in radiosensitivity between the endothelium of small vessels and that of large vessels are not yet entirely clear. One of the possible reasons may be related to the fact that greater degrees of endothelial change are seen in the small vessels of irradiated organs containing radiosensitive parenchymal cells and showing greater degrees of inflammatory response involving the vessels (congestion, edema) than in the small vessels of irradiated organs containing radioresistant parenchymal cells and showing lesser degrees of such inflammatory response. This suggests that some of the observed radiation-induced changes in the endothelium of the fine vasculature may depend on the degree of such inflammatory response, which in turn depends on the degree of destruction of parenchymal cells, which in turn depends on the relative radiosensitivity of the parenchymal cells in the organs under consideration.

Another possible reason for the difference in observed degree of endothelial effect between large and small vessels may be related to differences in the size of the vascular lumens. The lumens of fine blood vessels are much more easily occluded by various effects of radiation on endothelium than those of large blood vessels, and the integrity of the walls of small blood vessels is thereby likely to be much more jeopardized by small degrees of change in the endothelial lining. The production of similar degrees of initial radiation effect on the endothelium of large vessels with their large lumens involves much less immediate pathologic consequence to the vessels themselves.

Blood sinusoids, which are lined not by typical endothelial cells but by phagocytes, are also less sensitive to radiation than are the small blood vessels lined by typical endothelium. The phagocytic cells are considerably more radioresistant than the endothelial cells, and the lumens of sinusoids are usually considerably larger than those of the fine vasculature line by endothelium.

The radiation effects on capillaries reflect the early radiation-induced changes in endothelial cells that include degeneration, swelling, and necrosis. The swelling of endothelial cells may be due partly, or sometimes, to relatively direct or indirect damage to the endothelial cells themselves and sometimes to excessive contraction and/or shortening of the small vessels containing them. In either case this results in the bulging of endothelium into the small lumen, with narrowing or obstruction of the lumen and impedence of circulation. Necrosis or loss of the endothelial cells of the lining, which permits contact between the blood and the severely damage endothelium or subendothelial connective tissue, promotes the formation of thrombi which may occlude small lumens rapidly. With doses of degrees of vascular damage not large enough to prevent the active regeneration of endothelial cells, the remaining endothelial cells may proliferate in response to injury and may even overcompensate, with the result that there are increased numbers of endothelial cells and consequent narrowing or occlusion of the small lumens. Even without marked over compensatory regeneration of endothelial cells, an apparent increase in the number of endothelial cells at places along the course of vessels may result from the shortening of the length of vessels or from the formation of tortuous bends in vessels when they are reduced in extension. As a result of the radiation damage to the endothelium and/or the vascular response in the inflammation elicited by damaged parenchymal cells, there may occur hyperemia, blood congestion, and increased permeability of the endothelium. Blood congestion from any cause tends to promote increased permeability of the endothelium. As a consequence, blood fluid leaks out of the capillaries into the surrounding connective tissue or through the endothelial lining of the arterioles and venules into the subendothelial connective tissues and tunica media. If the increased permeability of fragility of the endothelium is marked, leukocytes and even erythrocytes may also pass in excessive numbers through the endothelium. In severe damage there may be fissuring of the walls of the small blood vessels, with the consequent development of punctate hemorrhages. Increases in perivascular fluid may exert external pressure on the walls of small blood vessels and may—especially in the case of vessels with thin, weak walls, such as capillaries and venules—compress them and impede blood flow.

The early changes after irradiation just described (i.e., swelling or an increase in the number of endothelial cells relatively or absolutely, thrombosis, vasoconstriction, and perivascular compression of small vessels) are all relatively rapid mechanisms by which blood flow may be impeded or vessels occluded. The slower mechanisms of occlusion or reduction of the fine vasculature and of blood flow involve the responses of connective tissue, which are discussed in the next section.

7 Histohematic Barrier

As a result of perivascular or subendothelial edema (early inflammatory phase) caused by radiation damage to small blood vessels, there may be increased interstitial colloid in the affected regions. Such regions become sites of fibroblastic activity and of a subsequent increase in the fibrillar density and amount of the interstitial connective tissue (later sclerotic phase). This process of cicatrization of fibrosis may then continue slowly and progressively for many years indefinitely, and may result in the gradual thickening of the vessel wall, the replacement of the muscular media of small vessels with connective tissue, and the narrowing, occlusion and obliteration of their lumens. This process of circatrization and scarring may be regarded as a process of secondary repair, i.e., replacement of damaged specialized tissue with less specialized tissue. Offhand, such a process of repair of vessels may seem to go too far, in that the end results seem much more deleterious than the initial damage. However, it is possible that, in the absence of sufficient capacity for primary repair (recovery to the typical normal state) the process of secondary repair of vessels may be inherently self-perpetuating, i.e., causing progressively further damage as a stimulus to its own continuation. In this regard, although the initial interstitial edema may disappear, edema may recur from time to time as the fibrous connective tissue becomes denser and increases in amount.

These responses of interstitial and vascular connective tissue are more marked, more permanent, and more progressive as the radiation dose is increased. All these changes are nonspecific (not unique to radiation). The interstitial fibrosis and the fibrosis of small blood vessels constitute a premature increase in the *histohematic connective tissue barrier* (the barrier between the blood and the dependent parenchymal tissue cells) through which diffusions of nutrients and gases must take place, and a premature advance in the development of arteriolocapillary fibrosis, both of which are progressive processes in "normal" aging. These vasculoconnective tissue changes are also seen to increase in association with a variety of diseases.

The advancement of cicatrization of the fine blood vessels by irradiation involves the gradual replacement of the muscle tissue of the small arteries by fibrous tissue, a tissue that is less resilient and less resistant to stress. Even during early periods after irradiation, the weakening of the walls of irradiated small arteries is manifest in their greater susceptibility to necrosis caused by hypertension.

Radiation-induced advancement of progressive fibrosis of the fine vasculature leads eventually to premature narrowing and obliteration of vascular lumens and usually to a reduction in the total extent of fine vasculature or a reduction in its effective function. Although there is some recovery by way of neovascular regeneration, there is usually a net loss of fine vasculature after irradiation. The reason for the distinction between the reduction of fine vasculature and the reduction of its effective function is that under certain critical conditions of dose in certain organs the damage to fine vasculature may be followed not simply by its partial recovery through regeneration, but by supra neovascularization. In such instances, however, the stimulation for the supravascularization seems to reside in the presence of marked interstitial fibrosis, or an increase in the histohematic connective tissue barrier, which reduces markedly the functional capacity of the fine vasculature. In other words, supravascularization in the presence of a marked increase in the histohematic barrier may be associated with reduced function of the fine vasculature (Rubin et al. 1960). Under other circumstances, fibrillogenesis (fibrous barrier formation) has been shown experimentally to inhibit capillary regeneration (Van den Brenk 1959).

8 Distribution of Radiation Effects on Small Vessels at Early Times After Irradiation is Subtle and Inconspicuous

Furthermore, these *changes are spotty in their distribution along the course of the vessels, rather than uniform and continuous.* Consequently, in any one histologic tissue section, thorough and competent examination of the fine vessels may reveal relatively few sites of prominent change even when many of the small vessels may be affected at one or another point along their course. It is obvious that a focal narrowing or occlusion of an arteriole supplying a capillary network, especially if the occlusion is distal to the last effective collateral channel of blood supply, may be all that is necessary to disrupt the blood supply to tissues dependent upon the portion of the capillary bed in question. With progression of the vascular damage and the cicatrization process with passing time, more and more points along the course of the affected small blood vessels may show degenerative and fibrotic changes, so that more and more sections of small blood vessels per unit area of sectioned tissue may reveal changes and the changes may become more obvious.

Marked changes in dependent tissues can be caused by the radiation induced changes in fine vasculature and interstitial connective tissue, despite their seeming subtlety and relative inconspicuousness. The amount of damage to dependent tissues caused by interference with their blood supply and gas and nutrient exchange with the blood depends upon the rate and degree of reduction of the blood supply and the increase in the histohematic connective tissue barrier and upon the rapidity and degree of success with which these factors are compensated by the establishment, if any, of collateral circulation or neovascular formation. If the blood supply is rapidly and completely shut off by changes such as vascular thrombosis, then the resulting destruction of dependent tissue may be massive and rapid. Less complete or slowly progressive obstruction of the blood supply or increase in the histohematic barrier, as in the case with slowly progressive arteriolocapillary fibrosis and interstitial fibrosis, causes a more gradual atrophy of dependent tissues.

These changes in the fine vasculature and connective tissue are also of fundamental importance to dependent tissues because of the consequent lowering of their resistance to further injury, stress, or functional demands and because of the consequent reduction of the regenerative powers of the fine vasculature itself as well as the dependent tissues. The rate and type of recovery of radiation-damage tissues depend to a large extent on the local blood circulation and on the condition of the histohematic barrier. Even in the case of slowly progressive arteriolocapillary and interstitial fibrosis, the obstructive nature of these changes and the instability and reduced resiliency and regenerative capacity of the affected fine vasculature may so compromise the vasculature that the dependent tissues or organs may succumb to added injury, stress, or functional demands, and undergo acute necrosis long after irradiation. Fibrotic arterioles and telangiectatic capillaries are easily disrupted under additional stresses.

As indicated previously, these changes in the fine vasculature and interstitial connective tissue play a prime role in the production of chronic or delayed lesions in dependent tissues after irradiation, regardless of the relative radiosensitivity of the dependent parenchymal tissues or cells and their inherent regenerative capacity. For example, large blood vessels, considered as organs, may not show the early radiation changes observable in their fine vasculature (vasa vasorum), but they may show lesions later as a result of progressive changes in the vasa vasorum and the added or continued stress placed upon these organs, such as hypertension or perhaps even the continuous normal pressure of the blood.

A factor of prime importance in the resistance or susceptibility of irradiation tissues and organs to the development of delayed radiation-induced lesions of serious clinical significance is the ability retained by the irradiated fine vasculature to regenerate and remodel under conditions of added injury or stress. Additional injury or stress that is either so mild or so localized as to require no extensive vascular remodeling, may be adequately resisted or repaired. However, more marked or more diffuse injury or stress, such as might result from diffuse infection and inflammation (which may require for repair a marked generalized hyperemia and considerable vascular remodeling without hindrance of the ability of the vascular endothelium by an increased fibrillar connective tissue barrier) may not be adequately resisted or repaired and necrosis may result. *Infection or diffuse trauma of irradiated organs in which the fine vasculature has been reduced and in which regeneration of the fine vasculature is inhibited by an increase in the histohematic fibrous barrier is often a precipitating factor in delayed radionecrosis of such organs. Delayed radionecrosis resulting partly from such complications may occur at any time, depending upon the degree of devitalization of the supporting tissues, which in turn depends upon dose.*

The consequences of similar degrees of damage to the fine vasculature and increased interstitial fibrous tissue vary among dependent tissues and organs of different types according to their activities, specialization, degree of dependence on blood supply, reserve of vasculature, degree if collateral circulation, capacity for vascular regeneration, and the functional demands placed upon their circulatory apparatus.

9 Microcirculation

Relationships between Cell/Tissue Renewal Kinetics and "the microvasculature response is faster and earlier in normal tissues that renew rapidly and is slower in, as well as later in, slow renewal tissues" (Rubin and Casarett 1968). It is important to understand which normal tissues parenchymal cells are considered to have rapid or slow renewal kinetics as well as the radiation sensitivity as a function of cell cycle kinetics.

The epithelial tissues that line mucosal surfaces in the upper aerodigestive passages, gastrointestinal (GI) tract, urinary system, and bone marrow are examples of rapid renewal tissues. These tissues tend to have uncommitted or committed stem cell compartments that rapidly proliferate and differentiate. Slow renewal tissues are characterized by a parenchymal cell compartment that turns over slowly, but often has the capacity to respond by reverting to a stem cell and regenerating or repopulating the lost parenchymal cells.

Examples of tissues that are conditionally proliferative include liver after partial resection, bone following fracture, microcirculation in wound healing, endocrine glands following increased trophic hormone, and bone marrow (protected areas) following irradiation of a large segment. Many adult organs have little or no capacity to restore their parenchymal cells, that is, proliferation occurs primarily early in life and is fixed. Examples of this type of tissue or organ are the central nervous system (CNS), heart, kidney, and muscle, in which lost cells are replaced by fibrosis.[3]

10 Rapid Cell Renewal Kinetics

10.1 Gastrointestinal Mucosal Epithelium

The rapidly dividing epithelium of the alimentary system varies throughout; the most rapid cell turnover is the small intestine, then stomach pylorus, followed by oral cavity and anus, then the esophagus and colon, and stomach cardia (Table 1) (Bertalanffy and Lau 1962).

From the view of cell kinetics, the time of appearance of mucositis in small intestine, and then oral cavity mucositis, followed by esophagus, then stomach, and colorectum is explained.

The rapidly dividing epithelium of the digestive system undergoing mitotic linked death triggers an early inflammatory response in which the microvascular system of this organ plays a critical role. The early ICAM expression arrests lymphocytes, macrophages, and neutrophils and allows their penetration through the capillary wall inciting the reactive mucositis or dermatitis. In contrast, slowly dividing cellular systems, the first tissue to respond is the microcirculation as in the heart or liver where diffuse capillary microthrombosis occurs. The volume effect in parallel organs may reflect the damage to the percentage of the microvasculature injured and in turn the functional units lost.

It is important to note that expression of mucositis is related to cell kinetics and the lifetime of the mature epithelial cell. Thus, gastrointestinal mucositis precedes oropharyngeal and colorectal mucositis. It is important to note that most epithelial-lined tissues are hollow organs and the fine vasculature is distinct and separate from the epithelial surface. The small arteriole often thickens its muscular wall and if the closure of its lumen is rapid and sudden, the tissues as gut undergoes necrosis (hypofractionation, single long dose). Alternatively, if the closure is slow and gradual (none hyperfractionated) then the altered microcirculation leads to a slower fibrogenic response. The damage extends from mucosa to the fine smooth muscle of the digestive lumen tube wall and leads to strictures rather than ulceration and perforation.

Table 1 "Turnover times" of the epithelial cells of the alimentary tract of the rat[a]

Cell population	Turnover time (Days)
Digestive system	
Lip	14.7
Oral cavity	
Buccal mucosa	4.3
Tongue surface	
Superior	4.9
Inferior	7.7
Esophagus	
At thyroid gland level	8.8
At cardiac junction	11.6
Stomach	
Cardia	9.1
Body	
Surface epithelium	2.9
Glands	6.4
Pslorus	
Surface epithelium	1.9
Glands	1.8
Small intestine	
Duodenum	1.6
Jejunum	1.3
Ileum	1.4
Large intestine	
Colon	10.0
Rectum	6.2
Anus	4.3

[a] From (Bertalanffy and Lau 1962) published by Academic Press Inc

The epithelium of skin is distinct and separate from the capillary loops in the papillary layer of the dermis. The fine small arteriole is vulnerable to large single doses or hypo/large fraction regimens. The volume effect first described by Patterson, then Van Essen is a micro-circulatory effect since there is no rationale for skin tolerance to change with volume. Again, rapid closure induces ulceration and necrosis versus slow closure that leads to obliteration of the capillary dermis, shortening of loops, and scarring leading to sinusoidal telangiectaisia and contractures.

The rapid renewing epithelium of other hollow organs behave similarly and include the lining of the upper respiratory system and larynx, the lining of the urinary system from renal pelvis, ureters, to urinary bladder. A major difference between upper respiratory and upper digestive systems is the presence of bone and cartilage which maintain respiratory lumen in paranasal sinuses, nasopharynx, larynx, and trachea. Fibrosis does not lead to stenosis of these structures. However, bone and cartilage are vulnerable to necrosis in these tissues when the vasculature is compromised. High dose radiation of the larynx or bronchi can and do result in chondronecrosis.

11 Slow Renewal Kinetics

The microcirculation alterations in slow renewal kinetic tissues and organs is the predominant factor in the expression of late effects. Since the parenchymal cell compartment is not rapidly proliferating the mitotic linked cell death is a late event often with no detectable acute phase, that is, only a late manifestation occurs clinically. This absence of an acute clinical phase of effect, and then an unexpected late adverse effect occurring is one of the main concerns of radiation treatment. The classic illustrations of radiation injury to the microvasculature is the dominant mechanism that drives the expression of radiation reaction in these organs.

- *CNS. Brain and Spinal Cord*: The central nervous system is a complex organ; however, permanent damage to neuronal tissues is largely due to injury of the fine vasculature of the spinal cord and brain. The classic Boron Neutron capture study in which radiation was delivered solely to the vessel wall because of alpha particles released without irradiating the nervous tissue reproduced the classic pattern of radiation injury of the central nervous system. Although the capillary network (blood–brain barrier) is the vulnerable target, the medium-size cerebral arteries can occlude, analogous to coronary arteries. Numerous studies in our and other laboratories established the cerebral and spinal cord capillary vasculitis as the mechanism for necrosis and hemorrhaging associated with cerebral and spinal cord necrosis. The neuroendocrine apparatus consists of a rich sinusoidal network in the hypothesis and pituitary stalk and gland. The vasculature is the vulnerable structure rather than neuroendocrine cells. The occlusion of the hypophysis-pituitary sinusoidal network can lead to infarction and necrosis leading to an empty sella syndrome (Fig. 4) (Rubin and Casarett 1966).
- *Heart*: The classic illustrations are in the heart, the musculoskeletal system, the kidneys, and the nervous system. The classic cardiac radiation experiments of Stewart and Fajardo established the fine microvasculature as the radiation target cell rather than the cardiac myocytes. In contrast, adriamycin vacuolated the cardiomyocyte and spread the capillary bed. A diffuse microthrombosis of the myocardial capillary network resulted in diffuse radiation-induced cariomyopathy over time. Since cardiac hypertrophy compensates initially for reduced ejection fraction but heart failure eventually occurs over time, especially if the whole heart volume was treated. Of interest is the vulnerability of other structures especially the coronary arteries. Radiation of coronary arteries was the first recognized and perhaps the largest artery that radiation accelerates atherosclerosis, i.e., 3 mm lumen to 1 mm in size as it descends on the heart wall. The first such evidence was detected in young females with Hodgkin's Lymphoma who developed coronary thrombosis when they reached adulthood. Subsequently, its appearance decades later was manifested in breast cancer survivors but limited to left rather than right side tangential chest irradiation. The mesothelial cell lining the pericardium rather than the heart endothelium can be more vulnerable in the sudden appearance of pericardial effusion, most often at 5–6 months, i.e., increase in capillary permeability of the visceral layer of pericardium. Another adverse late event is calcification of the chorda tendinae of valves due to obliteration of the

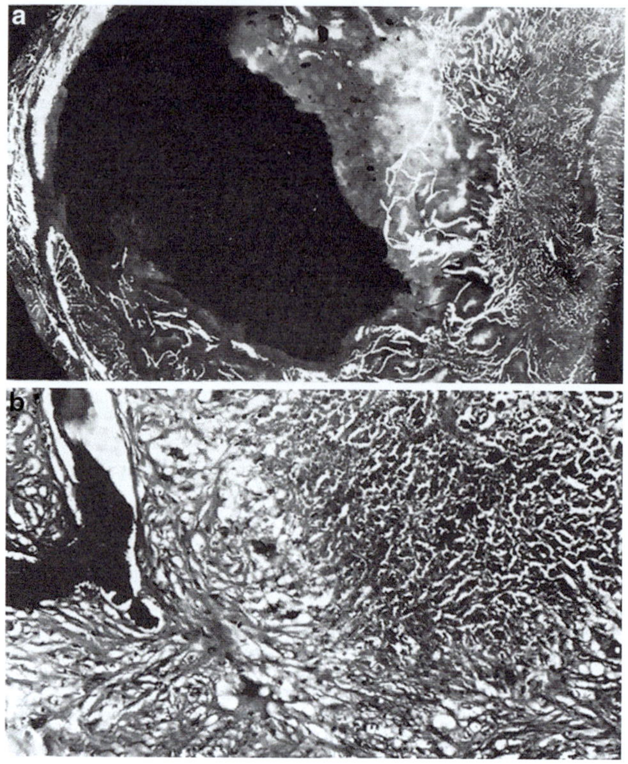

Fig. 4 **a** Microorganism of a nonregressing irradiated Walker tumor shows preservation of ample vasculature in the original zone of viable tumor (×10). The tumor cells appear to be degenerating at the completion of a 6000 R dose, but the vasculature remains intact despite the higher doses used in their phase. The lumens are narrowed, giving the lead-filled capilaries a thinned out appreance, but the dilatation of the channels in the totally necrotic area suggests patency of vessels but stagnation of flow. **b** Histologic section shows persistence of vessels in zones of fibrosis and giant cells to the left with some persistence of tumor foci to the right (×100) (From Rubin and Casarett 1966)

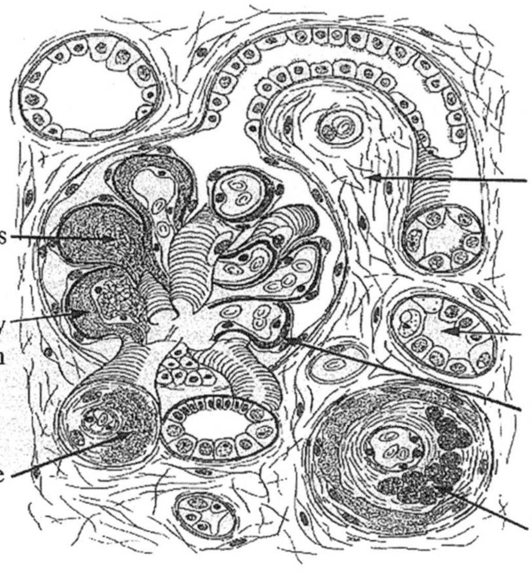

Fig. 5 The radiation response in the renal parenchyma. The responsive cell types are in the endothelium and epithelium. There is fibrinoid and hyaline accumulation associated with endothelial swelling in the afferent arterioles, which may spread beneath the glomerular capillary endothelium. the basement membrane thickens. Vascular compromise promotes thromboses, possibly leading to infarct. The tubular epithelium presents a variable picture, but there is some degree of interstitial fibrosis. As the vascular compromise develops, larger vessels may be affected, with focal necrosis and accumulations of foamy histiocytes. (With Permissions from (White 1975))

fine capillaries in the chorda tendinae leading to valve stenosis or regurgitation. The valves per se are not radiation vulnerable but obliteration of the fine capillaries and in turn the fine musculature at the base of the chorda tendinae renders them incompetent due to fibrosis and calcification of the valve. The calcification is due to a slow necrosing turned sclerosing reaction.

- *Kidney*: The major focus of change is in the arteriolar-glomerular region rather than the tubular epithelium, with the cortical rather than the medullary tubules being involved; this involvement usually follows vascular alterations (Fig. 5). In a classic study by Glatstein and colleagues, radiation-induced lesions were shown to occur as a progressive replacement of capillary walls leading to glomerular sclerosis, followed by tubular atrophy. Larger arteries were not affected, although blood flow was reduced significantly and was still variable 2–3 months after irradiation. The evidence suggests that a functional lesion occurs in the glomerular capillaries, preceding tubular depletion. However, both elements are affected according to Hoopes and coworkers, who proposed that multiple target sites exist for radiation, offering the best explanation for the observed clinical syndromes (Fig. 5) (White 1975).
- *Liver*: Whole liver irradiation results in "veno" occlusive disease unlike most organs in which the arteriole occlusion is the predominant lesion. The reason is in its embryonic origin from the vitelline veins from the yolk sac which develops into a network of venous liver sinusoids and become the hepatic portal network draining the gut. The venous capillary sinuses predominate as compared to the hepatic artery, arterioles, and capillaries which parallels the biliary duct system and are not significant or intimate to the function of the liver lobule and its hepatocytes. Thus, central vein thrombosis and congestion leads to a Budd Chiari syndrome as the irradiated liver decompensates.
- *Lung*: The major physiologic feature of the respiratory system is to oxygenate blood. Thus radiation acts on the acinar and alveolar capillary bed in contrast to the bronchial artery which bronches and parallels the dividing decremental bronchial tree. The endothelial cell is an early responding cell and its veno-occlusive pattern is similar to irradiated liver, i.e., VOD. The congestion that results leads to an increase in capillary permeability and diopedesis of RBCs (smallest circulating cell) as compared to the larger neutrophils and later reacting Type II pneumocytes. Radiation pneumonitis is an alveolitis which accounts for its geometric shape similar to radiation beam shapes and high dose isodose regions rather than its bronchial or major vascular anatomy as in infectious pneumonitis or embolism/infarction respectively.
- *Musculoskeletal*: Adult bone is a slow renewal system and responds to irradiation in a clinically occult fashion. There is no overt reaction except an initial increase in blood flow which is followed as the dose increases and over time into a sharp decrease in blood flow. The

Table 2 Site of microvascular injury

Organ	Site of microvascular injury
Skin	Capillaries in papillary layer increase permeability, loss of tufting, telangiectasia, neoformation of capillaries, vascular occlusions
Skin grafts	Inhibit neovascularization, increase permeability new vessels once formed, obliterated vessels in cicatrization of capillaries
Oral Cavity	Arteriolar capillary fibrosis, telangiectasia, increase HHB
Esophagus	Submucosal thickening of smooth muscle, vascular connective tissue change lead to necrosis
Stomach	Coagulation necrosis of epithelium, hyperemia, and dilation capillaries
Small intestine	Degenerative change microvasculature, endarterites obliterations of ?p.220
Large intestine	+ thickening of smooth muscle media, inflamed cells in adventitia with necrosis
Rectum	Intrinsic versus extrinsic reaction (p.208), oliterative endoarteritis
Salivary glands	Inflammation, locular adiposis, obiterative endoarteritis
Liver	Central vein of lobule thrombosis p. 274 obliterated central v. p.314
Kidney	Arteriolonephrosclerosis, glomerular tufts of/erent arterioles (p.317) rapid endothelial swelling and proliferation, slower thickening walls arte./vein hypertension
Bladder	Increased HHB, hyalinization of arteriole wall, endarteritis obliterans (p.302/3)
Ureter	Stenosis
Testis	Vascular sclerosis arteriolar p. 385 replacement fibrosis
Ovary	Vascular sclerosis
Breast	Fibroatrophy of fat
Lung	Capillary permeability, thickening septa fibrosis, displace capillaries Pl 456 damage to fine vasculature, capillaries, arterioles, venules

With Permissions from (Rubin and Casarett 1966; Fajardo 2001)

sclerosis of the capillary network leads to increase in bone sclerosis, necrosis, and fracture. If bone is exposed, (i.e., the mandible in the oral cavity), infection and osteomyelitis and then osteonecrosis occurs. Pelvis fractures lines in high dose overlap of pelvic field seams, can be insidious and crippling. Radiation due to overlapping of fields of the chest wall can lead to sclerosis, necrosis, and non-healing fractures of ribs.

- *Muscle*: The striated musculature can withstand large doses of fractionated or protracted radiation. Slow loss of supporting vasculature can lead to fibroartrophy but skeletal muscle seldom undergoes necrosis. Striated muscle has no regenerative capacity but can hypertrophy when challenged by exercise such as weight lifting. Irradiated muscle loses its capacity to respond and hypertrophy.

In summary, the relationship of the exact site of injury in the microvasculature apparatus varies. The specific characteristic histopathologic-induced lesions are well documented by Fajardo. The specific site in the microcirculation of each major organ is tabulated in Table 2 (Rubin and Casarett 1966; Fajardo 2001).

12 Special Topics/Effects

12.1 Skin Grafts

Skin graft experimentation in a porcine model correlated reactions in skin versus the status of the microcirculation beds. That is, the radiation response in the epidermis reflected the age or healing of the capillary bed under full or split thickness grafts.

- Immediate radiation within 24–48 h of the graft resulting in graft necrosis since this is the time for neovascularization and capillary buds are extremely radiosensitive to small doses of radiation.
- Early radiation at 2–3 weeks post grafting resulted in an acute severe reaction since the graft is supervascularized for 1–6 months as compared to normal skin.
- Late radiation of well-healed skin graft resulted in delayed response as compared to normal skin due to fibrosis and retraction subcutaneously as compared to normal skin. However, if the well healed grafted skin reacted it underwent necrosis due to its more limited microcirculation.

12.2 Supralethal

A vigorous acute effect in these tissues is followed by a late effect and has been appropriately referred to as a consequential effect. Excessive high doses of radiation can lead to superlethal adverse effects. That is, the microcirculation undergoes an obliterative vasculitis causing severe tumor hypoxia while simultaneously necrosing the normal tissue site. In head and neck cancers, Andrews extrapolated standard fractionation schedules to total doses of 100 Gy in 10 weeks. Numerous head and neck cancers persisted while the normal tissue site underwent total necrosis, i.e., advanced tongue and floor of the mouth, i.e., intrinsic and extrinsic musculature (striated muscle) necrosed due to thrombosis of the lingual arteriolar network. Similar patterns of liquidification of necrotic normal tissues occurred with high dose protracted continuous irradiation with cancer persistence of head and neck cancers.

12.3 Miscalculation High Dose

The lack of an early warning skin reaction of high dose miscalculation error in this megavoltage era is a challenge even for an astute clinician. Experience with medical–legal mishaps due to errors in calculation of dose are different in patterns and time of reaction due to beam quality. Mistakes in the kilovoltage era were readily apparent because of earlier acute reaction or persistence of the severe acute reactions into a chronic non-healing late effect, usually of skin or mucosa. Mistakes in the megavoltage era are unremarkable clinically in that no acute reaction of skin and even mucosa may occur despite daily, weekly, and total doses that are twice normal, i.e., 4.0 Gy daily to 20 Gy weekly and 100–120 Gy to total dose. The overdosed breast skin reaction occurs after completion of treatment and then undergoes liquefaction necrosis followed by complete obliteration of mammary glands. Now healing occurs with eventual and with persistent skin ulceration and underlying rib necrosis. A larynx mucosa reacts as anticipated at weeks but the mucositis persists, and then vocal cord cartilage necrosis results, requiring laryngectomy for survival. With superficial or low kilovoltages (200–400kv), of very high dose overexposures, the skin reaction is immediate. That is, blistering response due to increased capillary permeability and total disruption of the microvasculature. Necrosis follows requiring resection.

12.4 Arterial Restenosis

Following angioplasty and stenting of coronary arteries, restenosis of the lumen often occurs. Endolumenal catheters with a brachytherapy radiation source was designed to deliver high doses to the stented site. The concept was based on the use of irradiation for keloids, due to later thrombosis at stent site resulting in acute coronary thrombosis. This use of radiation for benign conditions was replaced by drug impregnated stents.

Arteriovenous malformations in the brain can be treated with high dose stereotactic radiation surgery if not feasible surgically. Doses range in the 15–30 Gy, in a single fraction and endothelial obliteration occurs gradually in 1–3 years. Levels of 90 % and high have been reported, particularly for A-V-M nidus is less than 4 cm^3.

References

Bertalanffy FD, Lau C (1962) Cell renewal. Int Rev Cytol 13:357–366

Fajardo LF (1989) The unique physiology of endothelial cells and its implications in radiobiology. Front Radiat Ther Oncol 23:96–112

Fajardo LF (1998) The endothelial cell is a unique target of radiation: an overview. In: Rubin DB (ed) The radiation biology of the endothelium. CRC Press, Boca Raton, pp 1–12

Fajardo L, Berthrong M, Anderson R (2001) Radiation Pathology. Oxford University Press, New York, pp 3–155

Ross M et al (2003) Histology: a text and atlas with cell and molecular biology, 4th edn. Lippincott Williams & Wilkins, p 340

Rubin P, Casarett G (1966) Microcirculation of tumors. II. The supervascularized state of irradiated regressing tumors. Clin Radiol 17:346–355

Rubin P, Casarett GW (1968) Clinical Radiation Pathology. Philadelphia, WB Saunders

Rubin P, Casarett GW, Grise J (1960) The vascular pathophysiology of an irradiated graft. Amer J Roentgenol 83:1097–1104

Van den Brenk HA (1959) The effect of ionizing radiations on capillary sprouting and vascular remodelling in the regenerating repair blastema observed in the rabbit ear chamber. Am J Roentgenol Radium Ther Nucl Med 81(5):859–884

White DC (1975) An atlas of radiation histopathology. US Energy Research and Development Administration, Oak Ridge, p 177

Molecular Mechanisms of Radiation Induced Injury

Isabel L. Jackson, Phil Rubin, Caroline Hadley, and Zeljko Vujaskovic

Contents

Abstract

Radiation-induced normal tissue injury represents a major impediment to the successful achievement of the desired clinical outcome from radiation therapy (RT) for cancer patients; usually improved local control, reduced risk for disease reoccurrence, and increased survival. Complications associated with RT can result in diminished quality of life and carries the potential for severe debilitating disease. The development of normal tissue protectors/radiomitigators is dependent on improved understanding of the molecular mechanisms associated with the development of acute and long-term RT-induced tissue toxicity. The following chapter provides a comprehensive review of the current state of knowledge with respect to those mechanisms underlying radiation-induced normal tissue pathologies. Future scientific endeavors will build upon this groundwork to delve deeper into the mechanistic understanding of disease onset and progression and develop new agents that can be translated from bench to bedside to reduce the risk for RT-induced complications.

In memory of George Casarett

I. L. Jackson · Z. Vujaskovic
Division of Translational Radiation Sciences, Department of Radiation Oncology, University of Maryland School of Medicine, Baltimore, MD 21201, USA

P. Rubin (✉)
Department of Radiation Oncology, University of Rochester School of Medicine and Dentistry, 601 Elmwood Ave, Box 647Rochester, NY 14642, USA
e-mail: oncophilip@gmail.com; oncophilip@earthlink.net

C. Hadley
Baylor University School of Medicine, Houston, Texas 77030, USA

1 Introduction

Advancements in cancer treatment have led to an increase in the number of cancer survivors, a population that now exceeds 11 million people. For the majority of individuals diagnosed with cancer, radiation therapy will play an important role in their treatment. Over the next several decades, the number of cancer survivors will continue to grow and as a result, so too will the number of patients exhibiting the late effects of radiation damage to healthy tissue.

The late effects of radiation exposure range from mild to severe and may last for several weeks or many years following radiotherapy. Depending on the anatomic location of

P. Rubin et al. (eds.), *ALERT – Adverse Late Effects of Cancer Treatment*, Medical Radiology. Radiation Oncology,
DOI: 10.1007/978-3-540-72314-1_4, © Springer-Verlag Berlin Heidelberg 2014

the tumor and treatment field, side effects can include mucositis, pneumonitis/fibrosis, or erectile dysfunction, among others. Unfortunately, the relative risk of normal tissue complications limits the maximum effective radiation dose that can be delivered to optimize tumor cytotoxicity, achieve local tumor control, and improve survival. This is of particular relevance for cancer types that continue to be associated with poor five-year cancer-free survival, such as lung cancers. In cancers of the lung, dose escalation or combined treatment regimens have the potential to increase survival but the exquisite radiosensitivity of the lungs puts patients at a greater risk for unacceptable treatment-related complications, such as pneumonitis and/or fibrosis. Further complicating matters is the inability to accurately predict which patients are at greater risk for developing normal tissue toxicity. In recent years, a number of clinicians and basic science researchers have worked to identify specific predictors of normal tissue toxicity, but to date, no single biomarker or gene polymorphism has been identified which can be associated with individual risk (Fleckenstein et al. 2007; Azria et al. 2008; Kelsey et al. 2011; Kong et al. 2008). The ability to identify predictive markers or develop effective protective strategies to prevent, mitigate, and/or treat radiation injury is impeded by the fact that the mechanisms driving radiation-induced normal tissue toxicity remain unclear. Therefore, improving our knowledge of the pathophysiological mechanisms associated with normal tissue toxicity could lead to therapeutic interventions that spare normal tissue from radiation damage without negating the cytotoxic effect of radiation on tumors.

Before advances can be made in elucidating the mechanisms underlying radiation injury, a thorough understanding of classical radiation biology is imperative. It is impossible to move forward without knowing where we have been. Thus, this chapter will focus on radiation chemistry, the cellular effects of radiation at the molecular level, and cell types involved in facilitating radiation injury, with a particular focus on lung injury.

2 "Target Cell Theory" of Radiation Injury

The initial ionizing event lasts for just milliseconds, yet, the damage caused by radiation is propagated for weeks to years after the initial exposure. How and why this occurs has been the basis for a number of research studies over the past several decades. It appears that the early and late effects of radiation injury are driven by a cascade of downstream events at the molecular and cellular level initiated at the time of exposure (Fig. 1).

At the time of irradiation, the production of hydroxyl radical due to radiolytic hydrolysis of water can lead to single or double stranded breaks within the DNA. Single stranded breaks are more easily repaired and rarely cause lethal injury to the cell where as double stranded breaks often cause cell death either due to apoptosis or mitotic catastrophe. The classical, "target cell theory" of radiation-injury suggested that organ-specific sequelae are a result of a threshold level of cell death within a target cell population. The target cell theory suggested that the so-called "latent period" between the time of exposure and the development of symptomatic injury was the direct result of the proliferation kinetics of a critical cell population required for proper tissue function. Based on this, the timing and expression of injury could be considered a result of the proliferation kinetics of the irradiated tissue (Michalowski 1986). Thus, organs with a rapidly renewing stem cell compartments (i.e., gastrointestinal tissue) would develop injury earlier than tissues characterized by well-differentiated cell populations (i.e., lung).

How cells recognize and respond to injury may influence the tissue response to radiation (McBride et al. 2004) Although only a few cells may be directly targeted by the ionizing event, bystander effects on non-irradiated cells have been observed up to 1 mm away by Brenner and colleagues (Belyakov et al. 2005). In the lung, as well as other "late responding tissues", the relevance of the target cell theory has been challenged in recent years. Based on work performed over the past several decades implicating a wide range of dynamic signaling events determining whether a cell lives or dies and communication of the trauma to surrounding tissues, it is becoming clear that the tissue response to radiation is driven by a dynamic tissue response that begins at the time of irradiation and continues throughout the course of disease progression.

3 Role of Free Radical Species and Redox Signaling in Radiation Response

Ionizing radiation directly damages DNA leading to genomic instability and cell death through apoptosis or mitotic catastrophe (O'Neill and Wardman 2009). Investigators evaluating radiation effects on DNA have found that high linear energy transfer results in "clustered DNA lesions" which are inefficiently repaired and are thus thought to be biologically relevant to the acute and delayed effects associated with radiation exposure (O'Neill and Wardman 2009). The ionizing event also results in formation of reactive oxygen species (ROS), however the levels generated by therapeutic doses of radiation are negligible compared to those generated by aerobic metabolism (Ward 1994). Within hours of the initial ionizing exposure, there is a robust activation of secondary sources of oxidative stress leading to persistent production of free radical species that

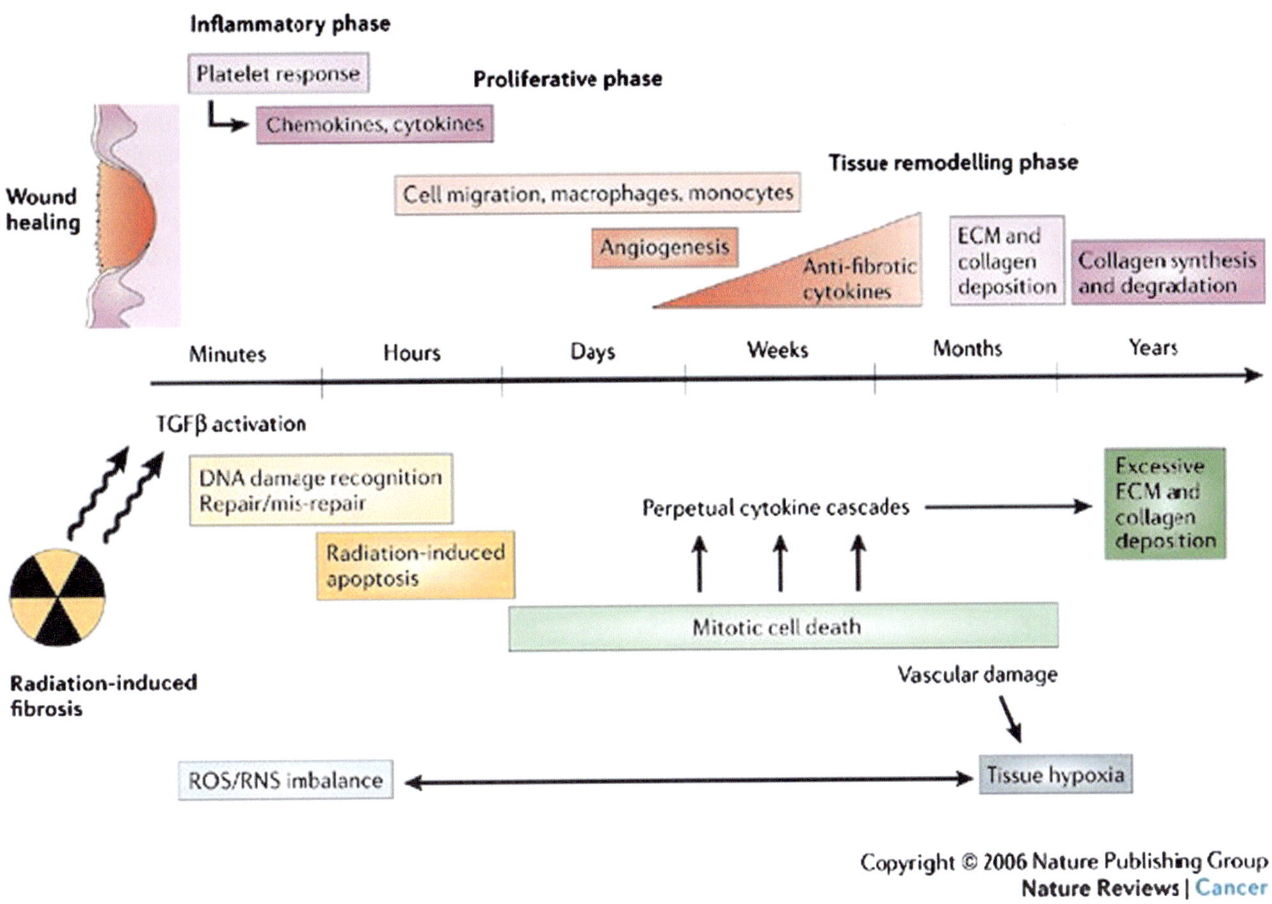

Fig. 1 Simplified schematic diagram of the molecular events underlying development of normal tissue toxicity following radiation exposure (Bentzen 2006)

can participate in cell signaling. A number of transcription factors and pro-inflammatory/pro-fibrogenic molecules, such as NFκB, HIF-1α, and TGF-β, are sensitive to changes in the redox status of the cell. As the level of free radical production is thought to be beyond the capacity of the cell's antioxidant defense mechanisms to eliminate them, the imbalance between free radicals and antioxidants leads to chronic upregulation of transcription factors, growth factors, and cytokines involved in radiation injury (Robbins and Zhao 2004; Benderitter et al. 2007; Zhao et al. 2007). The environment of chronic oxidative stress results in oxidative damage to DNA leading to chromatin remodeling and altered gene expression, chronic protein activation/inactivation, and oxidation/peroxidation of membrane lipids that can result in changes in cell signaling (Mikkelsen and Wardman 2003). The ability of potent superoxide dismutase (SOD)-like compounds and other antioxidants to mitigate radiation-induced injury is further evidence that redox-regulated signaling plays a substantial role in the development of radiation injury (Epperly et al. 1999a, b, 2002; Gauter-Fleckenstein et al. 2007, 2010; Rabbani et al. 2005, 2007; Vujaskovic et al. 2002; Rosenthal et al. 2011).

While the exact mechanism through which radiation-induced free radical production affects the activity of signal transduction pathways and transcription factors within the irradiated tissue is not clear, it is well known that many signaling mechanisms and gene expression pathways are sensitive to changes in intracellular oxidation/reduction status (Mikkelsen and Wardman 2003) leading to changes in signal transduction, transcription factor activation, and gene expression (Mikkelsen and Wardman 2003; Reboucas 2010; Zhang and Hogg 2005). It is theorized that the increase in ROS/RNS production in the early radiation response may result in oxidative modification of macromolecules participating in signal transduction pathways, resulting in signaling changes that perpetuate tissue injury over time (Reboucas 2010).

4 Biological Sources of ROS/RNS and the Role of Oxidative Stress in Radiation-Induced Tissue Injury

It is hypothesized that the initial ionizing event is followed by a ROS/RNS mediated signaling cascade through downstream activation of metabolic sources of prooxidant production. This includes mitochondria, nitric oxide synthases, and oxidoreductase enzymes, most notably the family of NADPH oxidases.

Non-phagocytic cells predominantly generate ROS/RNS through activity of the cell membrane-associated family of NADPH oxidases (von Lohneysen et al. 2010). A number of NADPH oxidase family members exist and have remarkably varied activation mechanisms and tissue distribution. For example, endothelial cells express Nox1, Nox2 ($gp91^{phox}$), Nox4, and Nox5 isoforms; whereas vascular smooth muscle cells express the Nox1, Nox4, and Nox5 isoforms (Lassegue and Griendling 2010). NADPH oxidase-derived superoxide anion ($O_2^{\cdot -}$) is involved in vascular maintenance and regulation of vascular smooth muscle tone under physiological conditions (Bengtsson et al. 2003). However, pathological overproduction of $O_2^{\cdot -}$ by NADPH oxidases may participate in radiation injury by activating redox-sensitive signaling pathways involved in inflammation and fibrosis. Collins-Underwood et al. (2008) found that increased expression of NADPH oxidase subunits (Nox4, $p22^{phox}$, and $p47^{phox}$) following in vitro irradiation of rat brain microvascular endothelial cells was associated with a pro-inflammatory response. In these studies, elevated intracellular generation of ROS, activation of the pro-inflammatory transcription factor NFκB, and expression of vascular adhesion molecules ICAM-1 and PAI-1 could be prevented by inhibition of NADPH oxidase (Collins-Underwood et al. 2008).

Nox4 is especially interesting as recent studies have shown TGF-β1 induced cell death to be dependent upon Nox4-derived H_2O_2 (Carnesecchi et al. 2011). Nox4 is a unique isoform as it produces H_2O_2 rather than $O_2^{\cdot -}$ due to an extra 23-amino acid sequence in its E-loop (Takac et al. 2011). In recent studies by Zhang et al. (2012), Nox4 expression was colocalized with increased PTEN expression, which correlated to a progressive and persistent increase in cell death between 24 h and 6 months after whole thorax irradiation. The increase in PTEN expression coincided with downregulation of Akt signaling.

4.1 Amplification of Existing ROS/RNS

Production of ROS/RNS by NADPH oxidases or dysfunctional mitochondria can be amplified by the reaction of nitric oxide and superoxide anion to form peroxynitrite ($ONOO^-$), a potent free radical species that has been implicated in proteoglycan degradation and matrix turnover (Cernanec et al. 2007). Depletion of NO through its rapid conversion to $ONOO^-$ or superoxide mediated inactivation of key components of the NO signaling pathway may also contribute to vasoconstriction observed after radiation (Ward et al. 1983; Fleckenstein et al. 2007).

4.2 Factors Affecting ROS/RNS Production by Theses Sources

It is well known that TGF-β, a ubiquitous cytokine activated by radiation, and angiotensin II exert upstream influence over NADPH oxidase activation. The use of angiotensin converting enzyme (ACE) inhibitors to mitigate radiation pneumonitis/fibrosis and nephropathy has been an active area of research primarily conducted by Moulder and colleagues (Ghosh et al. 2009). Pre-clinical studies using a rat model have shown that clinical doses of Captopril (34 mg/kg/day) improve survival and restore vascular reactivity in irradiated lung (Ghosh et al. 2009). The equally protective ability of both thiol and non-thiol containing ACE inhibitors suggests that free radical scavenging is not the primary mechanism of action for mitigation of radiation toxicity. Possible mechanisms include inhibition of AngII-mediated activation of NADPH oxidase and/or effects on blood pressure (Moulder et al. 2002). The role of blood pressure in reducing radiation-induced injury is supported by preclinical studies showing that a diet high in sodium ameliorates radiation nephropathy ostensibly through inhibition of ACE activity (Moulder et al. 2002). The reduction in nephropathy was only observed when a high sodium diet was initiated before the onset of nephropathy; it was not an effective treatment of existing nephropathy (Zhang and Rabbani 2012).

It is of note that the protective role of ACE inhibitors in preclinical models has, to date, not translated to the clinic. Wang and Anscher performed a retrospective study to determine the development and onset of radiation pneumonitis, determined by the NCI common toxicity criteria and CT imaging, in 213 patients treated for lung cancer with thoracic irradiation from 1994 to 1997 (Wang et al. 2000). In this study, the authors found the incidence and onset of radiation pneumonitis among patients taking ACE inhibitors (captopril, benazepril, enalapril, lisinopril, quinapril, or fosinopril) for hypertension was not significantly different than those who were not on ACE inhibitors (Wang et al. 2000). Thus, it remains unclear whether the mitigating effect of ACE inhibitors in preclinical models will translate to the clinic.

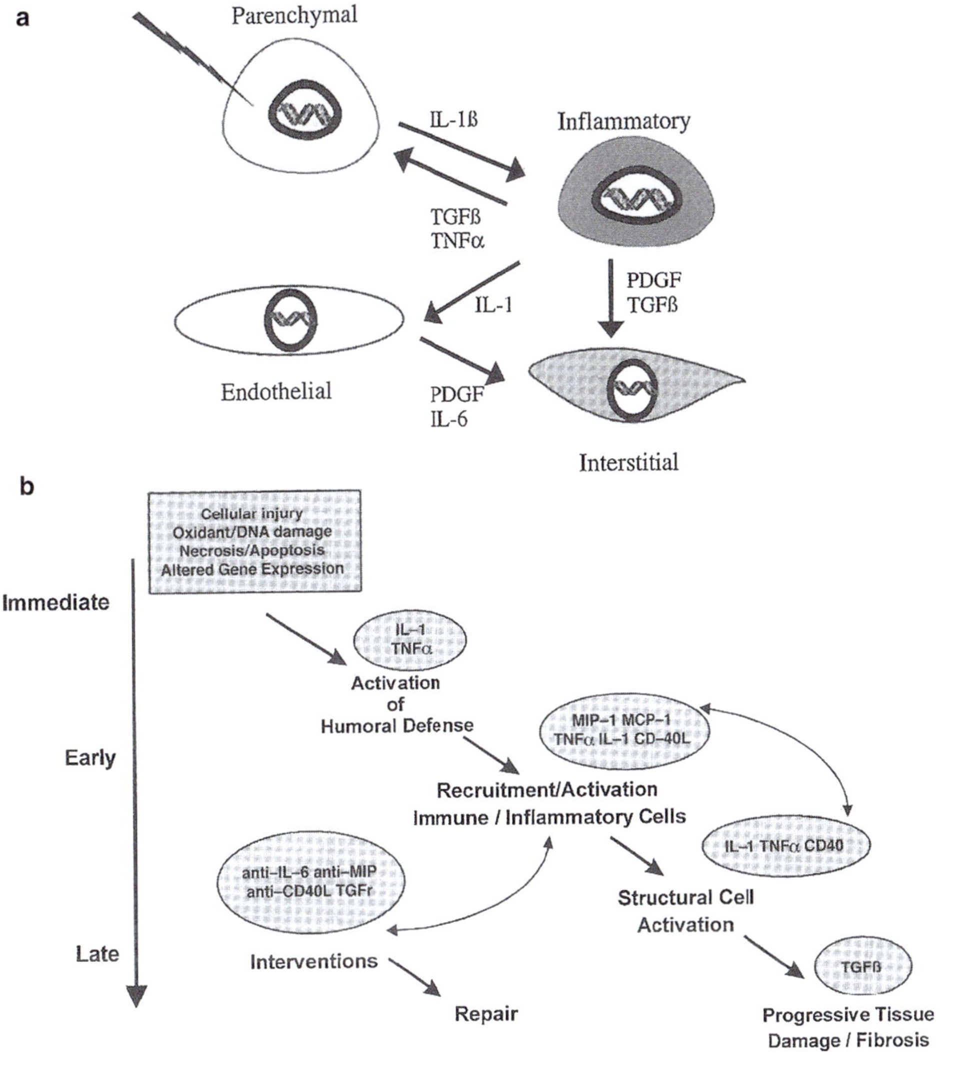

Fig. 2 **a** Suggested chain of events beginning with the initial injury to the primary target cell—the parenchymal cell—and culminating in activation of the interstitial cells (e.g., fibroblasts) to lay down extracellular matrix. **b** Hypothetical pathway indicating the chain of events from initial injury to the final late effect (e.g., fibrosis) (With permission from Rubin and Williams 2001)

5 The "Perpetual Cytokine Cascade" After Radiation Exposure

Within the first week following exposure to radiation, there is a decrease in inflammatory cells followed by an increase in neutrophils and lymphocyte accumulation that quickly returns to normal. Over time, fluctuations in inflammatory cell subsets infiltrating the irradiated tissue can be observed. The "perpetual cascade of cytokines" in the lungs after thoracic irradiation was first proposed by Rubin et al. 1995 which demonstrated an absence of a "latent period" at the molecular and cellular level in late responding tissues.

Our group has helped to pioneer the use of increasingly sophisticated molecular biologic methods to assess and analyze late effects in normal tissue (LENT). In so doing, we have extended the paradigm o the clinical pathologic course of events following irradiation or chemotherapy from target cells per se to include and emphasize the intercellular communication. In our current paradigm, during the course of LENT induction, the so-called cytokine cascade can be considered to involve four basic cell components in tissues or organs—the parenchymal cell, the inflammatory cell, the endothelial cell, and the interstitial cell. These are illustrated in Fig. 2a, are a few of the pro-inflammatory and profibrotic cytokines that are thought to be expressed concurrently (Rubin and Williams 2001).

An intercellular conversation is initiated at the moment of irradiation, when injury to cell components occurs (e.g., membrane, cytoplasmic body, or DNA), which leads to altered gene expression. This reaction is often in the form of an immediate release of cytokine mRNA; in time, this reaction may provoke a series of downstream events through cell signaling, which is illustrated in Fig. 2b. Through signal transduction, the receptor cells are activated; such activation may result in as little as additional or sequential cytokine expression or it can lead to proliferation or production of extracellular matrix proteins, depending on the species of receptor cell. In the specific case of the receptor cell being a fibroblast, activation of the collagen gene, which has been seen within 24 h of injury, can persist for days, weeks, or even months. This extended persistence may continue until the pathologic or clinical expression of injury is manifested (Rubin and Williams 2001).

Using a mixture of molecular biologic techniques and in vivo/in vitro assays, a number of in-field effects can be appreciated. The release of cytokines occurs shortly after irradiation and persists until the pathologic and clinical expression of late effects, and there is an arbitrary temporal division of cytokine expression:

- Immediate: first 24 h after injury
- Early: days to ~8 weeks post injury
- Late: 3–6 months post injury.

This scenario can be seen to correlate and give further credence to the postulated shape of the clinical pathologic course of events. The potential to use cytokines to alter the therapeutic ratio favorably is of great interest to clinicians in the protocol design of new clinical trials.

The most predominant cytokines involved in inflammation appear to be IL-1α/β, IL-6, TNF-α, and TGF-β (Rubin et al. 1995; Chiang et al. 1997; Herskind et al. 1998; Rube et al. 2004; Brush et al. 2007), however the pattern and timing of cytokine expression appears to vary among studies (Hill 2005), as well as among animal models. The variation of cytokine expression in response to radiation between mouse strains may present one possible mechanism for the observed difference in strain sensitivity and response to radiation. Likewise, baseline differences in the number and types of resident inflammatory cell types among strains as well as genetic differences in leukocyte recruitment may contribute to the variation in radiation response. For example, fibrosing strains have a higher ratio of active to latent TGF-β than non-fibrosing strains (Franko et al. 1997). Epperly et al. (1999) found a time dependent progression in pathological fibrosis coincided with increased IL-1 mRNA levels and a biphasic wave of TGF-β expression during the development of fibrotic disease in C57BL/6 J mice (Epperly et al. 1999). However, targeting cytokine production has not been completely effective in improving survival and respiratory function, nor has any single circulating cytokine been identified as a potential biomarker for susceptibility to development of radiation-induced injury.

Cytokines expressed in irradiated tissue, such as interleukins, monocyte chemoattractant protein-1, and keratinocyte chemoattractant (KC), are consistent with what one would expect based on the inflammatory cell infiltrates found in the tissue and in circulating plasma. Inflammatory cells accumulate in irradiated tissue due to persistent upregulation of vascular adhesion markers (Epperly et al. 2002; Son et al. 2006; Muller et al. 2006; Jaal and Dorr 2005; Ikeda et al. 2000; Olschowka et al. 1997; Gaugler et al. 1997). Targeting inflammatory cell recruitment through inhibition of vascular adhesion molecules, specifically ICAM-1, reduces the number of infiltrating inflammatory cells and blocks the development of fibrosis in irradiated lungs of C57BL/6 mice (Hallahan et al. 2002; Hallahan and Virudachalam 1997). Although the impact of systemically blocking ICAM-1 on acute and chronic inflammation is significant, there is no improvement in respiratory function or survival among non-treated and treated animals exposed to radiation (Hallahan et al. 2002). This suggests an underlying cause for radiation pneumonitis/fibrosis, which impacts animal survival, distinct from inflammation alone.

5.1 Transforming Growth Factor-Beta 1

TGF-β1 is a multipotent cytokine that activates transcriptional regulators and signal transducers involved in cellular proliferation, immunosuppression, extracellular matrix remodeling and inhibition of matrix degradation, chronic inflammatory disease, and angiogenesis (Flanders 2004; Lewis et al. 1999). TGF-β is secreted as an inactive polypeptide by virtually all cells, including fibroblasts, epithelial cells, macrophages, and others. Free radicals produced during radiation can activate TGF-β, which can then bind the TGF-β type II receptor (Ehrhart et al. 1997) setting off a phosphorylation cascade that transduces the signal from the cell membrane to the nucleus (Flanders 2004; Roberts 1999). Interestingly, it has recently been shown that the Smad2/3 phosphorylation cascade downstream of TGF-β1 is dependent on Nox4 signaling further suggesting a critical role of redox signaling in propagating fibrosis (Amara et al. 2010).

Franko and colleagues 1997 found differential expression of TGF-β latency associated peptide (LAP) in the lungs of C57LJ and C3HeB/FeJ mice after irradiation (11 and 18 Gy respectively). In the C57L/J mice, a significantly greater proportion of macrophages and uninvolved tissue expressed TGF-β LAP as compared to lesions with acute/intense inflammation and fibrosis. Cells positive for LAP within the areas of intense inflammation were predominantly macrophages and Type II Pneumocytes. This was in contrast to C3HeB/FeJ, a non-fibrosing mouse strain, which showed significantly higher levels of latent TGF-β (Franko et al. 1997). Since TGF-β is secreted as an inactive molecule bound to the extracellular matrix by its LAP, the results of Franko suggest Type II pneumocytes and macrophages are the predominant producers of TGF-β following radiation in fibrosing mouse strains (C57L background).

Studies by Epperly et al. (1999) found decreased early onset of TGF-β, IL-1, and TNF-α mRNA levels in irradiated lung following intratracheal administration of a manganese-

SOD plasmid/liposome complex correlated with improved median survival time. It is important to note that at the time of death, TGF-β levels were not significantly different among groups. Several studies using pharmacologic inhibitors to TGF-β or components of its signal transduction pathway have the ability to significantly reduce radiation fibrosis and improve lung function, indicating that unregulated TGF-β is a mediator of fibroproliferative disease (Flanders 2004; Anscher et al. 2008; Biswas et al. 2007; Nishioka et al. 2004; Xavier et al. 2004).

6 Vascular Dysfunction Following Ionizing Radiation

It has long been acknowledged that the vascular endothelium may be an important target of ionizing radiation. Indeed, several studies have shown both gastrointestinal toxicity and xerostomia to be influenced by endothelial cell damage. Ionizing radiation can disrupt the structural integrity of the vascular architecture resulting in endothelial cell damage, barrier breakdown, leakage, and edema (Anscher et al. 2005; Martin et al. 2000; Stone et al. 2004). As a consequence of the disruption in vascular function, hypoxic regions can develop in the under-perfused tissue. Indeed, one of the key pathophysiological consequences of vascular injury after radiation is the development of tissue hypoxia. Tissue hypoxia can recruit inflammatory cells, where they are then activated to undergo the respiratory burst. Not only does this increase oxidative stress, but also further contributes to tissue hypoxia as oxygen is required for the respiratory burst in phagocytic cells. One of the primary cell types recruited by hypoxia is the macrophage. Jackson et al., demonstrated that macrophages incubated under hypoxic conditions exhibit a redox-dependent increase in TGF-β production and the hypoxia-inducible factor-1 alpha (HIF-1α) product VEGF (Jackson et al. 2007).

HIF-1α has observed in lung tissue as early as one day after radiation. The ability of free radical scavenging to inhibit stabilization of HIF-1α has implicated ROS/RNS as a critical activator of HIF transcriptional activity (Pouyssegur and Mechta-Grigoriou 2006; Li et al. 2007). The consequences of HIF stabilization in irradiated healthy tissue likely include greater endothelial dysfunction, enhanced vascular hyperpermeability, formation of temporary fibrin matrices, and angiogenesis (van Hinsbergh et al. 2001; van Hinsbergh 2001a, b; Semenza 2000). Vascular leakage and fibrin deposition facilitate the formation of new vessels (van Hinsbergh et al. 2001) through establishment of a provisional fibrin matrix which provides a stable scaffold for HIF-1α mediated inflammatory and endothelial cell migration and vessel sprouting (Haroon et al. 1999). Under physiological conditions, HIF has a relatively short half-life of less than 5 min (Wang et al. 1995; Huang et al. 1998). However, under hypoxia, or in the event of oxidative/nitroxidative modification of protein residues in the oxygen dependent domain, the alpha subunit of HIF is stabilized and translocated to the nucleus where it forms a heterodimer with its constitutively expressed HIF-1β subunit. The HIF heterodimer binds to the hypoxia response element (HRE) of a wide variety of genes regulating cell proliferation, migration, pH, apoptosis, energy metabolism, and most importantly, angiogenesis (Brahimi-Horn et al. 2005).

Vujaskovic et al. showed an increase in expression of the HIF product vascular endothelial growth factor (VEGF) between the time of radiation exposure and development of symptomatic disease in a rat model of radiation-induced lung injury (Fleckenstein et al. 2007). Under physiological conditions, VEGF levels decline as tissues undergo reoxygenation/reperfusion and immature vessels tend to regress while healthy vasculature remains unaffected by the change in VEGF (Dorr et al. 2000). The involvement of VEGF in vascular pruning is a relatively new concept. Under pathological conditions, VEGF remains elevated resulting in little to no vessel regression, increased stimulation of neovascularization, and long-term irregularities in perfusion (Dorr et al. 2000), which have been observed in radiation studies. Perfusion imaging of normal tissue after radiation demonstrates vascular dysfunction almost immediately coinciding with a transient decrease in perfusion, increased edema, and elevated expression of HIF-1α and TGF-β (Ward et al. 1983; Fleckenstein et al. 2007). The vascular network renormalizes for a brief period of time, before progressively deteriorating beginning around the time of the initial onset of hypoxia and continuing until the development of histological and functional disease (Ward et al. 1983; Fleckenstein et al. 2007). Spatial distribution and density patterns of VEGF mRNA following the onset of radiation-induced spinal cord injury show that transient expression of VEGF at the legion border correlates with a local increase in blood vessel density (Bartholdi et al. 1997).

One of the leading producers of HIF after radiation appears to be macrophages. In addition to being one of the primary producers of oxidative stress after radiation, macrophages are known to be a source of pro-angiogenic stimuli (HIF-1α) (Lewis et al. 1999). Macrophages are closely associated with areas of inadequate perfusion and low partial oxygen pressure (Lewis et al. 1999), thus, it is not surprising that macrophage accumulation coincides with a decrease in perfusion and an increase in tissue hypoxia following irradiation (Fleckenstein et al. 2007).

In normal tissue, the number of macrophages significantly increases within several days to weeks post-radiation(Fleckenstein et al. 2007). Macrophage accumulation within the residual alveolar space and interstitium appears prior to the onset of functional damage and is associated with a surge in cytokine activity (Vujaskovic et al. 2002; 2001). Activated macrophages can secrete pro-angiogenic (HIF) (Kureshi et al. 1994) and fibrogenic growth factors (TGF-β) to induce the formation of granulation tissue containing myofibroblasts and neovessels (Frangogiannis 2006). In radiation induced late brain injury, macrophages were found to be a prominent histological feature in 5 out of 6 tissue biopsies studied by Kureshi and colleagues (1994). Under physiological conditions, macrophages respond to injured tissue to facilitate wound healing and return the environment to homeostatic levels. However, for reasons that remain unclear, in irradiated normal tissue, the healing response is aberrant and furthers the escalation of injury.

Interestingly, in a recent study, O'Brien et al. (2005) identified differential apoptosis among alveolar macrophages in C3H/HeJ, which develop an acute pneumonitis, and "fibrosis prone" C57BL/6 J mice, which the authors hypothesized could explain the disparity between inflammatory response between these strains.

The HIF-1α product, carbonic Anhydrase-9 (CA-9), is frequently used as molecular marker for imaging of hypoxia because of its colocalization with HIF-1α in tumor tissue. CA9 is a chimeric enzyme that catalyzes the hydration of carbon dioxide to bicarbonate ion to maintain an alkaline intracellular pH (Pouyssegur et al. 2001). Altered expression of CA9 in hypoxic regions suggests that these regions may possess metabolic alterations, although the specific changes involved have not been investigated. Evidence of HIF-1α upregulation in hypoxia driven pathologies including radiation induced normal tissue injury could support the hypothesis that cellular metabolism is altered following radiation, especially when combined with the observed mitochondrial dysfunction and nonoxidative synthesis of ATP.

7 Multimodality or Multidisciplinary Treatment

All cytotoxic treatment modalities utilized in the treatment of cancers share common proinflammatory and profibrotic pathways.

Surgery: with the initial incision through the final excision of the cancer, a similar cascade of cytokines are induced in tissues and organs traumatized by surgery. After the acute inflammatory phase, the induction of fibrotic scarring follows, resulting in infiltrates of immune cells (neutrophils, lymphocytes, and macrophages releasing cytokines that stimulate fibroblasts or progenitor cells that differentiate into myofibroblasts. Myofibroblasts produce collagens and metalloproteinases needed for collagen degradation. The ultimate surgical scar is hypocellular as myofibroblasts and inflammatory cells undergo apoptosis. Similar cell-cytokine cascades to radiation mediate and drive the initial inflammatory process to fibrogenesis and complete the scarring process (Yarnold et al. 2010).

Chemotherapy: can induce endocrine, paracrine, and autocrine cytokine cell signaling utilizing similar pathways as radiation. Cells sense signals from both extracellular and intracellular environments as well as other cells. Most signals are initiated by ligands and are sensed by cell membrane receptors which stimulate the formation of multiprotein complexes. These in turn generate small molecule messengers that control the inflammatory and fibrogenic tissue responses. Although pathways induced are depicted as linear, nearly all pathways induced are very interconnected and pleotrophic forming networks that allow dynamic cellular responses resulting in cell death either in mitosis or apoptosis. Thus, the inflammatory and fibrogenic responses parallel those of the other modalities in eradicating cancers producing adverse acute and LENT. Molecular targeted interventions that can block specific signals/cytokines may be applicable to other modalities (DeVita et al. 2011).

8 Conclusion

The development of radiation-induced tissue injury begins with an ionizing event that results in direct damage to DNA but also initiates a cascade of events on the cellular and molecular level that proceeds during a period of clinically occult injury. One of the effects of the propagation of the initial insult is a disruption of the balance between oxygen derived free radicals and antioxidants. This imbalance results in oxidative damage to DNA, lipids, and proteins within the affected tissues causing increased apoptosis of cells as well as altering signaling pathway activity. Changes in cell signaling can result in increased vascular contractility and permeability, angiogenesis, and inflammatory monocyte migration and inflammation, all of which contribute to development of acute and latent tissue injury. Because many of the changes that contribute to radiation-induced tissue injury are the result of a signaling cascade initiated by overproduction of ROS/RNS, it is unlikely that modification or elimination of any one event can alter the overall process of progressive radiation injury. The injury is self-perpetuating in nature and is, therefore, more likely to be mitigated by interventions which broadly interfere with the propagation of radiation damage.

References

Amara N, Goven D, Prost F et al (2010) NOX4/NADPH oxidase expression is increased in pulmonary fibroblasts from patients with idiopathic pulmonary fibrosis and mediates TGFbeta1-induced fibroblast differentiation into myofibroblasts. Thorax 65(8): 733–738

Anscher MS, Chen L, Rabbani Z et al (2005) Recent progress in defining mechanisms and potential targets for prevention of normal tissue injury after radiation therapy. Int J Radiat Oncol Biol Phys 62(1):255–259

Anscher MS, Thrasher B, Zgonjanin L et al (2008) Small molecular inhibitor of transforming growth factor-beta protects against development of radiation-induced lung injury. Int J Radiat Oncol Biol Phys 71(3):829–837

Azria D, Ozsahin M, Kramar A et al (2008) Single nucleotide polymorphisms, apoptosis, and the development of severe late adverse effects after radiotherapy. Clin Cancer Res 14(19): 6284–6288

Bartholdi D, Rubin BP, Schwab ME (1997) VEGF mRNA induction correlates with changes in the vascular architecture upon spinal cord damage in the rat. Eur J Neurosci 9(12):2549–2560

Batinic-Haberle I, Reboucas JS, Spasojevic I (2010) Superoxide dismutase mimics: chemistry, pharmacology, and therapeutic potential. Antioxid Redox Signal 13(6):877–918

Belyakov OV, Mitchell SA, Parikh D et al (2005) Biological effects in unirradiated human tissue induced by radiation damage up to 1 mm away. Proc Natl Acad Sci U S A 102(40):14203–14208

Benderitter M, Isoir M, Buard V et al (2007) Collapse of skin antioxidant status during the subacute period of cutaneous radiation syndrome: a case report. Radiat Res 167(1):43–50

Bengtsson SH, Gulluyan LM, Dusting GJ et al (2003) Novel isoforms of NADPH oxidase in vascular physiology and pathophysiology. Clin Exp Pharmacol Physiol 30(11):849–854

Bentzen SM (2006) Preventing or reducing late side effects of radiation therapy: radiobiology meets molecular pathology. Nat Rev Cancer 6(9):702–713

Biswas S, Guix M, Rinehart C et al (2007) Inhibition of TGF-beta with neutralizing antibodies prevents radiation-induced acceleration of metastatic cancer progression. J Clin Invest 117(5):1305–1313

Brahimi-Horn C, Mazure N, Pouyssegur J (2005) Signalling via the hypoxia-inducible factor-1alpha requires multiple posttranslational modifications. Cell Signal 17(1):1–9

Brush J, Lipnick SL, Phillips T et al (2007) Molecular mechanisms of late normal tissue injury. Semin Radiat Oncol 17(2):121–130

Carnesecchi S, Deffert C, Donati Y et al (2011) A key role for NOX4 in epithelial cell death during development of lung fibrosis. Antioxid Redox Signal 15(3):607–619

Cernanec JM, Weinberg JB, Batinic-Haberle I et al (2007) Influence of oxygen tension on interleukin 1-induced peroxynitrite formation and matrix turnover in articular cartilage. J Rheumatol 34(2):401–407

Chiang CS, Hong JH, Stalder A et al (1997) Delayed molecular responses to brain irradiation. Int J Radiat Biol 72(1):45–53

Collins-Underwood JR, Zhao W, Sharpe JG et al (2008) NADPH oxidase mediates radiation-induced oxidative stress in rat brain microvascular endothelial cells. Free Radic Biol Med 45(6): 929–938

DeVita VT, Lawrence TS, Rosenburg SA et al (eds) (2011) In: Devita, Hellman, and Rosenberg's Cancer: principles and practice of oncology, vol. 5, 9th edn. Lippincott Williams & Wilkins, Philadelphia 5: pp 57–67

Dorr W, Baumann M, Herrmann T (2000) Radiation-induced lung damage: a challenge for radiation biology, experimental and clinical radiotherapy. Int J Radiat Biol 76(4):443–446

Ehrhart EJ, Segarini P, Tsang ML et al (1997) Latent transforming growth factor beta1 activation in situ: quantitative and functional evidence after low-dose gamma-irradiation. Faseb J 11(12): 991–1002

Epperly MW, Bray JA, Krager S et al (1999a) Intratracheal injection of adenovirus containing the human MnSOD transgene protects athymic nude mice from irradiation-induced organizing alveolitis. Int J Radiat Oncol Biol Phys 43(1):169–181

Epperly MW, Travis EL, Sikora C et al (1999b) Manganese [correction of Magnesium] superoxide dismutase (MnSOD) plasmid/liposome pulmonary radioprotective gene therapy: modulation of irradiation-induced mRNA for IL-I, TNF-alpha, and TGF-beta correlates with delay of organizing alveolitis/fibrosis. Biol Blood Marrow Transpl 5(4):204–214

Epperly MW, Defilippi S, Sikora C et al (2002) Radioprotection of lung and esophagus by overexpression of the human manganese superoxide dismutase transgene. Mil Med 167(2 Suppl):71–73

Flanders KC (2004) Smad3 as a mediator of the fibrotic response. Int J Exp Pathol 85(2):47–64

Fleckenstein K, Gauter-Fleckenstein B, Jackson IL et al (2007a) Using biological markers to predict risk of radiation injury. Semin Radiat Oncol 17(2):89–98

Fleckenstein K, Zgonjanin L, Chen L et al (2007b) Temporal onset of hypoxia and oxidative stress after pulmonary irradiation. Int J Radiat Oncol Biol Phys 68(1):196–204

Frangogiannis NG (2006) Targeting the inflammatory response in healing myocardial infarcts. Curr Med Chem 13(16):1877–1893

Franko AJ, Sharplin J, Ghahary A et al (1997) Immunohistochemical localization of transforming growth factor beta and tumor necrosis factor alpha in the lungs of fibrosis-prone and "non-fibrosing" mice during the latent period and early phase after irradiation. Radiat Res 147(2):245–256

Gaugler MH, Squiban C, van der Meeren A et al (1997) Late and persistent up-regulation of intercellular adhesion molecule-1 (ICAM-1) expression by ionizing radiation in human endothelial cells in vitro. Int J Radiat Biol 72(2):201–209

Gauter-Fleckenstein B, Fleckenstein K, Owzar K et al (2007) Comparison of two Mn porphyrin-based mimics of superoxide dismutase in pulmonary radioprotection. Free Radic Biol Med 44(6):982–989

Gauter-Fleckenstein B, Fleckenstein K, Owzar K et al (2010) Early and late administration of MnTE-2-PyP5 + in mitigation and treatment of radiation-induced lung damage. Free Radic Biol Med 48(8):1034–1043

Ghosh SN, Zhang R, Fish BL et al (2009a) Renin-Angiotensin system suppression mitigates experimental radiation pneumonitis. Int J Radiat Oncol Biol Phys 75(5):1528–1536

Ghosh SN, Wu Q, Mader M et al (2009b) Vascular injury after whole thoracic x-ray irradiation in the rat. Int J Radiat Oncol Biol Phys 74(1):192–199

Hallahan DE, Virudachalam S (1997) Intercellular adhesion molecule 1 knockout abrogates radiation induced pulmonary inflammation. Proc Natl Acad Sci U S A 94(12):6432–6437

Hallahan DE, Geng L, Shyr Y (2002) Effects of intercellular adhesion molecule 1 (ICAM-1) null mutation on radiation-induced pulmonary fibrosis and respiratory insufficiency in mice. J Natl Cancer Inst 94(10):733–741

Haroon ZA, Lai TS, Hettasch JM et al (1999) Tissue transglutaminase is expressed as a host response to tumor invasion and inhibits tumor growth. Lab Invest 79(12):1679–1686

Herskind C, Bamberg M, Rodemann HP (1998) The role of cytokines in the development of normal-tissue reactions after radiotherapy. Strahlenther Onkol 174(Suppl 3):12–15

Hill RP (2005) Radiation effects on the respiratory system. BJR Suppl 27:75–81

Huang LE, Gu J, Schau M et al (1998) Regulation of hypoxia-inducible factor 1alpha is mediated by an O2-dependent degradation domain via the ubiquitin-proteasome pathway. Proc Natl Acad Sci U S A 95(14):7987–7992

Ikeda Y, Ito M, Matsuu M et al (2000) Expression of ICAM-1 and acute inflammatory cell infiltration in the early phase of radiation colitis in rats. J Radiat Res (Tokyo) 41(3):279–291

Jaal J, Dorr W (2005) Early and long-term effects of radiation on intercellular adhesion molecule 1 (ICAM-1) expression in mouse urinary bladder endothelium. Int J Radiat Biol 81(5):387–395

Jackson IL, Chen L, Batinic-Haberle I et al (2007) Superoxide dismutase mimetic reduces hypoxia-induced O2*-, TGF-beta, and VEGF production by macrophages. Free Radic Res 41(1):8–14

Kelsey CR, Jackson L, Langdon S et al (2011) A polymorphism within the promoter of the tgfbeta1 gene is associated with radiation sensitivity using an objective radiologic endpoint. Int J Radiat Oncol Biol Phys 82(2):e247–e255

Kong FM, Ao X, Wang L et al (2008) The use of blood biomarkers to predict radiation lung toxicity: a potential strategy to individualize thoracic radiation therapy. Cancer Control 15(2):140–150

Kureshi SA, Hofman FM, Schneider JH et al (1994) Cytokine expression in radiation-induced delayed cerebral injury. Neurosurgery 35(5):822–829; discussion 829–830

Lassegue B, Griendling KK (2010) NADPH oxidases: functions and pathologies in the vasculature. Arterioscler Thromb Vasc Biol 30(4):653–661

Lewis JS, Lee JA, Underwood JC et al (1999) Macrophage responses to hypoxia: relevance to disease mechanisms. J Leukoc Biol 66(6):889–900

Li F, Sonveaux P, Rabbani ZN et al (2007) Regulation of HIF-1alpha stability through S-nitrosylation. Mol Cell 26(1):63–74

Martin M, Delanian S, Sivan V et al (2000) Radiation-induced superficial fibrosis and TGF-alpha 1. Cancer Radiother 4(5):369–384

McBride WH, Chiang CS, Olson JL et al (2004) A sense of danger from radiation. Radiat Res 162(1):1–19

Michalowski A (1986) The pathogenesis of the late side-effects of radiotherapy. Clin Radiol 37(3):203–207

Mikkelsen RB, Wardman P (2003) Biological chemistry of reactive oxygen and nitrogen and radiation-induced signal transduction mechanisms. Oncogene 22(37):5734–5754

Moulder JE, Fish BL, Cohen EP (2002) Dietary sodium modification and experimental radiation nephropathy. Int J Radiat Biol 78(10):903–911

Muller K, Kohn FM, Port M et al (2006) Intercellular adhesion molecule-1: a consistent inflammatory marker of the cutaneous radiation reaction both in vitro and in vivo. Br J Dermatol 155(4):670–679

Nishioka A, Ogawa Y, Mima T et al (2004) Histopathologic amelioration of fibroproliferative change in rat irradiated lung using soluble transforming growth factor-beta (TGF-beta) receptor mediated by adenoviral vector. Int J Radiat Oncol Biol Phys 58(4):1235–1241

O'Brien TJ, Letuve S, Haston CK (2005) Radiation-induced strain differences in mouse alveolar inflammatory cell apoptosis. Can J Physiol Pharmacol 83(1):117–122

Olschowka JA, Kyrkanides S, Harvey BK et al (1997) ICAM-1 induction in the mouse CNS following irradiation. Brain Behav Immun 11(4):273–285

O'Neill P, Wardman P (2009) Radiation chemistry comes before radiation biology. Int J Radiat Biol 85(1):9–25

Pouyssegur J, Mechta-Grigoriou F (2006) Redox regulation of the hypoxia-inducible factor. Biol Chem 387(10–11):1337–1346

Pouyssegur J, Franchi A, Pages G (2001) pHi, aerobic glycolysis and vascular endothelial growth factor in tumour growth. Novartis Found Symp 240:186–196 (discussion 196–188)

Rabbani ZN, Anscher MS, Folz RJ et al (2005) Overexpression of extracellular superoxide dismutase reduces acute radiation induced lung toxicity. BMC Cancer 5:59

Rabbani ZN, Batinic-Haberle I, Anscher MS et al (2007) Long-term administration of a small molecular weight catalytic metalloporphyrin antioxidant, AEOL 10150, protects lungs from radiation-induced injury. Int J Radiat Oncol Biol Phys 67(2):573–580

Robbins ME, Zhao W (2004) Chronic oxidative stress and radiation-induced late normal tissue injury: a review. Int J Radiat Biol 80(4):251–259

Roberts AB (1999) TGF-beta signaling from receptors to the nucleus. Microbes Infect 1(15):1265–1273

Rosenthal RA, Fish B, Hill RP et al (2011) Salen Mn complexes mitigate radiation injury in normal tissues. Anticancer Agents Med Chem 11(4):359–372

Rube CE, Wilfert F, Palm J et al (2004) Irradiation induces a biphasic expression of pro-inflammatory cytokines in the lung. Strahlenther Onkol 180(7):442–448

Rubin P, Williams J (eds) (2001) Clinical oncology: a multidisciplinary approach for physicians and students, 8th edn. Elsevier, Philadelphia, p 899, Figure 34-2ab

Rubin P, Johnston CJ, Williams JP et al (1995) A perpetual cascade of cytokines postirradiation leads to pulmonary fibrosis. Int J Radiat Oncol Biol Phys 33(1):99–109

Semenza GL (2000) Oxygen-regulated transcription factors and their role in pulmonary disease. Respir Res 1(3):159–162

Son EW, Rhee DK, Pyo S (2006) Gamma-irradiation-induced intercellular adhesion molecule-1 (ICAM-1) expression is associated with catalase: activation of Ap-1 and JNK. J Toxicol Environ Health A 69(24):2137–2155

Stone HB, Moulder JE, Coleman CN et al (2004) Models for evaluating agents intended for the prophylaxis, mitigation and treatment of radiation injuries. Report of an NCI workshop, 3–4 Dec, 2003. Radiat Res;162(6):711–728

Takac I, Schroder K, Zhang L et al (2011) The E-loop is involved in hydrogen peroxide formation by the NADPH oxidase Nox4. J Biol Chem 286(15):13304–13313

van Hinsbergh VW (2001a) NO or H(2)O(2) for endothelium-dependent vasorelaxation: Tetrahydrobiopterin makes the difference. Arterioscler Thromb Vasc Biol 21(5):719–721

van Hinsbergh VW (2001b) The endothelium: vascular control of haemostasis. Eur J Obstet Gynecol Reprod Biol 95(2):198–201

van Hinsbergh VW, Collen A, Koolwijk P (2001) Role of fibrin matrix in angiogenesis. Ann N Y Acad Sci 936:426–437

von Lohneysen K, Noack D, Wood MR et al (2010) Structural insights into Nox4 and Nox2: motifs involved in function and cellular localization. Mol Cell Biol 30(4):961–975

Vujaskovic Z, Anscher MS, Feng QF et al (2001) Radiation-induced hypoxia may perpetuate late normal tissue injury. Int J Radiat Oncol Biol Phys 50(4):851–855

Vujaskovic Z, Batinic-Haberle I, Rabbani ZN et al (2002) A small molecular weight catalytic metalloporphyrin antioxidant with superoxide dismutase (SOD) mimetic properties protects lungs from radiation-induced injury. Free Radic Biol Med 33(6): 857–863

Wang GL, Jiang BH, Rue EA et al (1995) Hypoxia-inducible factor 1 is a basic-helix-loop-helix-PAS heterodimer regulated by cellular O2 tension. Proc Natl Acad Sci U S A 92(12): 5510–5514

Wang LW, Fu XL, Clough R et al (2000) Can angiotensin-converting enzyme inhibitors protect against symptomatic radiation pneumonitis? Radiat Res 153(4):405–410

Ward JF (1994) DNA damage as the cause of ionizing radiation-induced gene activation. Radiat Res 138(Suppl 1):S85–S88

Ward WF, Solliday NH, Molteni A et al (1983) Radiation injury in rat lung II. Angiotensin-converting enzyme activity. Radiat Res 96(2):294–300

Xavier S, Piek E, Fujii M et al (2004) Amelioration of radiation-induced fibrosis: inhibition of transforming growth factor-beta signaling by halofuginone. J Biol Chem 279(15):15167–15176

Yarnold J, Brotons MC (2010) Pathogenetic mechanisms in radiation fibrosis. Radiother Oncol 97(1):149–161

Zhang Y, Hogg N (2005) S-Nitrosothiols: cellular formation and transport. Free Radic Biol Med 38(7):831–838

Zhang Y Zhang X, Rabbani ZN et al (2012) Oxidative stress mediates lung injury by inducing apoptosis. Int J Radiat Oncol Biol Phys 83(2):740–748

Zhao W, Diz DI, Robbins ME (2007) Oxidative damage pathways in relation to normal tissue injury. Br J Radiol 80(1):S23–31

Biodetection and Biointervention: Cytokine Pathways as a Rationale for Anti-cytokine Interventions Post-Radiation

Paul R. Graves, Isabel Jackson, Mitchell S. Anscher, Ross Mikkelsen, and Zeljko Vujaskovic

Contents

Abstract

Recent advances in our understanding of the molecular events underlying the pathogenesis of radiation-induced normal tissue injury has opened up the possibility of biologically based interventions to prevent, mitigate, or treat these complications. This work has also stimulated efforts to develop strategies to stratify patients according to risk of injury as a means to individualize therapy and improve the therapeutic ratio. Since many of the proteins involved in the pathogenesis of radiation injury, such as transforming growth factor ß, can be measured in the blood, researchers have begun to attempt to identify cytokine profiles that might identify patients at risk for normal tissue injury. This chapter summarizes the current state of this research and discusses approaches to mitigate or treat radiation injury that targets one or more of the molecular pathways involved in its pathogenesis.

1 Introduction

The tolerance of normal tissue surrounding tumors limits the maximum therapeutic dose of radiation that can be delivered to treat most malignancies (Milano et al. 2007). Many cancers present as large masses that require high doses of radiation to achieve local control or cure. However, physicians are forced to limit the total dose and volume irradiated due to the risk of life threatening or fatal complications. Consequently, cure rates for some of these malignancies, such as lung cancers or malignant brain tumors, are distressingly low. Recent advances in our understanding of the molecular events underlying the pathogenesis of radiation-induced normal tissue injury has opened up the possibility to use biologically based interventions to prevent, mitigate, or treat these complications. Likewise, these advances in knowledge have facilitated efforts to develop new strategies to stratify patients

M. S. Anscher (✉) · R. Mikkelsen
Department of Radiation Oncology, Virginia Commonwealth University School of Medicine, 401 College Street, P.O. Box 980058Richmond, VA 23298-0058, USA
e-mail: manscher@mcvh-vcu.edu

I. Jackson · Z. Vujaskovic
Department of Radiation Oncology, University of Maryland Medical Center, Greenbaum Cancer Center, 22 South Greene Street, Baltimore, MD 21201, USA

P. R. Graves
Department of Radiation Oncology, New York Methodist Hospital, 506 Sixth Street, Brooklyn, NY 11215, USA

P. Rubin et al. (eds.), *ALERT – Adverse Late Effects of Cancer Treatment*, Medical Radiology. Radiation Oncology, DOI: 10.1007/978-3-540-72314-1_5, © Springer-Verlag Berlin Heidelberg 2014

according to risk of radiation injury as a means to individualize therapy and improve treatment outcome and overall survival.

2 Molecular Mechanisms of Radiation Injury

The biologic response to ionizing radiation begins immediately after the first exposure with the generation of reactive oxygen/reactive nitrogen species (ROS/RNS) (Riley 1994). More recently, researchers have described how these immediate biochemical events rapidly triggered a series of genetic and molecular phenomena leading to clinically and histologically recognizable injury (Brach et al. 1991; Kharbanda et al. 1994, 1995, 1996a, b; Hong et al. 1995; Rubin et al. 1995; Barcellos-Hoff 1998; Hauer-Jensen et al. 1999; Vujaskovic et al. 2001; Hallahan et al. 2002; Brush et al. 2007). This response to radiation is dynamic and involves a number of mediators of inflammation and fibrosis produced by macrophages, epithelial cells, and fibroblasts. These events appear to be sustained for months to years beyond the completion of therapy; (Fu et al. 2001) however, the mechanisms underlying the development of delayed radiation injury, until recently, have remained unknown (Li et al. 2001; Vujaskovic et al. 2001).

The molecular processes responsible for radiation-induced normal tissue injury have been, perhaps, most extensively studied in the lung (Fig. 1). As previously stated, the initial tissue damage from radiation is generated by direct action of reactive oxygen species (ROS) on DNA. This interaction causes tissue injury including endothelial cell damage with an increase in permeability, edema, and fibrin accumulation in the extracellular matrix. Endothelial cell damage plays an important role in this process, and recent evidence suggests that the capillary endothelial cell may be the first cellular element to be damaged by RT (Paris et al. 2001). This is followed by an inflammatory response dominated by macrophage activation. Activated macrophages are known to be a rich source of proinflammatory and profibrotic cytokines that contribute to the recruitment and activation of additional cells directly involved in wound repair (Wynn 2008). The source of the macrophages that contribute to radiation-induced lung injury is an active area of investigation and it is possible that resident macrophages as wells as macrophages recruited from circulating monocytes play major roles in this process. Both vascular changes as well as an increase in oxygen consumption (due to macrophage activation) contribute to the development of hypoxia (Fleckenstein et al. 2007b). Hypoxia further stimulates production of ROS, proinflammatory, profibrogenic, and proangiogenic cytokines (Jackson et al. 2007). This perpetuates tissue damage leading to fibrosis via TGFß1 production and stimulates angiogenesis via vascular endothelial growth factor (VEGF) production. In an attempt to respond to the proliferative stimulus of VEGF, endothelial cells die due to previously accumulated radiation damage (Rodemann and Blaese 2007). Hypoxia therefore, continuously perpetuates a non-healing tissue response leading consequently to chronic radiation-induced injury (Vujaskovic et al. 2001; Anscher et al. 2005).

Many of the molecular mediators of normal tissue injury are proteins, which can be measured both in tissue and in blood. The ability to quantify the expression of these proteins, in the normal and diseased state, has led to attempts to use them as predictors of risk of normal tissue injury after radiation therapy (Anscher et al. 1993, 1994; Vujaskovic et al. 1997; Chen et al. 2001; De Jaeger et al. 2004; Gridley et al. 2004; Novakova-Jiresova et al. 2004). Until recently, each protein had to be quantified individually using methods such as antibody-based enzyme-linked immunosorbent assays (ELISA) or bioluminescence assays, which are laborious and time consuming (Kong et al. 1998). Advances in bioassay technology now permit researchers to quantify multiple proteins simultaneously from the same sample in a rapid and reproducible manner (Jones et al. 2002). This technology will greatly enhance the ability to construct protein expression profiles for individual patients and determine whether these patterns of protein expression can improve our ability to predict risk of injury from radiation therapy (Hart et al. 2004). Along these lines, blood and tissue banks stocked with samples from patients irradiated for various malignancies will become invaluable resources for normal tissue injury research.

3 The Importance of Transforming Growth Factor ß1 in Radiation-Induced Injury

The most widely studied potential mediator of radiation-induced normal tissue injury is Transforming Growth Factor-ß1 (TGFß1). TGFß1 has multiple functions that are important in the development of excess fibrous tissue, one of the hallmarks of late radiation injury. TGFß1 is a chemoattractant for fibroblasts and also promotes differentiation of immature fibroblasts into myofibroblasts, which leads to increased production of collagen and extracellular matrix (Rodemann and Bamberg 1995, 2007). TGFß1 also decreases production of matrix-specific proteases and increases production of protease inhibitors, resulting in decrease collagen degradation, with a net result of increased fibrous tissue formation (Hakenjos et al. 2000; Martin et al. 2000). In addition to being autocrine stimulated, TGFß1 production is also stimulated by hypoxia, which further

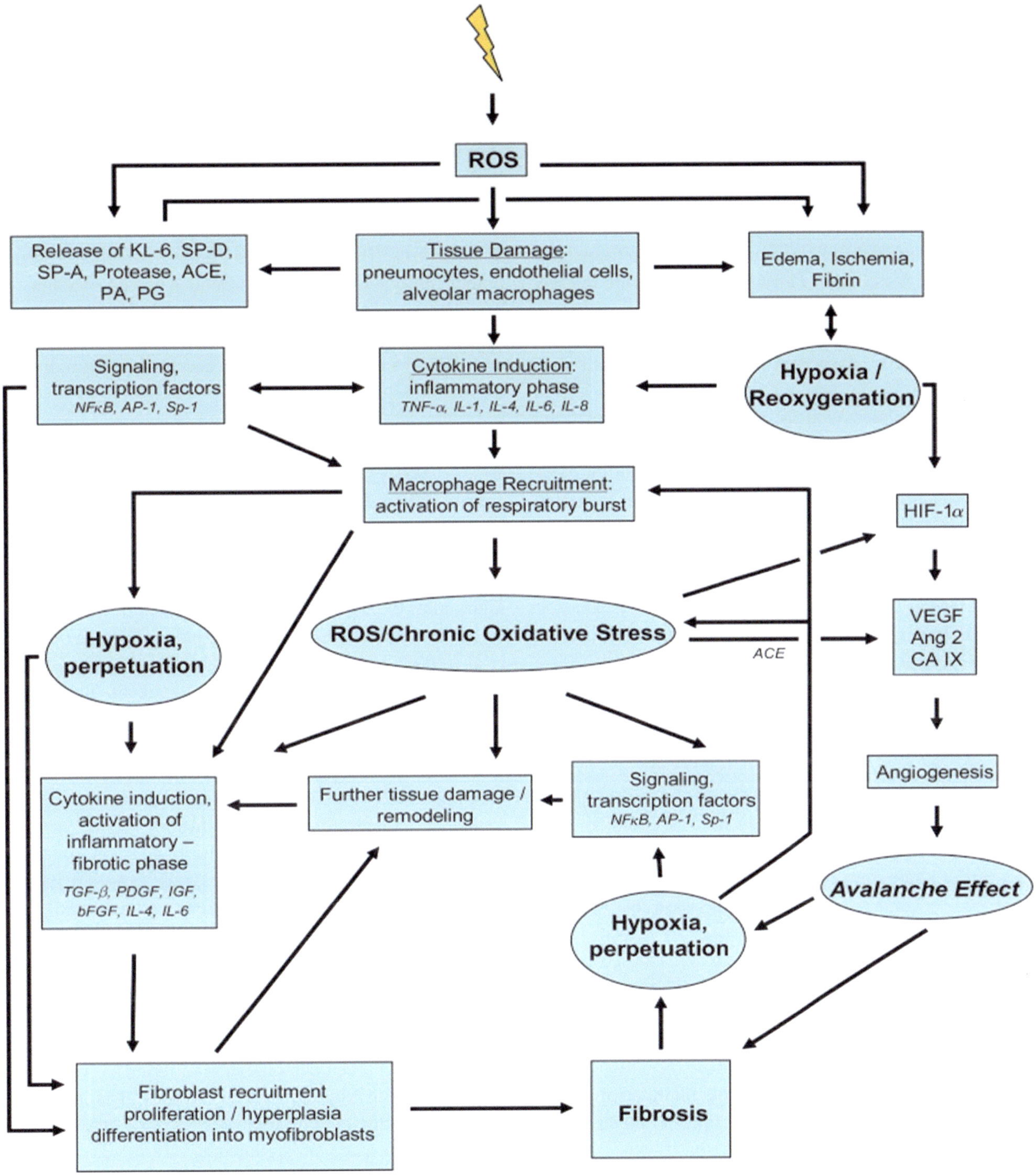

Fig. 1 Simplified model of processes involved in the pathogenesis of radiation-induced lung injury. As noted in the diagram, each event has the potential to influence several other processes. Exposure to ionizing radiation initiates a cascade of cytokines and growth factors. Proinflammatory cytokines promote an influx of macrophages and inflammatory cells, which are stimulated to produce ROS, proinflammatory and profibrotic cytokines. ROS serve as redox regulators of transcription factors, which further stimulate induction and activation of cytokines and growth factors. In addition, vascular changes, as well as an increase in oxygen consumption by activated macrophages, contribute to the development and perpetuation of hypoxia and chronic oxidative stress, leading to the non-healing tissue response of chronic radiation injury. ACE = angiotensin converting enzyme; PA = plasminogen activator; PG = prostaglandins; Ang2 = angiotensin II; CAIX = carbonic anhydrase IX, HIF = hypoxia inducible factor; PDGF = platelet derived growth factor; IGF = insulin-like growth factors; bFGF = basic fibroblast growth factor. [Reproduced with permission from Fleckenstein et al. (2007a)]

promotes collagen formation (Haroon et al. 2000; Moeller et al. 2004; Jackson et al. 2007).

Recent evidence confirms that TGFß1 is an important contributor to the pathogenesis of radiation-induced normal tissue injury. Rubin et al. (1992) reported that alveolar macrophages obtained from bronchial lavage specimens from irradiated rabbits demonstrated increased production and release of TGFß1 as compared to macrophages from normal lungs. These authors suggested that the fibroblast proliferation and extracellular matrix production found after irradiation are controlled by growth factors that are released from parenchymal cells following radiation exposure. Anscher et al. (1990) demonstrated that TGFß1 expression increased in a dose-dependent manner in the liver of rats following irradiation and that this increase in TGFß1 expression correlated with the extent of connective tissue production. Barcellos-Hoff (1995; Barcellos-Hoff and Dix 1996) has shown that free radicals produced during exposure to ionizing radiation can directly activate the latent form of TGFß1 which is sequestered in the extracellular matrix. It is likely that direct activation of TGFß1 from ionizing radiation contributes to the observed increase in TGFß1 levels 24 h post-radiation exposure (Fleckenstein et al. 2007b). Likewise, TGFß1 mRNA has also been shown to be elevated following radiation (Rube et al. 2000, 2004). Thus, radiation therapy can both increase local expression, as well as TGFß1 activation, resulting in increased fibrosis in irradiated tissues. As further evidence to support the role of TGFß1 in radiation injury, mice lacking Smad 3 (part of the TGFß1 signal transduction pathway) have been shown to be resistant to radiation-induced fibrosis (Flanders et al. 2002), suggesting that targeting the TGFß1 pathway might be a useful strategy to prevent radiation injury.

Indeed, several studies support the idea that reducing TGFß1 production may be one strategy to reduce normal tissue damage from radiation. Anscher and colleagues demonstrated that administration of a neutralizing TGFß1 antibody reduced radiation-induced macrophage accumulation, alveolar wall thickness, and TGFß1 activation in the lungs of rats (Anscher et al. 2006). More recently, a follow up study showed that a small molecule inhibitor of TGFß1 reduced breathing frequencies, lung fibrosis, inflammatory response, and TGFß1 activity in irradiated rats (Anscher et al. 2008).
A similar conclusion was obtained by inhibiting integrin signaling in the lung, an important activator of the TGFß1 pathway (Munger et al. 1999). It was shown that integrin alpha(v) beta6-deficient mice were completely protected from radiation-induced fibrosis (Puthawala et al. 2008).

Local activation of TGFß1 in tissues may also be an important component in sustaining the process of abnormal wound healing long after the exposure to radiation has ended. For example, active TGFß1 both recruits and activates macrophages to secrete inflammatory and fibrogenic cytokines, including TGFß1 itself (Ashcroft 1999; Roberts et al. 2001). This auto-induction is important in maintaining levels of TGFß1 in wound healing. Following radiation, however, this process contributes to overproduction of collagen and inhibition of epithelial cell proliferation, increased local oxygen consumption by activated macrophages, and decreased oxygen delivery due to microvasculature injury creating a hypoxic environment (Li et al. 2001). These combined factors perpetuate normal tissue injury. In addition, sustained overproduction of TGFß1 may contribute not only to chronic fibrosis, but may also reduce the effectiveness of cancer therapies (Biswas et al. 2007) and contribute to the development of radiation-induced malignancy (see below).

4 Using Plasma TGFß1 Levels to Predict Injury Risk

Plasma TGFß1 levels recently has been used to try and identify patients at risk for the development of normal tissue injury after exposure to chemotherapy and/or radiotherapy. In patients who develop radiation-induced lung injury, Fu et al. (2001) found sustained elevations in plasma TGFß1 level for as long as 2 years after treatment. In contrast, patients who did not develop symptomatic lung injury did not exhibit sustained elevations in circulating plasma TGFß1. In another patient study, it was shown that TGFß1 blood plasma levels increased during the period of radiation treatment and also became significantly higher 4 weeks after radiotherapy (Kim et al. 2009). In addition, of several cytokines measured, only TGFß1 levels showed a correlation with the symptomatic occurrence of radiation pneumonitis (Kim et al. 2009). Recently, it was also shown that elevated levels of plasma TGFß1 during radiation therapy was predictive of radiation-induced lung toxicity in patients with non-small-cell lung cancer (Zhao et al. 2009). In animal experiments, long-term overexpression and activation of TGFß1 have been demonstrated in tissue as well (Johnston et al. 1995; Vujaskovic et al. 2002a). Thus, elevations in plasma TGFß1 months after radiation exposure appear to reflect the presence of significantly dysregulated wound healing in the irradiated tissues. In contrast, the absence of sustained elevations of circulating TGFß1 levels appear to reflect a more normal wound healing process. Thus, prolonged elevations of plasma TGFß1 following radiation exposure may be a useful means to identify patients at risk for late radiation-induced injury. Other investigators, however, have not found plasma TGFß1 to be a reliable identifier of patients at increased risk for normal tissue injury after cancer therapy (Barthelemy-Brichant et al. 2004; De Jaeger et al. 2004; Novakova-Jiresova et al. 2004). These

Table 1 Summary of the function of candidate proteins for profiling

Protein	Function
IL-1ß	Inflammation, growth factor expression
IL-5	Proinflammatory
IL-6	Proinflammatory, decrease apoptosis of activated lung fibroblasts
IL-7	Proinflammatory
IL-8	Angiogenesis, leukocyte chemotaxis, and collagen synthesis
IL-10	Anti-inflammatory (decrease TNFα production, decrease upregulation of endothelial cell adhesion molecules)
IL-13	Proinflammatory
MCP-1	Inflammation, chemoattraction of monocytes
MIP-1alpha	Antiproliferative
PDGF BB	Angiogenesis, recruit smooth muscle cells
VEGF	Angiogenesis and increased vascular permeability
EGF	Epithelial cell motility, mitogenicity, and differentiation
EGFR	Receptor for EGF, initial component of EGF signaling pathway
NFkappaB	Pleotrophic gene transcription responses
HIF-1	Transcription factor for genes regulating angiogenesis
TGF-alpha	Cell motility and proliferation
FGF 2	Angiogenesis and fibroblast proliferation
MMP-1	Degradation of collagen and extracellular matrix proteins
MMP-2	Matrix remodeling, growth factor release
MMP-3	Matrix remodeling, growth factor release
MMP-13	Matrix remodeling, growth factor release
SMAD 2/3	Signal transduction in the TGFß pathway
IGF-1R	Binding of IGF-1 (re-epithelialization and granulation tissue formation)
TNF-alpha	Growth factor expression, inflammation, matrix production, and remodeling
TGFß1	Profibrotic, immunosuppression, angiogenesis, and metastasis

discrepancies may be due to a number of factors, including differences in techniques used to measure TGFß1, differences in patient populations under study, differences in tumor type and burden, and the fact that these studies contain relatively small numbers of patients with treatment-related injury, thus the power to detect a difference between groups is not large (Anscher and Kong 2005).

5 The Role of Other Cytokines in Radiation-Induced Injury

A growing body of evidence points toward a complex web of protein interactions as being important in the pathogenesis of radiation injury (see Table 1 and Fig. 1). For example, Huang et al. (2002) have found that IL-7, a cytokine that enhances T cell function and IFN-γ production, inhibits both TGFß1 production and signaling, and protects against the development of bleomycin-induced pulmonary fibrosis. Fedorocko et al. (2002) showed that radiation exposure could increase cytokine production both directly (IL-6, TNF-α) and indirectly (GM-CSF), either by locally acting paracrine or endocrine effects or as a result of systemic effects of early proinflammatory mediators such as IL-1 or TNF-α. There is no doubt that protein production is a dynamic process, which will change as a result of cancer treatment. Hong et al. (2003) have documented temporal and spatial changes in the expression of proinflammatory cytokines (TNF-α, IL-1α, and IL-1ß) following thoracic irradiation in mice. Given the impact that radiation has on the expression of these and other proteins in tissue and that these changes in tissue protein expression might be reflected in changes in plasma protein levels, it is reasonable to postulate that it may be possible to quantify an individual patient's inflammatory status by measuring candidate protein levels in the blood.

6 Using Other Markers to Predict Radiation-Induced Injury

In addition to TGFß1, several other proteins have been studied in humans to evaluate their potential as biomarkers for radiation-induced injury. Most of this work has been carried out in the lung. Of these, the most promising include interleukins (IL) 1α, IL-6, IL-8, IL-10, Krebs von den Lungen protein (KL-6, which is expressed mainly on type II pneumocytes and bronchiolar epithelial cells), soluble intracellular adhesion molecule (sICAM)-1, and surfactant proteins A and D (Kohno et al. 1992; Ishii and Kitamura 1999; Chen et al. 2001; Goto et al. 2001; Sasaki et al. 2001; Takahashi et al. 2001; Gridley et al. 2004; Hara et al. 2004, 2005; Chen et al. 2005; Matsuno et al. 2006). Of these, KL-6 is the most extensively studied, and has most consistently been correlated with the risk of radiation-induced lung injury (Fleckenstein et al. 2007a). As with TGFß1, more prospective studies with larger patient numbers will be required to confirm its value as a predictive marker for lung injury.

7 Chronic Inflammation as a Mediator of Radiation Injury

Epidemiologic evidence has also suggested a correlation between chronic inflammation and the development of malignancy at the inflamed site. Recent evidence points to a prolonged and progressive period of oxidative stress following the initial ionizing event in the development of radiation-induced lung injury. The underlying mechanism involves recruitment of inflammatory cells, as well as the expression of multiple mediators of inflammation, including cytokines, chemokines, and enzymes. Proinflammatory cytokines, such as the interleukins and tumor necrosis factor α, cause an influx of inflammatory cells and fibroblasts into the microenvironment (Johnston et al. 2004; Rube et al. 2005). These cells, primarily macrophages (Rubin et al. 1992; Vujaskovic et al. 2000), become stimulated to produce reactive oxygen species and additional proinflammatory and profibrotic cytokines (Fleckenstein et al. 2007a) (Fig. 1).

It is well established that tissue hypoxia is a potent stimulator of macrophage proliferation and activation. Fleckenstein et al. (Fleckenstein et al. 2007b) found a biphasic decrease in pulmonary perfusion following hemithoracic irradiation in rats, which correlated to the development of hypoxia, macrophage infiltration, and increased oxidative stress. Furthermore, in vitro studies lend support to the authors hypothesis that hypoxia stimulates TGFß1 and VEGF production by macrophages in an SOD-inhibitable manner.

Reactive oxygen species (ROS) functionally regulate transcription factors that also influence expression and activation of cytokines and growth factors (Sun and Oberley 1996). Furthermore, ROS play an important role in intracellular signaling, including activation of HIF-1a, NFkB, TGFß1, and a variety of other molecules found to play a role in radiation-induced injury (Schmidt-Ullrich et al. 2000). Over the past several decades, it has been shown that the free radical scavenging ability of endogenous antioxidants, most notably superoxide dismutase (SOD), acts as a cell-based protective mechanism. As the role of chronic oxidative stress in the development of radiation-induced lung injury has emerged, several investigators have attempted to restore the critical balance between chronic oxidative stress and antioxidant capacity through exogenous delivery of SOD. Several preclinical studies have shown mimics of SOD or liposomal-based delivery of SOD can mitigate injury when given after radiation and may even treat radiation-induced normal tissue injury once clinical symptoms become apparent (Epperly et al. 1999, 2000, 2008; Rabbani et al. 2007; Gautcr-Fleckenstein et al. 2008, 2010; Borrelli et al. 2009). Thus, SOD-based therapy may hold potential therapeutic value in the treatment of radiation-induced lung injury.

Recent evidence suggests the importance of ROS/RNS generated by macrophages and tumor cells in the processes of initiation and progression of malignancy (Wink et al. 1998; Fukumura et al. 2006; Ridnour et al. 2006; Hirst and Robson 2007). Thus, it is likely that many, if not all, of the proteins involved in the development of radiation-induced normal tissue inflammation and fibrosis might also be involved in the generation of radiation-induced malignancy. In support of this idea, recently it has been shown that the SOD mimetic, MnTE-2-PyP (5+), a potent catalytic scavenger of reactive oxygen species that exhibited the ability to reduce radiation-induced lung injury (Gauter-Fleckenstein et al. 2008, 2010), also reduced tumor growth in a mouse model (Rabbani et al. 2009).

8 Candidate Proteins for Predicting Radiation Injury

While many proteins have been implicated in the pathogenesis of radiation-induced injury, few have been evaluated as possible predictors of predisposition to such injury. At the present time, not every protein implicated in inflammation, wound healing, fibrogenesis, or radiation response can be detected in the blood, owing to the lack of

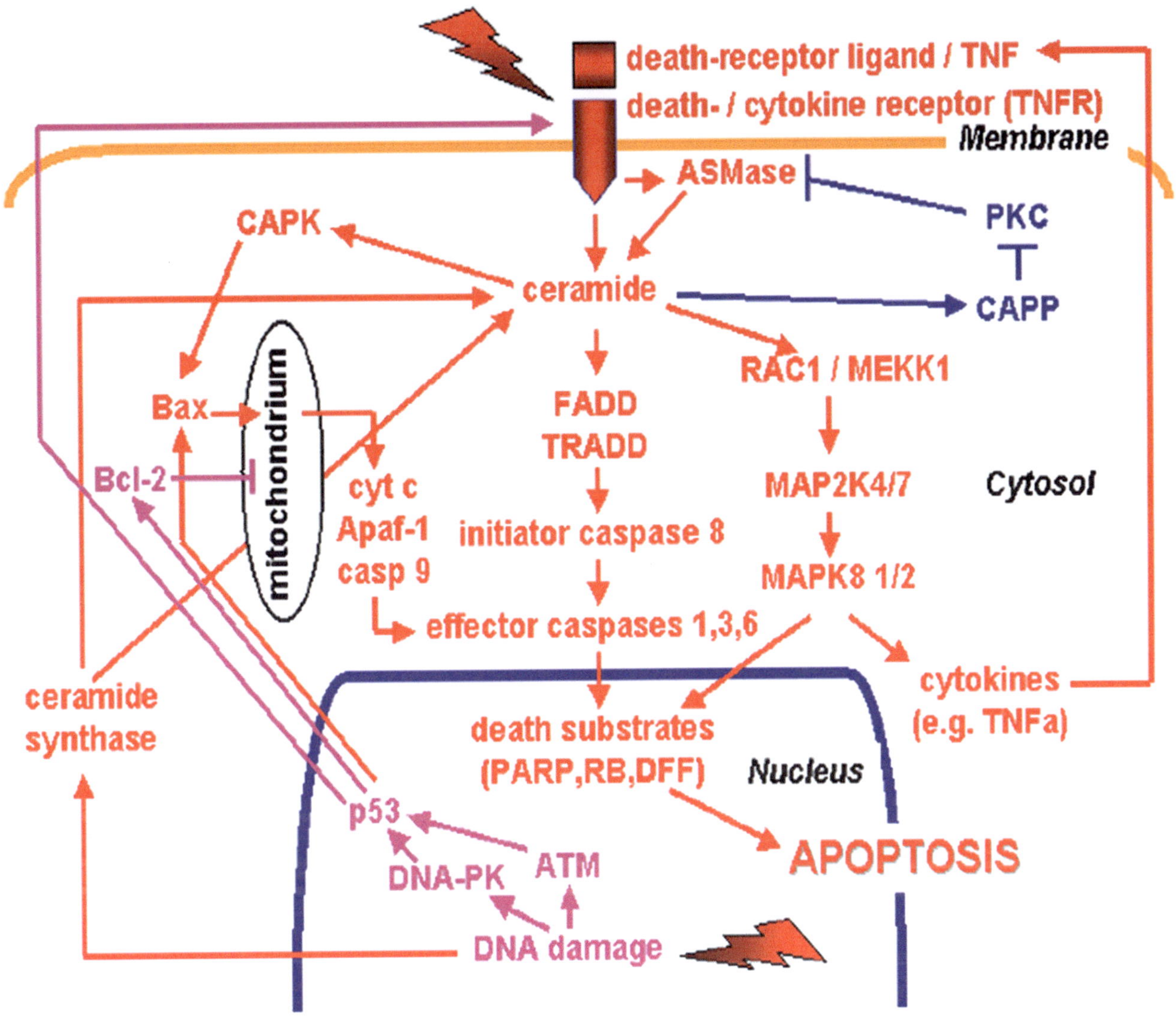

Fig. 2 DNA damage-independent and dependent pathways of endothelial cell apoptosis. The primary apoptotic response to ionizing radiation in the endothelial cells is DNA damage independent and is mediated through radiation-induced activation of acid sphingomyelinase (ASMase) and the generation of ceramide. Ceramide mediates the activation of the MAPK8 pathway, the mitochondrial pathway, or the death receptor pathway. The second source of ceramide occurs via production of DNA double-strand breaks and activation of ceramide synthase. *CAPK* ceramide-activated protein kinase, *PKC* protein kinase C, *TNF* tumor necrosis factor, *BAX* bcl-2 associated protein X, *BAD* bcl-2 antagonist of cell death, *cyt* cytochrome, *casp* caspase, *PARP* poly(adenosine-5′-diphosphate-ribose) polymerase, *RB* retinoblastoma protein [Reproduced with permission from Rodemann and Blaese (2007)]

availability of reliable antibodies to these proteins. Thus, it is not yet possible to screen for alterations in expression of every potential candidate protein. In addition, multiple proteins and signaling pathways are involved in these processes, and reliable antibodies are not available to target every individual protein involved in each pathway. Nevertheless, the list of proteins below represent components of the major mechanisms and pathways currently thought to be involved in the response of cells to radiation (Schmidt-Ullrich 2003; Tsoutsou and Koukourakis 2006). This approach is likely to detect a profile of protein expression associated with an increased risk of radiation injury, if in fact one exists. The role of each of these candidate proteins, relevant to radiation injury, is summarized in Table 1.

9 Strategies and Potential Targets for Intervention

There are three primary approaches to intervention in the injury process, depending upon the timing of intervention relative to radiation exposure, and whether or not injury has developed (Moulder and Cohen 2007). These approaches are: protection or prophylaxis, mitigation, and treatment.

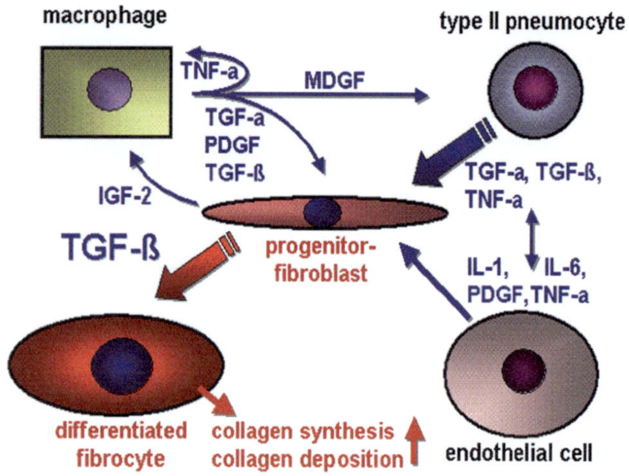

Fig. 3 The interaction between multiple cells, mediated via cytokines, in the process of connective tissue remodeling. [Reproduced with permission from Rodemann and Blaese (2007)]

Protection refers to treatments given before and/or during radiation. This is the most common strategy utilized in the clinic today and is illustrated by the use of the free radical scavenger amifostine in the prevention of injury following radiation to the head and neck (Brizel et al. 2000). Mitigation refers to therapies started after radiation exposure, but before overt injury is expressed, as exemplified by the use of angiotensin converting enzyme inhibitors to prevent renal injury (Moulder et al. 2003). Treatment refers to interventions begun after overt injury develops, an example of which would be the use of vitamin E and pentoxifylline to treat established radiation soft tissue fibrosis (Delanian et al. 2003) or the use of SOD mimics to treat symptomatic radiation-induced lung injury in rats (Gauter-Fleckenstein et al. 2010).

As we learn more about the specific molecular pathways involved in the process of radiation injury (Figs. 1, 2, 3), more targeted therapies are being studied as approaches to the prevention of radiation injury. Given the importance of the TGFß1 pathway in the pathogenesis of radiation injury, several investigators have demonstrated the efficacy of blocking TGFß1 in preventing radiation injury in animals (Flanders et al. 2002; Rabbani et al. 2003; Anscher et al. 2006, 2008). These agents, to date, have not been utilized in humans for this purpose. TGFß1 has also been demonstrated to work through Smad-independent pathways (Bierie and Moses 2006) and targeting one or more of these pathways may also prove to be an effective approach to prevention of radiation-induced injury. For example, one of these alternative pathways involves signaling via PI3-kinase and cAbl (Kharbanda et al. 1996a). The use of imatinib, which targets cAbl, has been shown to reduce the severity of bleomycin-induced lung injury (Daniels et al. 2004). In addition to TGFß1, other pathways have been demonstrated to be viable targets to inhibit the development of radiation-induced injury (Delanian et al. 1994; Hallahan and Virudachalam 1997; Adawi et al. 1998; Epperly et al. 1998; Arango et al. 2001; Kang et al. 2002; Vujaskovic et al. 2002b). Examples include reducing the level of TNFα expression using an antisense oligonucleotide strategy which reduced radiation-induced injury in mice (Zhang et al. 2008). In another approach, administration of the tyrosine kinase receptor inhibitor, Gefitinib, significantly reduced fibrosis scores and collagen levels at 5 months post-irradiation (Wang et al. 2008). The use of agents to scavenge free radicals to reduce oxidative/nitrosative stress has also been employed. In addition to the delivery of SOD itself or its mimetics, additional antioxidants have been examined. Taurine, which has been shown to exhibit antioxidant properties and inhibit TGFß1 mRNA expression, was shown to reduce lung tissue damage and hydroxyproline levels in mice (Robb et al. 2009). Genistein, an isoflavone found in soy with antioxidant and anti-inflammatory properties, reduced micronuclei formation and macrophage accumulation in mouse lungs after radiation (Para et al. 2009). Continuous administration of flaxseed to mice over $\sim$5 months after radiation reduced lipid oxidation at 3 weeks and lung fibrotic index at 4 months post-irradiation (Lee et al. 2009). In human studies, berberine, an alkaloid of herbal origin that exhibits anti-inflammatory activity and reduces the level of TGFß1, was shown to decrease radiation-induced lung injury and improve pulmonary function (Liu et al. 2008). Finally, the use of cerium oxide nanoparticles, which possess free radical scavenging properties, were found to be effective in reducing lung injury (Colon et al. 2009). Given the redundancy and crosstalk between these multiple pathways, it is likely that strategies to prevent radiation injury may require agents that target multiple pathways simultaneously, or combinations of multiple agents with more specific targets.

An example of a class of drugs, which target multiple cellular pathways, and might prove beneficial in the struggle to prevent radiation-induced normal tissue injury, are the statins. As noted above, vascular damage is an important component in the pathogenesis of radiation-induced injury. Vascular damage is important in the phenotype of RT-induced rectal injury, where telangiectatic vessels are often responsible for the bleeding characteristic of this condition. The cholesterol lowering agents HMG coA reductase inhibitors (statins) have been demonstrated to reduce the risk of myocardial infarction, in part, through their vascular protective effects, which are not dependent on changes in serum cholesterol levels. In vitro, statins have been shown to protect human endothelial cells from ionizing radiation (Gaugler et al. 2005; Boerma et al. 2006; Nubel et al. 2006). Multiple mechanisms appear to be involved, including attenuation of extracellular stress responses (Rikitake et al. 2001; Morikawa et al. 2002), downregulation of chemokines and chemokine receptors (Waehre et al. 2003), and by exerting anti-inflammatory and anti-thrombotic effects (Undas et al. 2002; Perez-Guerrero et al. 2003; Shi et al. 2003; Boerma et al. 2006) on these cells. In vivo, lovastatin has been shown to reduce radiation-induced normal tissue damage in mice (Ostrau et al. 2009). Lovastatin administration attenuated radiation-induced activation of NFkB, the expression of cell adhesion molecules, and the proinflammatory and profibrotic marker genes including TNFα, IL-6, TGFß1, and type I and type III collagens. Lovastatin also reduced radiation-induced thrombocytopenia (Ostrau et al. 2009).

10 Conclusion

Radiation-induced normal tissue injury is a frequent clinical problem that can result in considerable morbidity and limits the dose of radiation that can be used in the treatment of a variety of malignancies. Cytokines and their pathways represent promising targets for predicting responses to radiotherapy and also for therapeutic intervention. While considerable progress has been made in understanding the role of cytokines in radiation-induced tissue injury, more studies are needed to develop safe and effective means of preventing and treating radiation injuries. Future studies will need to focus on determining predictive factors associated with radiation injury and the pathways responsible for perpetuating tissue injury. Much work remains to be done, however, particularly in the areas of mitigation and treatment (Vujaskovic et al. 2002b) and additional human studies will be required to identify the most effective agents and approaches to this complex problem. Successful strategies could be implemented in the clinic and offer improved treatment outcomes to the population of patients who are most likely to develop late effects.

References

Adawi A, Zhang Y, Baggs R et al (1998) Blockade of CD40-CD40 ligand interactions protects against radiation- induced pulmonary inflammation and fibrosis. Clin Immunol Immunopathol 89(3):222–230

Anscher MS, Chen L, Rabbani Z et al (2005) Recent progress in defining mechanisms and potential targets for prevention of normal tissue injury after radiation therapy. Int J Radiat Oncol Biol Phys 62(1):255–259

Anscher MS, Crocker IR, Jirtle RL (1990) Transforming growth factor-beta 1 expression in irradiated liver. Radiat Res 122(1):77–85

Anscher MS, Kong FM (2005) In regard to De Jaeger et al.: significance of plasma transforming growth factor-beta levels in radiotherapy for non-small-cell lung cancer (Int J Radiat Oncol Biol Phys 2004;58:1378–1387). Int J Radiat Oncol Biol Phys 61(4):1276–1277

Anscher MS, Murase T, Prescott DM et al (1994) Changes in plasma TGF beta levels during pulmonary radiotherapy as a predictor of the risk of developing radiation pneumonitis. Int J Radiat Oncol Biol Phys 30(3):671–676

Anscher MS, Peters WP, Reisenbichler H et al (1993) Transforming growth factor beta as a predictor of liver and lung fibrosis after autologous bone marrow transplantation for advanced breast cancer. N Engl J Med 328(22):1592–1598

Anscher MS, Thrasher B, Rabbani Z et al (2006) Antitransforming growth factor-beta antibody 1D11 ameliorates normal tissue damage caused by high-dose radiation. Int J Radiat Oncol Biol Phys 65(3):876–881

Anscher MS, Thrasher B, Zgonjanin L et al (2008) Small molecular inhibitor of transforming growth factor-beta protects against development of radiation-induced lung injury. Int J Radiat Oncol Biol Phys 71(3):829–837

Arango D, Ettarh RR, Holden G et al (2001) BB-10010, an analog of macrophage inflammatory protein-1alpha, protects murine small intestine against radiation. Dig Dis Sci 46(12):2608–2614

Ashcroft GS (1999) Bidirectional regulation of macrophage function by TGF-beta. Microbes Infect 1(15):1275–1282

Barcellos-Hoff M (1998) How do tissues respond to damage at the cellular level? The role of cytokines in irradiated tissues. Radiat Res 150(Suppl):S109–S120

Barcellos-Hoff M, Dix T (1996) Redox-mediated activation of latent transforming growth factor-ß1. Mol Endocrinol 10:1077–1083

Barcellos-Hoff MH (1995). Redox mechanisms for activation of latent TGF-β. In: 43rd annual meeting of the Radiation Research Society

Barthelemy-Brichant N, Bosquee L, Cataldo D et al (2004) Increased IL-6 and TGF-beta1 concentrations in bronchoalveolar lavage fluid associated with thoracic radiotherapy. Int J Radiat Oncol Biol Phys 58(3):758–767

Bierie B, Moses HL (2006) Tumour microenvironment: TGFbeta: the molecular Jekyll and Hyde of cancer. Nat Rev Cancer 6(7):506–520

Biswas S, Guix M, Rinehart C et al (2007) Inhibition of TGF-beta with neutralizing antibodies prevents radiation-induced acceleration of metastatic cancer progression. J Clin Invest 117(5):1305–1313

Boerma M, Burton GR, Wang J et al (2006) Comparative expression profiling in primary and immortalized endothelial cells: changes in gene expression in response to hydroxy methylglutaryl-coenzyme A reductase inhibition. Blood Coagul Fibrinolysis 17(3):173–180

Borrelli A, Schiattarella A, Mancini R et al (2009) A recombinant MnSOD is radioprotective for normal cells and radiosensitizing for tumor cells. Free Radic Biol Med 46(1):110–116

Brach MA, Hass R, Sherman ML et al (1991) Ionizing radiation induces expression and binding activity of the nuclear factor kappa B. J Clin Invest 88(2):691–695

Brizel DM, Wasserman TH, Henke M et al (2000) Phase III randomized trial of amifostine as a radioprotector in head and neck cancer. J Clin Oncol 18(19):3339–3345

Brush J, Lipnick SL, Phillips T et al (2007) Molecular mechanisms of late normal tissue injury. Semin Radiat Oncol 17(2):121–130

Chen Y, Hyrien O, Williams J et al (2005) Interleukin (IL)-1A and IL-6: applications to the predictive diagnostic testing of radiation pneumonitis. Int J Radiat Oncol Biol Phys 62(1):260–266

Chen Y, Rubin P, Williams J et al (2001) Circulating IL-6 as a predictor of radiation pneumonitis. Int J Radiat Oncol Biol Phys 49(3):641–648

Colon J, Herrera L, Smith J et al (2009) Protection from radiation-induced pneumonitis using cerium oxide nanoparticles. Nanomedicine 5(2):225–231

Daniels CE, Wilkes MC, Edens M et al (2004) Imatinib mesylate inhibits the profibrogenic activity of TGF-beta and prevents bleomycin-mediated lung fibrosis. J Clin Invest 114(9):1308–1316

De Jaeger K, Seppenwoolde Y, Kampinga HH et al (2004) Significance of plasma transforming growth factor-beta levels in radiotherapy for non-small-cell lung cancer. Int J Radiat Oncol Biol Phys 58(5):1378–1387

Delanian S, Baillet F, Huart J et al (1994) Successful treatment of radiation-induced fibrosis using liposomal Cu/Zn superoxide dismutase: clinical trial. Radiother Oncol 32(1):12–20

Delanian S, Porcher R, Balla-Mekias S et al (2003) Randomized, placebo-controlled trial of combined pentoxifylline and tocopherol for regression of superficial radiation-induced fibrosis. J Clin Oncol 21(13):2545–2550

Epperly M, Bray J, Kraeger S et al (1998) Prevention of late effects of irradiation lung damage by manganese superoxide dismutase gene therapy. Gene Ther 5(2):196–208

Epperly MW, Bray JA, Krager S et al (1999) Intratracheal injection of adenovirus containing the human MnSOD transgene protects athymic nude mice from irradiation-induced organizing alveolitis. Int J Radiat Oncol Biol Phys 43(1):169–181

Epperly MW, Defilippi S, Sikora C et al (2000) Intratracheal injection of manganese superoxide dismutase (MnSOD) plasmid/liposomes protects normal lung but not orthotopic tumors from irradiation. Gene Ther 7(12):1011–1018

Epperly MW, Dixon T, Wang H et al (2008) Modulation of radiation-induced life shortening by systemic intravenous MnSOD-plasmid liposome gene therapy. Radiat Res 170(4):437–443

Fedorocko P, Egyed A, Vacek A (2002) Irradiation induces increased production of haemopoietic and proinflammatory cytokines in the mouse lung. Int J Radiat Biol 78(4):305–313

Flanders KC, Sullivan CD, Fujii M et al (2002) Mice lacking Smad3 are protected against cutaneous injury induced by ionizing radiation. Am J Pathol 160(3):1057–1068

Fleckenstein K, Gauter-Fleckenstein B, Jackson IL et al (2007a) Using biological markers to predict risk of radiation injury. Semin Radiat Oncol 17(2):89–98

Fleckenstein K, Zgonjanin L, Chen L et al (2007b) Temporal onset of hypoxia and oxidative stress after pulmonary irradiation. Int J Radiat Oncol Biol Phys 68(1):196–204

Fu X, Huang H, Bentel G et al (2001) Predicting the risk of symptomatic radiation-induced lung injury using both the physical and biologic parameters V(30) and transforming growth factor beta. Int J Radiat Oncol Biol Phys 50(4):899–908

Fukumura D, Kashiwagi S, Jain RK (2006) The role of nitric oxide in tumour progression. Nat Rev Cancer 6(7):521–534

Gaugler MH, Vereycken-Holler V, Squiban C et al (2005) Pravastatin limits endothelial activation after irradiation and decreases the resulting inflammatory and thrombotic responses. Radiat Res 163(5):479–487

Gauter-Fleckenstein B, Fleckenstein K, Owzar K et al (2008) Comparison of two Mn porphyrin-based mimics of superoxide dismutase in pulmonary radioprotection. Free Radic Biol Med 44(6):982–989

Gauter-Fleckenstein B, Fleckenstein K, Owzar K et al (2010) Early and late administration of MnTE-2-PyP(5+) in mitigation and treatment of radiation-induced lung damage. Free Radic Biol Med 48:1034–1043

Goto K, Kodama T, Sekine I et al (2001) Serum levels of KL-6 are useful biomarkers for severe radiation pneumonitis. Lung Cancer 34(1):141–148

Gridley DS, Bonnet RB, Bush DA et al (2004) Time course of serum cytokines in patients receiving proton or combined photon/proton beam radiation for resectable but medically inoperable non-small-cell lung cancer. Int J Radiat Oncol Biol Phys 60(3):759–766

Hakenjos L, Bamberg M, Rodemann H (2000) TGF-ß1-mediated alterations of rat lung fibroblast differentiation resulting in the radiation-induced fibrotic phenotype. Int J Radiat Biol 76(4):503–509

Hallahan DE, Geng L, Shyr Y (2002) Effects of intercellular adhesion molecule 1 (ICAM-1) null mutation on radiation-induced pulmonary fibrosis and respiratory insufficiency in mice. J Natl Cancer Inst 94(10):733–741

Hallahan DE, Virudachalam S (1997) Intercellular adhesion molecule 1 knockout abrogates radiation induced pulmonary inflammation. Proc Natl Acad Sci USA 94(12):6432–6437

Hara R, Itami J, Komiyama T et al (2004) Serum levels of KL-6 for predicting the occurrence of radiation pneumonitis after stereotactic radiotherapy for lung tumors. Chest 125(1):340–344

Haroon ZA, Raleigh JA, Greenberg CS et al (2000) Early wound healing exhibits cytokine surge without evidence of hypoxia. Ann Surg 231(1):137–147

Hart J, Rabbani Z, Pizzo S et al (2004) Cytokine profiling to predict radiation-induced lung injury. Int J Radiat Oncol Biol Phys 60(1 Suppl):S238

Hart JP, Broadwater G, Rabbani Z et al (2005) Cytokine profiling for prediction of symptomatic radiation-induced lung injury. Int J Radiat Oncol Biol Phys 63(5):1448–1454

Hauer-Jensen M, Kong FM, Fink LM et al (1999) Circulating thrombomodulin during radiation therapy of lung cancer. Radiat Oncol Investig 7(4):238–242

Hirst DG, Robson T (2007) Nitrosative stress in cancer therapy. Front Biosci 12:3406–3418

Hong JH, Chiang CS, Campbell IL et al (1995) Induction of acute phase gene expression by brain irradiation. Int J Radiat Oncol Biol Phys 33(3):619–626

Hong JH, Jung SM, Tsao TC et al (2003) Bronchoalveolar lavage and interstitial cells have different roles in radiation-induced lung injury. Int J Radiat Biol 79(3):159–167

Huang M, Sharma S, Zhu LX et al (2002) IL-7 inhibits fibroblast TGF-beta production and signaling in pulmonary fibrosis. J Clin Invest 109(7):931–937

Ishii Y, Kitamura S (1999) Soluble intercellular adhesion molecule-1 as an early detection marker for radiation pneumonitis. Eur Respir J 13(4):733–738

Jackson IL, Chen L, Batinic-Haberle I et al (2007) Superoxide dismutase mimetic reduces hypoxia-induced O2*-, TGF-beta, and VEGF production by macrophages. Free Radic Res 41(1):8–14

Johnston C, Piedboeuf B, Baggs R et al (1995) Differences in correlation of mRNA gene expression in mice sensitive and resistant to radiation-induced pulmonary fibrosis. Radiat Res 142:197–203

Johnston CJ, Williams JP, Elder A et al (2004) Inflammatory cell recruitment following thoracic irradiation. Exp Lung Res 30(5):369–382

Jones LP, Zheng HQ, Karron RA et al (2002) Multiplex assay for detection of strain-specific antibodies against the two variable regions of the G protein of respiratory syncytial virus. Clin Diagn Lab Immunol 9(3):633–638

Kang S, Rabbani Z, Folz R et al (2002) Overexpression of extracellular superoxide dismutase protects mice from radiation induced lung injury. Int J Radiat Oncol Biol Phys 54(2):78

Kharbanda S, Bharti A, Pei D et al (1996a) The stress response to ionizing radiation involoves c-Abl-dependent phosphorylation of SHPTP1. Proc Natl Acad Sci USA 93(14):6898–6901

Kharbanda S, Ren R, Pandey P et al (1995) Activation of the c-Abl tyrosine kinase in the stress response to DNA-damaging agents. Nature 376(6543):785–788

Kharbanda S, Saleem A, Datta R et al (1994) Ionizing radiation induces rapid tyrosine phosphorylation of p34cdc2. Cancer Res 54(6):1412–1414

Kharbanda S, Saleem A, Yuan ZM et al (1996b) Nuclear signaling induced by ionizing radiation involves colocalization of the activated p56/p53lyn tyrosine kinase with p34cdc2. Cancer Res 56(16):3617–3621

Kim JY, Kim YS, Kim YK et al (2009) The TGF-beta1 dynamics during radiation therapy and its correlation to symptomatic radiation pneumonitis in lung cancer patients. Radiat Oncol 4:59

Kohno N, Hamada H, Fujioka S et al (1992) Circulating antigen KL-6 and lactate dehydrogenase for monitoring irradiated patients with lung cancer. Chest 102(1):117–122

Kong F-M, Anscher M, Jirtle R (1998). Tumor marker protocols: plasma transforming growth factor beta, a plasma tumor marker. In: Hannausek M, Walaszek Z (eds) Methods in molecular medicine. Humana Press, Inc., Totowa, pp 417–430

Lee JC, Krochak R, Blouin A et al (2009) Dietary flaxseed prevents radiation-induced oxidative lung damage, inflammation and fibrosis in a mouse model of thoracic radiation injury. Cancer Biol Ther 8(1):47–53

Li Y-Q, Ballinger J, Nordal R et al (2001) Hypoxia in radiation-induced blood-spinal cord barrier breakdown. Cancer Res 61:3348–3354

Liu Y, Yu H, Zhang C et al (2008) Protective effects of berberine on radiation-induced lung injury via intercellular adhesion molecular-1 and transforming growth factor-beta-1 in patients with lung cancer. Eur J Cancer 44(16):2425–2432

Martin M, Lefaix J-L, Delanian S (2000) TGF-ß1 and radiation fibrosis: a master switch and a specific target? Int J Radiat Oncol Biol Phys 47(2):277–290

Matsuno Y, Satoh H, Ishikawa H et al (2006) Simultaneous measurements of KL-6 and SP-D in patients undergoing thoracic radiotherapy. Med Oncol 23(1):75–82

Milano MT, Constine LS, Okunieff P (2007) Normal tissue tolerance dose metrics for radiation therapy of major organs. Semin Radiat Oncol 17(2):131–140

Moeller BJ, Cao Y, Vujaskovic Z et al (2004) The relationship between hypoxia and angiogenesis. Semin Radiat Oncol 14(3):215–221

Morikawa S, Takabe W, Mataki C et al (2002) The effect of statins on mRNA levels of genes related to inflammation, coagulation, and vascular constriction in HUVEC. Human umbilical vein endothelial cells. J Atheroscler Thromb 9(4):178–183

Moulder JE, Cohen EP (2007) Future strategies for mitigation and treatment of chronic radiation-induced normal tissue injury. Semin Radiat Oncol 17(2):141–148

Moulder JE, Fish BL, Cohen EP (2003) ACE inhibitors and AII receptor antagonists in the treatment and prevention of bone marrow transplant nephropathy. Curr Pharm Des 9(9):737–749

Munger J, Huang X, Kawakatsu H et al (1999) The integrin avß6 binds and activates latent TGFß1: a mechanism for regulating pulmonary inflammation and fibrosis. Cell 96:319–328

Novakova-Jiresova A, Van Gameren MM, Coppes RP et al (2004) Transforming growth factor-beta plasma dynamics and post-irradiation lung injury in lung cancer patients. Radiother Oncol 71(2):183–189

Nubel T, Damrot J, Roos WP et al (2006) Lovastatin protects human endothelial cells from killing by ionizing radiation without impairing induction and repair of DNA double-strand breaks. Clin Cancer Res 12(3 Pt 1):933–939

Ostrau C, Hulsenbeck J, Herzog M et al (2009) Lovastatin attenuates ionizing radiation-induced normal tissue damage in vivo. Radiother Oncol 92:492–499

Para AE, Bezjak A, Yeung IW et al (2009) Effects of genistein following fractionated lung irradiation in mice. Radiother Oncol 92:500–510

Paris F, Fuks Z, Kang A et al (2001) Endothelial apoptosis as the primary lesion initiating intestinal radiation damage in mice. Science 293(5528):293–297

Perez-Guerrero C, Alvarez de Sotomayor M, Jimenez L et al (2003) Effects of simvastatin on endothelial function after chronic inhibition of nitric oxide synthase by L-NAME. J Cardiovasc Pharmacol 42(2):204–210

Puthawala K, Hadjiangelis N, Jacoby SC et al (2008) Inhibition of integrin alpha(v)beta6, an activator of latent transforming growth factor-beta, prevents radiation-induced lung fibrosis. Am J Respir Crit Care Med 177(1):82–90

Rabbani ZN, Anscher MS, Zhang X et al (2003) Soluble TGFb type II receptor gene therapy ameliorates acute radiation-induced pulmonary injury in rats. Int J Radiat Biol Oncol Phys (in press)

Rabbani ZN, Batinic-Haberle I, Anscher MS et al (2007) Long-term administration of a small molecular weight catalytic metalloporphyrin antioxidant, AEOL 10150, protects lungs from radiation-induced injury. Int J Radiat Oncol Biol Phys 67(2):573–580

Rabbani ZN, Spasojevic I, Zhang X et al (2009) Antiangiogenic action of redox-modulating Mn(III) meso-tetrakis(N-ethylpyridinium-2-yl)porphyrin, MnTE-2-PyP(5+), via suppression of oxidative stress in a mouse model of breast tumor. Free Radic Biol Med 47(7):992–1004

Ridnour LA, Thomas DD, Donzelli S et al (2006) The biphasic nature of nitric oxide responses in tumor biology. Antioxid Redox Signal 8(7–8):1329–1337

Rikitake Y, Kawashima S, Takeshita S et al (2001) Anti-oxidative properties of fluvastatin, an HMG-CoA reductase inhibitor, contribute to prevention of atherosclerosis in cholesterol-fed rabbits. Atherosclerosis 154(1):87–96

Riley PA (1994) Free radicals in biology: oxidative stress and the effects of ionizing radiation. Int J Radiat Biol 65(1):27–33

Robb WB, Condron C, Moriarty M et al (2009) Taurine attenuates radiation-induced lung fibrosis in C57/Bl6 fibrosis prone mice. Ir J Med Sci 179:99–105

Roberts AB, Piek E, Bottinger EP et al (2001) Is Smad3 a major player in signal transduction pathways leading to fibrogenesis? Chest 120(1 Suppl):43S–47S

Rodemann HP, Bamberg M (1995) Cellular basis of radiation-induced fibrosis. Radiother Oncol 35(2):83–90

Rodemann HP, Blaese MA (2007) Responses of normal cells to ionizing radiation. Semin Radiat Oncol 17(2):81–88

Rube CE, Uthe D, Schmid KW et al (2000) Dose-dependent induction of transforming growth factor beta (TGF-beta) in the lung tissue of fibrosis-prone mice after thoracic irradiation. Int J Radiat Oncol Biol Phys 47(4):1033–1042

Rube CE, Uthe D, Wilfert F et al (2005) The bronchiolar epithelium as a prominent source of pro-inflammatory cytokines after lung irradiation. Int J Radiat Oncol Biol Phys 61(5):1482–1492

Rube CE, Wilfert F, Palm J et al (2004) Irradiation induces a biphasic expression of pro-inflammatory cytokines in the lung. Strahlenther Onkol 180(7):442–448

Rubin P, Finkelstein JN, Shapiro D (1992) Molecular biology mechanisms in the radiation induction of pulmonary injury syndromes: interrelationship between the alveolar macrophage and the septal fibroblast. Int J Radiat Oncol Biol Phys 24:93–101

Rubin P, Johnston CJ, Williams JP et al (1995) A perpetual cascade of cytokines post irradiation leads to pulmonary fibrosis. Int J Radiat Oncol Biol Phys 33:99–109

Sasaki R, Soejima T, Matsumoto A et al (2001) Clinical significance of serum pulmonary surfactant proteins a and d for the early detection of radiation pneumonitis. Int J Radiat Oncol Biol Phys 50(2):301–307

Schmidt-Ullrich RK (2003) Molecular targets in radiation oncology. Oncogene 22(37):5730–5733

Schmidt-Ullrich RK, Dent P, Grant S et al (2000) Signal transduction and cellular radiation responses. Radiat Res 153(3):245–257

Shi J, Wang J, Zheng H et al (2003) Statins increase thrombomodulin expression and function in human endothelial cells by a nitric oxide-dependent mechanism and counteract tumor necrosis factor alpha-induced thrombomodulin downregulation. Blood Coagul Fibrinolysis 14(6):575–585

Sun Y, Oberley LW (1996) Redox regulation of transcriptional activators. Free Radic Biol Med 21(3):335–348

Takahashi H, Imai Y, Fujishima T et al (2001) Diagnostic significance of surfactant proteins A and D in sera from patients with radiation pneumonitis. Eur Respir J 17(3):481–487

Tsoutsou PG, Koukourakis MI (2006) Radiation pneumonitis and fibrosis: mechanisms underlying its pathogenesis and implications for future research. Int J Radiat Oncol Biol Phys 66(5):1281–1293

Undas A, Brozek J, Musial J (2002) Anti-inflammatory and anti-thrombotic effects of statins in the management of coronary artery disease. Clin Lab 48(5–6):287–296

Vujaskovic Z, Anscher M, Feng Q-F et al (2001) Radiation-induced hypoxia may perpetuate late normal tissue injury. Int J Radiat Oncol Biol Phys 50(4):851–855

Vujaskovic Z, Down JD, van Waarde MA et al (1997) Plasma TGFbeta level in rats after hemithoracic irradiation. Radiother Oncol 44(1):41–43

Vujaskovic Z, Batinic-Haberle I, Rabbani Z et al (2002a) A small molecular weight catalytic metalloporphyrin antioxidant with superoxide dismutase (SOD) mimetic properties protects lungs from radiation-induced injury. Free Radic Biol Med 33(6):857

Vujaskovic Z, Feng QF, Rabbani ZN et al (2002b) Radioprotection of lungs by amifostine is associated with reduction in profibrogenic cytokine activity. Radiat Res 157(6):656–660

Vujaskovic Z, Marks L, Anscher M (2000) The physical parameters and molecular events associated with radiation-induced lung toxicity. Sem Radiat Oncol 10(4):296–307

Waehre T, Damas JK, Gullestad L et al (2003) Hydroxymethylglutaryl coenzyme a reductase inhibitors down-regulate chemokines and chemokine receptors in patients with coronary artery disease. J Am Coll Cardiol 41(9):1460–1467

Wang C, Abe S, Matsuda K et al (2008) Effects of gefitinib on radiation-induced lung injury in mice. J Nippon Med Sch 75(2):96–105

Wink DA, Vodovotz Y, Laval J et al (1998) The multifaceted roles of nitric oxide in cancer. Carcinogenesis 19(5):711–721

Wynn TA (2008) Cellular and molecular mechanisms of fibrosis. J Pathol 214(2):199–210

Zhang M, Qian J, Xing X et al (2008) Inhibition of the tumor necrosis factor-alpha pathway is radioprotective for the lung. Clin Cancer Res 14(6):1868–1876

Zhao L, Wang L, Ji W et al (2009) Elevation of plasma TGF-beta1 during radiation therapy predicts radiation-induced lung toxicity in patients with non-small-cell lung cancer: a combined analysis from Beijing and Michigan. Int J Radiat Oncol Biol Phys 74(5):1385–1390

Quantitative/Objective Analyses of RT-Induced Late Normal Tissue Injury Using Functional Imaging

Jiho Nam, Mike E. Robbins, and Lawrence B. Marks

Contents

J. Nam · L. B. Marks (✉)
Department of Radiation Oncology, University of North Carolina at Chapel Hill, Campus Box 7512, Chapel Hill, NC 27599, USA
e-mail: marks@med.unc.edu

J. Nam
Department of Radiation Oncology, Pusan National University, Yangsan, 626-770, South Korea

M. E. Robbins
Departments of Radiation Oncology, Brain Tumor Center of Excellence, Wake Forest School of Medicine, Winston-Salem, NC 27157, USA

Abstract

There are several ways to score normal tissue injury. Imaging is an attractive tool since it allows for an objective assessment of normal tissue changes in vivo. Regional changes in tissue structure/function, detected by imaging, can be related to the different radiation doses delivered to different regions. This approach has been used for several organs, and for some, there is a clear dose–response relationship for changes in normal tissue (e.g., lung density or perfusion). Further, degree/extent of changes in regional imaging may be associated with changes in global organ function. Future improvements in imaging (e.g., more functional versus structural assessments) will afford additional opportunities for studies to better understand RT-induced normal tissue injury.

1 Introduction

The study of radiation therapy (RT)-induced normal tissue injury is challenging. Radiation dose distributions are complex, and the clinical endpoints used to describe injury are often nonspecific and difficult to quantify. Imaging is an attractive tool to address some of these challenges. The complex dose distributions afforded by modern therapy (e.g., multifield conformal therapy or intensity modulated RT) deposits variable doses to different regions of normal tissues. Imaging allows investigators to assess for different degrees of changes in different regions of organs, and then relate these regional changes to regional doses. Further, imaging is usually easily quantifiable, providing an objective assessment of regional effects.

There are several ways to score normal tissue injury, and imaging should be considered in the context of other types of metrics (Table 1). The incidence of injury is highly dependent on the type of endpoint selected. For most clinical situations, the rate of imaging changes is higher than

P. Rubin et al. (eds.), *ALERT – Adverse Late Effects of Cancer Treatment*, Medical Radiology. Radiation Oncology,
DOI: 10.1007/978-3-540-72314-1_6, © Springer-Verlag Berlin Heidelberg 2014

Table 1 Types of endpoints used to assess normal tissue injury

	Objective	Subjective
Regional	Imaging (e.g., CT-defined increases in tissue density, or reduced perfusion)	Symptoms from local effects (e.g., Pain or bleeding from a local ulceration)
Global	Laboratories (e.g., Declines in creatinine clearance, pulmonary function tests, anemia)	Symptoms of global function (e.g., Shortness of breath, fatigue)

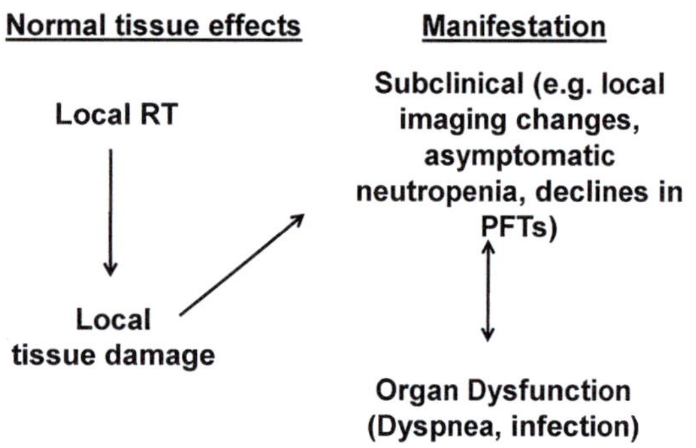

Fig. 1 Relation between RT induced normal tissue effects and subclinical and/or clinical manifestation

the rate of abnormalities in other types of metrics. Thus, imaging might be considered as the most sensitive means to assess injury, and some might say that it is *too* sensitive (since most patients with imaging-only defined normal tissue effects are asymptomatic). Indeed, there are many patients who have been made unnecessarily concerned due to abnormal radiologic findings post-RT. A good understanding of the high frequency of RT-induced imaging changes is also needed since these findings can be misinterpreted as recurrent disease (e.g., a patient irradiated for breast cancer develops nodularity ['rule out tumor'] in the anterior ipsilateral superior lung that is due to apical scarring from the supraclavicular RT field).

Changes in imaging are often seen well before the more clinically-meaningful symptoms/signs are manifest. In this regard, there is some hope that imaging changes might be early surrogate markers of longer term toxicities. However, the association between acute imaging changes and later functional changes is not clear for many organs. Further, degree/extent of changes in regional imaging may be associated with changes in global organ function (Fig. 1).

In this chapter we will review the data for several organs that relates local dose to local imaging changes, as well as the association between these local imaging changes and more meaningful functional changes.

2 Lung Injury

Symptomatic pulmonary injury following RT for cancers in and around the thorax is common, occurring in ~5–35 % of patients. The early phase of RT-induced lung injury [radiation pneumonitis (RP)] usually presents within 6 months of RT, and is commonly characterized by cough and dyspnea (Theuws et al. 1998). Late fibrotic injury usually evolves and becomes clinically manifested ≥6 months post-RT, and is characterized by progressive dyspnea, radiologic findings, and possible mortality (Theuws et al. 1998; Goethals et al. 2003). For patients treated for lung cancer, ~5–35 % will develop symptomatic lung injury, and 50–100 % develop radiologic evidence of lung injury (the majority of which are asymptomatic) (Anscher et al. 2003; Marks 1994; Graham et al. 1999; Marks et al. 2000; Fan et al. 2001; Fu et al. 2001). Similarly, for patients treated for breast cancer, 0–34 % may develop symptomatic lung injury, and 0–63 % of patients may develop radiologic changes (Dorr et al. 2005; Cazzaniga et al. 1998; Kuhnt et al. 1998; Rotstein et al. 1990; Schratter-Sehn et al. 1993; Lind et al. 2006b).

Review of radiation-induced lung injury by several investigators using various noninvasive imaging techniques has been previously described in detail (Evans et al. 2007; Kocak et al. 2007). In brief, nuclear medicine imaging provides a sensitive means to assess regional lung function. Investigators from the Netherlands Cancer Institute (NKI), Princess Margaret Hospital (PMH), and Duke University have related changes in regional perfusion/ventilation [via single photon emission computed tomography (SPECT)] and/or tissue density [via computed tomography (CT)] to the 3D radiation dose map. There is a clear association between regional dose and changes in regional perfusion/ventilation/density. Further, there appears to be an association, albeit weak, between the integrated response (e.g., the sum of changes in regional perfusion) and changes in whole lung function (Fan et al. 2001a, b; Seppenwoolde et al. 2004).

Recent reports have focused on radiation-induced lung injury in the context of stereotactic radiosurgery. In a study of 31 patients receiving stereotactic radiosurgery for primary or metastatic lung lesions, Aoki et al. noted asymptomatic increases in CT density 2–6 months post-RT, and later fibrotic reactions at 6–15 months post-RT (Aoki et al. 2004). While all 31 patients developed radiographic changes, no patients developed severe symptoms (e.g., Grade ≥2 or requiring steroids). When follow-up CTs were compared to the dose distribution on the treatment planning CT, investigators observed that the minimal dose for the development of CT-defined changes in lung tissue ranged

Table 2 Summary of studies reporting RT-induced lung injury: imaging and symptoms

Author, year	Number of cases	Disease site	Radiographic follow up	Radiologic endpoint	Rate	Clinical endpoint	Rate
CT/Radiographs							
Mah et al. 1987	54	Lung, Breast, Hodgkin's disease	6 months	↑ Lung density	36/54 (67 %)	RP	10/54 (19 %)
Rotstein et al. 1990	33	Breast	9 months	↑ Lung density	24/33 (73 %)	Cough/ Dyspnea	13/33 (39 %)
Polansky et al. 1980	37	Breast	0.7–10 years	↑ Radiopacity	16/37 (43 %)	–	0/37 (0 %)
Allavena et al. 1992	75	Hodgkin's disease	3–10 years	↑ Radiopacity	12/75 (16 %)	–	0/45 (0 %)
Marks et al. 2000	184	Lung, Breast, Lymphoma	24 months	↑ Lung density	162/259 (63 %)	Dyspnea	34/175 (19 %)
SPECT/Scintigraphies							
Allavena et al. 1992	75	Hodgkin's disease	3–10 years	↓ Perfusion	29/45 (64 %)	–	0/45 (0 %)
Boersma et al. 1996	25	Lymphoma	18 months	Dose-dependent reductions in perfusion/ventilation and partial recovery	25/25 (100 %)	RP	4/25 (16 %)
Theuws et al. 2000	110	Breast, Lymphoma	48 months	Dose-dependent reductions in perfusion/ventilation and partial recovery	110/110 (100 %)	–	–
Seppenwoolde 2000	106	Lung, Breast, Lymphoma	3 months	Dose–effect relation for perfusion and CT density	25/25 (100 %)	–	–
Marks et al. 2000	184	Lung, Breast, Lymphoma	24 months	↓ Perfusion	168/230 (81 %)	Dyspnea	34/175 (19 %)
Woel et al. 2002	79	Lung, Lymphoma, Breast, Other thoracic tumors	~65 months	Progressive Dose-dependent reductions in regional perfusion	79/79 (100 %)	–	–
Ogasawara et al. 2002	9	Lung	7.6 months	↓ and defective perfusion	9/9 (100 %)	Acute RP/ RT fibrosis	–
Tokatli et al. 2005	20	Breast	1 year	↓ Lung clearance	10/10 (100 %)	Mild RP	2/20 (10 %)
Zhang et al. 2010	123	Lung, Lymphoma, Breast, Other thoracic tumors	0.1–12 years	Dose-dependent reduction in serial perfusion scans Progress up to ~18 months	123/123 (100 %)	–	–
MRI							
Yankelevitz et al. 1994	10	Lung	3.5 years	↑ Signal intensity on T1 and T2 weighted images	10/10 (100 %)	–	–
Ogasawara et al. 2002	9	Lung	7.6 months	Asymmetric enhancement on dynamic perfusion MR	9/9 (100 %)	Acute RP/ RT fibrosis	–
Muryama et al. 2004	40	Lung, Esophagus	None (pre RT image)	↑ Vascular resistance on Velocity-encoded cine MR in patients with RP	–	RP	9/40 (23 %)
Ireland et al. 2010	5	Lung	1 and 3 months	↓ ^{3}He-MRI ventilation	3/3 (100 %)	–	–
PET							
Hicks et al. 2004	73	Lung	38 months	↑ FDG uptake	55/73 (75 %)	–	–
Guerrero et al. 2007	36	Esophagus	1.3 months	Linear relation between radiation dose and normalized FDG uptake	36/36 (100)	–	–
Hart et al. 2007	101	Esophagus	3–12 weeks	Linear relation between radiation dose and normalized FDG uptake	–	≤Grade 2 CTC symptoms	63/101 (62 %)

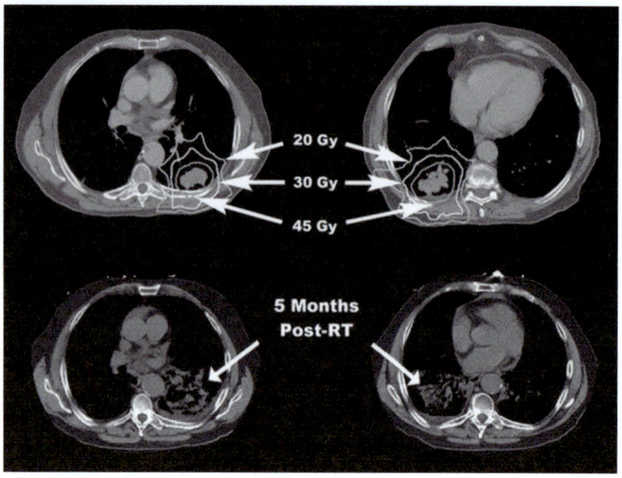

Fig. 2 Patient with synchronous bilateral lung lesions treated with radiosurgery. Follow-up CTs at 5 months post-RT showed significant increased in tissue density. Adapted with permission from Hubbs (2008)

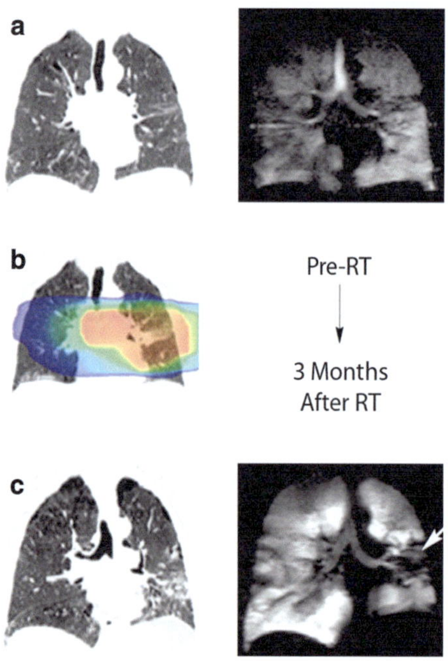

Fig. 3 Coronal lung CT images (*left*) and corresponding ventilation images based on hyperpolarized helium-3 MRI (*right*). The pre-RT images are on the *top* **a** and the three-month post-RT images are on the *bottom* **c**. The RT dose distribution is shown on the coronal CT image in the *middle* **b**. Note the reduced regional ventilation seen on the post-RT image (*arrow* in **c**. Reproduced with permission from Ireland et al. (2010)

from 16 to 36 Gy. Figure 2 illustrates the pre- and post-RT change in CT for a patient treated at Duke with radiosurgery for synchronous pulmonary lesions.

Contrast-enhanced magnetic resonance imaging (MRI) may also be used to describe perfusion characteristics of various phases of RT-induced lung injury (Ogasawara et al. 2002). Several studies from Japan suggest MRI can detect RT-induced lung injury in animal models. In the clinical setting, Yankelevitz et al. and Ogasawara et al. used MRI to study perfusion characteristics of RT-induced lung injury (Table 2) (Ogasawara et al. 2002; Yankelevitz et al. 1994). In a recent study by Muryama et al., velocity-encoded cine (VEC) MRI was used to investigate whether pulmonary arterial flow as a function of time could be used to predict RP (Muryama et al. 2004). Using hyperpolarized helium-3 MRI technique, Ireland et al. demonstrated the feasibility of detecting ventilation changes between pre- and post-RT in the patients with non-small cell lung cancer (Fig. 3).

A recent study from M.D. Anderson noted dose dependent changes in regional FDG-PET activity in 101 patients assessed 3–12 weeks post-RT for esophageal cancer (Hart et al. 2007). Further, the severity of these regional inflammatory changes appeared to be significantly correlated to the probability of symptoms.

Data from several studies regarding radiographic changes in the lung following thoracic RT, seen on SPECT, CT, MRI, and positron emission tomography (PET), are summarized in Table 2, and comparisons of the imaging characteristics of the several imaging modalities are in Table 3. Figs. 4, 5, 6 illustrate some of these imaging findings and correlation to dose.

There have been several attempts to relate the extent/severity of the imaging abnormalities to changes in global lung function [e.g., changes in pulmonary function tests (PFTs) or the development of symptoms]. For example, investigators at Duke and the Netherland Cancer Institute related the sum of the regional perfusion changes (i.e., the integrated response) to changes in PFTs. In general, there are associations, but these associations are not that strong (Fig. 7).

3 Heart Injury

RT to the thorax may induce both early and late cardiac effects if portions of the heart are included in the radiation field. Patients with breast cancer and Hodgkin's disease are particularly at risk for developing late myocardial damage, due to their longevity and possibly also due to the frequent use of anthracycline-containing chemotherapy. In general, one has to wait at least 10 years post-treatment to see these effects manifest clinically (Darby et al. 2005). The use of radiologic methods may allow for the early detection of treatment-associated dysfunction. Recent studies have investigated the incidence of cardiac effects on patients receiving RT for lung and esophageal RT. There are some preliminary data available on newer imaging technologies such as cardiac MRI and PET to assess RT-induced cardiac

Table 3 Comparisons of various imaging modalities used to evaluate radiation-induced lung injury

	CT	MR	PET	SPECT
Imaging techniques	Non-contrasted imaging.	T1, T2 weighted, dynamic perfusion, velocity-encoded cine image	18FDG-PET	Perfusion or ventilation scans
Image findings	Increase in lung density	Increased signal intensity Decrease pulmonary artery acceleration time	Increase FDG uptake value	Reductions in both perfusion and/or ventilation
Reported frequency of abnormal findings (%)	~60–70 % (Marks et al. 2000; Rotstein et al. 1990; Allavena et al. 1992; Mah et al. 1987; Polansky et al. 1980)	~100 % (Ogasawara et al. 2002; Yankelevitz et al. 1994; Muryama et al. 2004)	~75–100 % (Hart et al. 2007; Guerrero et al. 2007; Hicks 2004)	~64–100 % (Marks et al. 2000; Seppenwoolde et al. 2004; Ogasawara et al. 2002; Allavena et al. 1992; Boersma et al. 1996; Theuws et al. 2000; Tokatli et al. 2005; Woel et al. 2002; Zhang et al. 2010)
Follow-up times assessed	Median 24 months (range, 6–120)	Median 7.6 months (range, 0–42)	Median 1.3 months (range, 1–38)	Median 21 months (range, 3–120)
Dose/Volume dependency*	Yes	NA	Yes	Yes
Pros	Easy, Fast, Simple Images lung and surrounding soft tissue	Sensitive Images lung and surrounding soft tissue	Sensitive, Maybe useful to discriminate recurrence from normal tissue changes	Abundant clinical data, sensitive
Cons	Limited functional data	Expense	Expense	Low resolution and many artifacts

injury in patients with thoracic cancers. However, the vast majority of available data regarding the imaging of RT-induced heart injury uses SPECT myocardial perfusion imaging in patients with breast cancer and Hodgkin's disease.

3.1 SPECT

SPECT scans provide a noninvasive assessment of myocardial perfusion and function (changes in wall motion and left ventricular ejection fraction). Scans taken in the early years following RT may be able to assess for the subclinical damage. The incidence of perfusion defects appears to be related to the volume of left ventricle irradiated and largely persist up to 6 years after RT in patient irradiated for breast cancer (Fig. 8) (Marks et al. 2003, 2005; Prosnitz et al. 2007). Perfusion defects have been associated with wall motion abnormalities (Marks et al. 2005; Prosnitz et al. 2007; Yu et al. 2003; Seddon et al. 2002), and possibly episodes of acute pericarditis (Seddon et al. 2002), but their clinical implications are unclear. Relatively large perfusion defects associated with coronary artery disease may cause reductions in ejection fraction.

Data from several studies relating radiographic changes in the heart, as seen on SPECT, in patients treated for breast cancer and Hodgkin's disease, and preliminary data from studies in esophageal and lung cancer, are shown in Table 4. The rates of perfusion defects were plotted in Fig. 9 according to the follow up duration. Unlike the data for breast cancer, the results as assessed by SPECT for esophageal and lung cancer, are limited and somewhat mixed. It may be more difficult to draw conclusions about the incidence of RT-induced cardiac injury in this group of patients as many may have pre-existing heart disease and associated related risks. Further, additional follow-up may be needed.

There is some concern that the abnormalities detected on SPECT may be due to attenuation artifacts related to RT-induced scarring of the breast/chest-wall; i.e., RT causes pericardial scarring that may lead to an "artificial" defect in the anterior myocardium. However, a recent study reported that the soft tissue density changes in these patients are

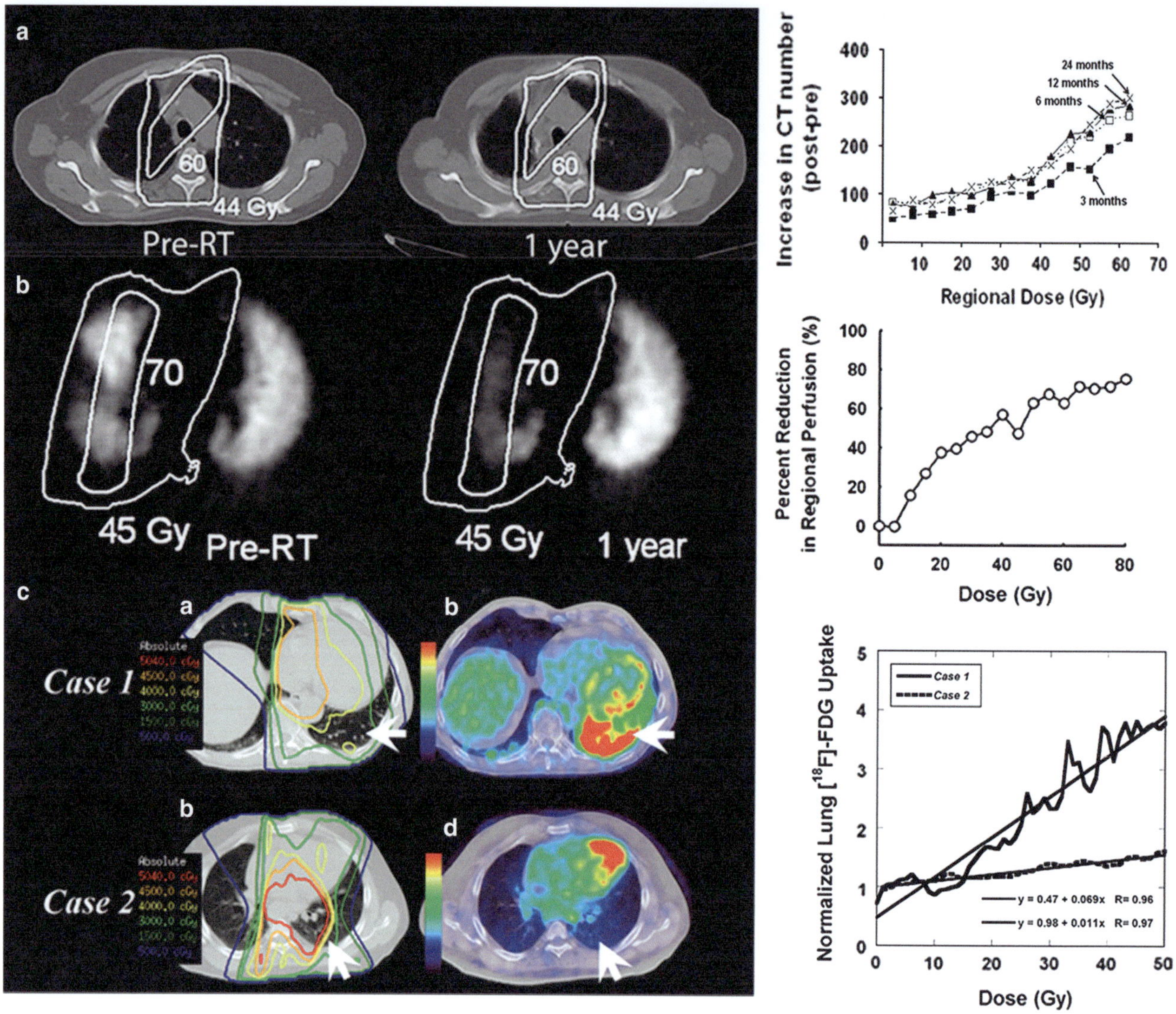

Fig. 4 Pre- and post-RT lung CT (**a**, from Duke) (Ma et al. 2010), SPECT perfusion scans (**b**, from Duke) (Zhang 2010), and FDG-PET images (**c**, from M.D. Anderson) (Guerrero et al. 2007). For each image pair, the associated isodose lines are shown. On the *right* side are dose response curves for changes in regional density, perfusion, and metabolic activity. For the CT images, the dose response curves for longer post-RT time intervals are shown, without the corresponding images. Reproduced with permission from Ma et al. (2010), Zhang et al. (2010), Hubbs (2008), and Guerrero et al. (2007)

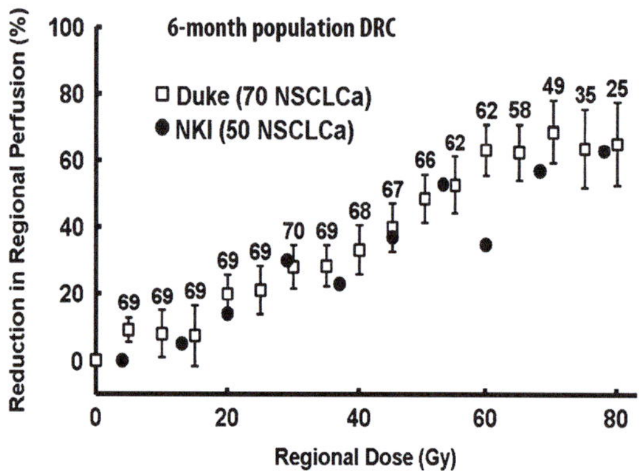

Fig. 5 Population dose response curves for RT-induced reductions in regional perfusion are shown from Duke and the Netherlands Cancer Institute. Adapted from Munley (2001)

typically modest and thus were unlikely to cause "artifactual" perfusion defects (Lawrence et al. 2010).

3.2 MRI

Nuclear medicine imaging provides both qualitative and quantitative information about regional and global cardiac function (Hardenbergh et al. 2001), and has been suggested to be a sensitive means to assess myocardial injury in patients with coronary artery disease (Li and Deshpande 2001; Hundley et al. 2003). MRI provides assessments of myocardial wall thickness and, with delayed hyper-enhancement, allows direct visualization of myocardial

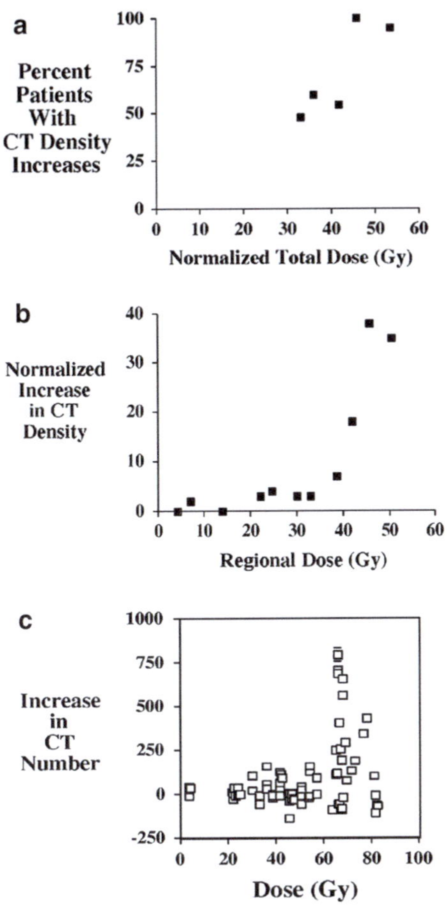

Fig. 6 Data from three centers (**a** Princess Margaret; **b** NKI; **c** Duke) relating changes in CT density to regional lung doses, data taken from Mah et al. (1994), Boersma et al. (1994), and Levinson et al. (1998)

injury/fibrosis, and is more sensitive in assessing subendocardial injury. Both MRI and the nuclear medicine techniques provide information regarding wall motion and ejection fraction, but MRI has better spatial resolution and thus may be more accurate (Wagner et al. 2005; Cuocolo et al. 2005; Schaefer et al. 2004). Conversely, quantification of myocardial perfusion is better developed with SPECT than with MRI (Cuocolo et al. 2005; Schaefer et al. 2004). While SPECT images only the left ventricle, MRI affords the possibility to assess global cardiac function.

Cardiac MRI has been applied to the study of RT-induced cardiac disease for a small number of patients with lung cancer. In a preliminary abstract (Lind et al. 2006a), there were no apparent changes in 13 evaluable patients 2–6 months post-RT. In patients who were treated with mediastinal RT for Hodgkin's disease, cardiac MR performed 20–28 years post-RT noted perfusion deficits in 68 % of patients, and other abnormal findings (e.g., decreased ejection fraction, hemodynamic valvular dysfunction, etc.) in ~50 % patients (Fig. 10) (Machann et al. 2011).

3.3 Cardiac PET

There is increased interest in the use of cardiac PET to provide a map of regional myocardial perfusion. PET has been suggested as having improved resolution and accuracy as compared to SPECT, in addition to allowing patients shorter exam times while similar to SPECT, only having the capability of imaging the left ventricle (Chua et al. 2006). A case report noted an increased FDG uptake within cardiac regions receiving ≥25 Gy approximately 4 years earlier (Zophel et al. 2007). The patient was asymptomatic and had a normal ECG (Fig. 11).

4 Brain Injury

Symptomatic brain injury from radiotherapy is relatively common and likely underestimated due to limited lifespan of the majority of treated patients and the subtlety of findings (Armstrong et al. 1993; Meyers and Weitzner 1995; Weitzner and Meyers 1997; Giovagnoli and Boiardi 1994; Archibald et al. 1994). Neurocognitive alterations can range from subtle cognitive dysfunction, such as mild short-term memory loss 1–6 months after treatment, to global irreversible/progressive neuropsychological deficits such as personality change and an overt decrease in IQ >6 months post RT (Hoppe-Hirsch et al. 1995; Merchant et al. 2005; Crossen et al. 1994; Taphoorn and Klein 2004). Different manifestations of RT-induced brain injury varying in their time of onset and in their clinical and/or radiologic characteristics (e.g., acute, early delayed, and late delayed effects) were illustrated in Fig. 12 (Tofilon and Fike 2000). The situation is further complicated by neurotoxic effects of the tumor as well as effects of surgery and/or chemotherapy.

The changes in normal brain following therapy for brain tumors is often complex. For example, it can be challenging to differentiate changes in normal brain tissue post-RT from recurrent disease. Nevertheless, several studies suggest that imaging is a reasonable way to differentiate these entities (Table 5). In addition, the clinical implications of often-subtle radiologic findings can be uncertain, and thus imaging may over-estimate the risks of RT. The post-RT imaging findings, and their association (or lack there of) with clinical findings, for several modalities are summarized below.

4.1 SPECT

SPECT (single photon emission computed tomography) can illustrate changes in blood flow following RT. A Japanese study by Araki et al. utilized Xenon 133 SPECT to evaluate

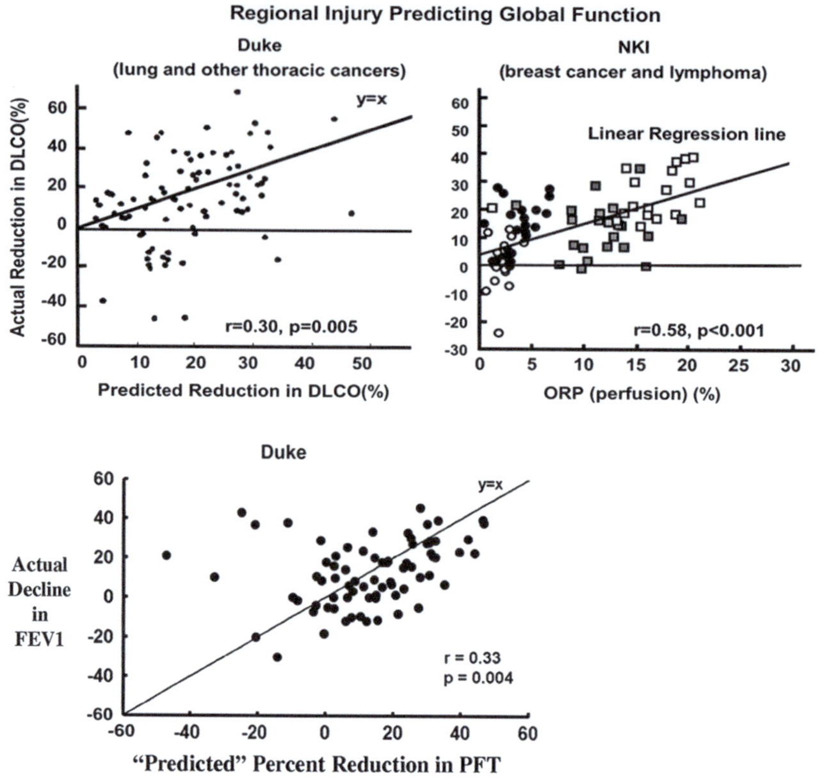

Fig. 7 Association between the regional perfusion changes and the changes in pulmonary function tests adapted from the studies from Duke and Netherland Cancer Institute. Adapted from Fan et al. (2001) and Theuws (1998a, b)

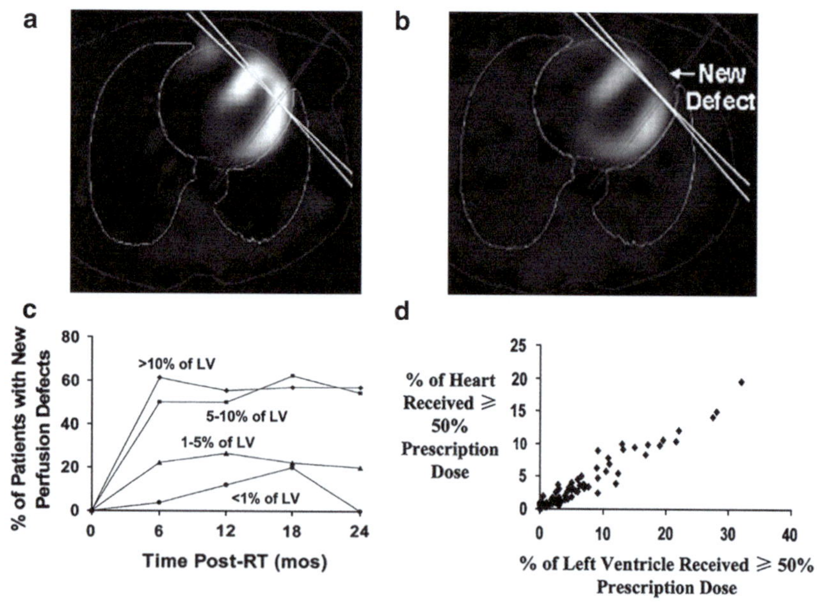

Fig. 8 SPECT cardiac perfusion scan images pre-RT **a** and 6 months post-RT **b** Note a new perfusion defect in the left ventricle which was partly included inside the tangential fields (*indicated*). As the volume of the left ventricle irradiated increases, the fraction of patients with new perfusion defects increases **c**. The irradiated left ventricle volume was highly correlated with the irradiated total cardiac volume **d**. Reproduced with permission from Marks et al. (2005)

changes in mean cerebral blood flow of non-tumor bearing areas in 40 patients as compared with 40 normal volunteers (Araki et al. 1990). Mean blood flow *increased* during therapy in some patients, compared to normal controls. At 3 months post-RT, significant *reductions* in blood flow were seen in three patients.

Table 4 Summary of studies using myocardial perfusion scintigraphy to assess for RT-induced cardiac injury in patients with thoracic malignancies

*Author, year affiliation, (reference)	Years of RT	Number of cases	Median time to radiographic follow-up	Subgroup	Incidence of perfusion defects (%)	
Breast cancer—retrospective						
Gyenes et al. 1994 Sweden	1971–1976	37	18.4	Left-sided photons or electrons	25	(5/20)
			19 years	Right-sided photons or electrons	0	(0/17)
Gustavsson et al. 1999 Sweden	1978–1983	90	13 years	Left-sided RT	12	(4/34)
				Right-sided or no RT	4	(2/56)
Hojris et al. 2000 Denmark	1982–1990	16	7.9 years	Left-sided electrons	44	(4/9)
				No RT	57	(4/7)
Cowen et al. 1998 France	1987–1993	17	8.4 years	Left-sided photons	0	(0/17)
Seddon et al. 2002 United Kingdom	1987–1995	36	6.7 years	Left-sided photons	71	(17/24)
			8.3 years	Right-sided photons	17	(2/12)
Sioka et al. 2011, Greece	1998–2010	131	3.3 years	Left-sided photons	54	(15/28)
				Right-sided photons	44	(8/18)
				No RT	33	(28/85)
Breast cancer—prospective						
Gyenes et al. 1996 Sweden	1993–1994	12	1.1 years	Left-sided photons	100	(4/4)
				Left-sided electrons	25	(2/8)
#Marks et al. 2005 Duke University	1998–2001	114	0.5 year	Left-sided photons	27	(21/77)
			1 year		29	(16/55)
			1.5 years		38	(13/34)
			2 years		42	(11/26)
#Prosnitz et al. 2007 Duke University	1998–2006	44	3 years	Left-sided photons	38	(3/8)
			4 years		58	(7/12)
			5 years		67	(4/6)
			6 years		67	(2/3)
Other disease sites						
Savage et al. 1990 University of Rochester		16	9.3 (2.5–21.5) years	Lymphoma	6	(1/16)
Gustavsson et al. 1990 Sweden)		26	15 (4–20) years	Lymphoma	61	(14/23)
Maunoury et al. 1992 France	1978–1988	31	7 (3–11) years	Lymphoma	84	(21/25)
Glanzmann et al. 1998 Switzerland	1964–1992	112*	13.7 (1.9–31.5) years	Lymphoma	7	(7/100)
Girinsky et al. 2000 France		49	75 (28–208) months	Lymphoma	78	(32/41)
Heidenreich et al. 2007 Stanford University	1964–1994	294	6.5 (4.0–8.4) years	Lymphoma	12	(32/274)
Gayed et al. 2006 MDACC	2005–2006	51	3 months	Esophageal cancer	54	(14/26)
				No RT	16	(4/25)
Lind et al. 2006a Karlinska Institute	–	13	2, 6 months	Lung Cancer	–	–*

Adapted with permission from Prosnitz et al. (2007)

Some patients overlap, incidence of new perfusion defects listed

*at least one patient with a new perfusion abnormality. Limited data in available abstract

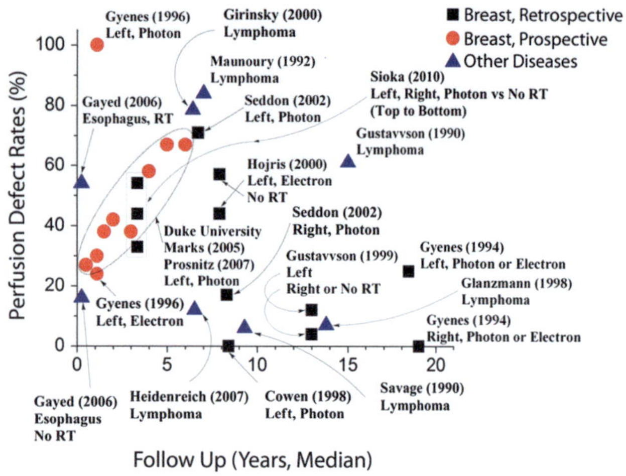

Fig. 9 Scatter plot of the rates of perfusion defects extracted from the reported studies using myocardial perfusion scintigraphy to assess RT induced cardiac injury in patients with thoracic malignancies. The incidence of perfusion defects does not consistently increase over time

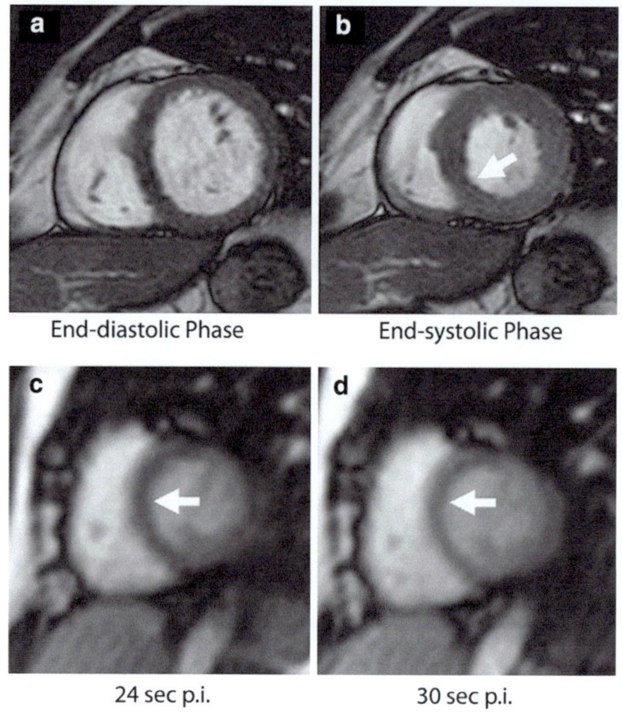

Fig. 10 Magnetic resonance images of the heart in patients treated with the mediastinal irradiation for Hodgkin's disease > 20 years previously. **a** and **b** illustrates hypokinesia (i.e., note that the wall thickness of indicated area is thinner than other region on end-systolic phase) in short-axis steady-state free precession cine image. **c** and **d** are stress and rest perfusion images, respectively, illustrating hypointensities (*arrows*) noting reduced perfusion. Reproduced with permission from Machann et al. (2011)

Harila-Saari et al. studied 25 patients with acute lymphoblastic leukemia (ALL) treated with either intrathecal (IT) chemotherapy or RT. SPECT perfusion defects were noted in 11/25 (44 %); eight of whom received chemotherapy alone and three who received cranial RT (Harila-Saari et al. 1997). The degree of SPECT abnormality has not been associated with neuropsychologic changes post-RT.

4.2 PET

There are limited data regarding the effects of RT on glucose metabolism in the brain assessed via FDG-PET and clinical symptoms, and the available data are contradictory. Kahkonen et al. evaluated 40 long term survivors of ALL half of whom received methotrexate and cranial RT (Kahkonen et al. 2000). No major differences were found in regional glucose metabolism in various defined cortical and subcortical anatomical areas for irradiated versus nonirradiated groups. Pre-RT imaging was not available in these patients. Munley et al. retrospectively evaluated eight patients with both pre- and post-RT FDG-PET imaging (Munley et al. 1999). There were no changes in regional metabolic activity in areas of brain receiving doses up to 50 Gy. Above 50 Gy, the effects varied, one with PET activity decreasing in one, and increasing in others, to varying degrees. Both of these studies were very small.

Mineura et al. reported on seven patients studied with ^{15}O-PET before and after RT for gliomas (Mineura et al. 1988). One month post-RT, there were increases in PET-defined regional blood flow in the contralateral gray matter felt to be normal tissue by CT. At longer time points, there

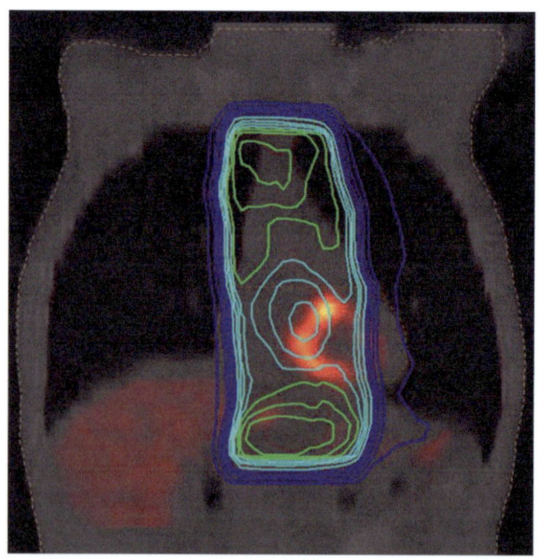

Fig. 11 FDG uptake was increased in the myocardium included in the prior RT fields. Note that the distribution did not correspond to coronary artery territories. Microvascular or myocardial effects might be responsible for the imaging changes. Reproduced with permission from Zöphel et al. (2007)

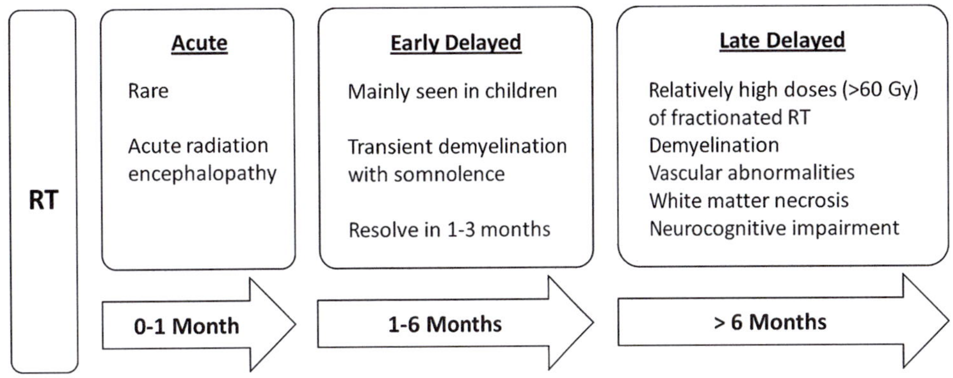

Fig. 12 RT induced brain injury and the characteristics according to the onset duration of clinical manifestation

were significant decreases in blood flow from pretreatment with later studies. Hahn et al. performed a prospective study in patients undergoing therapeutic brain RT. Patients had brain imaging (FDG- and ^{15}O-PET) and neurocognitive testing planned to be performed pre-RT and at 3 weeks and 6 months post-RT. Eleven patients were enrolled, with seven subjects completing the 3-week, and six subjects completing the 6-month follow-up imaging studies. Six subjects also completed follow-up neuropsychological testing. Three weeks and 6 months post-RT images revealed reductions in FDG uptake in regions of the brain receiving >40 Gy in comparison to pre-treatment scans (Hahn et al. 2005). The ^{15}O-PET showed increases (<10 %) at 3 weeks in relative regional blood flow in brain regions receiving greater than 30 Gy, but less at the 6-month follow-up studies (Fig. 13). There were significant correlations between decreases in FDG uptake and several neurocognitive endpoints associated with problem solving, cognitive flexibility, and global measures of psychopathology.

4.3 MRI

MRI is an essential tool for the evaluation of tumor and normal tissue characteristics, providing detailed information of either anatomic or pathologic structural changes as well as microstructural events. Various MRI techniques are available and widely adapted in cancer diagnosis. It is also an attractive tool for the differential diagnosis of post-treatment changes and tumor progression with both graphical appearances and quantifiable numeric parameters.

4.3.1 Diffusion Tensor Imaging

White matter changes (e.g., demyelination or axonal injury) after brain RT were reported in the studies using DTI techniques. Several DTI indices were tested for the analysis of RT-induced imaging changes relating to clinical manifestation (i.e., neurocognitive dysfunction). These objective parameters can be easily generated on a voxel-by-voxel matrix in the specific brain region of interest (Fig. 14).

Several preclinical and clinical studies were reported to address the normal brain changes using DTI. A Prospective study from University of Michigan revealed progressive post-RT changes in the genu and splenium areas of the corpus callosum (Nagesh et al. 2008b). A total of 25 brain tumor patients were evaluated in the study. Initially, in the high dose region, dose dependent demyelination was observed. After 6 months follow-up, diffuse demyelination was also noted in both high dose and lower dose areas.

A pediatric study showed similar results. Post-treatment survivors of childhood brain tumors were studied to compare DTI changes with neurocognitive function changes. Decreases in IQ test scores were significantly correlated with changes in DTI indices after age and RT dose adjustment (Khong et al. 2006).

RT-induced injury to a certain area (e.g., hippocampus) in the brain may cause long-term deficits in the specific neurocognitive function (e.g., memory loss, learning ability). From a preliminary study, decreased values of FA (Fractional anisotropy) in the para-hippocampal cingulum 1 month after whole brain irradiation were observed. These findings suggest that DTI indices can be used as a biomarker for monitoring patients treated with hippocampal sparing brain RT (Fig. 15) (Nagesh et al. 2008a).

In general, DTI is suitable for the detection of early changes in the white matter integrity after brain RT. Association between the DTI indices and the neurocognitive function changes needs to be studied further with longer follow up and prospective setting.

4.3.2 MR Perfusion Imaging

RT-induced vascular damage may lead to increased permeability in the brain normal tissues. Perfusion MR imaging can detect these early changes by tracing the intravenously injected contrast-enhancing pharmaceuticals. The movement of pharmaceuticals can be calculated as a value of a transfer

Table 5 Radiographic changes to the brain after irradiation

Author, year affiliation, (reference)	Number of cases	Radiographic follow-up	Post-RT radiographic response/outcome
SPECT			
*Araki et al. 1990 Gifu University, Japan	40	3 months	↑ mean blood flow during RT, ↓ in blood flow in 3 RT patients post-RT
Harila-Saari et al. 1997 Oulu university central hospital, Finland)	25	Varied (9–13 months)#	Defects in 44 % (11/25) – 8 Chemo Alone, 3 RT Alone Impairment in neuropsychological functioning in 19/22 (86 %) No significant difference intelligence testing between normal versus abnormal SPECT
Diffusion weighted (DW)—MRI			
Hein et al. 2004, Norris Cotton Cancer Center	18	1–3 years intervals	ADC ratios and means significantly ↓ for recurrent versus nonrecurrent lesions
Asao et al. 2005, Kumamota University	17	–	Marked hypointensity (67 %, [8/12]), in lesions due to RT-injury versus recurrent tumor Maximal ADC values significantly ↓ for recurrent versus nonrecurrent lesions
Diffusion tensor image (DTI)			
Khong et al. 2006	30	1 year–	Percent difference in fractional anisotropy (ΔFA %) significantly correlated with IQ
Nagesh et al. 2008b, University of Michigan	25	6 months	Progressive post-RT changes in the genu and splenium of the corpus callosum Dose dependent demyelination initially in the high dose region. After 6 months follow up, diffuse demyelination in both high and low dose areas
^{1}HMRSI			
Virta et al. 2000, NIH	9	0.5–10.5 years	Widespread chemical changes in white matter after RT
Chong et al. 2001, Singapore general hospital	18	Mean 4.6 years (range 3.0–9.6 years)	↓ NAA in RT-induced temporal lobe changes Cr levels relatively more stable than Cho or NAA levels Cho levels may be increased, normal, or reduced
Zeng et al. 2007 Shandong University, (MRS and DW-MRI)	55	2 months intervals (1.5–12 months) 3–4 months intervals (12-36 mos)	Cho/NAA, Cho/Cr, and ADC ratios and means significantly ↓ in regions of RT-injury versus recurrent tumor MRS with DW MRI correctly classified 96.4 % of subjects as recurrence or RT-Injury (100 % correct for RT-Injury group)
Plotkin et al. 2004 Germany, (I-IMT SPECT ^{1}HMRS)	25	9.7 months	I-IMT SPECT significantly ↑for recurrent disease versus treatment related changes SPECT yielded more favorable results in differentiating recurrent tumor versus post-RT changes
Matulewicz et al. 2006 Maria Sklodowska-Curie Memorial Cancer Center, Poland	100	2 years	Oscillations in Cho/NAA and Cho/Cr ratios seen in 8 month cycles Maxima in Cho/NAA and Cho/Cr ratios seen 2 months after RT
Sundgren et al. 2009 University of Michigan	11	6 months	↓NAA/Cr and Cho/Cr ratios at 3 weeks during RT and 1 month and 6 months after RT
PET			
Hahn et al. 2005, Duke University	11	3 weeks; 6 months	↓ FDG uptake

* Data extracted from Abstract
\# Radiographic follow-up not distinguished between patients with and without RT. Follow-up time measured from end of systemic therapy or RT
Abbreviations: Apparent diffusion coefficient (ADC), N-acetyl-aspartate (NAA), Diffusion-weighted (DW), Creatine (Cr), Choline (Cho)

constant or K_{trans}. High K_{trans} value means the increased vascular permeability (i.e., extravasation of contrast-enhancing materials). Changes in blood plasma volume, expressed as *Vp*, also provide a useful information. *Vp* is sensitive to the RT dose. *Vp* value increases with higher RT dose delivered during RT and then decreases after RT.

Cao et al. reported, using dynamic contrast-enhanced MRI, early vascular changes may be a predictor of delayed changes

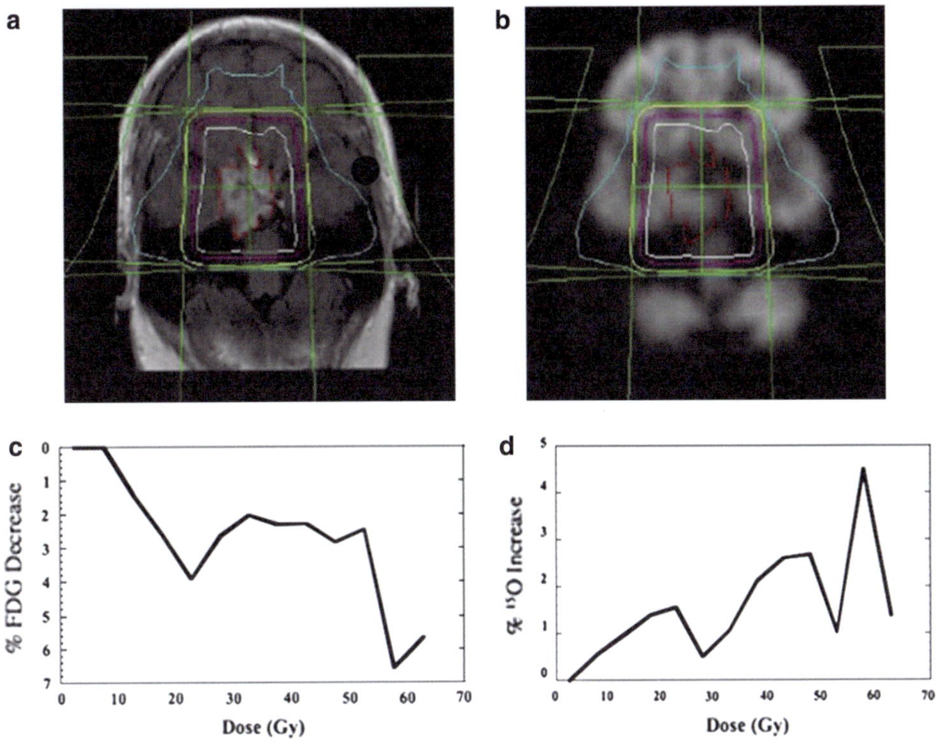

Fig. 13 Coronal CT image of brain **a** and registered with 2-deoxy-2-[^{18}F]-D-glucose positron emission tomography image **b** with three-dimensional radiation dose distribution shown on each image. Lower panel images represent the volume-weighted population average percentage of changes in FDG uptake (**c**) and ^{15}O-H_2O value (**d**), respectively. Reproduced with permission from Hahn et al. (2005)

in neurocognitive functions (e.g., verbal learning and total recall). Vascular volumes and blood–brain barrier permeability increased during RT and then decreased after RT. Six months after RT, changes in verbal learning scores and recall scores were significantly correlated with vascular volumes and permeability during RT (Fig. 16) (Cao et al. 2009).

4.3.3 MR Proton Spectroscopy

MR proton spectroscopy (MRS) provides unique information about metabolic status in tissues. Proton MRS is a noninvasive technique to, (i) interrogate metabolic distributions in the brain (Gillies and Morse 2005; Hoehn et al. 2001), (ii) differentiate radiation necrosis from brain tumor progression (Chong et al. 2002; Schlemmer et al. 2002), and (iii) serve as a indicator of neurotoxicity following experimental (Chan et al. 2009; Herynek et al. 2004) and clinical brain irradiation (Chan et al. 2001; Esteve et al. 1998; Lee et al. 2004; Sundgren et al. 2009; Virta et al. 2000; Walecki et al. 1999). Metabolites detected in brain tissue include choline-containing compounds, creatine, glutamate, lactate, *N*-acetylaspartate (NAA), myoinositol (mI), and taurine. The concentration of each of these metabolites can be mapped from 2D or 3D spectroscopic images having a voxel size of 0.7–1 cm^3. The metabolite, NAA is predominantly a neuronal marker, and decreases are associated with neuronal damage and dysfunction secondary to radiation. Choline is associated with cell membrane synthesis and/or increased metabolic turnover; it is elevated in both tumors and inflammatory processes. Creatine is a marker of energy metabolism with relatively constant concentrations throughout the brain (Sundgren and Cao 2009), while mI is a glial cell marker and has been used as an indicator of myelin breakdown (Pasantes-Morales et al. 2000). Changes in concentration of these metabolites are associated with tumor and/or normal brain tissue changes.

Many clinical studies of MRS focus on differentiating radiation necrosis and tumor progression. Currently, there are limited numbers of clinical and preclinical studies of normal brain tissue changes after RT. Herynek et al. reported decreases in creatine and NAA after Gamma Knife irradiation to the rat brain (Herynek et al. 2004). Chan et al. using 7T MRS, studied changes in concentrations of choline, glutamate, lactate, and taurine 1 year after RT to rats' brain (Chan et al. 2009). Atwood et al. reported similar results. They suggested a potential relationship between RT-induced brain injury and neurocognitive dysfunction (Fig. 17) (Atwood et al. 2007).

Chan et al. reported that MRS was able to detect decreasing NAA/Cr and Cho/Cr ratio in childhood ALL survivors treated with IT chemotherapy and prophylactic cranial irradiation with long-term follow up (up to 19 years) (Chan et al. 2001). Similar findings were noted in a recent prospective study performed in University of Michigan. MRS from 11 adult patients with low grade glioma or

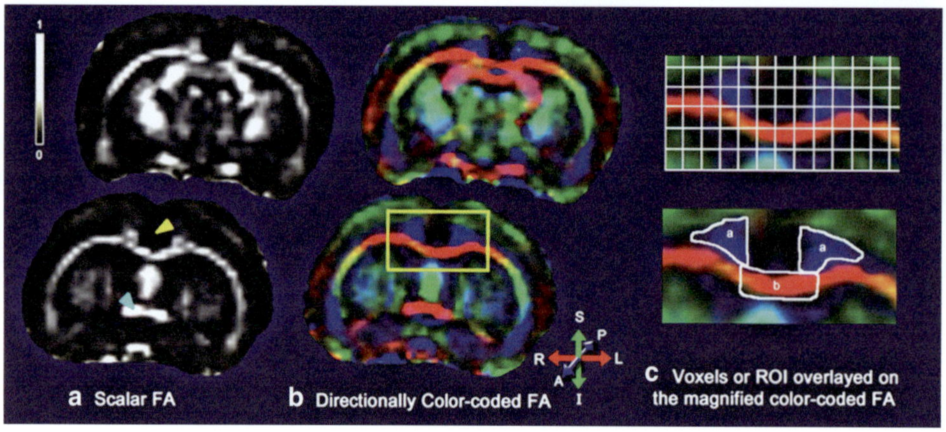

Fig. 14 DTI images of coronal brain slices of a rat. **a** Fractional Anisotropy values represent water diffusion characteristics within a voxel. **b** FA value can be translated as a direction of flow (*color coded*). **c** Voxel analysis of the specific region of the brain for comparison of individual areas. Reproduced with permission from Robbins et al. (2012)

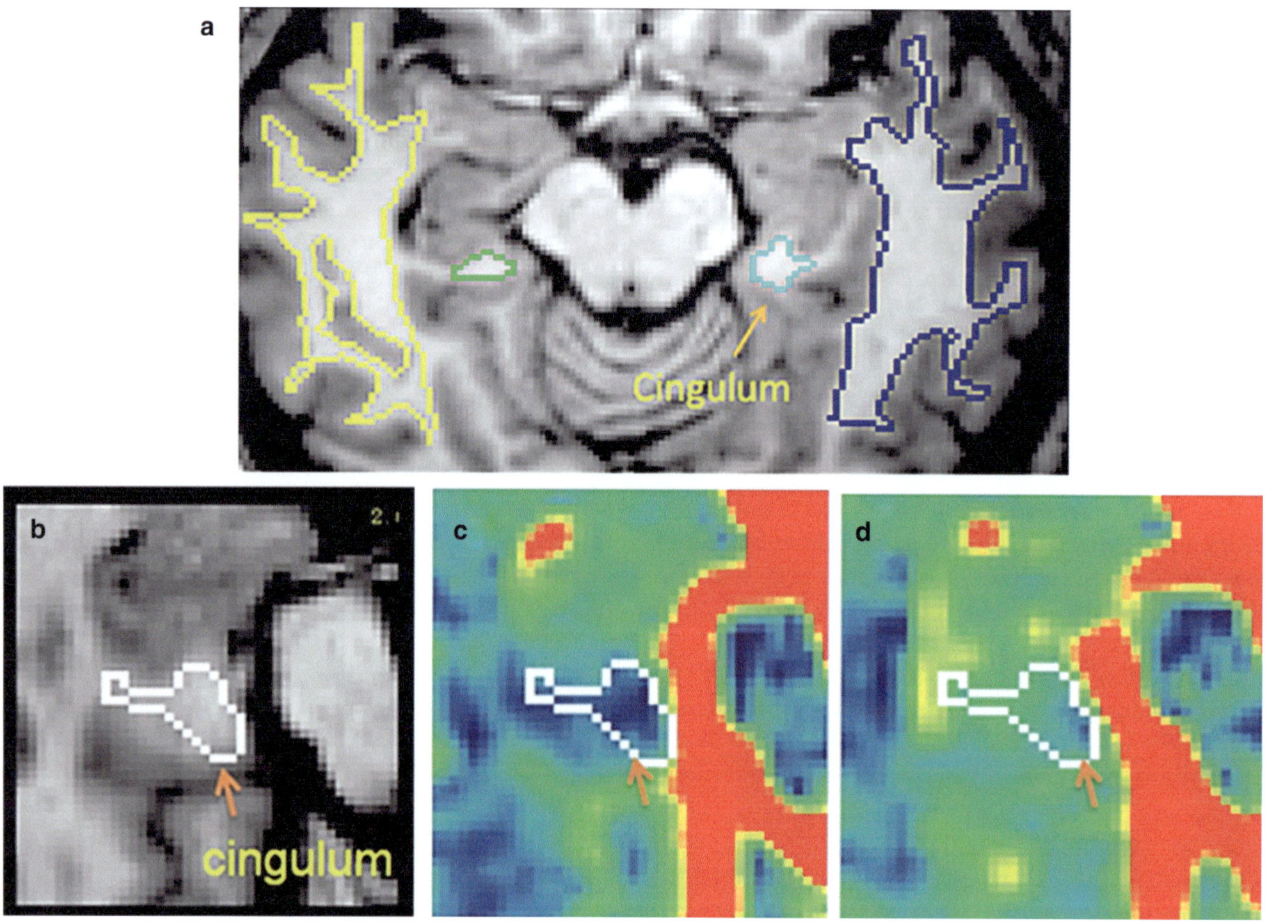

Fig. 15 DTI images of the brain treated with whole brain irradiation. **a** MR T1-weighted axial image of the region including parahippocampal cingulum [*right* side (*green*) and *left* (*light blue*)]. Each side of temporal lobe white matter was also indicated with *yellow* (*right*) and *blue* (*left*) colors, respectively. **b** Baseline pre-RT image of the parahippocampal cingulum (*white*). **c** Pre-RT DTI map of parahippocampal white matter showing greater diffusion characteristics (i.e., perpendicular diffusivity, $\lambda_\perp$) along with white matter fiber tract. **d** 1 month after RT, increase in $\lambda_\perp$ (*brighter color*) represents early demyelination in the parahippocampal cingulum. Reproduced with permission from Robbins et al. (2012)

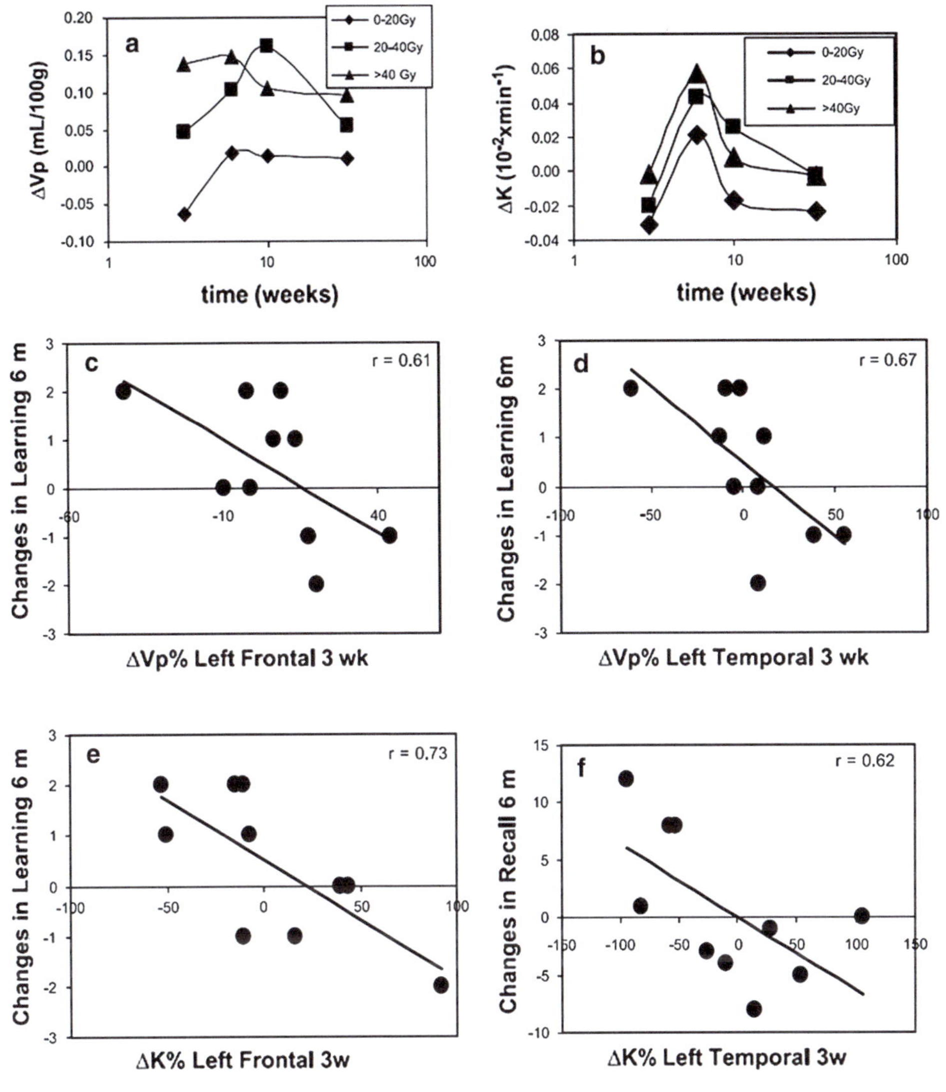

Fig. 16 Vascular volume (*Vp*) and blood brain barrier permeability (*K*) changes according to the different RT dose intervals (**a**, **b**). Note that increase in vascular volume at high dose region during RT. Changes in neurocognitive function test scores (learning score and recall score) 6 months after RT appear to be correlated with changes in ΔVp and ΔK during RT (**c**–**f**). Reproduced with permission from Cao et al. (2009)

benign brain tumors demonstrated decreases in NAA/Cr and Cho/Cr ratios from 3 weeks to 6 months following RT (Fig. 18) (Sundgren et al. 2009).

5 Liver Injury

Previous RT techniques limited the utility of radiation to the liver, due to the liver's low whole organ tolerance. Data from studies dating back to the 1960s indicated that with doses to the whole liver up to 30–35 Gy using standard fractionation resulted in a 5 % risk of radiation-induced liver disease (RILD), while smaller volumes of the liver could tolerate higher doses (Dawson and Ten Haken 2005; Lawrence et al. 1995; Ingold et al. 1965; Reed 1966). With the advent of 3D conformal therapy and more recently intensity modulated radiation therapy (IMRT), it has become increasingly important to assess the impact RT-induced liver injury. Radiologic changes are often evident on irradiated livers prior to, or even in the absence of, clinical symptoms (Lawrence et al. 1995; Kwek et al. 2006). Such imaging changes have been reported 6 months to 6 years post-RT (Dawson and Ten Haken 2005; Lawrence et al. 1995; Cao et al. 2007) (Table 6).

5.1 CT Perfusion Studies

Investigators at the University of Michigan have used CT to detect RT-induced liver injury. CTs obtained 2–3 months post-RT revealed low attenuation within irradiated areas in of 74 % of 31 patients studied. Using CT-based perfusion imaging, Cao et al. assessed the relationship between local radiation dose and changes in regional portal vein perfusion, similar to perfusion imaging studies of the lung and heart post-RT from other institutions noted above (Cao et al.

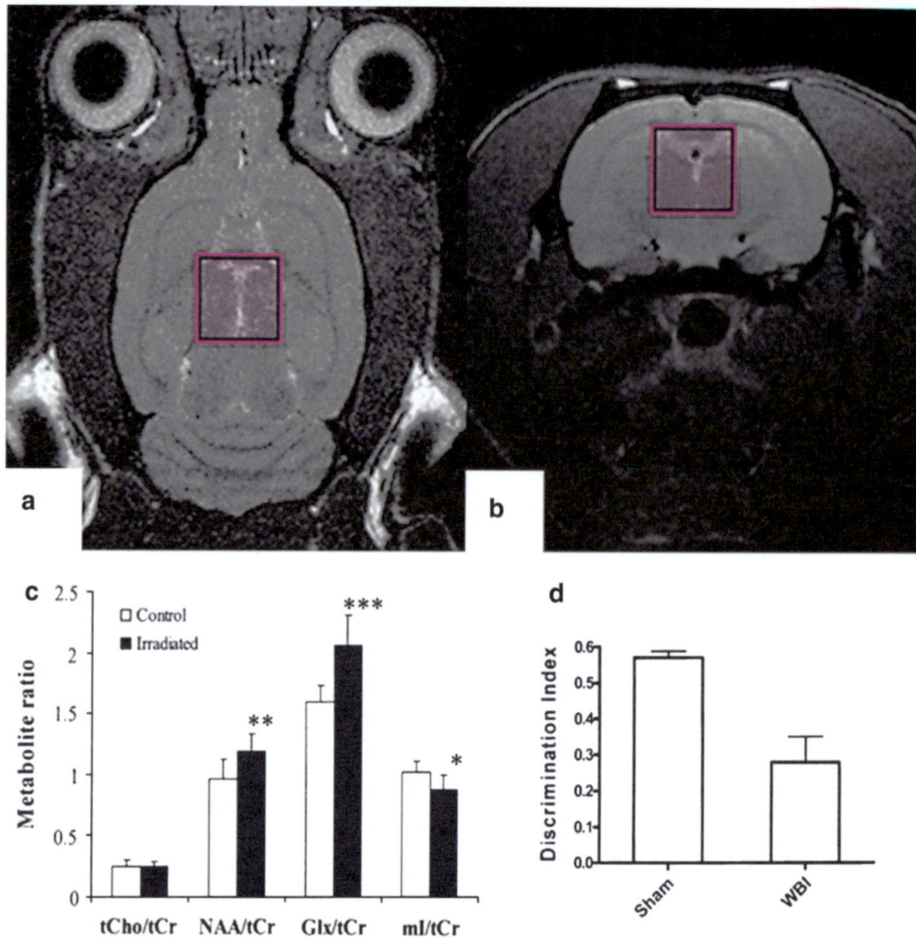

Fig. 17 T2-weighted MR images of rat brain with a 5 × 5 × 5 mm voxel region of interest to measure the concentration of specific metabolites using MRS: **a** coronal image and **b** axial image. Significant metabolites changes (**c**) and reduced cognitive function (**d**) after 52 and 54 weeks of whole brain irradiation, respectively (*, **, and, *** represent statistically significant results; p-values are less than 0.01). Reproduced with permission from Atwood et al. (2007)

2007). In ten patients with unresectable primary or metastatic hepatic tumors, reductions in regional portal vein perfusion ~1.5 and 3 weeks into treatment (i.e., *during* RT) were related to changes in perfusion at 1 month post-RT (Figs. 19, 20). Conceivably, one may be able to alter therapy based on normal tissue changes noted early-on during a proposed course of therapy, thereby individualizing therapy.

Munden et al. noted new CT liver abnormalities in 40 % (8/20) of patients ~8 (range 5–11) weeks post-IMRT for mesothelioma (Munden et al. 2005). The abnormalities were in the liver periphery, corresponding to the regions receiving >45 Gy. All patients with CT-defined abnormalities were asymptomatic and had normal liver function tests. For those patients with limited additional follow-up, the majority of the abnormalities resolved, however additional data with longer follow-up is warranted.

5.2 MRI

MRI also provides a noninvasive method of imaging the RT-induced liver disease. On conventional MR images, irradiated liver tissues show T1-weighted hypointensity and T2-weighted hyperintensity, potentially due to increased water content (Yankelevitz et al. 1992; Onaya et al. 2001). However, severe hepatic fibrosis can cause hypointensity on T2-weighted images that have been observed in irradiated patients with Budd-Chiari syndrome (Mori et al. 2002).

Special MR imaging techniques may provide a more precise differential diagnosis of radiation-induced hepatic injury. In gadolinium-enhanced dynamic studies, the irradiated liver parenchyma show early hyperintensity that become more prominent and persists at the end of the dynamic studies (Onaya et al. 2001). Recent study using Gd-EOB-DTPA (gadolinium ethoxybenzyl diethylenetriaminepentaacetate) in patients treated with interstitial brachytherapy to metastatic liver disease show hepatic injury after small volume single-fraction irradiation (Fig. 21) (Seidensticker et al. 2011). Superparamagnetic iron oxide-enhanced (SPIO) MR imaging may also be a sensitive modality for early and late radiation-induced liver injury (Fig. 22) (Mori et al. 2000; 2002; Nohara et al. 1997; Yoshiokaa et al. 2000).

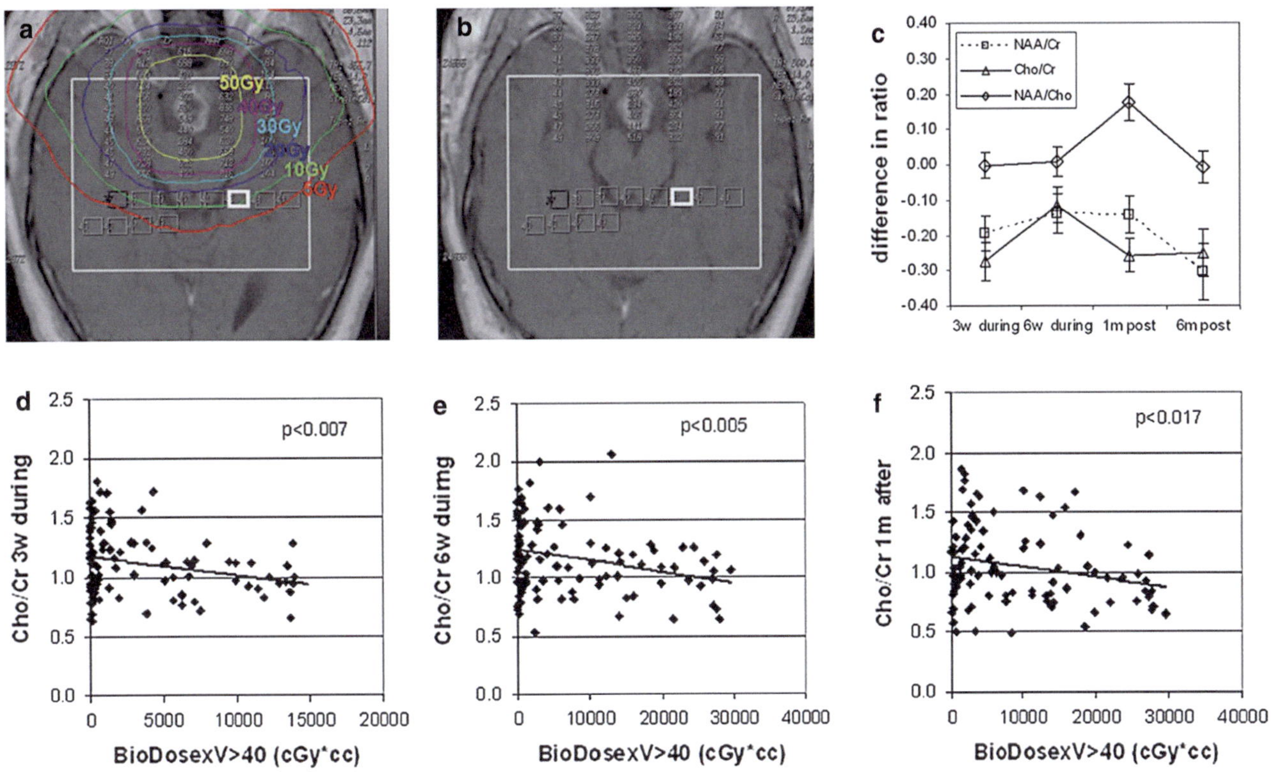

Fig. 18 MR images before (**a**) and 6 months after RT (**b**). Radiation dose distribution was overlaid (**a**). VOIs for MRS study were shown with *larger white box* (**a**) and individual VOIs for spectral analysis with *smaller white box* (**b**). Changes in ratios of NAA/Cr, Cho/Cr, and NAA/Cho at different time interval were plotted (**c**). **d–f** represent the relationships between radiation dose/volume and the changes of Cho/Cr ratio before and following completion of RT. Reproduced with permission from Sundgren et al. (2009)

5.3 PET

A study from M.D. Anderson reported hepatic radiation injury using FDG-PET in patients with distal esophageal cancer treated with chemoradiation. Abnormal FDG uptake in the irradiated liver was found in 19 % of the patients (Fig. 23) (Iyer et al. 2007). However, CT images demonstrated atrophy and density changes of irradiated liver in 58 % of the same patients group. Among those patients with increased FDG uptake in the liver, an additional diagnostic work-up (i.e., biopsy) was frequently required for excluding metastatic disease.

6 Parotid Gland Injury

The parotid glands are often incidentally irradiated during therapy for head and neck tumors, and the resultant injury can impact speech, chewing, and swallowing (Hakim et al. 2004). There is growing interest in sparing parotid function with IMRT, which usually results in a markedly variable dose of RT being delivered to the different regions of the parotid. Radiologic techniques afford the possibility of quantitatively assessing dose-dependent changes in regional parotid function (Table 7).

6.1 SPECT and PET

The ability of the parotid to clear ^{11}C-methionine (a surrogate for salivary flow) was assessed in 12 patients 8–54 months (median 21 months) post-IMRT using PET imaging (Buus et al. 2004). There was a dose-dependent reduction in the clearance rate (Fig. 24), with a threshold for regional injury at about 16 Gy. A 50 % reduction (TD50) in function was estimated to be 30 Gy, with marked inter-patient variation in TD50 (ranged from 7 to 50 Gy). Similar work has also been done with SPECT, with abnormalities in SPECT images seen at doses as low as 10–15 Gy (Bussels et al. 2004; Van Acker et al. 2001). In a study from Medical University of Lübeck (Germany), significant alterations in radiotracer uptake in irradiated salivary glands of rabbits demonstrated that functional impairment could be assessed by scintigraphy as early as 24 h post-irradiation (Hakim et al. 2004).

Table 6 Imaging assessment of RT-induced liver disease

Author, year affiliation	Number of cases	Disease	RT technique median dose (range)	Follow-up	Radiologic changes	Clinical RT-hepatitis
CT						
Yamasaki et al. 1995, Michigan	31	Primary or metastatic hepatic tumors	High-dose conformal RT 59 Gy (48–73 Gy)	8–12 weeks intervals	74 %	6 %
Munden et al. 2005, MDACC	20	Mesothelioma	–	16 weeks range (3–116)	40 %	0 %
Cao et al. 2007 Michigan, (perfusion)	10	Primary or metastatic hepatic tumors	67.5 Gy (48–78 Gy)	1.5, 3 weeks during RT; 1 month post-RT	↓Regional Perfusion	–
Imada et al. 2010, Chiba University	43	Hepatocellular carcinoma	Carbon ion RT (48.0–79.5 GyE)	3, 6, 12 months	Changes in liver volume	–
PET/CT						
Iyer et al. 2007, MDACC	26	Distal esophageal cancer	3D-conformal RT 50.4 Gy	6 weeks post-RT	19 %	0 %
MRI						
Yankelevitz et al. 1992, Cornell	10	Hodgkins disease	–	2, 4, 6, 12 weeks	30 %	0 %
Onaya et al. 2001	32	Hepatocellular carcinoma	Proton (50-87 Gy)	22 months range (1–75)	35 %*	–
Yoshiokaa et al. 2000, University of Tsukaba	21	Hepatocellular carcinoma	Proton (40.5–72 Gy) Proton (68.8–72 Gy)	3–9 weeks 4–65 months	–	–
Eccles et al. 2009, Princess Margaret	11	Primary or metastatic hepatic tumors	6-fraction conformal RT mean 43.9 Gy (28.8–54 Gy)	1, 3, 6, 12, every six months interval	100 %	–
Seidensticker et al. 2011, University Magdeburg	23	Metastatic hepatic tumors	Interstitial brachytherapy	3 days, 6, 12, 24 weeks	100 %	0 %

*For post-contrast T_{1-} –weighted images

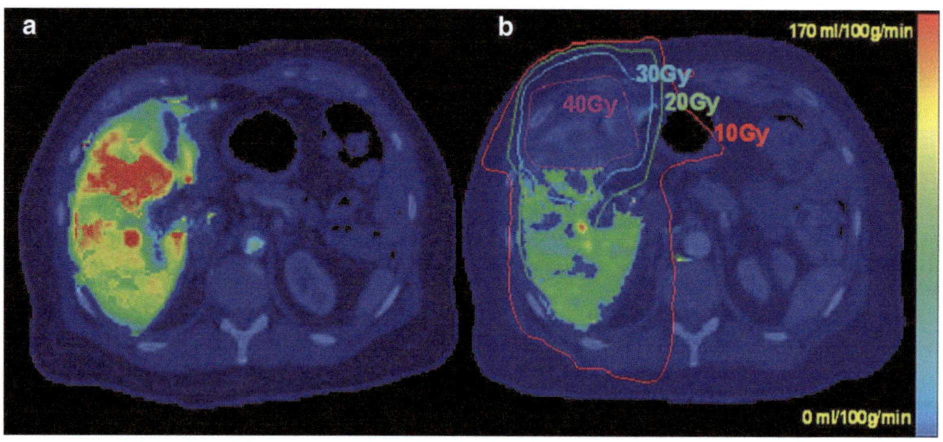

Fig. 19 CT images of radiation-induced hepatic venous perfusion changes. *Color-coded maps* represents portal vein perfusion status of pre-RT (**a**) and post-RT (after 46.5 Gy delivered) (**b**). Reproduced with permission from Cao et al. (2007)

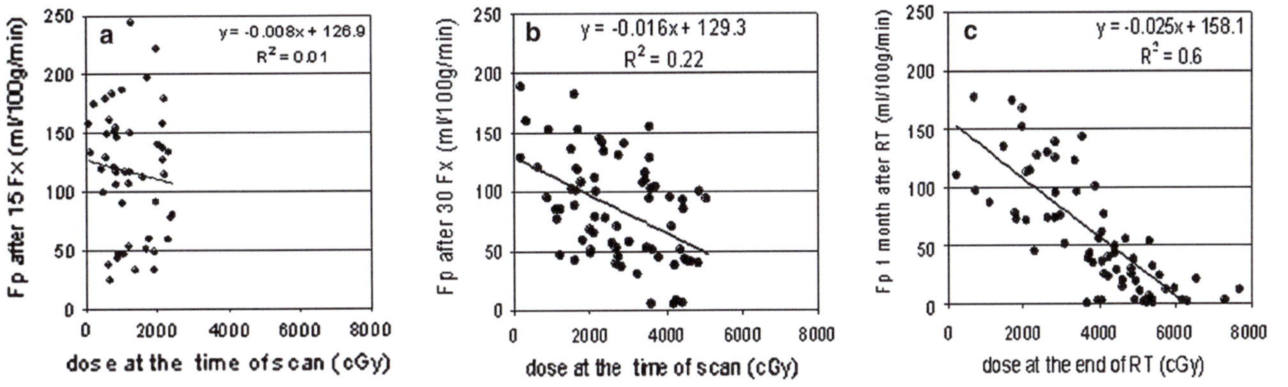

Fig. 20 Changes in portal venous perfusion according to RT dose received at the different time points (**a** 15 fractions; **b** 30 fractions; **c** one month following RT). *Scatter plots* showed the significant correlation between portal venous perfusion and regional RT dose. Reproduced with permission from Cao et al. (2007)

Fig. 21 Six weeks after irradiation of liver metastasis (indicated with *white arrow*), the hepatic injury of normal liver parenchyma (indicated with *black arrow*) is prominent in the region of higher radiation dose on T1-weight gradient echo with Gd-EOB-DTPA. Pre-RT (**a**) and 6 weeks Post-RT (**b**). Reproduced with permission from Seidensticker et al. (2011)

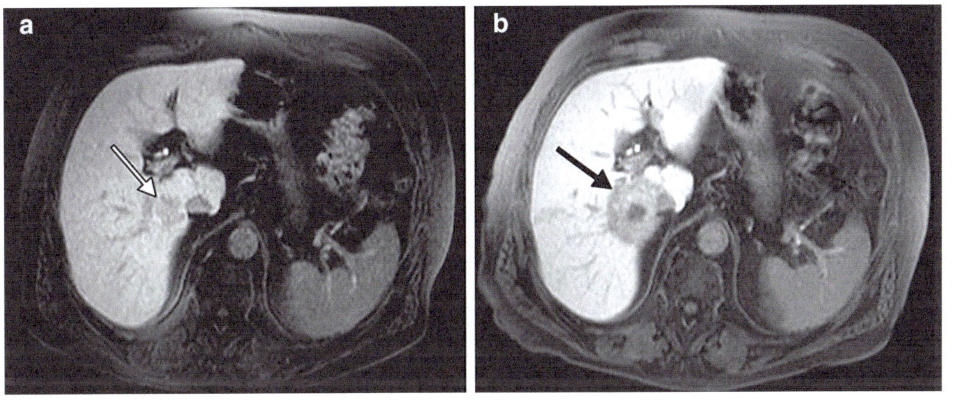

Fig. 22 MR images of a patient with hepatocellular carcinoma treated with 72 Gy proton beam RT. T2-weighted images with (**a**) or without (**b**) contrast enhancement using superparamagnetic iron oxide-enhanced technique show higher signal intensity in the previously irradiated area compared to the surrounding normal liver. Reproduce with permission from Yoshioka et al. (2000)

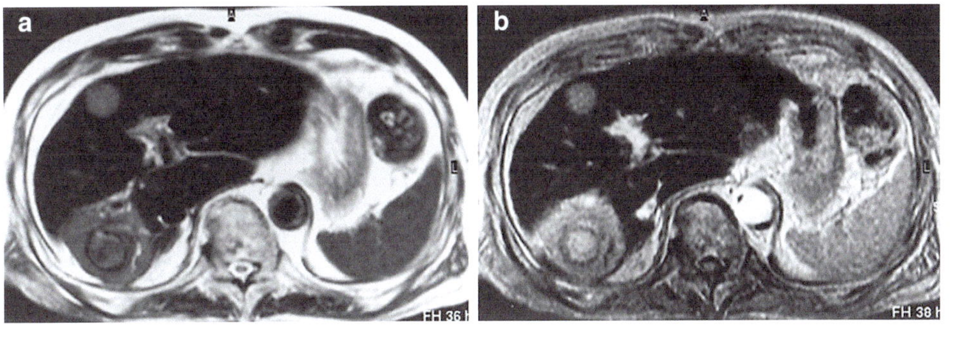

6.2 MRI

MRI has been used to evaluate salivary gland diseases, due to its excellent soft tissue contrast and the visualization of characteristic changes resulting from RT (Nomayr et al. 2001; Zhang et al. 2001). A reduction in MRI-defined apparent diffusion coefficients (ADC) has been noted in patients with RT-induced dysfunction as assessed by scintigraphy (Zhang et al. 2001).

High resolution MRI was used to evaluate the microstructural changes of parotid glands before and after RT (Kan et al. 2010). There were significant volume reductions

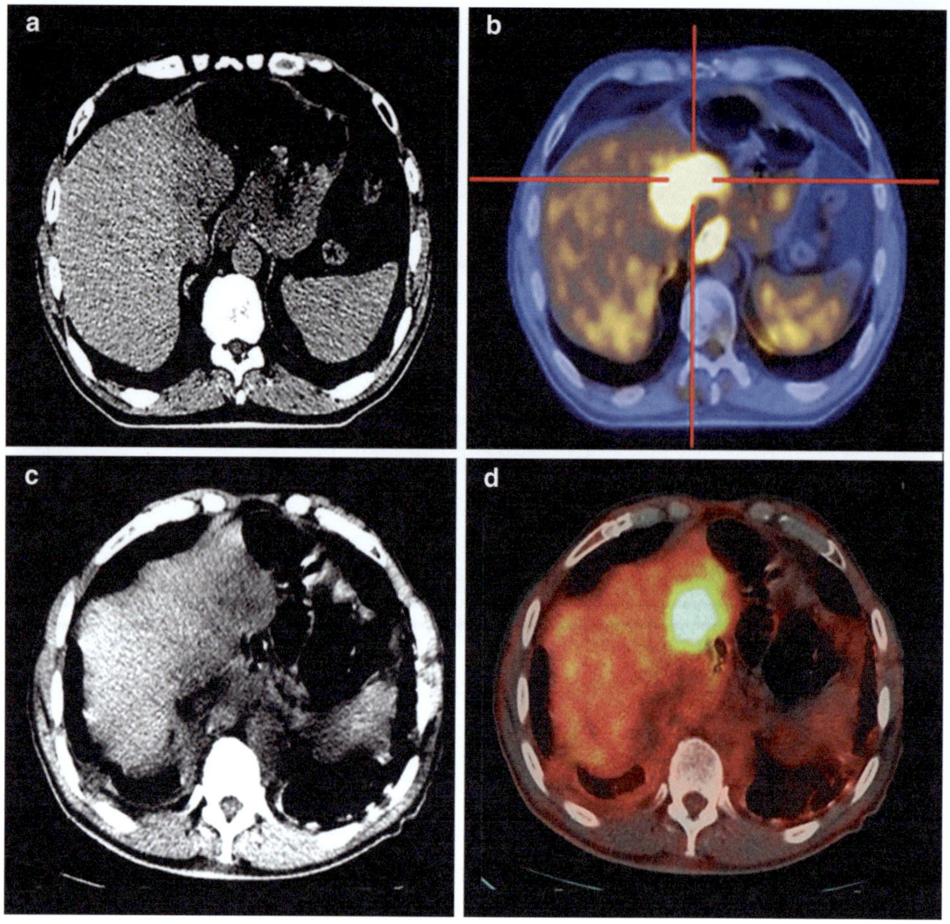

Fig. 23 **a** and **b** show CT and fused PET/CT images, respectively, from a patient with distal esophageal carcinoma, obtained after 6 weeks post-RT. Note the increased FDG uptake in the left lobe of the liver on fused PET/CT image and the well-demarcated low attenuation on axial nonenhanced CT image. **c** and **d** represent another patient with metastatic disease with similar images obtained 18 months post-RT. Reproduced with permission from Iyer et al. (2007)

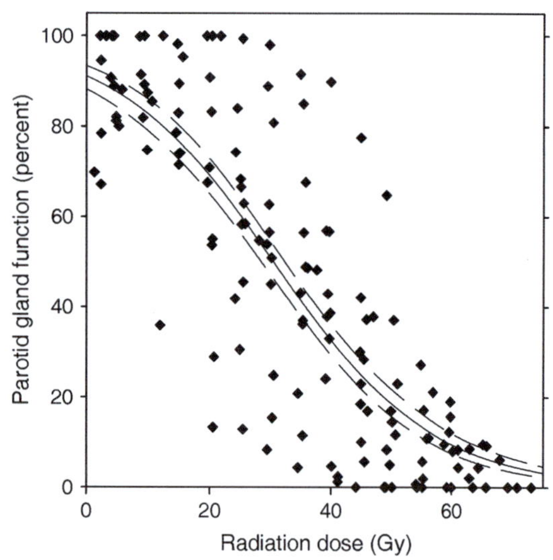

Fig. 24 Radiation dose response for *regional* parotid gland injury. Reductions in regional parotid function are measured in 12 patients, using dynamic PET to assess ^{11}C-methionine clearance (a surrogate for salivary flow). Data is obtained 8–54 months (median 21 months) post-IMRT. Reproduced with permission from Buus et al. (2006)

in the irradiated parotid gland and the decreased width of main duct following RT (Fig. 25). These changes were correlated with the regional radiation dose of the parotid gland (Fig. 26). Houweling et al. reported similar findings using 3T MRI with various MR protocols. A parameter v_e, the extra-vascular extra-cellular space per unit volume of tissue, was significantly increased on post-RT T1-weighted images (Fig. 27). There was a significant correlation between the radiation mean dose and the changes in T2-weighted signal (Houweling et al. 2011). Astreindou et al. noted abnormalities in the parotid gland ducts on 3D-MR sialography in patients irradiated for head and neck cancer. Visibility of the parotid ducts was reduced at 6 weeks post-RT (Fig. 28); after 6 months, some patients showed the visibility scores (Astreinidou et al. 2007).

Summary findings from several studies using various radiologic methods to assess RT-associated changes in the parotid gland are shown in Table 7.

7 Summary

Functional imaging can be used to quantitatively detect RT-induced normal tissue injury in a variety of organs. The data and images shown for the lung, heart, brain, liver, and parotid glands are intended to illustrate the concepts of how

Table 7 Radiologic changes in the parotid glands after RT

Author, year affiliation (reference)	Number of cases	Radiographic follow-up months post-RT median (range)	Type of radiographic study	Radiographic response/outcome
PET				
Buus et al. 2004 Denmark	8	6 months (minimum)	^{11}C-methionine PET	Metabolic clearance of ^{11}C-methionine in the parotid and submandibular glands decreased with increasing RT dose
#Buus et al. 2006, Denmark	12	21 months (8–54)	^{11}C-methionine PET	Dose–response analysis revealed a sigmoid relationship with a threshold dose of 16 Gy, and mean TD_{50}. of 30 Gy.
MRI				
Astreinidou et al. 2007, Utrecht	9	1.5 and 6 months	Magnetic-resonance sialography	Comparison of pre- and post-RT images revealed RT-induced decreases in visible of the parotid and submandibular ducts, at 1.5 months, but subsequent improvement at 6 months.
Nömayr et al. 2001, Germany	52	Within 24 months post-RT	MRI	RT-induced volume reduction of parotid
Zhang et al. 2001, Japan	21	1 month	MRI and Salivary gland scintigraphy (SGS)	Mean apparent diffusion coefficient (ADC) of dysfunctional parotids decreased by 23 % on diffusion-weighted imaging post-RT No significant change of ADCs of functional parotids
Kan et al. 2010, Japan	14	~3 weeks	High resolution MR	Decreased parotid gland volume and narrowing of main duct.
Houweling et al. 2011	18	6 weeks	3T MRI	Decreased parotid gland volume. Change in T2-weighted signal (i.e., increased intensity) was correlated with mean radiation dose.
Scitigraphy/SPECT				
Maes et al. 2002, Belgium	39	1 and 4 months	Salivary gland scintigraphy	The mean loss of SEF in the spared parotid was 67 % and 19 % in 1 and 4 months post-RT, respectively. Normal excretion function was regained in 75 % of the spared parotids.
Roesink et al. 2004, Utrecht	96	1.5 and 12 months	Salivary gland scintigraphy	Reduction in salivary excretion fractions (SEF) from 44.7 % to 18.7 % at 6 weeks and to 32.4 % at 12 months post-RT.
Hsiung et al. 2006, Taiwan	16	1 and 9 months	Salivary gland scintigraphy	Maximal excretion ratio dropped from 53.5 % to 10.7 %, and 23.3 % 1 and 9 months post-IMRT, respectively.
van Acker et al. 2001, Belgium	21	1 month	Salivary gland scintigraphy plus SPECT	Linear correlation between RT-induced changes in SEF on SGS-SPECT and RT dose
Bussels et al. 2004, Belgium	16	7 months (6–10)	Salivary gland scintigraphy plus SPECT	Median reduction in salivary excretion fractions (SEF) of 100 % (range 17–100 %) observed 7 months post-RT

Includes four of the same patients as the other Buus study

imaging can be used to better understand and study radiation-associated-normal tissue injury. There are similar, though lesser, data for other organs such as the submandibular gland, bone, and kidney that are not discussed. Imaging appears to be a powerful tool to objectively and quantitatively assess *regional* normal tissue injury. The degree of radiologically-defined *regional* normal tissue injury may be related to short/long-term clinically-meaningful endpoints (e.g., changes in global organ function), but further study is needed to better quantify this association. Additional work is needed to develop methods and standards to quantitatively score radiologic injury.

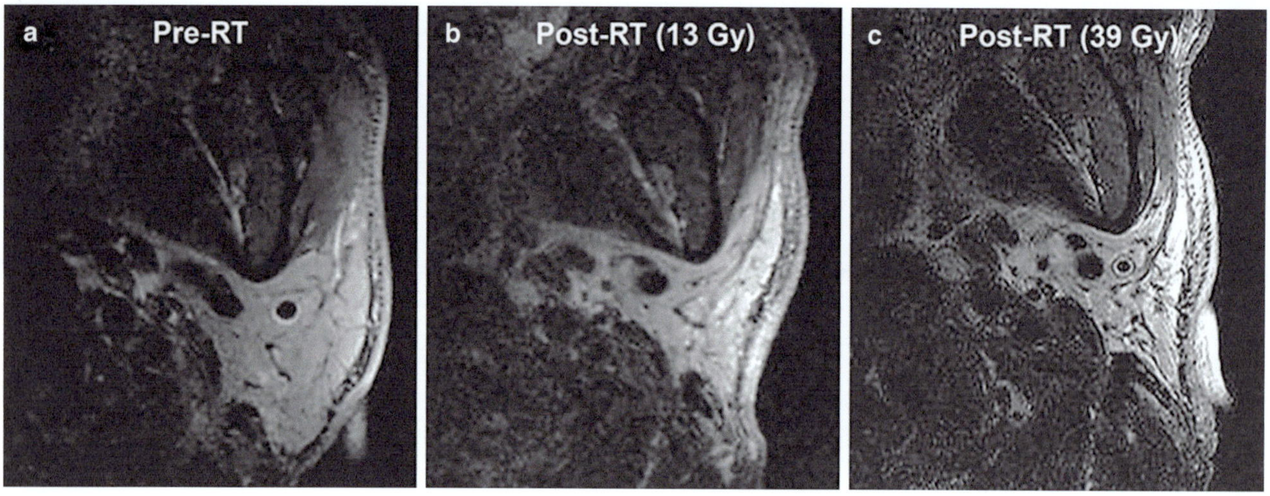

Fig. 25 High resolution MR images show the gradual volume reduction of the parotid gland according to the increase of the radiation dose. Significant narrowing (i.e., decreased signal intensity) of duct was also observed. Reproduced with permission from Kan et al. (2010)

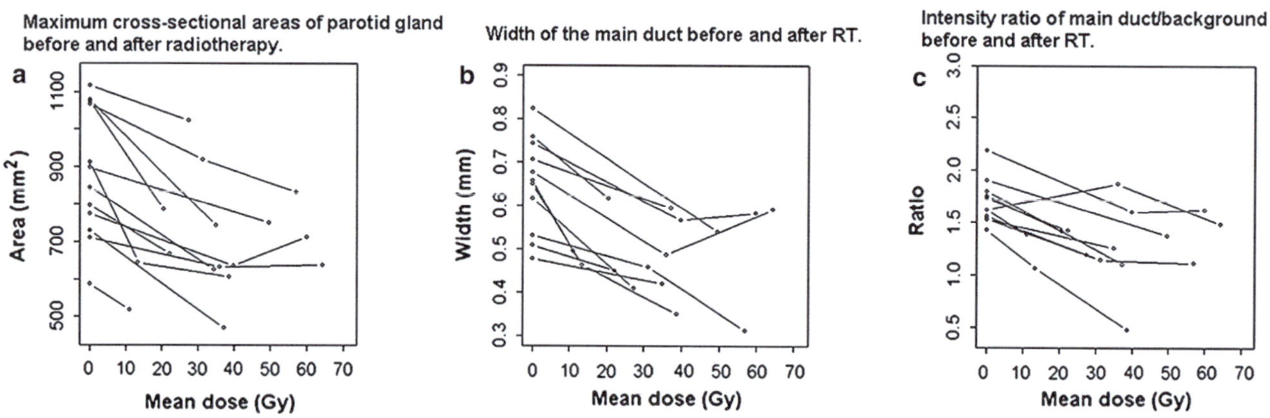

Fig. 26 RT induced parotid volume (**a**) and main duct (**b** and **c**) changes according to the mean radiation dose of the individual parotid gland. Reproduced with permission from Kan et al. (2010)

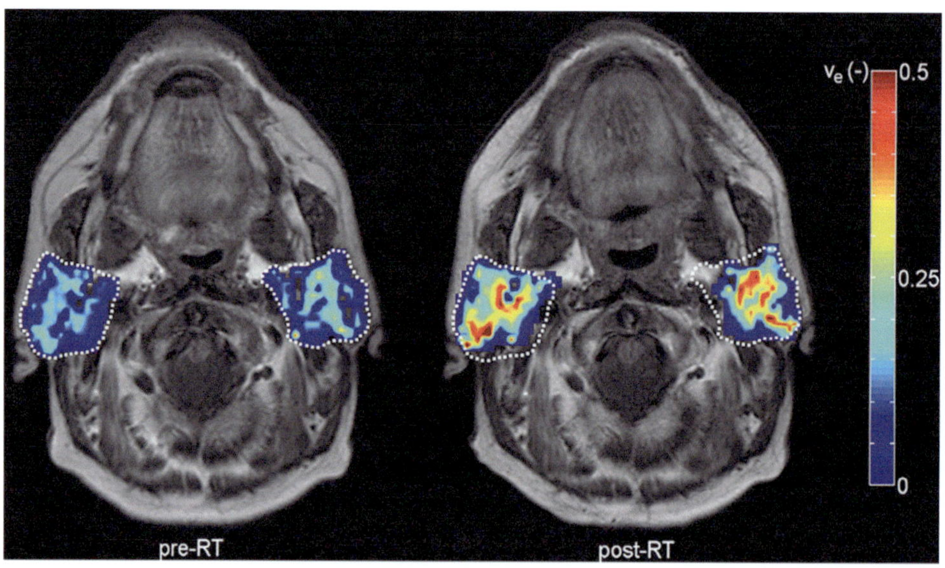

Fig. 27 T1-weighted MR images with the overlaid color-coded parameter v_e, showing post-RT change in both parotid glands. *Dotted lines* are pre-RT contours of both parotid glands. Reproduced with permission from Houweling et al. (2011)

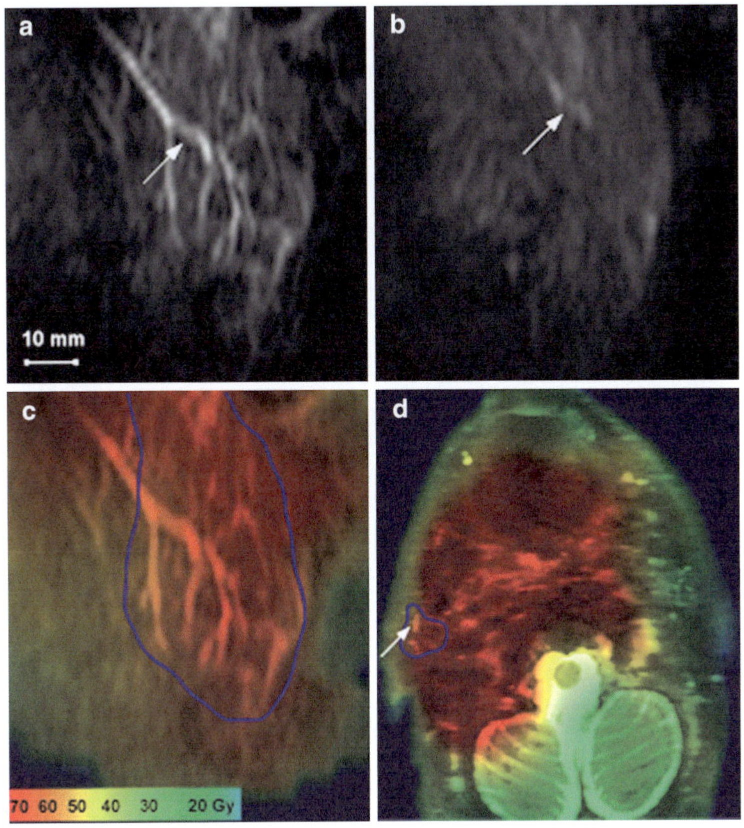

Fig. 28 MR sialogram of pre-RT (**a**) and 6 weeks post-RT (**b**) and superimposed radiation dose plan (**c** and **d**). *Arrows* indicates parotid ducts on the same position receiving the dose of 16 Gy. Reproduced with permission from Astreindou et al. (2007)

Acknowledgments Supported in part by grants NIH R01 CA69579, CA112593, CA122318, Department of Defense Grants 17-98-1-8071, BC010663, and a grant from the Lance Armstrong Foundation. Thanks to the University of North Carolina at Chapel Hill for PLUNC planning software. Portions of this document were adapted from Evans ES, Hahn C, Marks L et al. The role of functional imaging in the diagnosis and management of late normal tissue injury. Seminars in Radiation Oncology 17:72-80, 2007; Hubbs JL, Nam J, Zhou S, et al. Bioimaging in vivo discern the evolution of the late effects temporally and spatially. Cured II—Lent Cancer Survivorship Research and Education: Late Effects on Normal Tissues (Springer); and Imaging radiation-induced normal tissue injury, Mike E. Robbins, Judy K. Brunso-Bechtold, Ann M. Peiffer et al. Radiation Research in press.

References

Allavena C, Conroy T, Aletti P, Bey P, Lederlin P (1992) Late cardiopulmonary toxicity after treatment for Hodgkin's disease. Br J Cancer 65:908–912

Anscher MS, Marks LB, Shafman TD et al (2003) Risk of long-term complications after TFG-? 1-guided very-high-dose thoracic radiotherapy. Int J Radiat Oncol Biol Phys 56:988–995

Aoki T, Nagata Y, Negoro Y et al (2004) Evaluation of lung injury after three-dimensional conformal stereotactic radiation therapy for solitary lung tumors CT appearance. Radiology 230:101–108

Araki Y, Imao Y, Hirata T, Ando T, Sakai N, Yamada H (1990) Cerebral blood flow of the non-affected brain in patients with malignant brain tumors as studied by SPECT; with special reference to adverse effects of radiochemotherapy. No Shinkei Geka 18:601–608

Archibald YM, Lunn D, Ruttan LA et al (1994) Cognitive functioning in long-term survivors of high-grade glioma. J Neurosurg 80:247–253

Armstrong C, Mollman J, Corn BW, Alavi J, Grossman M (1993) Effects of radiation therapy on adult brain behavior: evidence for a rebound phenomenon in a phase 1 trial. Neurology 43:1961–1965

Asao C, Korogi Y, Kitajima M et al. (2005) Diffusion-weighted imaging of radiation-induced brain injury for differentiation from tumor recurrence. Am J Neuroradiol 26:1455–60

Astreinidou E, Roesink JM, Raaijmakers CP et al (2007) 3D MR sialography as a tool to investigate radiation-induced xerostomia: feasibility study. Int J Radiat Oncol Biol Phys 68:1310–1319

Atwood T, Payne VS, Zhao W et al (2007) Quantitative magnetic resonance spectroscopy reveals a potential relationship between radiation-induced changes in rat brain metabolites and cognitive impairment. Radiat Res 168:574–581

Boersma LJ, Damen EMF, de Boer RW et al (1994) Dose-effect relations for local functional and structural changes of the lung after irradiation for malignant lymphoma. Radiother Oncol 32:201–209

Boersma LJ, Damen EM, de Boer RW et al (1996) Recovery of overall and local lung function loss 18 months after irradiation for malignant lymphoma. J Clin Oncol 14:1431–1441

Bussels B, Maes A, Flamen P et al (2004) Dose-response relationships within the parotid gland after radiotherapy for head and neck cancer. Radiother Oncol 73:297–306

Buus S, Grau C, Munk OL, Bender D, Jensen K, Keiding S (2004) 11C-methionine PET, a novel method for measuring regional salivary gland function after radiotherapy of head and neck cancer. Radiother Oncol 73:289–296

Buus S, Grau C, Munk OL et al (2006) Individual radiation response of parotid glands investigated by dynamic 11C-methionine PET. Radiother Oncol 78:262–269

Cao Y, Platt JF, Francis IR et al (2007) The prediction of radiation-induced liver dysfunction using a local dose and regional venous perfusion model. Med Phys 34:604–612

Cao Y, Tsien CI, Sundgren PC et al (2009) Dynamic contrast-enhanced magnetic resonance imaging as a biomarker for prediction of radiation-induced neurocognitive dysfunction. Clin Cancer Res 15:1747–1754

Cazzaniga LF, Bossi A, Cosentino D et al (1998) Radiological findings when very small lung volumes are irradiated in breast and chest wall treatment. Radiat Oncol Investig 6:58–62

Chan YL, Roebuck DJ, Yuen MP et al (2001) Long-term cerebral metabolite changes on proton magnetic resonance spectroscopy in patients cured of acute lymphoblastic leukemia with previous intrathecal methotrexate and cranial irradiation prophylaxis. Int J Radiat Oncol Biol Phys 50:759–763

Chan KC, Khong PL, Cheung MM, Wang S, Cai KX, Wu EX (2009) MRI of late microstructural and metabolic alterations in radiation-induced brain injuries. J Magn Reson Imaging 29:1013–1020

Chong VF, Rumpel H, Fan YF, Mukherji SK (2001) Temporal lobe changes following radiation therapy: imaging and proton MR spectroscopic findings. Eur Radiol 11:317–324

Chong VF, Khoo JB, Chan LL, Rumpel H (2002) Neurological changes following radiation therapy for head and neck tumours. Eur J Radiol 44:120–129

Chua SC, Ganatra RH, Green DJ, Groves AM (2006) Nuclear cardiology: myocardial perfusion imaging with SPECT and PET. Imaging 18:166–177

Cowen D, Gonzague-Casabianca L, Brenot-Rossi I et al (1998) Thallium-201 perfusion scintigraphy in the evaluation of late myocardial damage in left-side breast cancer treated with adjuvant radiotherapy. Int J Radiat Oncol Biol Phys 41:809–815

Crossen JR, Garwood D, Glatstein E, Neuwelt EA (1994) Neurobehavioral sequelae of cranial irradiation in adults: a review of radiation-induced encephalopathy. J Clin Oncol 12:627–642

Cuocolo A, Acampa W, Imbriaco M, De Luca N, Iovino GL, Salvatore M (2005) The many ways to myocardial perfusion imaging. Q J Nucl Med Mol Imaging 49:4–18

Darby SC, McGale P, Taylor CW, Peto R (2005) Long-term mortality from heart disease and lung cancer after radiotherapy for early breast cancer: prospective cohort study of about 300,000 women in US SEER cancer registries. Lancet Oncol 6:557–565

Dawson LA, Ten Haken RK (2005) Partial volume tolerance of the liver to radiation. Semin Radiat Oncol 15:279–283

Dorr W, Bertmann S, Herrmann T (2005) Radiation induced lung reactions in breast cancer therapy: Modulating factors and consequential effects. Strahlenther Onkol 181:567–573

Eccles CL, Haider EA, Haider MA, Fung S, Lockwood G, Dawson LA (2009) Change in diffusion weighted MRI during liver cancer radiotherapy: preliminary observations. Acta Oncol 48:1034–1043

Esteve F, Rubin C, Grand S, Kolodie H, Le Bas JF (1998) Transient metabolic changes observed with proton MR spectroscopy in normal human brain after radiation therapy. Int J Radiat Oncol Biol Phys 40:279–286

Evans ES, Hahn CA, Kocak Z, Zhou SM, Marks LB (2007) The role of functional imaging in the diagnosis and management of late normal tissue injury. Semin Radiat Oncol 17:72–80

Fan M, Marks LB, Hollis D et al (2001a) Can we predict radiation-induced changes in pulmonary function based on the sum of predicted regional dysfunction? J Clin Oncol 19:543–550

Fan M, Marks LB, Lind P et al (2001b) Relating radiation-induced regional lung injury to changes in pulmonary function tests. Int J Radiat Oncol Biol Phys 51:311–317

Fan M, Marks LB, Lind P et al (2001c) Relating radiation-induced regional lung injury to changes in pulmonary function tests. Int J Radiat Oncol Biol Phys 51:311–317

Fu XL, Huang H, Bentel G et al (2001) Predicting the risk of symptomatic radiation-induced lung injury using both the physical and biologic parameters V30 and transforming growth factor ? Int J Radiat Oncol Biol Phys 50:899–908

Gayed IW, Liu HH, Yusuf SW et al (2006) The prevalence of myocardial ischemia after concurrent chemoradiation therapy as detected by gated myocardial perfusion imaging in patients with esophageal cancer. J Nucl Med 47:1756–1762

Gillies RJ, Morse DL (2005) In vivo magnetic resonance spectroscopy in cancer. Annu Rev Biomed Eng 7:287–326

Giovagnoli AR, Boiardi A (1994) Cognitive impairment and quality of life in long-term survivors of malignant brain tumors. Ital J Neurol Sci 15:481–488

Girinsky T, Cordova A, Rey A, Cosset JM, Tertian G, Pierga JY (2000) Thallium-201 scintigraphy is not predictive of late cardiac complications in patients with Hodgkin's disease treated with mediastinal radiation. Int J Radiat Oncol Biol Phys 48:1503–1506

Glanzmann C, Kaufmann P, Jenni R, Hess OM, Huguenin P (1998) Cardiac risk after mediastinal irradiation for Hodgkin's disease. Radiother Oncol 46:51–62

Goethals I, Dierckx R, De Meerleer G et al (2003) The role of nuclear medicine in the prediction and detection of radiation-associated normal pulmonary and cardiac damage. J Nucl Med 44:1531–1539

Graham MV, Purdy JA, Emami B et al (1999) Clinical dose-volume histogram analysis for pneumonitis after 3D treatment for non-small cell lung cancer (NSCLC). Int J Radiat Oncol Biol Phys 45:323–329

Guerrero T, Johnson V, Hart J et al. (2007) Radiation pneumonitis: local dose versus [18f]-fluorodeoxyglucose uptake response in irradiated lung. Int J Radiat Oncol *Biol* Phys 68:1030–1035

Gustavsson A, Eskilsson J, Landberg T et al (1990) Late cardiac effects after mantle radiotherapy in patients with Hodgkin's disease. Ann Oncol 1:355–363

Gustavsson A, Bendahl PO, Cwikiel M, Eskilsson J, Thapper KL, Pahlm O (1999) No serious late cardiac effects after adjuvant radiotherapy following mastectomy in premenopausal women with early breast cancer. Int J Radiat Oncol Biol Phys 43:745–754

Gyenes G, Fornander T, Carlens P, Rutqvist LE (1994) Morbidity of ischemic heart disease in early breast cancer 15–20 years after adjuvant radiotherapy. Int J Radiat Oncol Biol Phys 28:1235–1241

Gyenes G, Fornander T, Carlens P, Glas U, Rutqvist LE (1996) Myocardial damage in breast cancer patients treated with adjuvant radiotherapy: a prospective study. Int J Radiat Oncol Biol Phys 36:899–905

Hahn CA, Zhou S, Renee DH et al. (2005) Dose-dependent effects of radiation therapy on cerebral blood flow, metabolism and neurocognitive dysfunction. Int J Radiat Oncol *Biol* Phys 63:S67

Hakim SG, Jacobsen H, Hermes D et al (2004) Early immunohistochemical and functional markers indicating radiation damage of the parotid gland. Clin Oral Invest 8:30–35

Hardenbergh PH, Munley MT, Bentel GC et al (2001) Cardiac perfusion changes in patients treated for breast cancer with radiation therapy and doxorubicin: preliminary results. Int J Radiat Oncol Biol Phys 49:1023–1028

Harila-Saari AH, Ahonen AK, Vainionpaa LK et al (1997) Brain perfusion after treatment of childhood acute lymphoblastic leukemia. J Nucl Med 38:82–88

Hart JP, Guerrero T, Johnson V et al. (2007) Radiation pneumonitis: correlation of clinical toxicity with pulmonary [18f]-fluorodeoxyglucose uptake dose response. Int J Radiat Oncol *Biol* Phys 69:S155

Heidenreich PA, Schnittger I, Strauss HW et al (2007) Screening for coronary artery disease after mediastinal irradiation for hodgkin's disease. J Clin Oncol 25:43–49

Hein PA, Eskey CJ, Dunn JF, Hug EB (2004) Diffusion-weighted imaging in the follow-up of treated high-grade gliomas: tumor recurrence versus radiation injury. Am J Neuroradiol 25:201–209

Herynek V, Burian M, Jirak D et al (2004) Metabolite and diffusion changes in the rat brain after Leksell Gamma Knife irradiation. Magn Reson Med 52:397–402

Hicks RJ, Mac Manus MP, Matthews JP (2004) Early FDG-PET imaging after radical radiotherapy for non-small-cell lung cancer: inflammatory changes in normal tissues correlate with tumor response and do not confound therapeutic response evaluation. Int J Radiat Oncol Biol Phys 60:412–418

Hoehn M, Nicolay K, Franke C, van der Sanden B (2001) Application of magnetic resonance to animal models of cerebral ischemia. J Magn Reson Imaging 14:491–509

Hojris I, Sand NP, Andersen J, Rehling M, Overgaard M (2000) Myocardial perfusion imaging in breast cancer patients treated with or without post-mastectomy radiotherapy. Radiother Oncol 55:163–172

Hoppe-Hirsch E, Brunet L, Laroussinie F et al. (1995) Intellectual outcome in children with malignant tumors of the posterior fossa: influence of the field of irradiation and quality of surgery. Childs Nerv Syst 11:340–345; discussion 5–6

Houweling AC, Schakel T, van den Berg CAT et al (2011) MRI to quantify early radiation-induced changes in the salivary glands. Radiother Oncol: J Eur Soc Ther Radiol Oncol 100:386–389

Hsiung CY, Ting HM, Huang HY, Lee CH, Huang EY, Hsu HC (2006) Parotid-sparing intensity-modulated radiotherapy (IMRT) for nasopharyngeal carcinoma: preserved parotid function after IMRT on quantitative salivary scintigraphy, and comparison with historical data after conventional radiotherapy. Int J Radiat Oncol Biol Phys 66:454–461

Hubbs JL, Nam J, Hahn CA, Marks LB (2008) Bioimaging in vivo to discern the evolution of late effects temporally and spatially. In: Cured II LENT cancer survivorship research and education. Springer, pp 7–23

Hundley WG, Hamilton CA, Rerkpattanapipat P (2003) Magnetic resonance imaging assessment of cardiac function. Curr Cardiol Rep 5:69–74

Imada H, Kato H, Yasuda S et al (2010) Compensatory enlargement of the liver after treatment of hepatocellular carcinoma with carbon ion radiotherapy—relation to prognosis and liver function. Radiother Oncol 96:236–242

Ingold JA, Reed GB, Kaplan HS, Bagshaw MA (1965) Radiation hepatitis. Am J Roentgenol, Radium Ther Nucl Med 93:200–208

Ireland RH, Din OS, Swinscoe JA et al (2010) Detection of radiation-induced lung injury in non-small cell lung cancer patients using hyperpolarized helium-3 magnetic resonance imaging. Radiother Oncol 97:244–248

Iyer RB, Balachandran A, Bruzzi JF, Johnson V, Macapinlac HA, Munden RF (2007) PET/CT and hepatic radiation injury in esophageal cancer patients. Cancer Imaging 7:189–194

Kahkonen M, Metsahonkala L, Minn H et al (2000) Cerebral glucose metabolism in survivors of childhood acute lymphoblastic leukemia. Cancer 88:693–700

Kan T, Kodani K, Michimoto K, Fujii S, Ogawa T (2010) Radiation induced damage to microstructure of parotid gland: evaluation using high-resolution magnetic resonance imaging. Int J Radiat Oncol Biol Phys 77:1030–1038

Khong PL, Leung LH, Fung AS et al (2006) White matter anisotropy in post-treatment childhood cancer survivors: preliminary evidence of association with neurocognitive function. J Clin Oncol 24:884–890

Kocak Z SL, Sullivan DC, Marks LB (2007) The role of imaging in the study of radiation-induced normal tissue injury. In: Rubin P CL, Marks LB, Okunieff P (eds) Cured I—lent late effects of cancer treatment on normal tissue, 1st edn. Springer, New York, pp 37–45

Kuhnt T, Richter C, Enke H, Dunst J (1998) Acute radiation reaction and local control in breast cancer patients treated with postmastectomy radiotherapy. Strahlenther Onkol 174:257–261

Kwek JW, Iyer RB, Dunnington J, Faria S, Silverman PM (2006) Spectrum of imaging findings in the abdomen after radiotherapy. AJR Am J Roentgenol 187:1204–1211

Lawrence MV, Roper J, Bateman T et al. (2010) Can density changes of surrounding soft tissues cause post-RT cardiopulmonary perfusion defects? Int J Radiat Oncol *Biol* Phys 78:S47

Lawrence TS, Robertson JM, Anscher MS, Jirtle RL, Ensminger WD, Fajardo LF (1995) Hepatic toxicity resulting from cancer treatment. Int J Radiat Oncol Biol Phys 31:1237–1248

Lee MC, Pirzkall A, McKnight TR, Nelson SJ (2004) 1H-MRSI of radiation effects in normal-appearing white matter: dose-dependence and impact on automated spectral classification. J Magn Reson Imaging 19:379–388

Levinson B, Marks LB, Munley MT et al (1998) Regional dose response to pulmonary irradiation using a manual method. Radiother Oncol 48:53–60

Li D, Deshpande V (2001) Magnetic resonance imaging of coronary arteries. Top Magn Reson Imaging 12:337–348

Lind PA, Wennberg B, Gagliardi G et al (2006a) ROC curves and evaluation of radiation-induced pulmonary toxicity in breast cancer. Int J Radiat Oncol Biol Phys 64:765–770

Lind PA, Larsson T, Lidestahl A, Agren-Cronqvist A, Nygren A, Brodin O (2006b) 2497: Heart changes on MRI and SPECT after definitive radiation therapy in patients with lung cancer. Int J Radiat Oncol *Biol* Phys 66:S487

Ma J, Zhang J, Zhou S et al (2010) Regional lung density changes after radiation therapy for tumors in and around thorax. Int J Radiat Oncol Biol Phys 76:116–122

Machann W, Beer M, Breunig M et al (2011) Cardiac magnetic resonance imaging findings in 20-year survivors of mediastinal radiotherapy for Hodgkin's disease. Int J Radiat Oncol Biol Phys 79:1117–1123

Maes A, Weltens C, Flamen P et al (2002) Preservation of parotid function with uncomplicated conformal radiotherapy. Radiother Oncol 63:203–211

Mah K, Keane TJ, Van Dyk J, Braban LE, Poon PY, Hao Y (1994) Quantitative effect of combined chemotherapy and fractionated radiotherapy on the incidence of radiation-induced lung damage: A prospective clinical study. Int J Radiat Oncol *Biol* Phys 28:563–574

Mah K, Van Dyk J, Keane T, Poon PY (1987) Acute radiation-induced pulmonary damage: a clinical study on the response to fractionated radiation therapy. Int J Radiat Oncol Biol Phys 13:179–188

Marks LB (1994) The pulmonary effects of thoracic irradiation. Oncology (Williston Park, NY) 8:89–106; discussion 0, 3

Marks LB, Zhou S, Yu X (2003) The impact of irradiated left ventricular volume on the incidence of radiation-induced cardiac perfusion changes. Int J Radiat Oncol Biol Phys 57:S129

Marks LB, Fan M, Clough R et al (2000) Radiation-induced pulmonary injury: symptomatic versus subclinical endpoints. Int J Radiat Biol 76:469–475

Marks LB, Yu X, Prosnitz RG et al (2005) The incidence and functional consequences of RT-associated cardiac perfusion defects. Int J Radiat Oncol Biol Phys 63:214–223

Matulewicz L, Sokol M, Michnik A, Wydmanski J (2006) Long-term normal-appearing brain tissue monitoring after irradiation using proton magnetic resonance spectroscopy in vivo: statistical analysis of a large group of patients. Int J Radiat Oncol Biol Phys 66:825–832

Maunoury C, Pierga JY, Valette H, Tchernia G, Cosset JM, Desgrez A (1992) Myocardial perfusion damage after mediastinal irradiation for Hodgkin's disease: a thallium-201 single photon emission tomography study. Eur J Nucl Med 19:871–873

Merchant TE, Kiehna EN, Li C, Xiong X, Mulhern RK (2005) Radiation dosimetry predicts IQ after conformal radiation therapy in pediatric patients with localized ependymoma. Int J Radiat Oncol Biol Phys 63:1546–1554

Meyers CA, Weitzner MA (1995) Neurobehavioral functioning and quality of life in patients treated for cancer of the central nervous system. Curr Opin Oncol 7:197–200

Mineura K, Suda Y, Yasuda T et al (1988) Early and late stage positron emission tomography (PET) studies on the haemocirculation and metabolism of seemingly normal brain tissue in patients with gliomas following radiochemotherapy. Acta Neurochir (Wien) 93:110–115

Mori H, Yoshioka H, Ahmadi T, Saida Y, Ohara K, Itai Y (2000) Early radiation effects on the liver demonstrated on superparamegnetic iron oxide-enhanced T1-weighted MRI. J Comput Assist Tomogr 24:648–651

Mori H, Yoshioka H, Mori K et al (2002) Radiation-induced liver injury showing low intensity on T2-weighted images noted in Budd-Chiari syndrome. Radiat Med 20:69–76

Munden RF, Erasmus JJ, Smythe WR, Madewell JE, Forster KM, Stevens CW (2005) Radiation injury to the liver after intensity-modulated radiation therapy in patients with mesothelioma: an unusual CT appearance. AJR Am J Roentgenol 184:1091–1095

Munley MT, Marks LB, Strickland JL et al (1999) The effect of radiotherapy on brain metabolism using F-18 FDG PET imaging. Int J Radiat Biol 45:330–331

Munley MT, Marks LB Hardenbergh PH, Bentel G (2001) Functional imaging of normal tissues. Semin Radiat Oncol 11:28–36

Muryama S, Akamine T, Sakai S et al (2004) Risk factor of radiation pneumonitis: assessment with velocity-encoded cine magnetic resonance imaging of pulmonary artery. J Comput Assist Tomogr 28:204–208

Nagesh V, Tsien CI, Sundgren PC et al. (2008a) Diffusion tensor imaging as a biomarker for neurotoxicity of radiation. Int J Radiat Oncol *Biol* Phys 72:S529

Nagesh V, Tsien CI, Chenevert TL et al (2008b) Radiation-induced changes in normal-appearing white matter in patients with cerebral tumors: a diffusion tensor imaging study. Int J Radiat Oncol Biol Phys 70:1002–1010

Nohara C, Matsumine H, Suzuki K et al (1997) (Neurological CPC-59). A 65-year-old man with a history of gastric cancer who presented progressive loss of vision, memory loss and consciousness disturbance. No to shinkei = Brain and nerve 49:1041–1051

Nomayr A, Lell M, Sweeney R, Bautz W, Lukas P (2001) MRI appearance of radiation-induced changes of normal cervical tissues. Eur Radiol 11:1807–1817

Ogasawara N, Suga K, Karino Y, Matsunaga N (2002) Perfusion characteristics of radiation-injured lung on Gd-DTPA-enhanced dynamic magnetic resonance imaging. Invest Radiol 37:448–457

Onaya H, Itai Y, Ahmadi T et al (2001) Recurrent hepatocellular carcinoma versus radiation-induced hepatic injury: differential diagnosis with MR imaging. Magn Reson Imaging 19:41–46

Pasantes-Morales H, Franco R, Torres-Marquez ME, Hernandez-Fonseca K, Ortega A (2000) Amino acid osmolytes in regulatory volume decrease and isovolumetric regulation in brain cells: contribution and mechanisms. Cell Physiol Biochem 10:361–370

Plotkin M, Eisenacher J, Bruhn H et al (2004) 123I-IMT SPECT and 1H MR-spectroscopy at 3.0 T in the differential diagnosis of recurrent or residual gliomas: a comparative study. J Neuro oncol 70:49–58

Polansky SM, Ravin CE, Prosnitz LR (1980) Pulmonary changes after primary irradiation for early breast carcinoma. AJR Am J Roentgenol 134:101–105

Prosnitz RG, Hubbs JL, Evans ES et al (2007) Prospective assessment of radiotherapy-associated cardiac toxicity in breast cancer patients: analysis of data 3 to 6 years after treatment. Cancer 110:1840–1850

Reed GB Jr, Cox AJ Jr (1966) The human liver after radiation injury. A form of veno-occlusive disease. Am J Pathology 48:597–611

Robbins ME, Brunso-Bechtold JK, Peiffer AM, Tsien CI, Bailey JE, Marks LB (2012) Imaging radiation-induced normal tissue injury. Radiat Res 177(4):449–466

Roesink JM, Moerland MA, Hoekstra A, Van Rijk PP, Terhaard CH (2004) Scintigraphic assessment of early and late parotid gland function after radiotherapy for head-and-neck cancer: a prospective study of dose-volume response relationships. Int J Radiat Oncol Biol Phys 58:1451–1460

Rotstein S, Lax I, Svane G (1990) Influence of radiation therapy on the lung-tissue in breast cancer patients: CT-assessed density changes and associated symptoms. Int J Radiat Oncol Biol Phys 18:173–180

Savage DE, Constine LS, Schwartz RG, Rubin P (1990) Radiation effects on left ventricular function and myocardial perfusion in long term survivors of Hodgkin's disease. Int J Radiat Oncol Biol Phys 19:721–727

Seppenwoolde Y, Muller SH, Theuws JC et al. (2000) Radiation dose-effect relations and local recovery in perfusion for patients with non-small-cell lung cancer. Int J Radiat Oncol Biol Phys 47:681–690

Schaefer WM, Lipke CSA, Nowak B et al. (2004) Validation of QGS and 4D-MSPECT for quantification of left ventricular volumes and ejection fraction from gated 18F-FDG PET: comparison with cardiac MRI. J Nucl Med 45:74–79

Schlemmer HP, Bachert P, Henze M et al (2002) Differentiation of radiation necrosis from tumor progression using proton magnetic resonance spectroscopy. Neuroradiology 44:216–222

Schratter-Sehn AU, Schurawitzki H, Zach M, Schratter M (1993) High-resolution computed tomography of the lungs in irradiated breast cancer patients. Radiother Oncol 27:198–202

Seddon B, Cook A, Gothard L et al (2002) Detection of defects in myocardial perfusion imaging in patients with early breast cancer treated with radiotherapy. Radiother Oncol 64:53–63

Seidensticker M, Seidensticker R, Mohnike K et al (2011) Quantitative in vivo assessment of radiation injury of the liver using Gd-EOB-DTPA enhanced MRI: tolerance dose of small liver volumes. Radiat Oncol 6:40

Seppenwoolde Y, De Jaeger K, Boersma LJ, Belderbos JSA, Lebesque JV (2004) Regional differences in lung radiosensitivity after radiotherapy for non-small-cell lung cancer. Int J Radiat Oncol Biol Phys 60:748–758

Sioka C, Exarchopoulos T, Tasiou I et al (2011) Myocardial perfusion imaging with (99 m)Tc-tetrofosmin SPECT in breast cancer patients that received postoperative radiotherapy: a case-control study. Radiat Oncol 6:151

Sundgren PC, Cao Y (2009) Brain irradiation: effects on normal brain parenchyma and radiation injury. Neuroimaging Clin N Am 19:657–668

Sundgren PC, Nagesh V, Elias A et al (2009) Metabolic alterations: a biomarker for radiation-induced normal brain injury-an MR spectroscopy study. J Magn Reson Imaging 29:291–297

Taphoorn MJ, Klein M (2004) Cognitive deficits in adult patients with brain tumours. Lancet Neurol 3:159–168

Theuws JCM, Kwa SLS, Wagenaar AC et al (1998a) Dose-effect relations for early local pulmonary injury after irradiation for malignant lymphoma and breast cancer. Radiother Oncol 48:33–43

Theuws JCM, Kwa SLS, Wagenaar AC et al (1998b) Prediction of overall pulmonary function loss in relation to the 3-D dose distribution for patients with breast cancer and malignant lymphoma. Radiother Oncol 49:233–243

Theuws JC, Seppenwoolde Y, Kwa SL et al (2000) Changes in local pulmonary injury up to 48 months after irradiation for lymphoma and breast cancer. Int J Radiat Oncol Biol Phys 47:1201–1208

Tofilon PJ, Fike JR (2000) The radio response of the central nervous system: a dynamic process. Radiat Res 153:357–370

Tokatli F, Kaya M, Kocak Z et al (2005) Sequential pulmonary effects of radiotherapy detected by functional and radiological end points in women with breast cancer. Clin Oncol (R Coll Radiol) 17:39–46

van Acker F, Flamen P, Lambin P et al (2001) The utility of SPECT in determining the relationship between radiation dose and salivary gland dysfunction after radiotherapy. Nucl Med Commun 22:225–231

Virta A, Patronas N, Raman R et al (2000) Spectroscopic imaging of radiation-induced effects in the white matter of glioma patients. Magn Reson Imaging 18:851–857

Wagner A, Mahrholdt H, Kim RJ, Judd RM (2005) Use of cardiac magnetic resonance to assess viability. Current cardiology reports 7:59–64

Walecki J, Sokol M, Pieniazek P et al (1999) Role of short TE 1H-MR spectroscopy in monitoring of post-operation irradiated patients. Eur J Radiol 30:154–161

Weitzner MA, Meyers CA (1997) Cognitive functioning and quality of life in malignant glioma patients: a review of the literature. Psycho Oncol 6:169–177

Woel RT, Munley MT, Hollis D et al (2002) The time course of radiation therapy-induced reductions in regional perfusion: a prospective study with >5 years of follow-up. Int J Radiat Oncol Biol Phys 52:58–67

Yamasaki SA, Marn CS, Francis IR, Robertson JM, Lawrence TS (1995) High-dose localized radiation therapy for treatment of hepatic malignant tumors: CT findings and their relation to radiation hepatitis. AJR Am J Roentgenol 165:79–84

Yankelevitz DF, Knapp PH, Henschke CI, Nisce L, Yi Y, Cahill P (1992) MR appearance of radiation hepatitis. Clin Imaging 16:89–92

Yankelevitz DF, Henschke CI, Batata M, Kim YS, Chu F (1994) Lung cancer: evaluation with MR imaging during and after irradiation. J Thorac Imaging 9:41–46

Yoshiokaa H, Itai Y, Saida Y, Mori K, Mori H, Okumura T (2000) Superparamagnetic iron oxide-enhanced MR imaging for early and late radiation-induced hepatic injuries. Magn Reson Imaging 18:1079–1088

Yu X, Prosnitz RR, Zhou S et al (2003) Symptomatic cardiac events following radiation therapy for left-sided breast cancer: Possible association with radiation therapy-induced changes in regional perfusion. Clinical Breast Cancer 4:193–197

Zeng QS, Li CF, Liu H, Zhen JH, Feng DC (2007) Distinction between recurrent glioma and radiation injury using magnetic resonance spectroscopy in combination with diffusion-weighted imaging. Int J Radiat Oncol Biol Phys 68:151–158

Zhang L, Murata Y, Ishida R, Ohashi I, Yoshimura R, Shibuya H (2001) Functional evaluation with intravoxel incoherent motion echo-planar MRI in irradiated salivary glands: a correlative study with salivary gland scintigraphy. J Magn Reson Imaging 14:223–229

Zhang J, Ma J, Zhou S et al (2010) Radiation-induced reductions in regional lung perfusion: 0.1-12 year data from a prospective clinical study. Int J Radiat Oncol Biol Phys 76:425–432

Zophel K, Holzel C, Dawel M, Holscher T, Evers C, Kotzerke J (2007) PET/CT demonstrates increased myocardial FDG uptake following irradiation therapy. Eur J Nucl Med Mol Imaging 34:1322–1323

Biograding of Normal Tissue TNM Toxicity Taxonomy: Scoring the Adverse Effects of Cancer Treatment

Taxonomy and Classification are Attempts to Order the Chaos in Nature

Andy M. Trotti and Philip Rubin

Contents

A. M. Trotti (✉)
H. Lee Moffit Cancer Center Research Institute, 12902 Magnolia Drive, Tampa, FL 33612, USA
e-mail: andy.trotti@moffitt.org

P. Rubin
Department of Radiation Oncology, University of Rochester School of Medicine and Dentistry, 601 Elmwood Ave, Box 647Rochester, NY 14642, USA

Abstract

Although dramatic improvements in cancer survival statistics have occurred over the past 5 decades and are well documented in the literature, the same has not been true for detailing the unwanted incidental adverse effects following multimodal cancer treatment. The dramatic gains in 5-year survival has been compiled by cancer site in a SEER tabulation marking the passing of 50 % level for all cancers at the turn of this century. (American Cancer Society: Cancer Facts and Figures 1995). At issue and unresolved is the price for the success and how to best measure and grade these adverse toxicity effects which persist and progress over time detracting from the cancer survivor's quality of life.

1 Introduction and Overview: Genesis and Evolution

Although dramatic improvements in cancer survival statistics have occurred over the past 5 decades and are well documented in the literature, the same has not been true for detailing the unwanted incidental adverse effects following multimodal cancer treatment. The dramatic gains in 5-year survival has been compiled by cancer site in a SEER tabulation marking the passing of 50 % level for all cancers at the turn of this century. (American Cancer Society: Cancer Facts and Figures 1995). At issue and unresolved is the price for the success and how to best measure and grade these adverse toxicity effects which persist and progress over time detracting from the cancer survivor's quality of life.

The need for a grading system to assess treatment toxicities lagged behind the TNM classification of cancers. It was in the 1980's because of the increasing number of clinical trials sponsored by NCI and EORTC that a consolidation of numerous individual approaches by each specialty was initiated. The genesis of acute toxicity scoring versus late effect grading originated in a bipolar fashion.

P. Rubin et al. (eds.), *ALERT – Adverse Late Effects of Cancer Treatment*, Medical Radiology. Radiation Oncology,
DOI: 10.1007/978-3-540-72314-1_7, © Springer-Verlag Berlin Heidelberg 2014

Table 1 The Evolution of Toxicity Grading Systems (1979–1998)

System	Number of criteria	Number of organs	Modality	Phase
WHO (1979)	28	9	Chemo	Acute
CTC (1983)	18	13	Chemo	Acute
RTOG/EORTC-Acute (1984)	14	13	RT	Acute
RTOG/EORTC-Late (1984)	68	17	RT	Late
LENT/SOMA (1995)	140	13	RT	Late
CTC v2.0 (1998)	152	22	RT	Late
CTCAE v3.0 (2003)	260	22	All[a]	Acute
	370	All	All	Acute and late

WHO, World Health Organization; Chemo, chemotherapy; *RT*, radiation therapy
[a] Limited pediatric and surgical criteria

The NCI, CTEP recognized the need to uniformly score the toxic acute and subacute effects of chemotherapy. The Common Toxicity Criteria (CTC), first published in 1983, was concerned with the physiologic and functional endpoints, many of which are transitory and reversible (Miller et al. 1981). Then, version (2.0) attempted to incorporate the acute effects of other modalities as radiation and expanded 13–22 organ systems and the number of criteria incremented from 18 to 260 (Table 1) (Trotti et al. 2000; World Health Organization 1992).

The radiation oncology profession has traditionally been concerned with reporting late effects of cancer treatment and the RTOG in conjunction with EORTC introduced both the "Acute and Late Radiation Morbidity Scoring Criteria" simultaneously (Cox et al. 1995). A series of NCI sponsored workshops led to the introduction of more comprehensive system entitled: LENT ~ **L**ate **E**ffects **N**ormal **T**issue and SOMA criteria, representing **s**ubjective **S**ymptoms, **O**bjective findings and **MA**nagement features. The A referred to Analytic quantifiable parameters in the laboratory or imaging. With acceptance and joint publications on both sides of the Atlantic, RTOG/EORTC hope to standardize reporting of late effects. (Trotti 2002; Rubin et al. 1995a) Some of the guiding thoughts to reduce interobserver variability was to replace the commonly used four grades of 1 + mild, 2 + moderate, 3 + severe, 4 + life threatening with better descriptors with corresponding terms as occasional, intermittent, persistent and refractory, respectively, when referring to the expression of symptoms and signs, i.e., pain. Longitudinal clinical trials emphasizing correlation of symptoms and sign of toxicity with metrics and interventions are future goals. (Trotti and Rubin 2003).

The most recent collaboration sponsored by all modalities has resulted in a more comprehensive CTC v3.0, which includes more late effects criteria and is inclusive of all modalities (Available at: http://ctep.info.nih.gov/CTC3/ctc.htm. Accessed 1 April 2003; Trotti et al. 2003). However, the merging of late effect and acute effect criteria, although more comprehensive with 510 criteria, when specifying anatomic sites or other subclassifications, raises the number to 900 adverse effect criteria for grading. The need for a summary toxicity methodology and a global adverse effect score, inclusive of multiple organ systems, has yet to be defined, and is essential for outcomes reporting.

2 The Biologic Basis For Combining Acute and Late Criteria

The most prominent feature of CTCAE v3.0 is the merging of early and late effects criteria into a single uniform document and the development of criteria applicable to all modalities. The research support for the concept of a "biologic continuum" is based upon the original paradigm by Rubin and Casarett (Rubin and Casarett 1968) in which the clinical radiation pathophysiologic course of events incorporating the dynamic sequence of cellular events and tissue specific effects began at the moment of radiation exposure. The schema illustrated radiation effects, both the clinical and subclinical events, in each organ system, but noted that depending on its cell population and tissue organization would express radiation syndromes differently. The underlying pathophysiologic commonality was the obliteration of the normal tissues' fine microvasculature, whereas the time to clinical expression, the latent period, is related to stem cell depletion in either rapid or slow renewal system, i.e., acute versus chronic or early versus late effects. This paradigm was the first formalism linking acute and late effects as both a pathophysiologic and a clinical bio continuum. More recently, the molecular biologic events captured as a persistent cytokine cascade induced by radiation in a murine model has recapitulated the shape of the Rubin and Casarett tissue effect over time curves adding further to their validity (Rubin et al. 1995b). The arbitrary 90 day rule dividing early and late is no longer acceptable, since modalities overlap and are administered concurrently, and adjuvant chemotherapy is repeatedly cycled often for months and years. The use of a complex concurrent or hybrid sequential schedules undermines the usefulness of a simplistic temporally defined "early-late" construct.

Moreover, there is a growing recognition that surgery (Fedyk et al. 2001; Mercado et al. 2002) and chemotherapy (Petak and Houghton 2001) much like radiation lead to molecular events resulting in a perpetual cytokine, chemokine cascade and surgery induces wound healing responses that result in a inflammation, fibrogenesis, and neoangiogenesis leading to epithelial regeneration. This multimodal molecular cascade leads to and supports the biologic continuum model (Fig. 1).

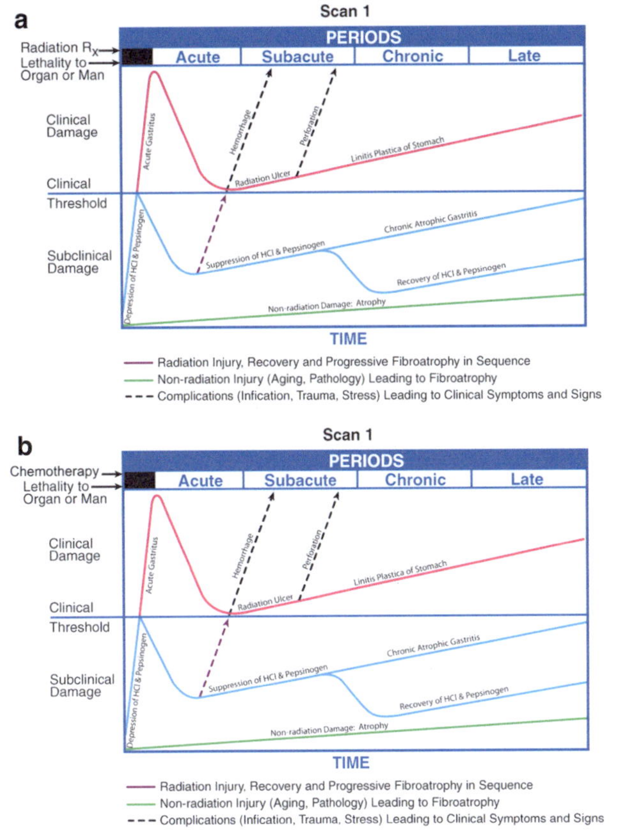

Fig. 1 The clinicopathologic course of events following irradiation can be complicated by the addition of chemotherapy. Similarly, chemotherapy can result in parallel set of events. **a** Classically, when radiation therapy precedes chemotherapy, the introduction of the second mode can lead to expression of subclinical damage or, when injury is present, to death. **b** The same is true if chemotherapy precedes radiation therapy. Reprinted with permission. (With permissions from Rubin & Casarett, 1968)

3 Standardization, and Statistical Reporting

Standardization of language requires use of the International Dictionary of Medical Terminology and commonly used disease codes, i.e., ICD 10 (World Health Organization 1992; International Statistical Classification of Diseases and Related Health Problems. 10th ed. American Psychiatric Publishing 1992) need to synchronized with both CTC and LENT-SOMA diagnoses. Thus, the descriptors of adverse effects language can become more uniform and will reduce interinvestigator variability. The introduction of quality of life scales to represent the patients' viewpoint is an important aspect of grading adverse effects. Another important aspect is the need to integrate CTC and LENT-SOMA more fully. The LENT-SOMA is based on anatomic terms consisting of 15–20 major systems with approximately 50–60 subsites and is compatible but not identical with the terminology of the TNM system (American Joint Committee on Cancer (AJCC) 2002). By contrast, the CTCAE v3.0 utilizes more physiologic and functional terms and clinical syndromes. There is as much concurrence and similarities as differences and a comparison of terms is presented in Table 2. The anatomical terminology reconciliation of the 3 systems is consistent with the International Anatomical Terminology (Terminologic Anatomica) approved in 1998 by the International Federation of the Association of Anatomists (Table 2). (Federative Committee on Anatomical Terminology (FCAT) 1998).

There is a large and growing literature assessing both the CTC systems and LENT-SOMA. Numerous clinical trials have been published often comparing these systems with other late toxicity grading criteria, particularly in Europe. The literature is equally divided between concordance and discordance in confirmation of their applicability. The majority of reports are retrospective and not prospectively designed to assess validation, especially for LENT-SOMA. Davidson et al. (2002, 2003a, b); Routledge et al. (2003); Hoeller et al. (2003); Fehlauer et al. (2003); Denis et al. (2003); Anacak et al. (2001); Tawfiq et al. (2000) However, more recently, direct comparison has been made utilizing CTC v3.0 and LENT-SOMA. Furthermore, recent analysis of a validation perspective clinical trial in variety of anatomic sites by RTOG confirms that LENT-SOMA is a superior instrument as to capturing late effects. Utilizing a technique of linguistic analysis there are 12 recurrent criteria that apply to grading most of the organ systems. The "shared" word descriptors for each grade which can be identified in both LENT-SOMA and CTC v3.0 allows for a "**concise grading dictionary**" of well defined lexicons which captures the essence of both systems. The **SOMA**tization of CTC v3.0 is shown in Table 3, which provides a more focused selection of criteria and should enable users to record toxicities more efficiently and accurately. The array of criteria relate to five categories: symptoms, physical findings, interventions to ameliorate, quality of life, or activities of daily living. Laboratory values and imaging studies are working in progress as to

Table 2 Anatomic-physiologic systems: hybrid nomenclature

Anatomic sites AJCC[a] TNM	LENT/ SOMA[b]	Physiologic systems CTC v3.0[c]
Central nervous system	(2)	Neurology
(Neuroendocrine[c])	(3)	Endocrine
Ophthalmologic sites	(6)	Ocular/Visual
Head and neck sites	(10)	Upper respiratory
Digestive system	(6)	Gastrointestinal
Major digestive glands	(5)	Hepato/Biliary/Pancreas
Thorax breast	(1)	
Lung	(1)	Pulmonary
Pleura	(1)	
(Heart[c])	(1)	Cardiac, Arrhythmia
(Vascular[c])	(1)	Vascular
Genitourinary sites	(7)	Renal/Genitourinary
		Male sexual reproduction
Gynecologic sites	(7)	Female sexual reproduction
Musculoskeletal	(2)	Musculoskeletal
Skin	(1)	Dermatology, Lymphatics
Lymphoid sites	(4)	Allergy, Immunology
Bone marrow	(1)	Blood, Bone marrow
		Hemorrhage, bleeding
		Infection, coagulation

[a] AJCC Cancer Staging Manual anatomic terms

[b] LENT/SOMA applies to the number of normal tissue sites and subsites that are graded for toxicity and are in parentheses

[c] NCI CTC v3.0 are the basis for the physiologic terms. There are a number of unique terms in CTC v3.0 as syndromes, second malignancies, growth and development that do not fit into a hybrid anatomic/physiologic systems nomenclature

correlations with gradations of toxicity and at this time should not override the other criteria when assigning grade.

4 Normal Tissue/Organ TNM Taxonomy for Adverse Effects of Cancer Treatment

4.1 TNM Language

There is logic for adopting the TNM nomenclature for normal tissue/organ adverse effects following cancer treatment. The TNM language was introduced to allow for consistency in the classification and staging of cancer. The adoption by the AJCC and the UICC 50 years ago has enabled oncologists worldwide to stratify patients, allow for multidisciplinary communication, better treatment decisions, and more accurate end results reporting. With a common language for cancer staging, cooperative oncology group protocols allowed for multimodal regimen to be designed and tested in clinical trials. The standardization of TNM staging nomenclature allows for evaluation and assessment of the literature. Therefore, a modification of this cancer nomenclature will be applied to normal tissue/organ toxicity.

4.2 General Rules

Philosophically, the TNM cancer classification is based on the premise that all malignant tumors progress from an early localized stage to a more disseminated later stage. The life cycle of all cancers shares in having a locus of origin in a normal tissue, which invades locally and advances to lymph nodes regionally and/or hematogenously to remote sites. In a parallel fashion, there is a similar life cycle for normal tissue reactions to multimodal cancer treatment. The normal tissues in which the cancer originated will be the target of surgery and radiation as well as targeted chemotherapy. The normal tissue structures and sites in the region (lymph nodes) are at risk and often have reactions to the aforementioned modalities, especially in concurrent regimens. Multiagent chemotherapy combinations are designed to diffuse the toxicity and can elicit systemic responses hematologically. Remote sites from the cancer can be affected, i.e., heart (Adriamycin), kidney (Cisplatinum), etc.

The practice of dividing cancer into "early versus late" was based on the progression from a localized stage to an advanced stage. In a parallel fashion adverse effects also progress from "acute to late". Just as cancer is staged before treatment, the normal tissues—structure and function—need to be noted for baseline values and the presence of co-morbidities.

The proper staging of cancer applies to accurate recording of the status of host normal tissues and serves a number of related objectives, such as:

a. Selection of a corrective therapeutic intervention
b. Estimation of eventual prognosis
c. Assistance in evaluation of results of the intervention
d. Facilitates exchange of data amongst investigators
e. Of special importance to cancer control is establishing the therapeutic ratio.

4.3 New Definitions of TNM Applied to Adverse Effects of Normal Tissue

The conceptual design of the $_{N}$TNM is similar to tumor spread into 3 compartments: primary tumor site, regional nodes, and systemic dissemination. The adverse effect of cancer treatment can be confined to the anatomic site of

Table 3 Somatization of CTCAE v3.0

	Mild grade 1+	Moderate grade 2+	Severe grade 3+	Life threatening grade 4+
S	Asymptomatic	Symptomatic usually	Persistent symptoms	Refractory symptoms
	Minimal symptoms	Marked symptoms	Intensive symptoms	Symptoms unresponsive to medication
O	Transient signs	Intermittent signs	Symptoms apparent	Advanced persistent signs
	Functionally intact	Function altered	Function impaired	Function collapsed
M	No interventions	Non-invasive intervention	Interventional radiology	Rad life saving surg
	Occasional medication	Continuous medication	Surgical correction	Intensive care unit
	Occasional non-narcotic	Regular non-narcotic	Occasional narcotic	Parenteral narcotic
A	Normal laboratory values	Abnormal laboratory	Very abnormal lab	Pailing lab values
	Borderline low,	Values,	Lab values not	Potentially lethal
	Correctable	Correctable	Correctable	BM <75 %
	BM cellularity <25 % decrease	B.M. cellularity >25–50 %	BM cellularity >50 %, <75 %	
ADL QOL	ADL regular	ADL Altered	ADL impaired	ADL extremely poor
	KPS 80–100	KP 60–75	KP 30–50	KP 10–25
	Fully ambulatory	Symptomatic, in bed <50 % day	Symptomatic, in bed >50 %	100 % bedridden

cancer origin or extend to involve other structures in the neighboring region or be a generalized or systemic toxic effect.

$_N$T = The normal **T**issue, anatomic structure, organ in which the cancer arose and spreads initially.

$_N$N = **N**eighboring or surrounding normal tissues or organs, viscera that are not involved by the tumor and in the regional nodal drainage zone.

$_N$M = Syste**M**ic effects that are generalized and include hematologic, hepatic toxicity, weight loss.

Progression of the adverse effect can be designated numerically and becomes the **operational taxonomy unit**.

4.4 Assigning the Grade for Progression

The progression of a malignancy over time is designated by the assignment of numbers 1, 2, 3, 4 as subscripts to T and N, the primary tumor and nodal compartments, respectively. In an analogous fashion, the translation of late effects into a scale that allows for progression over time is important. The general guidelines are in the construction of criteria.

The operational taxonomic unit (OTU) is the grade assigned as applied according to criteria in CTCAE v3.0 or LENT-SOMA which is 1 + Mild, 2 + Moderate, 3 + Severe, or 4 + Life threatening and will be determined by the degree of toxicity at each anatomic site, organ.

Grade 1 +: Asymptomatic, signs are minimal and not interfere with functional endpoints, nor impede mobility. Most often, management is restrained; interventions and medication are not required.

Grade 2 +: Symptomatic, moderate findings clinically or in laboratory, that may alter functional endpoints without impact on quality of life (QOL) or activities of daily living (ADL) Medications and interventions can be used and be useful.

Grade 3 +: Effects are indicative of severity of symptoms and signs, which persist over time, and disruption of mobility, working, and numerous functional endpoints. More serious intervention as hospitalization or surgery is often indicated.

Grade 4 +: Effects are potentially life threatening, catastrophic, disabling, and result in loss of limb, bowel, and organ function.

Some more important principles established in CTC v3.0 are equally applicable to this proposed $_N$T$_N$N$_N$M taxonomy:

- Acute and late effects merged in one system and applied with restrictive time applications
- The system applies equally to all modalities
- The duration or chronicity should be determined by serial longitudinal protocol studies.

When multiple normal structures are affected each will be evaluated separately and be given a **summary score**. When multiple normal structures are involved and then compiled, a **global toxicity** score is derived.

4.5 Classification According to Evidence for Certainty of Grade

As in cancer classification there are 4 types of classification depending on the diagnostic procedures and the relationship to the cancer treatment versus an intervention to manage the adverse effect. Clearly, the adverse normal tissue effect can be assessed before treatment, during and immediately after multimodal treatment.

a. **Clinical classification** is based on physical examination, imaging often with CT or MRI, endoscopy, and routine laboratory procedures. Minimal invasive procedures as needle aspiration are useful and allowable. Most baseline values for vital normal tissues and assessments of acute and subacute reactions to multimodal treatment are in this category $_{CN}$TNM.
b. **Pathologic classification** requires an invasive procedure and as in cancer staging an adverse chemoradiation effect may require a surgical intervention and resection. Even surgical handling of vasculocompromised tissues may precipitate a necrotizing reaction as in exploring adherent bowel at laparotomy. Such invasive procedures are usually performed after multimodal cancer treatment to rule out recurrent cancers, which can masquerade as a late effect. PET or SPECT, MRI/MRS are valuable for establishing radiation sequelae as a confirmatory tissue diagnosis is critical (Tawfiq et al. 2000; Bragg et al. 2002). Biopsies, especially generous ones, may precipitate severe necrosis and need to be done with caution.
c. **Retreatment classification** could apply to salvage cancer treatment as well as management intervention to ameliorate the adverse effect. Either sophisticated imaging as PET/SPECT or MRI/MRS can be of value to distinguish recurrence or persistence of cancer versus normal tissue necrosis (Tawfiq et al. 2000; Bragg et al. 2002) $_{RN}$TNM.
d. **Autopsy classification**: If a death is attributed to an adverse effect usually life threatening (4 +) and fatal (5 +), autopsy is mandatory to exclude incidental comorbidities. According to Fajardo et al. there are no pathognomic microscope features but certain constellation of radiation/chemotherapy stigmata and again ruling out cancer recurrence is essential (Husband and Reznek 1998) $_{AN}$TNM.
e. **Prefixes and suffixes** may be added for certain circumstances:

m suffix indicates multiple structures, sites and organs may express the adverse effect, i.e., $TN_{(m)}M$.

y prefix indicates evaluation performed during or following initial multimodal therapy, i.e., $_{yp}$TNM.

5 Summary Toxicity Grade

5.1 $_{N}$T $_{N}$N $_{N}$M Summary Grade

The expansion of CTC v3.0 approaches a thousand descriptors involving 15–20 major organ systems, which if divided into subsites (50–60) multiplies the elements and challenges investigators to offer a Summary Grade for reporting outcomes. LENT-SOMA has a similar complex and detailed compilation of criteria. This has often been circumnavigated by utilizing the abbreviated late effects scales of the RTOG/EORTC cooperative groups. The operational taxonomic unit (OTU) is the number assigned to the grade of toxicity; however, the adverse late effect can vary over time. The biocontinuum of acute/late effects has been confirmed both in the laboratory measuring function in the clinic with physiologic testing. There are numerous possibilities for selecting the OTU or summary grade of a specific organ system as a function of time in a longitudinal protocol (Fig. 2). When radiation is combined with chemotherapy, the variations in toxicity are illustrated as a function of time (Fig. 3) (Forestiere et al, 2003).

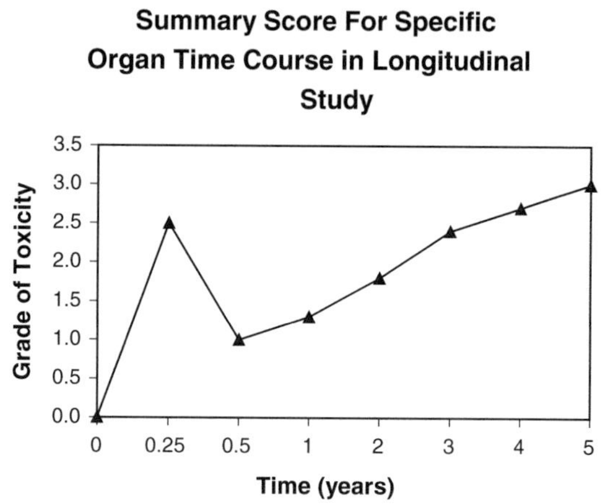

Fig. 2 Summary toxicity grade. The summary toxicity grade for a specific effect is a function of the grade of the effect over time. This can be recorded in 3 different parameters: (1) Maximal toxicity grade, (2) Average grade over time, (3) Area under the curve (grade x time). (with permission from Rubin et al. 2007)

5.2 Global Toxicity Score of Multiple Organs

Stage grouping is an important aspect of the staging of cancer and applies directly to adverse effects involving multiple sites. Because in cancer staging there are 4T's, 3 N's, and 2 M's, there are 24 possible combinations. To recluster TN into the four Stages I, II, III, and IV would be a challenge when adverse effects are collated in multiple normal tissues.

The global toxicity score would be the compilation of the summary grades for each normal tissue assessed. With more than one structure in each of the defined zones, i.e., $_{N}$T for site of cancer origin or

$_{N}$N for site of neighboring tissue

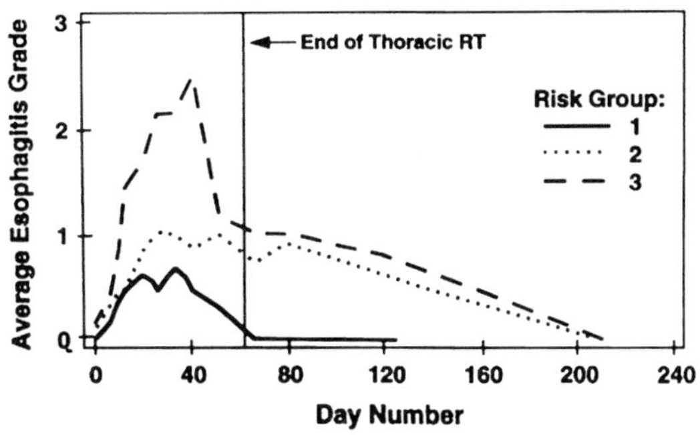

Fig. 3 The time course of acute and chronic esophagitis; Group 1 = standard thoracic RT alone or with induction chemotherapy, Group 2 = standard thoracic RT with concurrent chemotherapy, Group 3 = twice daily RT with concurrent chemotherapy. *With permission* (Forestiere et al. 2003)

$_N$M for systemic toxicities of system.

The recommendation is to score each summary grade as noted and then add the subscripts. Thus, the global toxicity is the sum of subscripts and creation of stage grouping similar to staging cancers.

Stage I = T1N1M1 or T2N1M0 or T3 N0M0
Total = 1–3
Stage II = T2N2M2 OR T3N1M0 OR T1N3M1
Total = 4–6
Stage III = T3N3M3 or T4N2M1 or T2N2 + 2M1
Total = 7–9
Stage IV = T4N4M4 or T3N2M1 or T2N2 + 2+3M1 + 2
Total = 10–16, or
Stage V Total > 16.

Obviously, these recommendations and generalizations will need compilation of data from clinical trials before an accurate global score can be arrived at.

5.3 Tame

TAME is a new reporting system to summarize toxicity burden of cancer treatment advocated by Trotti et al. consolidating traditional adverse event data into three risk domains: T (Toxicity, acute short-term): A (Adverse long-term late) and M (Mortality risk generated) and E (End results). TAME definitions use a new set of terms, definitions, endpoints and calculation algorithms (Trotti et al. 2007).

3.1 T = mean number of grade 3–4 acute events for a treatment regimen during a defined period of acute toxicity risk. Mean raw T values for a given treatment group can be calculated by taking the mean of all T scores generated from individual patient data (JPD). An IPD T score is derived by summing the number of high-grade (3 or 4) acute events reported on that individual for a defined acute-risk interval. Mean T scores, therefore, represent the range of acute effects reported by a typical patient, on average, over a defined acute-events interval. T scores from multiple acute-risk intervals (e.g., induction chemotherapy, radiotherapy, and early follow-up) can be added to derive an overall T value (e.g., $T_{\text{induction}} + T_{\text{radiotherapy}} + T_{\text{acute/recovery interval}} = T_{\text{overall}}$).

3.2 A = mean number of grade 3–4 late events for a treatment regimen during a defined late-toxicity risk period. The patient's A score is the number of high-grade events reported for that individual during the defined late-risk interval. Mean A scores, therefore, represent the number of late effects reported by a typical patient, on average, over a defined late-events interval. In principle, A scores from one or more late-risk intervals (e.g., years 1 + 2 + 3) can be added together to derive an overall A value (e.g., $A_{\text{3-year}}$).

However, for this preliminary work, we defined the late events interval as beginning with the 4-month follow-up visit and including all subsequent visits (until death or censoring) combined into a single late-risk interval).

3.3 M = risk of death attributed to cancer treatment during a given risk period. M is calculated as the cumulative incidence of death due toxicity, from study entry and up to 30 days after completion of cancer treatment, if the cause of death was attributed to treatment by the investigator.

3.4 E = end results.

All established methods for analyzing late-events data suffer from the inherent limitation of having small number of events. Traditional summary approaches to late events analysis include crude incidence and actuarial methods where all types of late events are consolidated into overall rates of high-grade injuries. These methods do not capture the duration of injuries and, therefore, tend to overestimate injury rates. An area-under-the-curve (AUC)-type approach is the only method that can measure average duration of an injury, but this method is applicable only to individual injury terms (e.g., fibrosis, necrosis). TAME methods can simultaneously summate multiple terms and have the potential to measure duration by summing adverse-event burden over multiple, smaller (e.g., every 3 months) risk intervals, thereby representing time factors in a more realistic manner (including duration via capture of onset and resolution) compared with traditional actuarial approaches (Fig. 4).

Traditional methods for summarizing adverse events systematically exclude important data, giving an inaccurate impression of the toxicity burden in complex multimodality trials. By contrast, T values use data on all high-grade adverse events. T values are proportional to the intensity of treatment, showing 500 % increase between treatment groups in acute toxicity burden in RTOG trials of head and neck cancer done during this study interval. TAME reporting provides a concise and uniform method to compare relative risk among treatment options (Trotti et al. 2007).

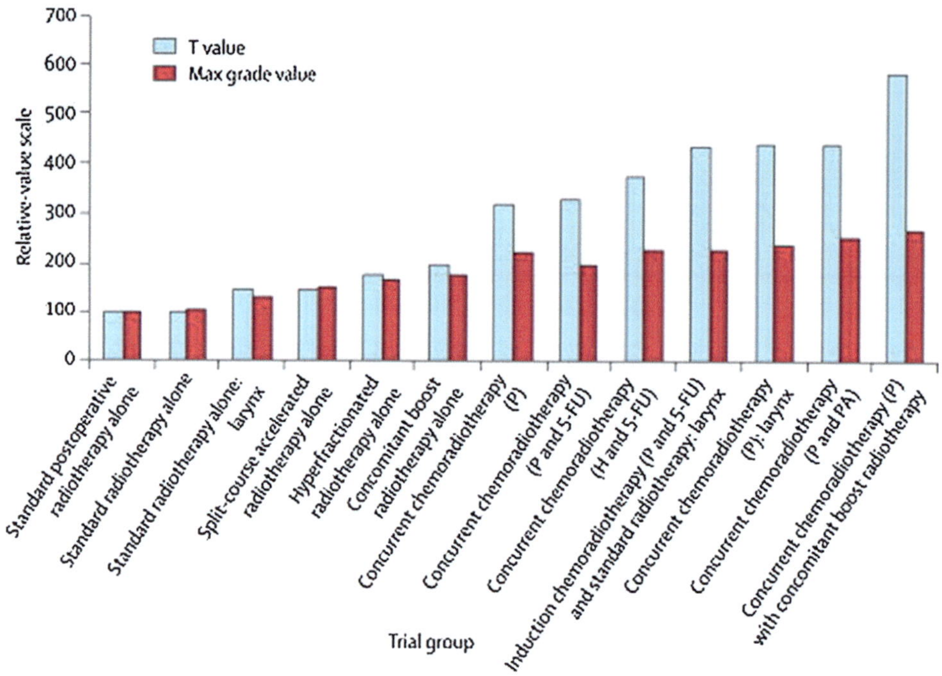

Fig. 4 The acute toxicity relative risk values (T) and relative max grade values for 13 head and neck cancer treatment groups ranked by relative risk (With permission from Trotti et al. 2007)

6 Therapeutic Ratio Determination and Decision Making

In summary, a compelling reason for developing a parallel TNM system of staging adverse effects of normal tissue is to determine therapeutic ratios. An excellent illustration is when there is no survival advantage in competitive multimodal treatment programs but one has less adverse effects. A recent report on advanced laryngeal cancers favored concurrent administration of cisplatinum and 5-fluorouracil followed by radiotherapy or surgery with primary endpoint being laryngeal preservation as well as local regional control, the latter being the same in other arm (Fajardo et al. 2001). Ideally, cure without complications is a function of cancer stage and the aggressiveness of the treatment. The classic figure of therapeutic ratio is a dose–response curve based on cancer control versus normal tissue injury with displacement to the left for cancer control and to the right for the normal tissue. The reality is the cancer control curves are displaced to the right as function of cancer stage and cancer treatment becomes more aggressive leading to more complications, displacing normal tissue effects to the left. Thus, toxicity of treatment often increases as the cancer stage advances and the therapeutic window is often closed.

References

American Cancer Society (1995) Cancer facts and figures. Atlanta, American Cancer Society

American Joint Committee on Cancer (AJCC) (2002) Cancer staging manual. 6th ed. Springer

Anacak Y, Yalman D, Ozsaran Z et al (2001) Late radiation effects to the rectum and bladder in gynecologic cancer patients: the comparison of LENT/SOMA and RTOG/EORTC late-effects scoring systems. Int J Radiat Oncol Biol Phys 50:1107–1112. http://ctep.info.nih.gov/CTC3/ctc.htm. Accessed 1 April 2003

Bragg DG, Rubin P, Hricak H (2002) Oncologic imaging, 2nd edn. WB Saunders Company, Philadelphia, PA

Cox JD, Stetz J, Pajak TF (1995) Toxicity criteria of the Radiation Therapy Oncology Group (RTOG) and the European Organization for Research and Treatment of Cancer (EORTC). Int J Radiat Oncol Biol Phys 31:1341–1346

CTCAE v3.0 (2003) Development of a comprehensive grading system for the adverse effects of cancer treatment. Semin Radiat Oncol 13(3):176–181

Davidson SE, Burns M, Routledge J et al (2002) Short report: a morbidity scoring system for clinical oncology practice: questionnaires produced from the LENT SOMA scoring system. Clin Oncol (R Coll Radiol) 14:68–69

Davidson SE, Burns MP, Routledge JA et al (2003a) The impact of radiotherapy for carcinoma of the cervix on sexual function assessed using the LENT SOMA scales. Radiother Oncol 68:241–247

Davidson SE, Burns MP, Routledge JA et al (2003b) Assessment of morbidity in carcinoma of the cervix: a comparison of the LENT SOMA scales and the Franco-Italian glossary. Radiother Oncol 69:195–200

Denis F, Garaud P, Bardet E et al (2003) Late toxicity results of the GORTEC 94–01 randomized trial comparing radiotherapy with concomitant radiochemotherapy for advanced-stage oropharynx carcinoma: comparison of LENT/SOMA, RTOG/EORTC, and NCI-CTC scoring systems. Int J Radiat Oncol Biol Phys 55:93–98

Fajardo LF, Berthrong M, Anderson RE (2001) Radiation pathology. Oxford University Press, USA

Federative Committee on Anatomical Terminology (FCAT) (1998) Terminologia Anatomica: International Anatomical Terminology. Stuttgart, Georg Thieme Verlag

Fedyk ER, Jones D, Critchley HO et al (2001) Expression of stromal-derived factor-1 is decreased by IL-1 and TNF and in dermal wound healing. J Immunol 166:5749–5754

Fehlauer F, Tribius S, Holler U et al (2003) Long-term radiation sequelae after breast-conserving therapy in women with early-stage breast cancer: an observational study using the LENT-SOMA scoring system. Int J Radiat Oncol Biol Phys 55:651–658

Forestiere AA, Goepfert H, Maor M et al (2003) Concurrent chemotherapy and radiotherapy for organ preservation in advanced laryngeal cancer. N Engl J Med 349:2091–2098

Hoeller U, Tribius S, Kuhlmey A et al (2003) Increasing the rate of late toxicity by changing the score? A comparison of RTOG/EORTC and LENT/SOMA scores. Int J Radiat Oncol Biol Phys 55:1013–1018

Husband JES, Reznek RH (1998) Imaging in oncology. ISIS Medical Media, Oxford

LENT SOMA scales all for anatomic sites. (1995). Int J Radiat Oncol Biol Phys 30;31(5):1049–1091

Mercado AM, Padgett DA, Sheridan JF et al (2002) Altered kinetics of IL-1, Il-1, and KGF-1 gene expression in early wounds of restrained mice. Brain Behav Immun 16:150–162

Miller AB, Hoogstraten B, Staquet M et al (1981) Reporting results of cancer treatment. Cancer 47:207–214

Movsas B (2003) Quality of life in oncology trials: a clinical guide. Semin Radiat Oncol 13:189–202

Petak I, Houghton JA (2001) Shared pathways: death receptors and cytotoxic drugs in cancer therapy. Pathol Oncol Res 7:95–106

Routledge JA, Burns MP, Swindell R et al (2003) Evaluation of the LENT-SOMA scales for the prospective assessment of treatment morbidity in cervical carcinoma. Int J Radiat Oncol Biol Phys 56:502–510

Rubin P (2001) Clinical Oncology, 8th edn. WB Saunders, Philadelphia, PA

Rubin P, Casarett GW (1968) Clinical Radiation Pathology. Saunders, Philadelphia, PA

Rubin P, Constine S, Fajardo L et al (1995a) Overview of Late Effects of Normal Tissues (LENT) scoring system. Int J Radiat Oncol Biol Phys 31:1041–1042

Rubin P, Constine LS, Marks L, Okunieff P (eds) (2007) Late Effects of Cancer Treatment on Normal Tissues: Cured I, Lent. Springer, Berlin Heidelberg, New York

Rubin P, Johnston CJ, Williams JP et al (1995b) A perpetual cascade of cytokines postirradiation leads to pulmonary fibrosis. Int J Radiat Oncol Biol Phys 33:99–109

Tawfiq N, Lagarde P, Stockle E, et al (2000) Conservative treatment of extremity soft tissue sarcomas. Functional evaluation using LENT-SOMA scales and Enneking scoring. Cancer Radiother (French) 4:421–7

Trotti A (2002) The evolution and application of toxicity criteria. Sem Radiat Oncol 12:1–3

Trotti A, Bentzen MS (2004) The need for adverse effects reporting standards in oncologyclinical trials. J Clinc Oncol 22:19–22

Trotti A, Rubin P (2003) Introduction. Sem Radiat Oncol 13:175

Trotti A, Byhardt R, Stetz J et al (2000) Common toxicity criteria: Version 2.0. an improved reference for grading the acute effects of cancer treatment: impact on radiotherapy. Int J Radiat Oncol Biol Phys 47:13–47

Trotti A, Colevas DA, Setser A et al (2003) CTCAE v3.0: Development of a comprehensive grading system for the adverse effects of cancer treatment. Semin Radiat Oncol 13:176–181

Trotti A, Pajak T, Gwede C, Paulus R, Cooper J, Forastiere A, Ridge J, Watkins-Bruner D, Garden A, Ang K, Curran W (2007) TAME: development of a new method for summarising adverse events of cancer treatment by the Radiation Therapy Oncology Group. Lancet Oncol 8(7):613–624. Pubmedid: 17543584

Werner-Wasik M, Pequignot E, Leeper D, Hauck W, Curran W Jr (2000) Predictors of severe esophagitis include use of concurrent chemotherapy, but not the length of irradiated esophagus: a multivariate analysis of patients with lung cancer treated with nonoperative therapy. Int J Radiat Oncol Biol Phys 48(3): 689–696

World Health Organization Icd 10 (1992) International Statistical Classification of Diseases and Related Health Problems. 10th ed. American Psychiatric Publishing

Understanding and Predicting Radiation-Associated Normal Tissue Injury: A Global and Historical Perspective

Michael T. Milano, Philip Rubin, and Lawrence B. Marks

Contents

M. T. Milano (✉) · P. Rubin
Department of Radiation Oncology, University of Rochester School of Medicine and Dentistry, 601 Elmwood Ave, Box 647 Rochester, 14642, NY, USA
e-mail: Michael_milano@urmc.rochester.edu

L. B. Marks
Department of Radiation Oncology, University of North Carolina, Chapel Hill, NC, USA

Abstract

Radiation injury to normal tissues has been recognized for many decades, and is dependent upon a multitude of factors, including radiation dose and fractionation and volume of tissue or organ exposed to radiation. Since the 1980s, technologic innovations in imaging, radiation planning and radiation delivery have allowed for more accurate quantification of dose delivery to tissues, which in turn has resulted in a burgeoning research effort to understand and quantify risks to normal tissues after radiation. This chapter will broadly discuss factors that potentially influence the risk of radiation-normal tissue injury, provide a framework for understanding the differences and similarities between organs in their response to radiation, and describe additional considerations that might be more relevant in the future. It also reviews the major efforts in past 2 decades, namely the 1991 Emami, Lyman et al. review and the recent 2010 QUANTEC reviews, which compiled published data, summarized this data, and provided recommended organ dose/volume constraints.

1 Introduction

The potentially toxic effects of radiation therapy on normal tissues have been recognized for decades. Normal tissues immediately adjacent to targets are at risk, as are normal tissues well displaced from the target that are nonetheless in the path of the treatment beam. Given the penetrating nature of therapeutic radiation beams, incidental irradiation of nontarget tissues is an unavoidable physical reality of modern external beam radiation therapy. The radiation treatment planning process is an attempt to deliver a therapeutic dose to the target tissues while "redistributing the dose" to normal tissues, in the hope of minimizing risks. The total elimination of risk is not possible. The physician therefore needs to have a firm understanding of the

P. Rubin et al. (eds.), *ALERT – Adverse Late Effects of Cancer Treatment*, Medical Radiology. Radiation Oncology,
DOI: 10.1007/978-3-540-72314-1_8, © Springer-Verlag Berlin Heidelberg 2014,

predictors for radiation-induced normal tissue injury. This knowledge helps to guide the decisions as to "where and how-much" radiation will be delivered to the different organs.

The art of radiation treatment planning largely involves the decisions on how to distribute the "undesired dose" within the surrounding normal tissue. This is largely accomplished by selecting desirable beam orientations, energies, and shapes. Other approaches to minimize dose deposition to the surrounding normal tissues include the use of compensators or segmented fields, modulated radiation beams (e.g., intensity-modulated radiation therapy—IMRT), improving targeting accuracy (i.e., image-guided radiotherapy [IGRT] and stereotactic body radiotherapy/stereotactic ablative radiotherapy [SBRT/SABR]) and/or using proton or other ion therapy. Even using the most modern radiation planning and delivery approaches, for a given geometric situation (i.e., tumor surrounding or partially surrounding a critical organ), often there is little that can be done to reduce suprathreshold dose delivery to critical organs without compromising target coverage.

Radiation Oncologists have long understood that the risk for radiation-associated normal tissue injury is dependent on a variety of factors, including:

1. The organ's inherent sensitivity to radiation (related to the cellular sensitivity as well as microscopic/macroscopic architecture/anatomy);
2. The volume of normal tissue irradiated;
3. Total radiation dose delivered;
4. The number of fractions delivered (i.e., dose per fraction);
5. The time interval during which the entire radiation course is delivered;
6. The dose rate for each fraction of the delivered radiation treatment;
7. Pre-existing medical conditions that may influence response (e.g., different levels of reserve).

There are also relatively rare known genetic factors (specifically DNA repair defects) that predispose patients to greater risks of radiation toxicity, and perhaps unknown host/genetic factors as well.

Most modern studies of radiation-associated normal tissue injury consider the dose/volume characteristics as the major determinant of risk. Prior to the wide-spread use of computer tomography (CT)-based radiation planning, the three dimensional (3D) dose distribution and the 3D anatomy were not as well understood. The wide-spread adoption of CT-planning, and modern radiation treatment planning software, has facilitated many dose/volume/outcome studies.

This chapter will broadly discuss several of the factors that influence the risk of radiation-normal tissue injury, provide a framework for understanding the differences and similarities between organs in their response to radiation, and describe additional considerations that might be more relevant in the future.

2 Factors that Influence the Risk of Radiation-Normal Tissue Injury

2.1 Inherent Cell Sensitivity, Tissue Architecture, and their Interaction

The underlying biological/physiological mechanism for radiation-induced normal tissue injury is not fully understood. Historically, radiation sensitivity was modeled with respect to inherent cell sensitivity. For example, Casarett postulated radiation sensitivity occurring along a spectrum, with uncommitted stem cells (i.e., skin and intestinal basal layers, hematopoietic blastic cells) and committed stem cells (intermediate hematopoietic cell) exhibiting relatively more radiation sensitivity than microcirculation, connective tissue, and stroma cells, reverting mature cells (i.e., liver, kidney, pancreas), and fixed mature cells (i.e., neurons) (Rubin and Casarett 1968). Similarly, Michalowski also postulated a spectrum of sensitivity with hierarchal stems cells and functional cells representing opposite ends of the spectrum (Michalowski et al. 1984). These models did not account for the heterogeneity of cells comprising most normal tissues, which generally include parenchymal cells with differing functions (i.e., alveolar cells and type II pneumocytes; or neurons and glial cells), connective tissue cells (i.e., fibroblasts), cells constituting the vascular supply, and hematopoietic cells. Broadly speaking, radiation damage may result from injury to the primary parenchymal cells (e.g., hepatocytes, neurons), injury to the supporting structures (e.g., vasculature, myelin) or a combination of mechanisms. Alternative mechanisms may also exist (e.g., modifications to local immunity). Since all organs have a vascular supply, all organs should be sensitive to vascular-mediated radiation-induced normal tissue injury. The vascular endothelial cells within small vessels are often considered the primary target for such injury. For many organs, there is a marked increase in risk of late effects when the prescribed dose exceeds approximately 60 Gy (with conventional fractionation). This observation is consistent with the hypothesis that a vascular injury might be the cause of such "high dose" injury.

Other organs demonstrate clinical dysfunction at far lower doses (e.g., the lung at approximately 30 Gy, the kidney at approximately 22 Gy, and the liver at approximately 33 Gy). This increased sensitivity maybe due to an inherent increased sensitivity of one or several of its critical components (e.g., parenchymal cells or supporting structures), or a reflection of its architecture—the manner in

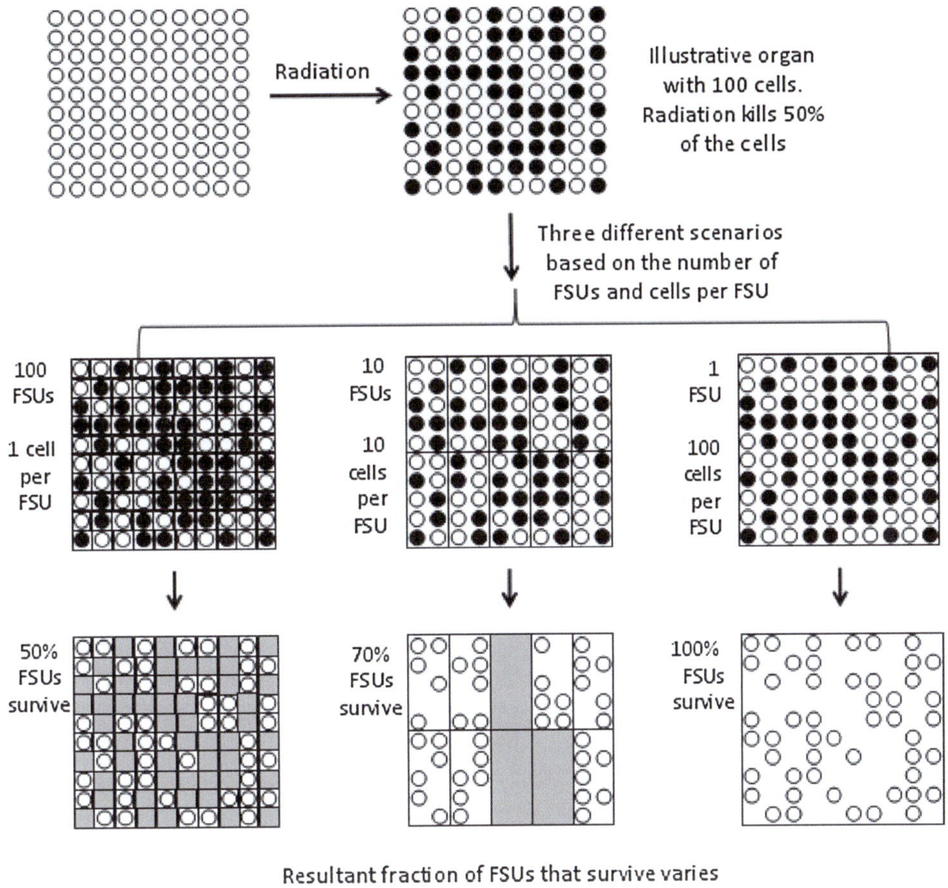

Fig. 1 A hypothetical idealized organ made up of 100 cells (*circles*), exposed to a dose of radiation that will kill (*black* cells) 50 % of the cells. For illustrative purposes, it is assumed that a FSU, represented by—*boxes*, becomes dysfunctional (*gray* filled *boxes*) if there are fewer than 5 cells remaining (i.e., if there are ≥5 cells remaining, then the FSU can be repopulated to be functional). Note how the number of FSU's that are functional after the radiation changes dramatically as the number of cells per FSU (and the total number of FSUs within the organ) changes. If there is 1 cell per FSU (*left* side), then 50 % of the FSU remain functional. If there are 100 cells per FSU (*right* side), then that FSU would remain functional. The middle panes reflect an intermediate of 10 cells per FSU, resulting in 70 % FSUs remaining functional (though conceptually this could range from 50–100 % depending on the distribution of damage to the 100 cells). Cell repopulation is not depicted in this figure

which the cells or vasculature within the organ are organized.

Two key concepts in the realm of tissue architecture include the functional subunit (FSU), and the manner in which these FSUs are 'connected to each other' to yield the overall organ function (e.g., parallel vs. series structure).

1. Functional subunit: The FSU is the minimum unit that can function independently of the remaining organ (Hall and Giaccia 2012; Marks 1996) originally described by Withers and Taylor (Withers and Taylor 1993). Irreparable damage to one subunit will render *only* that subunit dysfunctional. However, surrounding subunits will remain functional (in the absence of direct radiation damage to the surrounding FSUs). Further, any surviving cell (or minimum complement of cells) within a single FSU may repopulate its FSU, but not repopulate (or rescue from 'death') a surrounding FSU. The number of cells making up a FSU, therefore, has a profound impact on the organ sensitivity. (Fig. 1). At one extreme, if there is one FSU for the entire (hypothetical) organ, then that organ is relatively insensitive to radiation since one or just a few surviving cells can repopulate the entire organ. If there are very few cells per FSUs (at the extreme one cell per FSU), then the organ is much more sensitive to radiation. The tissue rescue unit concept (Hendry and Thames 1986) can be used to describe the minimum number of FSUs needed to maintain tissue/organ function.

Thus, the observed global sensitivity of an organ will depend on the inherent sensitivity of the target cells, as well as the number of target cells within a FSU. For example, in the kidney, each nephron has a proximal tubule, loop of Henle, and the distal tubule that are dependent on each other. One might consider the FSU to be the entire nephron,

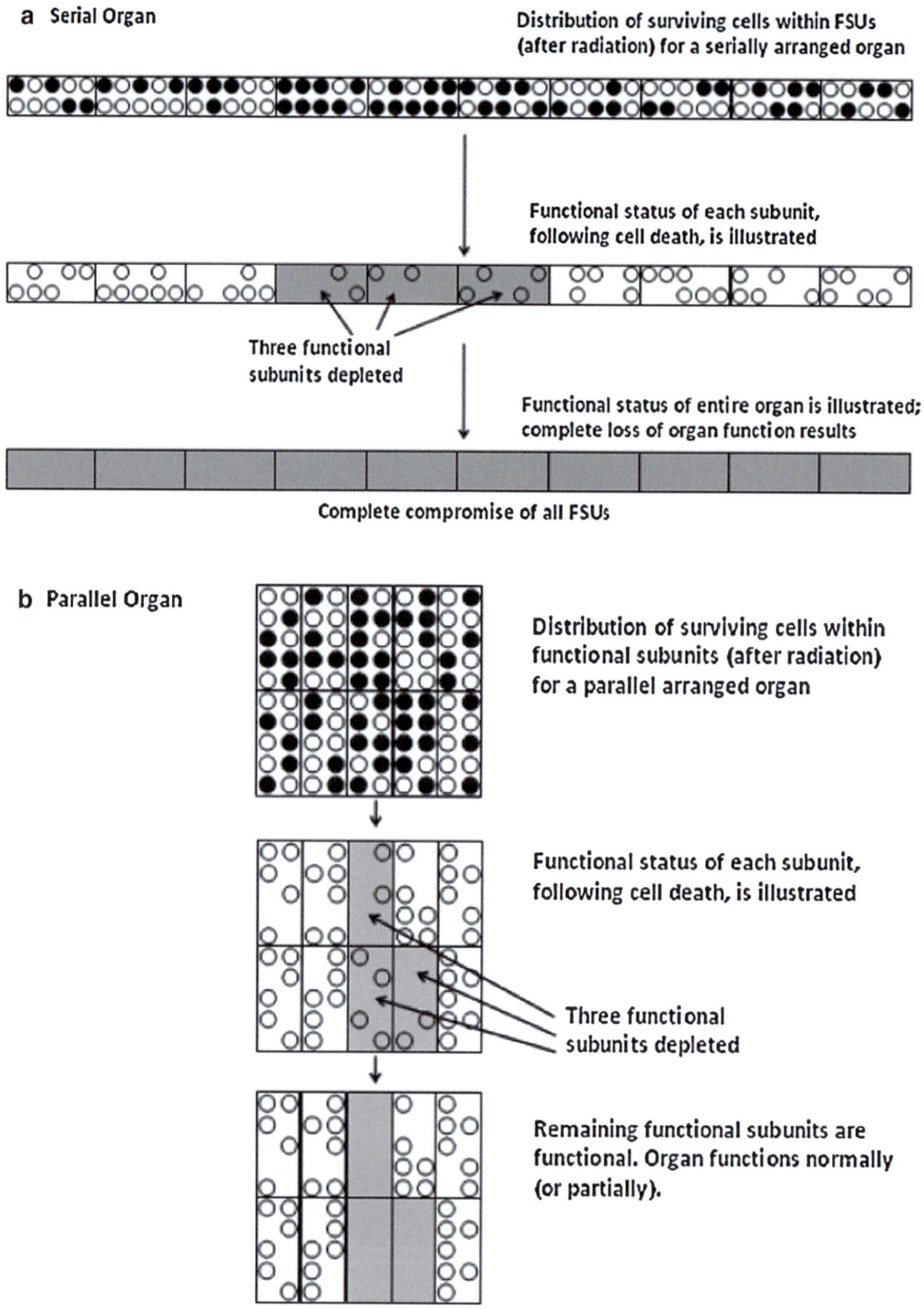

Fig. 2 Illustrative comparison of serial versus parallel organs. In this figure, the hypothetical example (depicted in Fig. 1) of 10 cells (*circles*) per functional unit (*square*) is shown, after radiation in which 50 % of cells are killed (*black circles*), and FSUs with five or more cells remain functional after radiation. Figure 2a shows an organ in which FSUs are arranged in series; the organ's function is dependent upon connectivity to its neighboring FSUs. For organs with FSUs arranged in series (**a**) damage to 1 or more FSUs (3 are damaged in figure) results in complete compromise of that component (i.e., loop of bowel, or region of spinal cord). For organs in which FSUs are arranged in parallel (**b**) damage to a portion of FSUs (3 shown in figure) results in partial, or no apparent, organ compromise. Repopulation within the FSUs is not shown

or more likely, the most sensitive subcomponent of the nephron (e.g., perhaps the arteriolar-glomerular interface). The relatively few number of cells per FSU might explain the sensitivity of the kidney to radiation, despite the large number of nephrons (or FSUs) within the kidney. FSUs are thus an often-useful construct, though it is not widely applicable to all organs. Even in the kidney, there are some inter-tubule dependencies. For example, the nephrons cannot concentrate urine without the concentration gradient created by the other nephrons globally.

2. Organizational structure between FSUs: A related consideration is the manner in which FSUs are 'connected to each other' to yield the overall organ function (Fig. 2). Normal organs can be broadly classified as having a parallel versus series architecture, analogous to electrical circuits (Hall and Giaccia 2012; Marks 1996; Withers and Taylor 1993). In parallel organs, regions of an organ can be damaged without necessarily impairing global organ function, since the other regions retain function. Just as a surgeon can remove regions of the lung, liver,

or kidney, without demonstrable impact on global organ function, large regions of these organs can be similarly irradiated to "locally-damaging" radiation doses. The global response of such "parallel organs" depends largely on the *volume* of organ affected. There is typically little effect on global function until a "critical volume" of the organ is affected, at which point global organ function can become compromised.

Conversely, in "series" organs, dysfunction of one region may render the entire organ dysfunctional. This might be the case for nerves, esophagus, intestines, or bronchi. For example, a stricture in one portion of the esophagus or bowel renders the region of esophagus or bowel both proximal and distal to that injury essentially nonfunctioning. The response of such series organs to radiation is most dependent on the maximum dose delivered to that organ (e.g., a focal hotspot in the spinal cord can cause major neurologic dysfunction).

2.2 Distribution of Function

The above discussion is idealized as many organs as typically *not* uniform. Thus, organs can be considered to have homogeneous versus heterogeneous function throughout. In homogeneous organs, different regions of the organ are relatively functionally equivalent. This might be the case for healthy lung, liver, and kidney. Nevertheless, even in these settings, there may be some regional differences in functional importance (e.g., a more favorable ventilation/profusion ratio in the lung bases versus lung apices). In other organs, variations in regional function are readily apparent (e.g., heart, brain). In these organs, the risk of radiation-associated injury is also related to the spatial distribution of radiation dose within the organ (e.g., "is the hot spot in the brain stem [critical] vs. the anterior tip of the temporal lobe [less important]). It may *not* be enough to know that 20 % of the organ is receiving >40 Gy; one may need also to know *which* 20 % of the organ is irradiated.

A good example of this phenomenon is the brain. In patients treated with radiosurgery, there is a nice relationship between the prescribed radiation dose, and the incidence of radiographic-defined radiation injury. For this endpoint, the risks are relatively similar in different regions of the brain. However, for the endpoint of symptomatic injury, the location of the effected region is critical (Flickinger et al. 2000).

Table 1 illustrates the association between the concepts of parallel versus series, and heterogeneous versus homogeneous function. Note that the distinctions are not always clear. Some organs may be considered parallel in some regards, but serial in others. For example, for the endpoint of stricture, the bowel may be considered a series organ. Conversely, for the endpoint of ulceration/bleeding, the organ may be considered parallel. These distinctions are imperfect. The different regions of small bowel are relatively homogeneous in function, but there are clearly regional differences. The entire digestive apparatus can be considered as a heterogeneous series (e.g., esophagus, stomach, intestines).

2.3 Different Paths, Different Organs, Same Outcomes

Different types of injuries can lead to the same clinical outcome. For example, damage to the alveoli (small FSUs organized in parallel), or damage to the trachea (a likely larger FSU organized in series) can both lead to shortness of breath. Similarly, adding another level of complexity, symptoms such as dyspnea can reflect lung injury, as well as heart injury, chest wall fibrosis, anemia, or any combination of the above. These realizations make the study of radiation-associated normal tissue injury even more complex and interesting.

In summary, one could then think of organs as being comprised of FSUs, which are arranged in parallel or series. The number of cells per FSU (as a theoretical construct) describes the inherent radiation sensitivity of the organs components, and the arrangement of the FSUs (parallel or series) describes how FSU damage from radiation impacts organ function. It should be recognized that the concept of a FSU describes a *model* used to explain differences in radiation sensitivity between organs. The notion that the FSU represents a separate functional unit, and that remaining cells within the FSU can repopulate the FSU in a sense is assigning two conflicting characteristics to the FSU cells: (Rubin and Casarett 1968) independent organ function and (Michalowski et al. 1984) progenitor cell differentiation to functional cells. The FSU construct also does not account for other important mediators of late effects, including small vessel vascular injury and inflammation. While all organs possess similar vascularity, conceivably, differences in radiation sensitivity between organs could reflect differences in vascular redundancy or angiogenesis after radiation. The inflammatory reaction after radiation to some extent is systemic, and therefore similar for all organs (as manifested by the release of serum cytokines). However, local inflammatory reactions, or inflammation in the setting of specific organ conditions may result in different susceptibilities to late effects. Figure 3 depicts the complicated multifaceted nature of late effects after radiation.

Table 1 Association between concepts of parallel versus series and heterogeneous versus homogeneous function

	Homogeneous	Heterogeneous
Parallel	Liver, Kidney, Lung, Alveoli (Gas Exchange)	Brain, lung with COPD, Heart, Spinal cord
Series	Small bowel, Nerve, Esophagus	Optic chiasm and nerves, Digestive Tract, Lung airways (gas conduction)

2.4 Other Confounding Factors

The study of radiation-associated normal tissue injury is also confounded by the increasing use of systemic agents for cancer therapy. Concurrent systemic agents (i.e., chemotherapy) with radiation are used for the treatment of many malignancies, to augment the effect of radiation. Incorporating chemotherapy into predictive models is challenging, as the dosing/schedules of these drugs vary, and there are often new agents being added into the mix. The exact timing of the drugs relative to the radiation treatment delivery likely impacts the degree of interaction. Furthermore, chemotherapy in the absence of radiation can result in late normal tissue effects (i.e., cardiotoxicity from anthracyclines). Often patients receive chemotherapy prior to or after radiation, and accounting for the possible interactions of these different therapies can be complicated. Likewise, prior surgical interventions can result in late complications, often resulting from post-surgical scarring and vascular disruption, as can direct effects from the tumor itself, presenting even more confounding variables.

The risk of delayed effects is further compounded by the possibility of "consequential late effects," which can develop from healing that occurs after a severe acute radiation reaction. For example, in a study from Duke, the major determinant of late esophageal stricture was the severity of the acute reaction (Ahn et al. 2005). Consequential late effects have also been described in the rectum and other organs with a brisk acute reaction (Fig. 3).

3 The Impact of Endpoint Selection

A variety of approaches can be taken to define and score radiation-associated normal tissue injury, and the approach taken will impact the reported injury *rate*. Endpoints might be broadly categorized as symptomatic/clinical (e.g., shortness of breath), imaging-based (e.g., changes on chest X-ray or CT), or analytic (e.g., reduction of pulmonary function tests or alterations in serum markers such as BUN and creatinine to assess renal function, liver enzymes, and albumin to assess liver function and TSH and thyroid hormone levels to assess thyroid function). The degree to which these different types of endpoints are related to each other is variable and organ-dependent. For example, endpoints of interest among patients undergoing thoracic radiation include shortness of breath (clinical), pulmonary function tests (analytic), and chest CT (imaging). Patients who have a decline in pulmonary function tests may be more likely to complain of shortness of breath compared to patients without a decline in pulmonary function tests. However, the presence of a change on radiographs may or may not be associated with the complaints of shortness of breath.

Furthermore, specific clinical endpoints may reflect either a regional injury (e.g., structure of the esophagus), or a global dysfunction (e.g., hepatic renal insufficiency). Most analytic endpoints are reflective of global organ function (e.g., liver function tests, creatinine, pulmonary function tests). There are some association between the different endpoints and their impact on global function, and their relationship with each other, and the organ's structure (parallel vs. series, and heterogeneous vs. homogeneous). For example, imaging typically can detect changes in *regional* structure/anatomy. Again in the lung, there is very good data that relates regional radiologic changes (in tissue density [CT] or blood perfusion) to regional radiation dose (Mah and Van Dyk 1988; Marks et al. 1997; Ma et al. 2009, 2010; Boersma et al. 1993). However, the degree to which the "average" regional radiographic change relates to the change in global function is far less clear. In several studies, the sum of regional injuries (or the average change in regional imaging) is only weakly related to changes in global function (Fan et al. 2001a, b; Seppenwoolde et al. 2004). Further, the relationship between the sum of regional injuries and changes in global function will necessarily relate to the *distribution of a function* within the organ (i.e., is the "global" function impacted equally by each region of the lung). Figure 4 depicts an example of the interaction between the various endpoints after radiation to the lung.

4 Tolerance Dose and Dose/Volume/ Outcome Considerations

4.1 Historical Background

4.1.1 Introduction: Historical Perspective, Background, and Significance

The need to precisely measure and quantify the radiation dose became evident with its discovery by Roentgen and the Curies. The early pioneers unwittingly exposed themselves to radiation in exploring its possible applications in medicine and ultimately realized that radiation resulted in adverse normal tissue reactions. The initial observation of skin erythema and alterations in blood/bone marrow

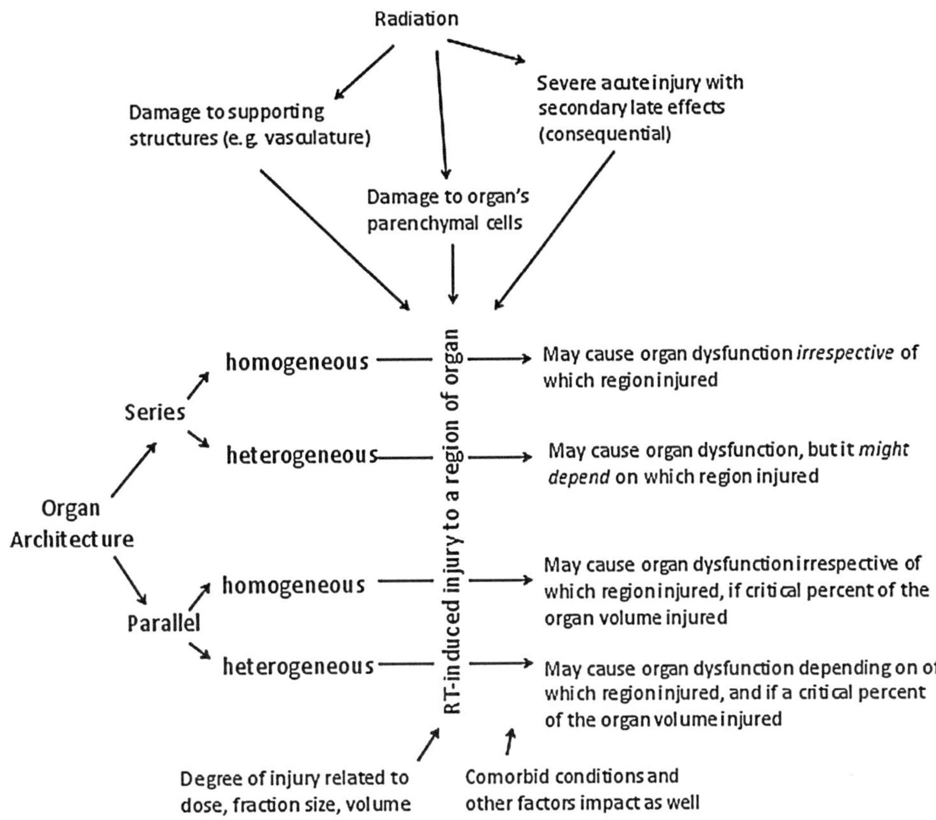

Fig. 3 There are many variables which impact development of late effects, as described in the text

translate in time to neoplasia, which proved fatal. Radiation claimed the lives of its researchers who became its "martyrs," sacrificing themselves to uncover its potential uses. Through decades of research, the benefits of therapeutic radiation were realized, and ultimately, the field of Radiation Oncology was born.

Radiation is a double-edged sword as a treatment modality in that it cures and injures simultaneously. In the early years of therapeutic radiation, with the use of relatively low energy radiation, skin toxicity was the primary dose-limiting factor. With the introduction of megavoltage radiation therapy, the radiocurability of a large variety of cancers became possible due to improved capability of delivering therapeutic dose to greater depth. Historically, radiation therapy fields/doses were selected empirically, based largely on experience. Physicians relied on clinical intuition to select field sizes/doses. They understood that these empiric guidelines were imprecise and did not fully reflect the underlying anatomy, physiology, and dosimetry.

4.1.2 Dose-Limiting Normal Tissues

With the widespread adoption of megavoltage radiation, there arose a need to better understand the tolerance of internal organs to radiation. The National Cancer Institute (NCI) mandated and sponsored research conferences to explore dose/time relationships to define "tumor lethal doses" and "normal tissue tolerance doses". Figure 5 depicts a hypothetical dose–response curves for tumor control and normal tissue complication; ideally the therapeutic dose is chosen to maximize tumor control while minimizing toxicity risks, as graphically demonstrated by the "uncomplicated tumor control" curve.

The biometric of normal tissue tolerance doses was initially described by Rubin and Casarett (Rubin and Casarett 1968, 1972) and remains a commonly used metric. The minimal tolerance doses, with respect to specified toxicity endpoints, were described by the $TD_{5/5}$ (i.e., the dose which results in a 5 % severe complication rate within 5 years) and the $TD_{50/5}$ (i.e., the dose that results in 50 % severe complication rate in 5 years). Radiation oncologists are often faced with the clinical dilemma whereby the optimum dose for tumor control exceeds the normal tissue dose tolerance of what are considered vital "dose limiting normal tissues". With the impetus of defining therapeutic ratios in RTOG protocols, Rubin, Phillips, et al. defined tolerance doses into three categories: (Rubin and Casarett 1968, 1972).

Class 1: Organs in which radiation lesions can be fatal or result in severe morbidity (See Table 5 in Chap. 2).

Class 2: Organs in which radiation lesions can result in moderate to mild morbidity, generally late effects are compatible with survival (see Table 6 in Chap. 2).

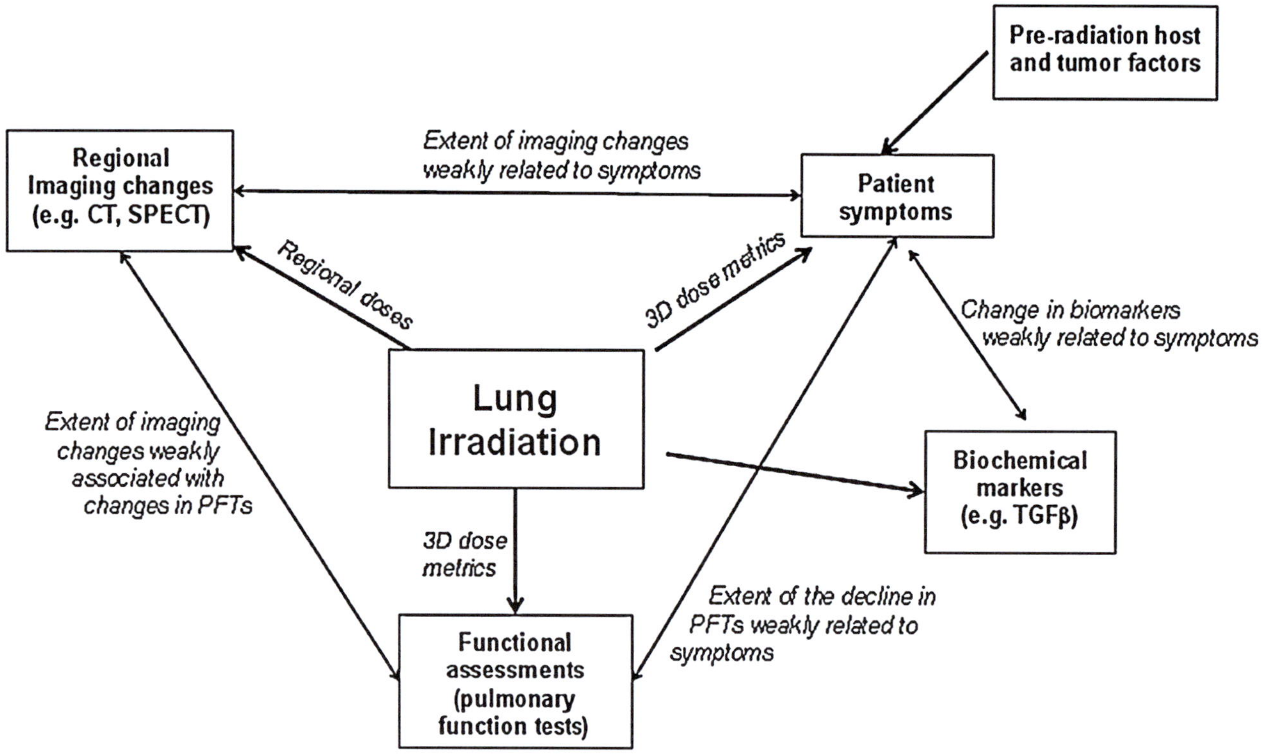

Fig. 4 A schematic representing the impact of localized radiation to the lung on global subjective and objective pulmonary function. *Regional* lung radiation is associated with reasonably well described dose-dependent *regional* imaging changes. The *sum* of *regional* injuries (perhaps reflected by the regional imaging changes) is weakly associated with changes in global lung function (e.g., pulmonary symptoms, objective declines in pulmonary function) or cytokine release. A similar construct could also be considered for the heart where there are also dose-dependent changes in *regional* myocardial perfusion, and where the presence/severity of these regional perfusion defects is perhaps weakly related to changes in regional function (e.g., regional wall motion) or global function (e.g., ejection fraction)

Class 3: Organs in which radiation lesions result in mild, transient, reversible effects, and in no morbidity (see Table 7 in Chap. 2).

4.1.3 Tolerance Volumes (Rubin et al.)

The concept of tolerance volume is defined in the same fashion as tolerance dose. The dose to a given volume or organ/tissue frequently proves to be more predictive of complication risks. It is possible to obliterate or lose a certain volume of a vital organ with suprathreshold doses, akin to surgical resection (i.e., stereotactic radiation surgery). Depending on the organ, loss of some volume may not affect organ survival because that organ can compensate for volume loss, up to a threshold volume, through regeneration or hypertrophy (i.e., liver) and/or remain, although impaired, within functional tolerance for survival (i.e., kidney or lung). Different organs demonstrate a range of tolerance volume (TV) parameters:

1. $TV_{5–25}$: 5–25 % of the organ volume irradiated above suprathreshold doses can result in a life-threatening or lethal complication.
2. $TV_{50–90}$: 50–90 % of the organ volume irradiated above suprathreshold doses can result in a life-threatening or lethal complication.

There are generally two levels of critical volume for dose-limiting vital organs. The gastrointestinal tract, proximal tracheal-bronchial airway, and central nervous system (CNS) can have disastrous outcomes after small volumes (TV 5–10 %) are exposed to doses exceeding $TD_{5–50}$. However, it is important to note that necrotic bowel and necrotic CNS foci can occasionally be resected successfully. For the majority of organs considered dose-limiting, such as bone marrow, lung, kidney, heart, and liver, high doses can be tolerated to relatively small volumes. Such organs may decompensate when more than 50 % of the total volume (as applied to paired organs) is exceeded and threaten survival.

The time when organ decompensation begins clearly depends on the compensatory regenerative mechanisms that come into play when significant organ volume loss occurs. The dose–response curve is not an absolute or fixed effect but varies as a function of volume (Fig. 6a). This is an

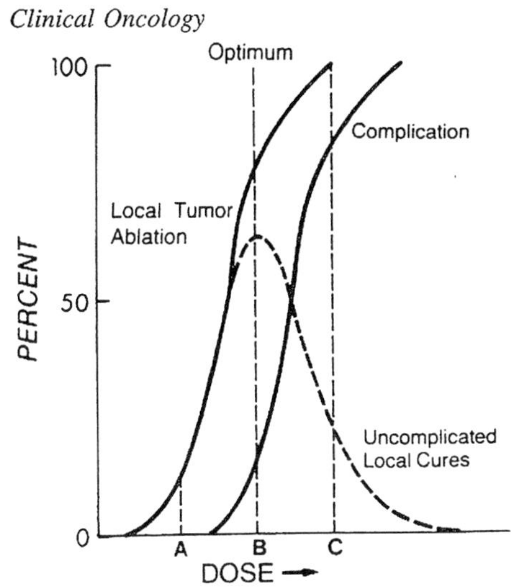

Fig. 5 The hypothetical dose–response curves for tumor control and normal tissue complication are shown, along with the associated curve for 'Uncomplicated Tumor Control", [From Rubin Clinical Oncology 8th edn. Treatment outcomes. Uncomplicated cures (*dashed lines*) are the desired result of treatment. This is illustrated as a function of the therapeutic ratio, i.e. the greater the separation between the tumor control (ablation) curve and the normal tissue complication curve, the greater the number of uncomplicated cures that will result. *A*, *B*, and *C* represent three different dose levels that if chosen, would lead to three diffrent outcomes. *A* would result in few tumor cures but no complications. *C* would lead to complicate cure in many cases, but virtually all patients would suffer complications. The optimal choice in this group of dose levels is *B*, which would result in the greatest number of cured patients without complications. (Adapted from Mendelsohn 1969 with permission)]

important concept because it describes why large doses can be delivered to partial volumes. For TD_5 and TD_{50}, the dose increases as the volume decreases.

4.1.4 Tolerance Dose/Volume/Injury Concept (Lyman and Wolbarst)

An important and insightful concept was developed by Lyman, in which the dose response curve is not an absolute or fixed effect but varies as a function of organ volume. A 3D construct allowed for a method of assessing complication probabilities from dose volume histograms (Fig. 6a) this concept provided the radiation oncologist with a guide as to varying the dose depending on volume (Fig. 6b). This concept applied to organ tolerance doses, was then published by Emami, Lyman et al. (discussed below).

4.1.5 Tolerance Volume: Focal/Global Injury

Marks (1996) related the concepts of focal and global injury to clinical endpoints. The diagram linking these factors for the bladder (as an example) is shown in Fig. 7. For many organs, either, or both, focal and global injury are most clinically relevant (Table 2).

4.1.6 Emami and QUANTEC: Summary of Normal Tissue Dose/Volume (Emami, Lyman et al., and Marks et al.)

In the late 1980s and early 1990s, 3D planning systems were providing clinicians with a plethora of information. A great promise of 3D treatment planning was quantitative correlates of doses/volumes with clinical outcomes. This promise was partly delivered; guidelines were needed to help physicians predict the relative safety of proposed treatment plans, although only limited data were available. In 1991, to meet this need, investigators pooled their clinical experience, judgment, and information regarding whole organ partial organ tolerance doses, and produced the "Emami and Lyman paper" (Emami et al. 1991). This report was, and remains, a landmark summary of decades—worth of data for a wide variety of organs, supplemented with expert opinion where data were lacking. While this paper is often criticized, it clearly stated the uncertainties and limitations in its recommendations, and it is widely admired for addressing a clinical need.

During the decades of the 1990s and 2000s, numerous studies reported associations between dose/volume parameters and normal tissue outcomes. Much of this was reviewed by Milano et al. in 2007 (Milano et al. 2007, 2008). In 2007, a joint task force of physicists and physicians was formed, with the support of ASTRO and AAPM, to summarize the available data in a format useful to clinicians and to update/refine the estimates provided by Emami, Lyman. The resulting quantitative analysis of normal tissue effects in the clinic (QUANTEC) review articles (published in a special issue of the *International Journal of Radiation Oncology, Biology, and Physics* in March, 2010) summarized the available data. A central goal of QUANTEC was to update and refine the estimates provided by Emami, Lyman et al. and summarize published information in a clinically useful manner (Marks et al. 2010a, b). A summary table from the Quantec effort is shown in Table 3.

A brief summary of historical landmarks described above, along with our opinion regarding the key contributions and shortcomings of these reviews, are provided in Fig. 8 and Table 4.

4.2 The Incorporation of 3D Dose/Volume Information into Clinical Guidelines

The study of radiation dose/volume/outcome was revolutionized with the advent of treatment planning computers and imaging software, which enabled appreciation of the 3D relationship of the delivered radiation dose relative to the underlying anatomy. The introduction of 3D treatment planning offered the promise of quantitative correlates of

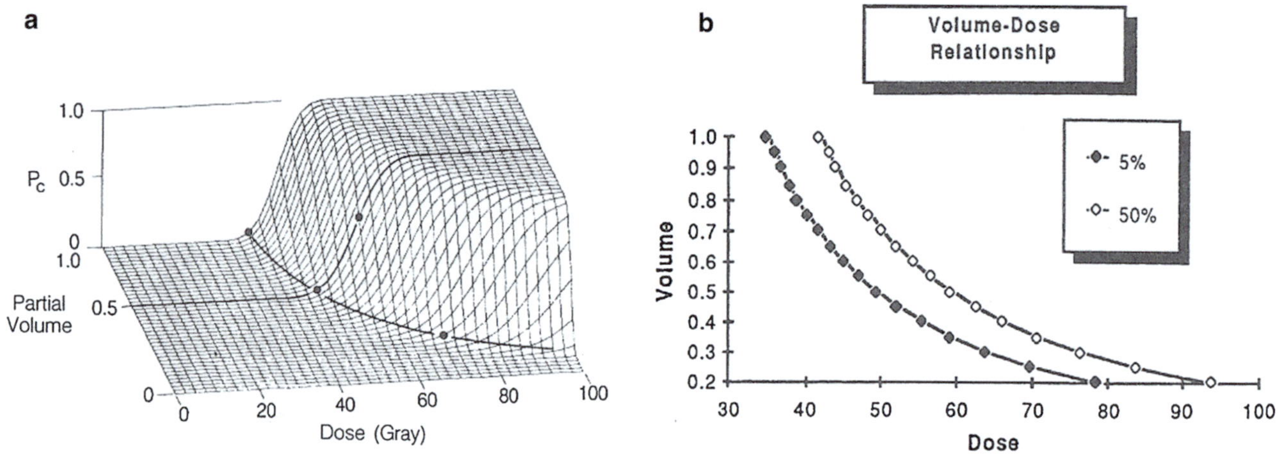

Fig. 6 Volume effect: (**a**) The dose response curve is not an absolute or fixed effect but varies as a function of volume. (**b**) For TD_5 and TD_{50}, the dose increases as the volume decreases. Note that the slope changes as more than 50 % of the whole organ is included. Small increments in dose, that is, 10–20 %, can prove to be lethal. From Rubin Clinical Oncology 8th edn. This important concept allows the radiation oncologist to give much larger doses to partial volumes. (From Lyman and Wolbrast 1987 with permission from Elsiever Science)

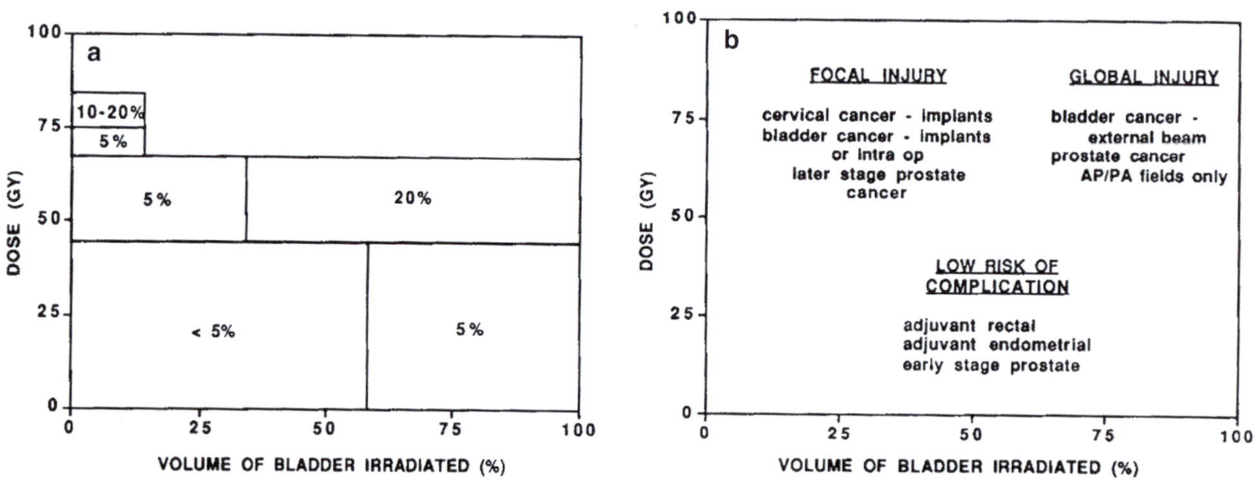

Fig. 7 A schematic diagram illustrating the dose-volume relationship to complications, using urinary bladder as an example. This is shown in two different ways in panels **a** and **b**. In panel **a**, the approximate overall serious complication rate is shown as a function of the dose delivered and volume exposed. The corresponding clinical situations are shown in panel **b**. Global bladder injury appears to occur when the total dose to the bladder exceeds 50–55 Gy. A focal bladder injury occurs when the dose to a portion of the bladder exceeds approximately 70–75 Gy, Marks (1995)

doses/volumes with clinical outcomes. Before the Emami and Lyman paper (Emami et al. 1991) was published in 1991, systematic dose/volume/outcome data to guide clinical decisions were limited. The Emami and Lyman paper provided a summary table where the risk of injury was related to the dose/volume received by any organ. While the authors reported the one-third and two-thirds partial organ tolerance doses, for the most part, the clinical experience which provided the basis for the these tolerance doses was based upon 2D radiation planning and delivery. For close to 20 years, the Emami and Lyman report was the basis for 3D radiation dose/volume prescriptions. The sixteen organ-specific QUANTEC papers, published in 2010, exhaustively, and systematically reviewed relevant studies of radiation dose-volume affects on normal tissue; Marks et al. produced a summary table of these reviews, providing evidenced-based dose-volume metrics for each of the reviewed organ sites (Marks et al. 2010b). Major differences between the Emami and Lyman paper and QUANTEC reviews are discussed below.

Table 2 Example clinically relevant focal and global endpoints for various organs

Organ	Focal endpoint	Global endpoint
Brain and cranial nerves	Focal weakness, blindness	Neurocognitive decline
Eye	Visual field cut	Acuity
Lung	Bronchial stricture	Dyspnea
Heart	Coronary stenosis	Pericarditis, reduced ejection fraction
Esophagus	Stricture, ulcer	
Bladder	Bleeding	Reduced capacity, urinary frequency
Bowel	Stricture, bleeding	Malabsorption
Kidney		Reduced renal clearance
Liver		Reduced hepatic function

4.3 Dose-Volume Histograms and Associated Figures of Merit

3D dose/volume data can be difficult for clinicians to readily digest. Visualizing isodose distributions are challenging and comparing competing distributions are almost impossible. Therefore, dose-volume histograms (DVH's; essentially 2D representations of the 3D data) were embraced as a rapid way to summarize the dose distribution. Note that DVH's discard information regarding the spatial character of dose as well as (usually) variations in fraction size.

Despite the marked data reduction in going from a 3D plan to a DVH, DVHs also remain challenging for clinicians to consider and compare. Therefore, it has become attractive to further data reduce, and extract 'figures of merit' from the DVH (Fig. 9). Examples include:

a. Vx reflects the volume of tissue (generally a percentage) receiving ≥X Gy. This is probably the most commonly used metric for parallel-type organs such as the lung and kidney. For these, as discussed above, the portions of the organ exposed to a "regionally-injuring" dose of radiation will become dysfunctional. Thus, the percent of the organ exposed to that dose is a useful parameter.
b. Dx reflects the minimum dose to the hottest x % (generally percentage of total volume) of tissue. This parameter is not widely used clinically. It might be most useful for parallel-type organs where the percent of an organ's function that can be lost is known (e.g., let's say 30 %). Then, if the D30 is less than the locally injuring dose, global organ function should remain. Similarly, for organs where an injury might be clinically manifest if there is a hotspot of a particular size, the Dx, where x is equal to that critical size, might be a useful parameter to predict outcomes.
c. Dmax is the maximum dose delivered to an organ, and is most useful for series organs. Dmax is analogous to Dx as the volume x decreases toward zero.
d. Mean dose is the simple arithmetic average of the dose to an organ. For parallel organs where there is a gradual dose response function for radiation-induced regional injury, the mean dose might reasonably correlate with outcomes.
e. More complex modeling has also been widely used to extract figures of merit that better reflect the entire DVH, rather than a single point (e.g., Dmax, Dx, Vx). These models will "sum up" the risk associated with each component of a DVH, and apply different methods of summing, depending on the type (or architecture/structure) of the organ. For example, for a series-structured organ, the high-dose region of the DVH might be most weighted more heavily in the "summing" while this is less strongly considered in a parallel-structured organ. Early work in this area lead to the Lyman, Kutcher Burman (LKB) model, and more recently the equivalent uniform dose (EUD) model, that both reduce a DVH to a single normal tissue complication probability (NTCP). These models and their relationships are summarized elsewhere (Marks et al. 2010b).

The Emami et al. report systematically used the same DVH-based construct across many organs; e.g., the TD 5/5 and TD 50/5 for the uniform irradiation of one-third, two-thirds, and the whole volume of an organ (Emami et al. 1991). This uniform approach enabled the application of "single unifying models" of dose/volume/outcome across organs. For example, the dose/volume/outcome estimates from Emami et al. were used by Lyman, Kutcher, Burman et al. (Burman et al. 1991; Kutcher et al. 1991; Lyman 1985) to generate a set of organ-specific model parameters. Such a uniform approach is attractive.

During the past two decades, many clinical dose/volume/outcome reports computed parameters for these "unifying models" [e.g., Ten Haken et al. (Chapet et al. 2005; Ten Haken et al. 1993, 2006)]. However, the majority of published clinical dose/volume/outcome data generated over the past two decades has used alternative approaches/models that appeared to be better suited to specific organs. Therefore, the dose/volume/outcome data available for the QUANTEC review was not of a uniform format. Outcomes across organs were correlated with a diverse array of dose/volume metrics (e.g., threshold volumes [Vx], threshold doses [Dx], mean doses). Therefore, the QUANTEC review included model-based parameters for just a few organs, and not always in a systematic fashion.

Table 3 QUANTEC Summary: Approximate Dose/Volume/Outcome Data for Several Organs Following Conventional Fractionation (Unless Otherwise Noted)*

Organ	Volume segmented	Irradiation type (partial organ unless otherwise stated)[†]	Endpoint	Dose (Gy), or dose/volume parameters[†]	Rate (%)	Notes on dose/volume parameters
Brain	Whole organ	3D-CRT	Symptomatic necrosis	Dmax <60	<3	Data at 72 and 90 Gy, extrapolated from BED models
	Whole organ	3D-CRT	Symptomatic necrosis	Dmax = 72	5	
	Whole organ	3D-CRT	Symptomatic necrosis	Dmax = 90	10	
	Whole organ	SRS (single fraction)	Symptomatic necrosis	V12 <5–10 cc	<20	Rapid rise when V12 > 5–10 cc
Brain stem	Whole organ	Whole organ	Permanent cranial neuropathy or necrosis	Dmax <54	<5	
	Whole organ	3D-CRT	Permanent cranial neuropathy or necrosis	D1-10 cc[‖] ≤59	<5	
	Whole organ	3D-CRT	Permanent cranial neuropathy or necrosis	Dmax <64	<5	Point dose <<1 cc
	Whole organ	SRS (single fraction)	Permanent cranial neuropathy or necrosis	Dmax <12.5	<5	For patients with acoustic tumors
Optic nerve/ chiasm	Whole organ	3D-CRT	Optic neuropathy	Dmax <55	<3	Given the small size, 3D CRT is often whole organ[‡‡]
	Whole organ	3D-CRT	Optic neuropathy	Dmax 55–60	3–7	
	Whole organ	3D-CRT	Optic neuropathy	Dmax >60	>7–20	
	Whole organ	SRS (single fraction)	Optic neuropathy	Dmax <12	<10	
Spinal cord	Partial organ	3D-CRT	Myelopathy	Dmax = 50	0.2	Including full cord cross-section
	Partial organ	3D-CRT	Myelopathy	Dmax = 60	6	
	Partial organ	3D-CRT	Myelopathy	Dmax = 69	50	
	Partial organ	SRS (single fraction)	Myelopathy	Dmax =13	1	Partial cord cross-section irradiated 3 fractions, partial cord cross-section irradiated
	Partial organ	SRS (hypofraction)	Myelopathy	Dmax = 20	1	
Cochlea	Whole organ	3D-CRT	Sensory neural hearing loss	Mean dose ≤45	<30	Mean dose to cochlear, hearing at 4 kHz
	Whole organ	SRS (single fraction)	Sensory neural hearing loss	Prescription dose ≤14	<25	Serviceable hearing
Parotid	Bilateral whole parotid glands	3D-CRT	Long term parotid salivary function reduced to <25% of pre-RT level	Mean dose <25	<20	For combined parotid glands[¶]
	Unilateral whole parotid gland	3D-CRT	Long term parotid salivary function reduced to <25% of pre-RT level	Mean dose <20	<20	For single parotid gland. At least one parotid gland spared to <20 Gy[¶]
	Bilateral whole parotid glands	3D-CRT	Long term parotid salivary function reduced to <25% of pre-RT level	Mean dose <39	<50	For combined parotid glands (per Fig. 3 in paper) [¶]
Pharynx	Pharyngeal constrictors	Whole organ	Symptomatic dysphagia and aspiration	Mean dose <50	<20	Based on Section B4 in paper

(continued)

Table 3 (continued)

Organ	Volume segmented	Irradiation type (partial organ unless otherwise stated)†	Endpoint	Dose (Gy), or dose/volume parameters†	Rate (%)	Notes on dose/volume parameters
Larynx	Whole organ	3D-CRT	Vocal dysfunction	Dmax <66	<20	With chemotherapy, based on single study (see Section A4.2 in paper)
	Whole organ	3D-CRT	Aspiration	Mean dose <50	<30	With chemotherapy, based on single study (see Fig. 1 in paper)
	Whole organ Whole organ	3D-CRT 3D-CRT	Edema Edema	Mean dose <44 V50 <27%	<20 <20	Without chemotherapy, based on single study in patients without larynx cancer**
Lung	Whole organ	3D-CRT	Symptomatic pneumonitis	V20 ≤ 30%	<20	For combined lung. Gradual dose response
	Whole organ	3D-CRT 3D-CRT 3D-CRT 3D-CRT 3D-CRT	Symptomatic pneumonitis	Mean dose = 7 Mean dose =13 Mean dose = 20 Mean dose = 24 Mean dose = 27	5 10 20 30 40	Excludes purposeful whole lung irradiation
Esophagus	Whole organ	3D-CRT	Grade ≥3 acute esophagitis	Mean dose <34	5–20	Based on RTOG and several studies
	Whole organ Whole organ Whole organ	3D-CRT 3D-CRT 3D-CRT	Grade ≥2 acute esophagitis Grade≥2 acute esophagitis Grade ≥2 acute esophagitis	V35 <50% V50 <40% V70 <20%	<30 <30 <30	A variety of alternate threshold doses have been implicated. Appears to be a dose/volume response
Heart	Pericardium Pericardium	3D-CRT 3D-CRT	Pericarditis Pericarditis	Mean dose <26 V30 <46%	<15 <15	Based on single study
	Whole organ	3D-CRT	Long-term cardiac mortality	V25 <10%	<1	Overly safe risk estimate based on model predictions
Liver	Whole liver - GTV Whole liver - GTV	3D-CRT or Whole organ 3D-CRT	Classic RILD‡‡ Classic RILD	Mean dose <30–32 Mean dose <42	<5 <50	Excluding patients with pre-existing liver disease or hepatocellular carcinoma, as tolerance doses are lower in these patients
	Whole liver - GTV Whole liver - GTV	3D-CRT or Whole organ 3D-CRT	Classic RILD Classic RILD	Mean dose <28 Mean dose <36	<5 <50	In patients with Child-Pugh A preexisting liver disease or hepatocellular carcinoma, excluding hepatitis B reactivation as an endpoint
	Whole liver -GTV Whole liver - GTV	SBRT (hypofraction) SBRT (hypofraction) SBRT (hypofraction) SBRT (hypofraction)	Classic RILD Classic RILD Classic RILD Classic RILD	Mean dose <13 Mean dose <18 Mean dose <15 Mean dose <20	<5 <5 <5 <5	3 fractions, for primary liver cancer 6 fractions, for primary liver cancer 3 fractions, for liver metastases 6 fractions, for liver metastases
	>700 cc of normal liver	SBRT (hypofraction)	Classic RILD	D_{max} <15	<5	Critical volume based, in 3–5 fractions
Kidney	Bilateral whole kidney‡ Bilateral whole kidney‡	Bilateral whole organ or 3D-CRT Bilateral whole organ	Clinically relevant renal dysfunction Clinically relevant renal dysfunction	Mean dose <15–18 Mean dose <28	<5 <50	
	Bilateral whole kidney‡	3D-CRT	Clinically relevant renal dysfuntction	V12 <55% V20 <32% V23 <30% V28 <20%	<5	For combined kidney

(continued)

Table 3 (continued)

Organ	Volume segmented	Irradiation type (partial organ unless otherwise stated)[†]	Endpoint	Dose (Gy), or dose/volume parameters[†]	Rate (%)	Notes on dose/volume parameters
Stomach	Whole organ	Whole organ	Ulceration	D100‖ D_{min}<45	<7	
Small bowel	Individual small bowel loops	3D-CRT	Grade ≥ 3 acute toxicity[§]	V15 <120 cc	<10	Volume based on segmentation of the individual loops of bowel, not the entire potential peritoneal space
	Entire potential space within peritoneal cavity	3D-CRT	Grade ≥ 3 acute toxicity[§]	V45 <195 cc	<10	Volume based on the entire potential space within the peritoneal cavity
Rectum	Whole organ Whole organ Whole organ Whole organ Whole organ	3D-CRT 3D-CRT 3D-CRT 3D-CRT 3D-CRT	Grade ≥ 2 late rectal toxicity Grade ≥ 3 late rectal toxicity, Grade ≥ 2 late rectal toxicity Grade ≥ 3 late rectal toxicity, Grade ≥ 2 late rectal toxicity Grade ≥ 3 late rectal toxicity, Grade ≥ 2 late rectal toxicity Grade ≥ 3 late rectal toxicity, Grade ≥ 2 late rectal toxicity Grade ≥ 3 late rectal toxicity,	V50 <50% V60 <35% V65 <25% V70 <20% V75 <15%	<15 <10 <15 <10 <15 <10 <15 <10 <15 <10	Prostate cancer treatment
Bladder	Whole organ	3D-CRT	Grade ≥ 3 late RTOG	Dmax <65	<6	Bladder cancer treatment. Variations in bladder size/shape/ location during RT hamper ability to generate accurate data
	Whole organ	3D-CRT	Grade ≥3 late RTOG	V65 ≤50 % V70 ≤35 % V75 ≤25 % V80 ≤15 %		Prostate cancer treatment Based on current RTOG 0415 recommendation
Penile bulb	Whole organ Whole organ Whole organ	3D-CRT 3D-CRT 3D-CRT	Severe erectile dysfunction Severe erectile dysfunction Severe erectile dysfunction	Mean dose to 95% of gland <50 D90[‖] <50 D60–70 <70	<35 <35 <55	

Abbreviations: 3D-CRT = 3-dimensional conformal radiotherapy, SRS = stereotactic radiosurgery, BED = Biologically effective dose, SBRT = stereotactic body radiotherapy, RILD = radiation-induced liver disease, RTOG = Radiation Therapy Oncology Group

* All data are estimated from the literature summarized in the QUANTEC reviews unless otherwise noted. Clinically, these data should be applied with caution. Clinicians are strongly advised to use the individual QUANTEC articles to check the applicability of these limits to the clinical situation at hand. They largely do not reflect modern IMRT. The figures and sections noted in the far right-hand column refer to the individual QUANTEC papers

† All at standard fractionation (i.e., 1.8-2.0 Gy per daily fraction) unless otherwise noted. Vx is the volume of the organ receiving ≥ x Gy. Dmax = Maximum radiation dose

‡ Non-TBI

§ With combined chemotherapy

‖ Dx = minimum dose received by the ''hottest'' x% (or x cc's) of the organ.D100 = minimum dose

¶ Severe xerostomia is related to additional factors including the doses to the submandibular glands

** Estimated by Dr. Eisbruch

†† Classic Radiation induced liver disease (RILD) involves anicteric hepatomegaly and ascites, typically occurring between 2 weeks and 3 months after therapy. Classic RILD also involves elevated alkaline phosphatase (more than twice the upper limit of normal or baseline value)

‡‡ For optic nerve, the cases of neuropathy in the 55 to 60 Gy range received ≈59 Gy (see optic nerve paper for details). Excludes patients with pituitary tumors where the tolerance may be reduced

Table 4 Historical overview of several summaries of dose/volume/outcome information

Report	Key contributions	Key shortcomings
Rubin, NCI contract	Introduced the concept of TD 5/5 and 50/5	Minimal dose/volume data
Rubin RTOG	Categorized organs into classes based on sensitivity	Minimal dose/volume data
Emami, 1991	Concise summary addressing most clinically meaningful endpoints in a uniform manner Based on available data and expert opinion	Dose/volume relationship based on limited data and, thus, much expert opinion
QUANTEC, 2010	Driven largely by the available 3D dose/volume/outcome data Systematic review addressing many challenges such as organ delineation and confounding factors such as chemotherapy	Since dose/volume/outcome data on all meaningful clinical outcomes are *not* available, the summary is not able to guide all clinical practice

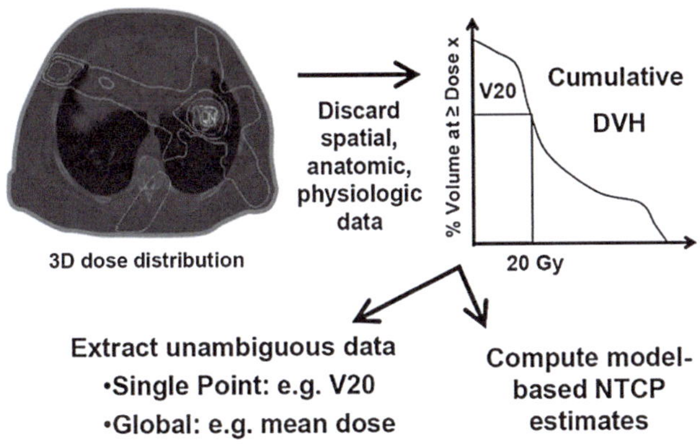

Fig. 8 The derivation of figures of merit from a complex 3D dose distribution that are then tested for correlation with normal tissue toxicity endpoints. From Marks (2010b)

4.4 Shortcomings of DVHs

1. The use of DVHs inherently assumes that all regions of an organ are of equal importance, and that function is distributed relatively uniformly throughout the organ. This may not be the case for many organs.
2. Further, even if the organ is of uniform structure throughout, the global structure of the organ may reduce the utility of DVHs. For example, in tubular structures (e.g., bowel), the circumferential and longitudinal nature of the radiation dose may be pertinent but is not considered.
3. Differences in fraction size are typically ignored when computing a DVH, though one can apply a mathematical "correction." However, there must be some a priori assumption that the impact of fraction size is understood in order to apply such a correction.
4. For patients that are treated with sequential groups of beams (i.e., boost treatment), there will be unique DVHs for each portion of therapy. Exactly how to combine these DVHs is unclear, especially if there have been anatomic changes between the sequential portions of therapy. Indeed, even if there is one plan used throughout treatment, anatomic changes might make the DVH inaccurate. Just "adding up DVHs" is often not possible. For parameters such as mean dose, one can simply "add up" the mean dose from sequential phases of therapy (assuming the volume remains constant). However, for parameters such as V20, one needs to fuse the 3D dose distributions from sequential phases of therapy to generate a 'composite plan' (and assume spatial consistency as well). Additional challenges occur since the fraction size within each region might be variable between the different portions of therapy.
5. There is a tendency to "over contour" critical structures, often to be "really sure" that fields are shaped to limit exposure and that set-up irregularities do not result in excess exposure. The resultant DVHs thus may not accurately reflect the dose/volume characteristics of the target tissues.
6. Threshold parameters of a DVH (e.g., V20) can often be manipulated by skilled planners, resulting in a "kink" in the DVH just below the constrained threshold limits (e.g., a high value of V15–18 with a low V20). For example, while the lung V20 is predictive of radiation pneumonitis in many studies (Marks et al. 2010c) lung volumes receiving at or below lower doses (i.e. V10 or V13) are also predictive, and thus striving for a specific dose metric such as lung V20, and ignoring the overall dose-volume distribution can lead to errors in judgment regarding toxicity risks.
7. The calculated dose distribution and DVHs are affected by the algorithms used to calculate dose (i.e., Monte Carlo calculation is often considered the 'gold standard'). In the presence of tissue inhomogeneities, there will be relatively greater discrepancies in the calculated dose distribution and DVHs between different planning algorithms (Vanderstraeten et al. 2006). As a result, interpreting the published dose tolerances, and using them as a guide to predict toxicity risks becomes more complicated. Differences between planning systems are

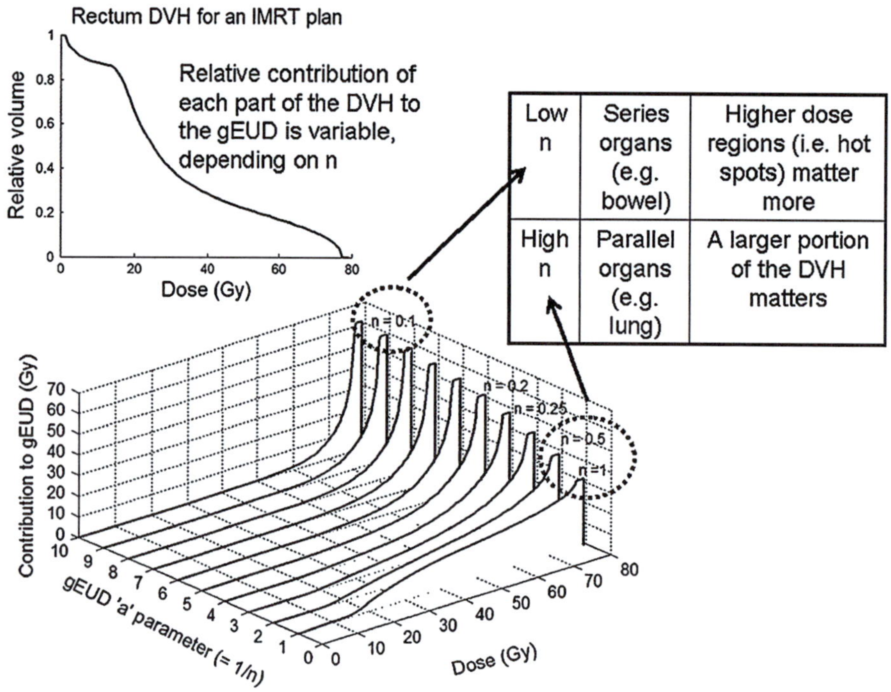

Fig. 9 Radiation planning software generates dose volume histograms (DVH) by tallying the 'point doses' delivered to each voxel of a contoured structure, and generating a cumulative histogram. The cumulative histogram depicts the number of voxels (plotted as *volume*) receiving a given dose or less. This graphical representation discards the anatomical spatial distribution of the dose delivered to the patient. Similarly, the dose metrics such as mean organ dose, or organ dose receiving 20 Gy or less (V20) does not account for how that dose is distributed in the organ. Likewise, computer based models which extract DVH data do not account for spatial distribution of dose. Reproduced with permission from Marks. (Marks et al. 2010b)

likely relatively modest compared to some of the other factors herein discussed.

8. As described in each of the QUANTEC reviews, there are potential challenges in defining a given organ's volume, which then impacts the DVHs and therefore interpretation of the DVH. Challenges include intra-fraction and inter-fraction organ motion, difficulty in defining anatomical borders of an organ, and differing opinions on how to define extent of an organ. There is also variability in the published literature in how a given organ is defined. For example, total lung is defined as lung minus GTV in some studies, and lung minus PTV in others (Marks et al. 2010c). These two lung definitions would result in substantially different lung dose metrics, particularly with relatively large PTVs. These discrepancies further complicate the interpretation and use of published dose tolerances.

5 Major Differences between the QUANTEC and Emami/Lyman Reviews

a. Emami et al. provided information for 26 organs, judged necessary to support protocols for "three dimensional treatment planning for high energy photons."(Emami et al. 1991) Conversely, the QUANTEC review was focused on organs for which the steering committee thought that there was meaningful dose/volume/outcome data (see Table 5).

b. The QUANTEC reviews had the benefit of 18 additional years of published data from which they could make their dose/volume/outcome estimates.

c. Emami et al. addressed a wide variety of clinical outcomes, and thus provides the reader with a set of dose/volume parameters for *essentially* all clinical situations. Conversely, the QUANTEC review was focused on endpoints where there was dose/volume/outcome data. In this regard, the Emami/Lyman tables are more complete. For example, consider the QUANTEC summary for the small bowel. A volume restriction is provided for the endpoint of acute grade ≥ 3 toxicity. No guidance is provided for late small bowel injury, as the authors did not believe that there was meaningful dose/volume/outcome data for late injury. This is a shortcoming of the QUANTEC review as it is not "complete." When evaluating a proposed 3D treatment plan, one obviously must consider both acute and late injury.

d. Emami et al. presented information in a systematic/uniform manner, facilitating inter-organ comparisons

Table 5 Comparison of the character/content of Emami et. al. and QUANTEC

Characteristic	Emami et. al.	QUANTEC
Number of organs	26	16
3D data available	Minimal	More/moderate (18-year interval)
Format of dose/volume limits	Uniform TD 5/5, 50/5 for 1/3, 2/3, 3/3	Non-uniform
Endpoints	Specific, complete	Specific, incomplete
Expert opinion	A lot	Much less
Impact of chemotherapy	Not explicitly discussed	Addressed individually for each organ

and model-based parameter estimates. The investigators generated an enlarged table wherein the doses that would be expected to cause a 5 % risk of injury with exposure 1/3, 2/3, 3/3 of an organ expected to cause 5 % risk of injury. This approach has definite appeal on many levels. It is a uniform format, and forced the investigators to address each organ in a similar manner. However, this paradigm might not be logical for some organs. For example, for some organs, in some situations, a 5 % of risk of injury is not clinically acceptable, such as the case with spinal cord irradiation. Similarly, it is challenging to consider radiation of 1/3, 2/3, 3/3 of small organs such as the retina, larynx. The QUANTEC reviews presented dose/volume/outcome data in the diverse manner in which they were available in the literature. The reviewers for each organ were free to select what they thought were the "optimal parameters" to consider. For example, in the lung, the threshold doses (e.g., V13, V20) as well as the mean dose, were both considered. For the penile bulb, the minimum dose received by the hottest 75 or 90 % of the organ was considered. Where this might make the QUANTEC reviews slightly more clinically relevant, it does make inter-organ comparisons more challenging.

e. One of the benefits of having a uniform dose/volume/outcome construct, as was done in Emami and Lyman, is that it readily lends itself to the calculation of parameters for a unified normal tissue complication probability (NPCP) modeling. Such modeling was done with the Emami and Lyman estimates. The QUANTEC reports did not also systematically include modeling-based information.

6 Challenges for Future Study

The study of dose/volume/outcome for normal tissues is somewhat hampered by inter- and intra-fraction motion. Almost all analyses, including the QUANTEC effort were based on 3D dose/volume parameters extracted from the treatment planning CT. Motion of various organs (e.g., rectum, bladder) between the time of planning and treatment clearly occur. One might argue that such motion should be "randomly distributed" and that therefore analyses based on these treatment planning-based dose/volume parameters would be valid. However, there might be some systematic errors relating to organ motion. Additionally, there can be motion of various organs during treatment (i.e., cardiac and respiratory-associated motion).

Normal tissue effects are highly dependent on fraction size. For a variety of organs, a lower dose per fraction has been associated with the reduction in risk of normal tissue injury. With modern 3D treatment planning techniques, in particular IMRT; the dose delivered to the regions of an organ may be highly variable. The consideration of dose/volume statistics that do not account for this variation in fraction size is a major potential shortcoming. Most DVH-based analyses do not "correct" for regional differences in fraction size. There are some notable exceptions however, where variations in fraction size are considered (Jin et al. 2010).

The impact of fraction size on late toxicity has typically been modeled using the linear quadratic model (Hall and Giaccia 2012). However, this model appears to be less accurate at high doses per fraction (Milano et al. 2008). Furthermore, the linear quadratic model, which is based upon in vivo measurements of cancer cell survival, does not necessary apply to normal tissues (Glatstein 2008, 2011). The emergence of novel technologies such as SBRT/SABR, IGRT, IMRT and 4-dimensional planning facilitate hypofractionated radiation delivery, via more accurate positioning and targeting. More accurate positioning allows reduction in PTV margins, coupled with the uniformly rapid dose gradient beyond the target (e.g., with SBRT), generally results in only a small volume of normal tissue exposed to hypofractionated radiation. However, the impact of hypofractionated radiation on small volumes of normal tissues is not well characterized (Milano et al. 2008; Benedict et al. 2010). Thus further efforts are needed to better understand the normal tissue response to hypofractionated radiation.

In the future, models predicting dose/volume injury will likely more consistently consider the underlying physiology and substructures of organs. Differences in regional importance (e.g., different regions of the heart maybe being more important, such as the coronary arteries or the left ventricle). The commonly used NTCP models are not necessarily physiologically based. The widely used Lyman-Kutcher, Berman model does not have a biologically physiologic underpinning.

Additional work is needed to better understand inter-patient differences in inherent radiation sensitivity. A variety of studies in the pre-clinical setting (bacteria, cell culture in animals) noted marked inter-variations in radiation sensitivity. Numerous studies have been trying to identify predictors of radiation sensitivity in humans. To date none of these have been widely found to be useful, though more recent studies provide reason to be more optimistic (as discussed in " BioPediatric Complexities of Growth and Development" by Rosenstein and coauthors).

Current models do not particularly consider potential interactions between organs. For example, the risk of pneumonitis has been particularly related to the dose/volume of the lung. It is certainly possible that there might be interactions between the lung and the heart for the endpoint of shortness of breath. There are similar interactions that may exist for the kidney and liver, retina and brain, and other organs that "share a function". Further investigation into organ–organ interaction is warranted.

The study of radiation-associated normal tissue injury has interested investigators for decades. Much progress has been made over the last 20 years, largely in the 'physical realm.' Additional technologies (e.g., gating, image-guided therapy) will provide some refinements in these physical advances. There is a huge need to gain further understanding of the biological underpinnings of radiation-associated normal tissue. This will hopefully improve our abilities to predict, prevent and treat radiation-associated normal tissue injury.

Acknowledgments Portions of this work are adapted from Milano et al. (2012) (in Gunderson and Tepper), Marks et al. (2010b) (QUANTEC review), and Rubin (1978) (Clinical Oncology Book)

References

Ahn SJ, Kahn D, Zhou S et al (2005) Dosimetric and clinical predictors for radiation-induced esophageal injury. Int J Radiat Oncol Biol Phys 61:335–347

Benedict SH, Yenice KM, Followill D et al (2010) Stereotactic body radiation therapy: the report of AAPM Task Group 101. Med Phys 37:4078–4101

Boersma LJ, Damen EM, de Boer RW et al (1993) A new method to determine dose-effect relations for local lung-function changes using correlated SPECT and CT data. Radiother Oncol 29:110–116

Burman C, Kutcher GJ, Emami B et al (1991) Fitting of normal tissue tolerance data to an analytic function. Int J Radiat Oncol Biol Phys 21:123–135

Chapet O, Kong FM, Lee JS et al (2005) Normal tissue complication probability modeling for acute esophagitis in patients treated with conformal radiation therapy for non-small cell lung cancer. Radiother Oncol J Eur Soc Ther Radiol Oncol 77:176–181

Emami B, Lyman J, Brown A et al (1991) Tolerance of normal tissue to therapeutic irradiation. Int J Radiat Oncol Biol Phys 21:109–122

Fan M, Marks LB, Hollis D et al (2001a) Can we predict radiation-induced changes in pulmonary function based on the sum of predicted regional dysfunction? J Clin Oncol 19:543–550

Fan M, Marks LB, Lind P et al (2001b) Relating radiation-induced regional lung injury to changes in pulmonary function tests. Int J Radiat Oncol Biol Phys 51:311–317

Flickinger JC, Kondziolka D, Lunsford LD et al (2000) Development of a model to predict permanent symptomatic postradiosurgery injury for arteriovenous malformation patients. Arteriovenous malformation radiosurgery study group. Int J Radiat Oncol Biol Phys 46:1143–1148

Glatstein E (2008) Hypofractionation, long-term effects, and the alpha/beta ratio. Int J Radiat Oncol Biol Phys 72:11–12

Glatstein E (2011) The omega on alpha and beta. Int J Radiat Oncol Biol Phys 81:319–320

Hall EJ, Giaccia AJ (2012) Radiobiology for the radiobiologist, 7th edn. Wolters Kluwer/Lippincott Williams & Wilkins, Philadelphia

Hendry JH, Thames HD (1986) The tissue-rescuing unit. Br J Radiol 59:628–630

Jin JY, Kong FM, Chetty IJ et al (2010) Impact of fraction size on lung radiation toxicity: hypofractionation may be beneficial in dose escalation of radiotherapy for lung cancers. Int J Radiat Oncol Biol Phys 76:782–788

Kutcher GJ, Burman C, Brewster L et al (1991) Histogram reduction method for calculating complication probabilities for three-dimensional treatment planning evaluations. Int J Radiat Oncol Biol Phys 21:137–146

Lyman JT (1985) Complication probability as assessed from dose-volume histograms. Radiat Res. (Supplement) 8:S13–S19

Lyman JT, Wolbrast AB (1987) Optimization of radiation therapy III: a method of assessing complication probabilities from dose-volume histograms. Int J Radiat Oncol Biol Phys 13:103

Ma J, Zhang J, Zhou S et al (2009) Association between RT-induced changes in lung tissue density and global lung function. Int J Radiat Oncol Biol Phys 74:781–789

Ma J, Zhang J, Zhou S et al (2010) Regional lung density changes after radiation therapy for tumors in and around thorax. Int J Radiat Oncol Biol Phys 76:116–122

Mah K, Van Dyk J (1988) Quantitative measurement of changes in human lung density following irradiation. Radiother Oncol 11:169–179

Marks LB, Carroll PR, Dugan TC, Anscher MS (1995) The response of the urinary bladder, urethra, and ureter to radiation and chemotherapy. Int J Radiat Oncol Biol Phys 31:1257–1280

Marks LB (1996) The impact of organ structure on radiation response. Int J Radiat Oncol Biol Phys 34:1165–1171

Marks LB, Munley MT, Spencer DP et al (1997) Quantification of radiation-induced regional lung injury with perfusion imaging. Int J Radiat Oncol Biol Phys 38:399–409

Marks LB, Ten Haken RK, Martel MK (2010a) Guest editor's introduction to QUANTEC: a users guide. Int J Radiat Oncol Biol Phys 76:S1–S2

Marks LB, Yorke ED, Jackson A et al (2010b) Use of normal tissue complication probability models in the clinic. Int J Radiat Oncol Biol Phys 76:S10–S19

Marks LB, Bentzen SM, Deasy JO et al (2010c) Radiation dose volume effects in the lung. Int J Radiat Oncol Biol Phys 76:S70–S76

Mendelsohn ML (1969) The biology of dose-limiting tissuses. In: Time and dose relationship in radiation biology as applied to radiotherapy, Brookhaven National Laboratory [BNL] Report 5023 (C-57), Brookhaven National Laboratory, Upton, p 54

Michalowski A, Wheldon TE, Kirk J (1984) Can cell survival parameters be deduced from non clonogenic assays of radiation damage to normal tissues? Br J Cancer Suppl 6:257–261

Milano MT, Constine LS, Okunieff P (2007) Normal tissue tolerance dose metrics for radiation therapy of major organs. Semin Radiat Oncol 17:131–140

Milano MT, Constine LS, Okunieff P (2008) Normal tissue toxicity after small field hypofractionated stereotactic body radiation. Radiat Oncol 3:36

Milano MT, Marks LB, Constine LS (2012) Survivorship and late effects. In: Gunderson LL, Tepper JE (eds) Clinical radiation oncology, 3rd edn. Churchill Livingstone, Philadelphia, PA

Rubin P (1978) Clinical oncology: a multidisciplinary approach for physicians and students, 5th edn. American Cancer Society, Inc

Rubin P, Casarett GW (1968) Clinical radiation pathology. W. B. Saunders, Philadelphia

Rubin P, Casarett GW (1972) A direction for clinical radiation oncology. In: Vaeth JM (ed) Frontiers of radiation therapy and oncology VI. University Park Press, Baltimore, pp 1–16

Seppenwoolde Y, De Jaeger K, Boersma LJ et al (2004) Regional differences in lung radiosensitivity after radiotherapy for non-small-cell lung cancer. Int J Radiat Oncol Biol Phys 60:748–758

Ten Haken RK, Lawrence TS, Dawson LA () Prediction of radiation-induced liver disease by Lyman normal-tissue complication probability model in three-dimensional conformal radiation therapy for primary liver carcinoma: in regards to Xu et al. (Int J Radiat Oncol Biol Phys 2006;65:189–195). Int J Radiat Oncol Biol Phys 66:1272; author reply 1272–1273

Ten Haken RK, Martel MK, Kessler ML et al (1993) Use of Veff and iso-NTCP in the implementation of dose escalation protocols. Int J Radiat Oncol Biol Phys 27:689–695

Vanderstraeten B, Reynaert N, Paelinck L et al (2006) Accuracy of patient dose calculation for lung IMRT: a comparison of Monte Carlo, convolution/superposition, and pencil beam computations. Med Phys 33:3149–3158

Withers HR, Taylor JM (1993) Critical volume model. Int J Radiat Oncol Biol Phys 25:151–152

Biotoxicity of Chemotherapy

Chunkit Fung and Kishan J. Pandya

Contents

Abstract

With successful treatment of many malignancies, long-term toxicities began to emerge and are becoming increasingly important in the growing number of cancer survivors. Research has begun to investigate management options to mitigate these chemotherapy-related toxicities without compromising the therapeutic outcomes. This chapter will discuss these late adverse effects based on organ system, including cardiotoxicity, pulmonary toxicity, nephrotoxicity, peripheral neuropathy, ototoxicity, reproductive toxicity, cognitive impairment, and risks of second malignant neoplasms. We will review the underlying pathophysiology of each of these long-term complications and will provide the most up-to-date evidence-based prevention, follow-up and monitoring guidelines. In the latter part of the chapter, we will review the current literatures regarding the molecular basis of germline genetic susceptibility to some of the late effects of chemotherapy, including peripheral neuropathy, ototoxicity and therapy-induced myeloid leukemia. This rapidly emerging field within cancer survivorship does not only provide invaluable insights and inform the development of therapeutic agents to target the underlying molecular pathway of these adverse effects, but it may also allow development of a risk-classification system that incorporates genetic markers to predict risks of chemotherapy-related side effects. The final part of this chapter will attempt to look at future research directions in the development of genetic markers as well as therapeutic agents to prevent or treat late-effects of chemotherapy.

1 Introduction

The field of cancer chemotherapy developed from the idea of chemical warfare. Toxic chemicals were developed for the explicit purpose of causing biological damage to the

C. Fung · K. J. Pandya (✉)
James P Wilmot Cancer Center,
University of Rochester Medical Center,
Rochester, USA
e-mail: Kishan_pandya@urmc.rochester.edu

P. Rubin et al. (eds.), *ALERT – Adverse Late Effects of Cancer Treatment*, Medical Radiology. Radiation Oncology,
DOI: 10.1007/978-3-540-72314-1_9, © Springer-Verlag Berlin Heidelberg 2014

enemy. Sulfur mustards were synthesized in 1854, but their vesicant properties were not described until 1887. Medical attention was focused on these properties on the skin, eyes, and respiratory tract during World War I. Serious systemic toxicities were recognized later on in the form of leucopenia.

Autopsies of those exposed to sulfur mustard showed bone marrow aplasia, lymphoid tissue dissolution, and gastrointestinal ulcerations. Biological and chemical effects of *nitrogen mustard* were studied between the two wars in secrecy. The marked cytotoxic effects on the lymphoid tissue led to studies on transplanted lymphosarcoma in mice, quickly leading to clinical trials in patients with lymphoid malignancies in 1942, beginning the era of cancer chemotherapy.

Targeting the metabolic pathways, antifolates produced the first dramatic, but short lived remissions in acute leukemias in 1948, and first cure of choriocarcinoma in 1963. In the ensuing decades, a variety of chemical agents were shown to have antitumor effects in animal models, and began to be tested in human malignancies. *Fluorouracil* was the first rationally designed drug that interfered with synthesis and function of nucleic acid in 1957. Natural products, derived mostly from plants, such as vinca alkaloids (e.g., *vincristine*), taxanes (e.g., *paclitaxel*), podophyllotoxins (e.g., *etoposide*), camptothecins (e.g., *irinotecan*), as well antibiotics derived from fungi such as *doxorubicin* along with miscellaneous agents such as the platinum compounds (e.g., *cisplatin*) are the mainstay of antineoplastic chemotherapy today.

The field of Medical Oncology emerged as a subspecialty of Internal Medicine in 1972, with a focus on maximizing the beneficial effects and minimizing the side effects of these agents which were by definition highly biotoxic, with a very narrow therapeutic index. A great deal of effort has been devoted to containing the acute side effects, such as nausea, vomiting and diarrhea, as well as myelosuppression, and is not the topic of this chapter. With successful treatments of many malignancies, long-term toxicities began to emerge, and efforts began to best mitigate those effects without compromising the therapeutic outcomes. This chapter will outline the late effects of chemotherapy based on organ systems, and will provide prevention, follow-up, and monitoring guidelines. It will also describe the use of pharmacogenomics for mitigation of biotoxicity of these agents, and attempt to look at future research directions in the development of genetic markers as well as therapeutic agents to prevent or treat late effects of chemotherapy.

2 Late Effects of Chemotherapy

2.1 Cardiotoxicity

Cardiotoxicity is a serious complication of numerous cytotoxic cancer agents and it frequently manifests many years after chemotherapy (Zuppinger and Suter 2010). These cardiovascular toxicities may include cardiomyopathy with or without overt congestive heart failure (CHF), endothelial dysfunction, and arrhythmias (Carver et al. 2007). Anthracyclines (daunorubicin, doxorubicin, and epirubicin) are perhaps the most well-known chemotherapeutics that cause CHF (Zuppinger and Suter 2010; Geiger et al. 2010; Yeh and Bickford 2009). Long-term cardiotoxicity has been described in other cytotoxic agents as well (Geiger et al. 2010; Yeh and Bickford 2009) such as alkylating agents (cyclophosphamide, ifosfamide, and cisplatin) and the newer targeted therapies (Zuppinger and Suter 2010; Geiger et al. 2010; Yeh and Bickford 2009), including monoclonal antibody-based tyrosine kinase inhibitors (bevacizumab and trastuzumab).

2.1.1 Types of Chemotherapeutic Agents

2.1.1.1 Anthracyclines

Since their introduction in the 1960s, anthracyclines have been an integral component of many cytotoxic regimens in both the pediatric and adult populations (Smith et al. 2010). *Doxorubicin* and *daunorubicin* are produced by the fungus *S. peucetius*, and *idarubicin* and *epirubicin* are synthetic derivatives. They all share a common structure of a tetracycline ring with quinine and hydroquinone moieties on adjacent rings that permit them to function as electron-accepting and -donating agents. *Mitoxantrone* is an anthrocenedione with less cardiac toxicity than the anthracyclines. Unfortunately, anthracyclines can cause cardiac dysfunction and this adverse effect is categorized into acute reversible and early- and late-onset chronic progressive cardiotoxicity (Yeh and Bickford 2009; Trachtenberg et al. 2011; Wouters et al. 2005). Cardiac damage caused by anthracyclines can manifest as either subclinical or clinical cardiotoxicity (van Dalen et al. 2009, 2010). The term subclinical cardiotoxicity is defined by various cardiac abnormalities, such as decreased left ventricular ejection fraction (LVEF), as confirmed by diagnostic tests in patients without symptoms (van Dalen et al. 2009, 2010) while clinical cardiotoxicity describes patients who experience symptoms of cardiac damage due to cardiac dysfunction (van Dalen et al. 2009, 2010). Common clinical manifestations of anthracycline-induced cardiotoxicity may include arrhythmias, electrocardiographic abnormalities, heart failure, or a myocarditis and pericarditis syndrome (Trachtenberg et al. 2011).

Incidence

Acute reversible anthracycline-induced cardiotoxicity occurs in <1 % of childhood cancer patients immediately after infusion of anthracyclines (Giantris et al. 1998) and is defined by a transient decrease in myocardial contractility with improvement after discontinuation of treatment (Wouters et al. 2005; Giantris et al. 1998). In a study of adult patients with lymphoma, Nousiainen et al. (2002) reported that the prevalence of subclinical cardiac damage is at 36 % during anthracycline therapy, as defined by more than 10 % decline in absolute ejection fraction units to a final LVEF of ≤50 %. Although discontinuation of therapy usually results in marked improvement, some patients nonetheless suffer permanent cardiac damage, especially for those who received higher cumulative doses of anthracyclines (Wouters et al. 2005). Furthermore, the risk of developing heart failure remains a lifelong threat as more cancer patients are now living longer due to recent advances in oncologic therapies (Zuppinger and Suter 2010; van Dalen et al. 2009, 2010). Kremer et al. (2001) reported that the risk of developing clinical heart failure remains elevated at approximately 5 % even at 15 years after anthracycline therapy for childhood cancer.

Early-onset chronic anthracycline-induced cardiotoxicity is defined by progressive depression of myocardial function within the first year after treatment and occurs in 1.6–2.1 % (Kremer et al. 2001; Krischer et al. 1997) of children treated with anthracyclines. Late-onset chronic progressive anthracycline-induced cardiotoxicity occurs at least 1 year after anthracycline therapy with a latency period when no cardiac dysfunction is detected and the patients have no symptoms (Giantris et al. 1998). Kremer et al. (2001) reported that the cumulative incidence of anthracycline-induced clinical heart failure in children after a mean follow-up time of 6.3 years is 2.8 % while Von Hoff et al. (1979) reported an incidence of 1.6 %. In adults with breast cancer, Meinardi et al. (2002) reported that the incidence of clinical heart failure is 30 % at a median of 37 months after adjuvant treatment with epirubicin and locoregional radiotherapy. Interestingly, the majority of adult patients who developed cardiotoxicity have a chronic dilated cardiomyopathy while the pediatric populations experience mainly a restrictive cardiomyopathy (Giantris et al. 1998).

The risk of cardiotoxicity increases with higher cumulative dose of anthracycline. Heart failure occurs in 3–5, 7–26, and 18–48 % of patients with cumulative doxorubicin dose of 400, 550, and 700 mg/m^2, respectively (Wouters et al. 2005; Von Hoff et al. 1979; Swain et al. 1997). In contrast, the incidence of heart failure for patients after epirubicin (0.9–3.3 %) or idarubicin (5–18 %) appears to be less (Yeh and Bickford 2009). Table 1 lists the maximum lifetime cumulative doses for various anthracyclines before risk of clinical cardiotoxicity becomes clinically significant. Aside from high cumulative dose of anthracyclines, other risk factors for development of cardiotoxicity include young children, elderly people, females, bolus administration and higher single doses of anthracyclines, history of radiotherapy, concomitant therapy with agents known to have cardiotoxic effects, and pre-existing cardiovascular disorders (Geiger et al. 2010; Trachtenberg et al. 2011; Von Hoff et al. 1979) (Table 2).

Table 1 Maximum lifetime cumulative doses of various anthracyclines (Zuppinger and Suter 2010)

Types of anthracyclines	Maximum lifetime cumulative doses mg/m^2
Daunorubicin	550–800
Doxorubicin	400–550
Epirubicin	900–1000
Idarubicin	150–225
Mitoxantrone	100–140

Adapted from Geiger and colleagues with permission

Two recent meta-analyses examined if different dosing schedules and various anthracycline derivates reduce cardiotoxicity. The risk of clinical heart failure is significantly lower with an infusion duration of 6 h or longer of anthracyclines as compared to a shorter duration (relative risk (RR) = 0.27; 95 % confidence interval (CI) 0.09–0.81; 5 studies; 557 patients) (van Dalen et al. 2009). However, the same authors (van Dalen et al. 2009) reported no statistically significant difference in the occurrence of clinical heart failure in patients treated with a doxorubicin peak dose of <60 mg/m^2 versus ≥60 mg/m^2 (RR = 0.65; 95 % CI 0.23–1.88; 2 studies; 4,146 patients), a liposomal doxorubicin peak dose of 25 mg/m^2 versus 50 mg/m^2 (No patients in either treatment groups developed clinical heart failure; 1 study; 48 patients), and an epirubicin peak dose of 83 mg/m^2 versus 110 mg/m^2 (RR = 0.97; 95 % CI 0.06–15.48; 1 study; 1,086 patients). Regarding the risk of cardiotoxicity with various anthracycline derivatives, only liposomal-encapsulated doxorubicin is found to be associated with a significantly lower rate of clinical heart failure when compared to conventional doxorubicin (RR = 0.20; 95 % CI 0.05–0.75; 2 studies; 521 patients) (van Dalen et al. 2010). No evidence for a significant difference in the occurrence of clinical heart failure exists between epirubicin versus doxorubicin of the same dose (RR = 0.36; 95 % CI 0.12–1.11; 5 studies; 1,036 patients) (van Dalen et al. 2010).

Table 2 Risk factors predisposing patients to anthracycline-associated cardiotoxicity (Zuppinger and Suter 2010; Carver et al. 2007)

Risk factors	Increased risk in case of
Age at diagnosis	Young (<4 years) and old age (>65 years)
Sex	Female
Rate and schedule of anthracycline administration	Rapid infusion resulting in high peak dose
Individual anthracycline dose	Higher daily dose
Cumulative anthracycline dose	Increased cumulative dose
Radiation therapy	Cumulative dose >30 Gy to the mediastinum or >5 Gy to the heart
Concomitant therapy	Trastuzumab, cyclophosphamide, bleomycin, vincristine, amsacrine, and mitoxantrone
Pre-existing cardiovascular disorders	Hypertension, coronary heart disease, valvular disorders, prior cardiotoxic treatment
Medical comorbidities	Diabetes, obesity, renal dysfunction, pulmonary disease, endocrinopathies, hypocalcemia and hypomagnesemia, sepsis, infection, thyrotoxicosis, alcohol, and pregnancy
Others	Trisomy 21 and African American ancestry

Adapted from Geiger and colleagues (Zuppinger and Suter 2010) and Trachtenberg and colleagues (Carver et al. 2007) with permission

Pathophysiology

The underlying mechanism of anthracycline-induced cardiotoxicity is complex and remains incompletely understood despite decades of research (Trachtenberg et al. 2011). Loss of myofibrils and cytoplasmic vacuolization caused by dilatation of the sarcoplasmic reticulum in cardiomyocytes are the most prominent histological features (Wouters et al. 2005). Oxidative stress caused by free radical formation is generally accepted as the main mechanism (Zuppinger and Suter 2010; Geiger et al. 2010; Yeh and Bickford 2009; Trachtenberg et al. 2011; Wouters et al. 2005). Reduction of the quinine moiety of anthracyclines to semiquinone generates reactive oxygen species that initiates a cascade of free radical formation (Trachtenberg et al. 2011), which causes damage to cells, cell membranes, and subcellular apparatuses (Trachtenberg et al. 2011; Wouters et al. 2005). Since cardiomyocytes have high oxidative metabolism as evidenced by the abundance of cardiac mitochondria (Trachtenberg et al. 2011) but with fewer natural antioxidants than other organs (Trachtenberg et al. 2011; Wouters et al. 2005), they are most susceptible to oxidative stress (Trachtenberg et al. 2011; Wouters et al. 2005). Furthermore, anthracyclines have a very strong affinity for cardiolipin, which is a phospholipid in the inner cell membrane of cardiac mitochondria that facilitates transport of anthracyclines (Trachtenberg et al. 2011; Wouters et al. 2005). This affinity leads to increased accumulation of anthracyclines inside cardiomyocytes (Trachtenberg et al. 2011; Wouters et al. 2005).

Other postulated mechanisms for anthracycline-induced cardiotoxicity include transcriptional changes in intracellular adenosine triphosphate (ATP) production in cardiomyocytes (Yeh and Bickford 2009); impaired formation of the myofilament protein known as titin in cardiac sarcomeres via calcium-dependent protease activation (Yeh and Bickford 2009; Trachtenberg et al. 2011); downregulation of transcription factors involved in sarcomere synthesis such as GATA4 (Trachtenberg et al. 2011); decrease in cardiac glutathione peroxidase activity (Yeh and Bickford 2009); depletion of cardiac stem cells (Trachtenberg et al. 2011); respiratory defects associated with mitochondrial DNA damage (Yeh and Bickford 2009; Trachtenberg et al. 2011), and impaired mitochondrial creatine kinase activity and function (Trachtenberg et al. 2011). Recently, Lyu et al. (2007) hypothesized that cardiotoxicity caused by doxorubicin may also be due to disruption of the activity of topoisomerase II beta.

2.1.1.2 Alkylating Agents

Drugs that contain reactive alkyl groups capable of forming covalent bonds with DNA are included in this group. Except cisplatin, these drugs were developed from nitrogen mustards, and their clinical use launched the era of cancer chemotherapy.

Incidence

Cyclophosphamide. No cardiotoxicity has been reported for low doses of cyclophosphamide (Floyd et al. 2005). However, acute cardiac toxicity has been described after high-dose cyclophosphamide (120–200 mg/kg) (Yeh and Bickford 2009; Floyd et al. 2005; Senkus and Jassem 2011), as commonly administered in high-dose conditioning regimens for bone marrow transplantation (Floyd et al. 2005). Clinical manifestations may include electrocardiogram changes (decreased amplitude of the QRS complex and nonspecific T wave of ST segment abnormalities), arrhythmias, conduction disorders, and hemorrhagic myopericarditis leading to pericardial effusion, tamponade, and death in some cases (Floyd et al. 2005; Senkus and Jassem 2011). While an asymptomatic transient decrease in ejection fraction has been reported that usually resolves over 3–4 weeks (Floyd et al. 2005), up to 28 % of patients may develop acute-onset fulminant heart failure after high-dose cyclophosphamide (Floyd et al. 2005). Risk of cardiotoxicity is increased with elderly patients, prior anthracycline or mitoxantrone therapy, and mediastinal radiation (Yeh and Bickford 2009; Floyd et al. 2005; Senkus and Jassem 2011).

Ifosfamide. Arrhythmias, ST-T wave changes, and CHF associated with left ventricular dysfunction have been reported for ifosfamide in a dose response manner, usually observed at doses greater than 6.25–10 g/m^2, and these toxicities are usually reversible with medical treatment (Floyd et al. 2005; Senkus and Jassem 2011). However, controversy exists regarding if concomitant administration of both ifosfamide and anthracyclines increases cardiotoxicity (Floyd et al. 2005).

Cisplatin. Acute cardiotoxicity of cisplatin includes supraventricular tachycardia, bradycardia, ST-T wave changes, left bundle branch block, acute ischemic events, myocardial infarction, and ischemic cardiomyopathy (Floyd et al. 2005; Senkus and Jassem 2011). Importantly, risk of cardiovascular diseases remains elevated many years after treatment with cisplatin (Senkus and Jassem 2011; Fung and Vaughn 2011). For instance, the risk of cardiovascular disease in long-term testicular cancer survivors who received cisplatin-based chemotherapy is approximately twofold greater than those treated with orchiectomy alone (Fung and Vaughn 2011). This increased risk of cardiovascular disease may be an indirect result of increased incidence of hypertension, hyperlipidemia, and metabolic syndrome observed in patients after cisplatin-based chemotherapy (Fung and Vaughn 2011).

Pathophysiology

The precise mechanism of cyclophosphamide-induced cardiotoxicity is unknown. Cyclophosphamide may cause endothelial capillary damage leading to extravasations of toxic metabolites resulting in damage to cardiomyocytes and hemorrhagic necrosis of the myocardium (Yeh and Bickford 2009; Floyd et al. 2005; Senkus and Jassem 2011). Ifosfamide may cause cardiotoxicity through a similar mechanism as cyclophosphamide due to their analogous structures (Yeh and Bickford 2009). Furthermore, ifosfamide can cause nephrotoxicity that results in delayed elimination of cardiotoxic metabolites along with disturbances of fluid, acid–base, and electrolyte homeostasis (Yeh and Bickford 2009; Floyd et al. 2005; Senkus and Jassem 2011).

Direct endothelial damage caused by cisplatin, as shown by elevations in von Willebrand factor, C-reactive protein, and soluble intercellular adhesion marker 1, may explain the increased risk of cardiotoxicity (Fung and Vaughn 2011). In addition, hypomagnesemia and hypokalemia resulting from cisplatin-induced nephrotoxicity may in turn lead to conduction abnormality and cardiac arrhythmias in the acute setting (Senkus and Jassem 2011).

2.1.1.3 Monoclonal Antibody-Based Tyrosine Kinase Inhibitors

Incidence

Trastuzumab. Trastuzumab, a recombinant DNA-derived humanized monoclonal antibody that selectively binds to the extracellular domain of the HER2 protein, is perhaps the best recognized targeted compound associated with a relatively high risk of cardiac complications (Floyd et al. 2005; Senkus and Jassem 2011). Various degrees of left ventricular systolic dysfunction, which occasionally leads to CHF, is the most common trastuzumab-related cardiac damage (Senkus and Jassem 2011). Improvement of symptoms usually occurs within 6 weeks after discontinuation of trastuzumab and its reinstitution is usually possible with resolution of symptoms (Senkus and Jassem 2011).

In the first landmark clinical trial that evaluated the efficacy and safety of trastuzumab by Slamon et al. (2001), New York Heart Association class III or IV cardiac dysfunction occurred in 27 % of the group given an anthracycline, cyclophosphamide, and trastuzumab; 8 % of the group given an anthracycline and cyclophosphamide alone; 13 % of the group given paclitaxel and trastuzumab; and 1 % of the group given paclitaxel alone. In more recent studies, however, the reported incidence of cardiac complications resulting from trastuzumab was lower with careful monitoring of cardiac function and avoidance of concomitant administration of anthracyclines (Senkus and Jassem 2011). The incidence of cardiac dysfunction ranges from 2 to 7 % when trastuzumab is used as monotherapy and 2–13 % when it is combined with paclitaxel (Yeh and Bickford 2009). More importantly, approximately 1 % of patient will ultimately develop symptomatic CHF (Hayes and Picard 2006).

A recent phase II trial by Rayson et al. (2011) examined the cardiac safety of adjuvant trastuzumab with liposomal doxorubicin in women with breast cancer. The incidence of cardiac toxicity or inability to administer trastuzumab due to cardiotoxicity was 18.6 % ($n = 11$) in the group with doxorubicin and cyclophosphamide followed by paclitaxel and trastuzumab compared to 4.2 % ($n = 5$) in the group that replaced doxorubicin with the liposomal formulation (Rayson et al. 2011). In a group of 30 patients with HER2-overexpressing metastatic breast cancer, Chia et al. (2006) reported that after treatment with liposomal doxorubicin and trastuzumab, no patient experienced symptomatic CHF; however, three patients experienced an asymptomatic absolute decline in LVEF of ≥15 % and all of them had previous exposure to anthracyclines.

Increased cumulative dose of trastuzumab does not appear to correlate with risk of cardiotoxicity. Risk factors for trastuzumab-induced cardiomyopathy are age >50 years, pre-existing cardiovascular disease and borderline LVEF, sequence of chemotherapy administration, mediastinal radiation and prior treatment with >300 mg/m^2 cumulative dose of anthracyclines (Yeh and Bickford 2009).

Bevacizumab. Bevacizumab is a recombinant humanized monoclonal antibody that binds to and inhibits the biologic activity of human vascular endothelial growth factor (VEGF) (Floyd et al. 2005). Hypertension and thromboembolic events are both well-recognized vascular toxicities of bevacizumab (Senkus and Jassem 2011). Hypertension occurs in 22–36 % of patients (Senkus and Jassem 2011) and this risk is increased 3 times with low dose and 7.5 times with high dose of bevacizumab as shown in a meta-analysis of 7 trials ($n = 1{,}850$) (Zhu et al. 2007). Incidence of arterial thromboembolic events is approximately 4–5 % (Senkus and Jassem 2011). When used alone, grade 2–4 left ventricular dysfunction developed in 2 % of patients (Floyd et al. 2005). Among patients who received concurrent anthracyclines, CHF occurred in 14 % of them and in 4 % of those who had prior exposure to anthracycline only (Floyd et al. 2005). Risk factors for bevacizumab-induced cardiovascular toxicity are age greater than 65 years and prior arterial thromboembolic events (Floyd et al. 2005).

Pathophysiology

HER2 protein is critical in the embryonic cardiogenesis and pathogenesis of cardiac hypertrophy (Yeh and Bickford 2009; Senkus and Jassem 2011) and it activates transcription factor AP-1 and nuclear kappa B factor, which are involved in the pathogenesis of cardiac hypertrophy and cellular response to stress respectively (Senkus and Jassem 2011). Inhibition of this pathway by trastuzumab leads to abnormal growth, repair, and survival of cardiomyocytes (Yeh and Bickford 2009) and it may also cause ATP depletion and contractile dysfunction of cardiomyocytes by disrupting the mitochondrial integrity through dysregulation of the BCL-X proteins (Yeh and Bickford 2009). Other proposed mechanisms include drug–drug interaction with anthracyclines; induction of immune-mediated destruction of cardiomyocytes; and an indirect consequence of trastuzumab-related effects outside the heart (Floyd et al. 2005).

The underlying mechanism for development of bevacizumab-induced CHF involves hypertension and inhibition of angiogenesis that causes reduction of myocardial capillary density, cardiac fibrosis, and global contractile dysfunction (Senkus and Jassem 2011). Inhibition of angiogenesis may also explain the increased risk of arterial thromboembolic events with bevacizumab (Yeh and Bickford 2009). Since VEGF is responsible for endothelial cell proliferation and survival, inhibition of VEGF decreases their capability to generate in response to trauma and causes defects in their lining that exposes subendothelial collagen, which subsequently activates tissue factor and increases the risk of thrombotic events (Yeh and Bickford 2009). Furthermore, inhibition of VEGF also leads to decreased concentrations of nitric oxide and prostacyclin and overproduction of erythropoietin that result in increased hematocrit and blood viscosity, all of which may predispose patients to risks of thromboembolism (Yeh and Bickford 2009).

2.1.2 Cardioprotective Interventions

Dexrazoxane, which is an EDTA-like chelator of iron (Geiger et al. 2010), is the most widely investigated agent for reducing anthracycline-induced heart failure (van Dalen et al. 2011). By removing iron from the anthracycline-iron complex or by binding to free iron, it prevents the formation of oxygen radicals, which are thought to be the main mechanism of anthracycline-induced cardiomyopathy (Wouters et al. 2005). A recent meta-analysis by van Dalen et al. (2011) reported that dexrazoxane is associated with lower risks of clinical heart failure (RR = 0.29; 95 % CI 0.20–0.41; 10 studies; 1,619 patients). Furthermore, no evidence was found for a difference in response rate or survival between the dexrazoxane and control groups in this meta-analysis (van Dalen et al. 2011).

Dexrazoxane is currently approved in the United States and the European Union (Geiger et al. 2010) and is usually administered after a cumulative dose of 300 mg/m^2 or at the beginning of an anthracycline-based chemotherapy (Geiger et al. 2010). The American Society of Clinical Oncology has published detailed guidelines regarding adjunctive use of dexrazoxane (Hensley et al. 2009) as summarized in Table 3. Aside from dexrazoxane, seven other agents, including N-acetylcysteine, phenethylamine, coenzyme Q10, a combination of vitamins E and C and N-acetylcysteine, L-carnitine, carvedilol, and amifostine, have been studied and demonstrated no cardioprotective effects (Hensley et al. 2009).

2.1.3 Cardiac Monitoring

Regular monitoring of heart function is important during chemotherapy with anthracyclines and trastuzumab (Yeh and Bickford 2009). Echocardiography and multi-gated acquisition (MUGA) scan are the most common non-invasive procedures performed to evaluate LVEF (Geiger et al. 2010; Yeh and Bickford 2009) in order to monitor and diagnose chemotherapy-induced cardiomyopathy (Yeh and Bickford 2009). While echocardiography can identify valvular, pericardial disease, and both systolic and diastolic dysfunction, MUGA scans primary detect decline in left ventricular dysfunction only (Yeh and Bickford 2009). Although endometrial biopsy remains the gold standard for diagnosis of cardiac dysfunction, its invasive nature has

Table 3 American society of clinical oncology guidelines for use of dexrazoxane in 2008 (Geiger et al. 2010)

Category	Recommendation
Breast cancer	
Initial use in patients with metastatic breast cancer	It is recommended that dexrazoxane not routinely be used for patients with metastatic breast cancer receiving initial doxorubicin-based chemotherapy
Delayed use in patients with metastatic breast cancer who have received more than 300 mg/m^2 of doxorubicin	It is suggested that the use of dexrazoxane be considered for patients with metastatic breast cancer who have received more than 300 mg/m^2 of doxorubicin in the metastatic setting and who may benefit from continued doxorubicin-containing therapy; treatment of patients who received more than 300 mg/m^2 in the adjuvant setting and are now initiating doxorubicin-based chemotherapy in the metastatic setting should be individualized, with consideration given to the potential for dexrazoxane to decrease response rates as well as decreasing the risk of cardiac toxicity; these patients were not included in the clinical trials of dexrazoxane
Use in patients receiving adjuvant chemotherapy for breast cancer	The use of dexrazoxane in the adjuvant setting is not suggested outside of a clinical trial
Other malignancies	
Use in adult patients with other malignancies	The use of dexrazoxane can be considered in adult patients who have received more than 300 mg/m^2 of doxorubicin-based therapy; caution should be exercised in the use of dexrazoxane in setting in which doxorubicin-based therapy has been shown to improve survival
Use in pediatric malignancies	There is insufficient evidence to make a recommendation for the use of dexrazoxane in the treatment of pediatric malignancies
Other anthracycline doses and schedules	
Use in patients receiving other anthracyclines or other anthracycline dose schedules	On the basis of the available data and extrapolations from the experience with doxorubicin plus dexrazoxane, the use of dexrazoxane may be considered for patients responding to anthracycline-based chemotherapy for advanced breast cancer and for whom continued epirubicin therapy is clinically indicated; data for using dexrazoxane with epirubicin for treatment of other cancers are limited; data are insufficient to make a recommendation regarding the use of dexrazoxane with other potentially cardiotoxic agents
Use in patients receiving high-dose anthracycline therapy	There are no new data addressing the use of dexrazoxane, and there are no new data regarding the clinical use of high-dose anthracyclines; thus, the panel has elected to delete this particular guideline statement, since its clinical relevance appears limited
Use in patients with cardiac risk factors	There is insufficient evidence on which to base a recommendation for the use of dexrazoxane in patients with cardiac risk factors or underlying cardiac cause
Monitoring therapy	
Termination of anthracycline therapy for patients receiving dexrazoxane	Patients receiving dexrazoxane should continue to undergo cardiac monitoring; after cumulative doxorubicin doses of 400 mg/m^2, cardiac monitoring should be frequent; the panel suggests repeating the monitoring study after 500 mg/m^2 and subsequently after every 50 mg/m^2 of doxorubicin; the panel suggests that the termination of dexrazoxane/doxorubicin therapy be strongly considered in patients who develop a decline in LVEP to below institutional normal limits or who develop clinical congestive heart failure
Dose of dexrazoxane	It is suggested that patients who are being treated with dexrazoxane receive dexrazoxane at a ratio of 10:1 with the doxorubicin dose, given by slow IV push or short IV infusion, 15–30 min before doxorubicin or epirubicin administration; a ratio of 10:1 with the epirubicin dose may be reasonable; however, it should be noted that the optimal dose ratio has not been determined

Adapted from Hensley and colleagues (Geiger et al. 2010) with permission

limited its use (Yeh and Bickford 2009). In addition, stress testing and dobutamine stress echocardiogram have also been studied extensively but with mixed reported value in their utility to enhance the diagnostic sensitivity for left ventricular dysfunction (Carver et al. 2007). Tables 4 and 5 summarize proposed respective guidelines for cardiac surveillance during doxorubicin (Schwartz et al. 1987) and trastuzumab (Keefe 2002) therapies.

Table 4 Guidelines for monitoring patients receiving doxorubicin (Yeh and Bickford 2009)

Normal baseline LVEF ≥50 %	Abnormal baseline LVEF <50 %
After cumulative dose of 250–300 mg/m^2: second examination of LVEF	Baseline LVEF ≤30 %: doxorubicin therapy should not be initiated
After cumulative dose of 400 mg/m^2 in patients with known cardiac risk factors and 450 mg/m^2 in absence of risk factors: third examination of LVEF with sequential monitoring of cardiac function before each subsequent dose thereafter	Baseline LVEF between 30–50 %: LVEF should be monitored before each dose of doxorubicin
Functional signs of cardiotoxicity and/or absolute decrease in LVEF ≥10 % associated with a decline to a level of overall LVEF ≤50 %: discontinue doxorubicin therapy	Absolute decrease in LVEF ≥10 % and/or overall LVEF ≤30 %: discontinue doxorubicin therapy

LVEF left ventricular ejection fraction

Adapted from Schwartz and colleagues (Yeh and Bickford 2009) with permission

Table 5 Proposed guidelines for the management of patients treated with trastuzumab (Smith et al. 2010)

		Action		
Physical status	LVEF	Trastuzumab	LVEF monitoring	Management
Asymptomatic[a]	↓ but normal	Continue	Repeat in 4 weeks	
	↓ >10 points but normal	Continue	Repeat in 4 weeks	Consider β-blockers
	↓ 10–20 points and LVEF >40 %	Continue	Repeat in 2–4 weeks *Improved: monitor *Not improved: stop trastuzumab	Treat for CHF
	↓ >20 points to <40 % or LVEF <30 %	Hold	Repeat in 2 weeks *Improved to >45 %: restart trastuzumab *Not improved: stop trastuzumab	Treat for CHF
Symptomatic[a]	↓ <10 points	Continue		Search for noncardiac pathology (e.g., anemia)
	↓ >10 points and LVEF >50 %	Continue	Repeat in 2–4 weeks *Stable or improved: continue trastuzumab *Worsened: stop trastuzumab	Treat for CHF
	↓ <30 points	Stop		Treat for CHF

LVEF left ventricular ejection fraction, *CHF* congestive heart failure

[a] Asymptomatic is defined by changes in heart rate (HR) (increase in HR by 10 beats per minute with baseline HR of <80 bpm or an increase by 20 bpm with baseline HR of ≥80 bpm) and/or weight (weight increase of ≥2 kg in 1 week) without symptoms of dyspnea on exertion. Symptomatic is defined by symptoms of dyspnea on exertion, pulmonary vascular congestion, or edema

Adapted from Keefe and colleagues (Smith et al. 2010) with permission

There is evidence that several biochemical markers, including elevations in troponin I (Cardinale et al. 2002, 2004) and B-type natriuretic peptide (BNP) (Nousiainen et al. 2002), may indicate early myocardial injury before development of left ventricular dysfunction. Therefore, there has been interest in serial measurements of BNP to detect changes in left ventricular function (Carver et al. 2007). However, no study has thus far validated this as a routine measurement or screening tool in this population (Carver et al. 2007).

2.2 Pulmonary Toxicity

A wide variety of chemotherapeutic agents has pulmonary toxicities (Carver et al. 2007; Limper 2004) as shown in Table 6. Onset of these adverse effects may be acute or insidious (Limper 2004), with some of them causing permanent lung damage in long-term cancer survivors (Limper 2004; Huang et al. 2011). Clinical manifestations include dyspnea, nonproductive cough, and fever, which may develop weeks to years after chemotherapy (Limper 2004).

Table 6 Chemotherapy agents associated with pulmonary toxicity (Trachtenberg et al. 2011; Wouters et al. 2005)

Class of chemotherapy	Agents
Antibiotics	Bleomycin
	Mitomycin C
Alkylating agents	Busulfan
	Cyclophosphamide
	Chlorambucil
	Procarbazine
Antimetabolites	Methotrexate
	Cytosine arabinoside
	Fludarabine
	Gemcitabine
Antimicrotubules agents	Docetaxel
	Paclitaxel
	Vinca alkaloids
Nitrosamines	Carmustine
Topoisomerase inhibitors	Etoposide

Aside from hilar lymphadenopathy that is commonly associated with methotrexate-induced lung injury, there is no characteristic radiographic pattern that is specific for other chemotherapy agents. Bleomycin and busulfan are the most relevant in terms of late effects and will be the main focus of this section.

2.2.1 Types of Chemotherapeutic Agents

2.2.1.1 Bleomycin

Bleomycin is an antibiotic mixture of two copper chelating peptides; fermentation products of *Streptococcus verticillus*, used in the curative treatment of lymphomas and testicular tumors.

Incidence

As many as 20 % of patients develop pulmonary disease after bleomycin (Limper 2004) and the mortality rate from bleomycin-induced pulmonary diseases reaches as high as 1 % (Limper 2004). Bronchiolitis obliterans, eosinophilic hypersensitivity, and interstitial pneumonitis are common bleomycin-related pulmonary disorders (Yousem et al. 1985). Unexplained nonproductive cough and dyspnea on exertion are frequently first signs of bleomycin-induced pneumonitis (BIP) (Comis 1990; Sleijfer 2001) followed by onset of fever, tachypnea, cyanosis, and dyspnea with progressive lung injury (Comis 1990; Sleijfer 2001).

There is a linear relationship between the cumulative dose of bleomycin and the incidence of pulmonary toxicity in animal models (Sleijfer 2001). Studies have shown that the incidence of BIP increases from 3 to 5 % with cumulative bleomycin dose <300 mg to 20 % with doses >500 mg (Fung and Vaughn 2011). Aside from cumulative dose of bleomycin, other risk factors that predispose patients to bleomycin-induced lung injury include mediastinal radiation, renal dysfunction, increased age, smoking, exposure to high-inspired oxygen concentration, and pre-existing pulmonary comorbidity (Carver et al. 2007; Fung and Vaughn 2011; Limper 2004). Concomitant administration of cyclophosphamide, vincristine, doxorubicin, and methotrexate with bleomycin has also been reported to increase risk of pulmonary fibrosis (Huang et al. 2011).

Pathophysiology

The primary mechanism for BIP is direct endothelial damage from bleomycin (Huang et al. 2011; Sleijfer 2001; Cooper et al. 1988), most likely caused by induction of cytokines and free radicals (Sleijfer 2001). These cytokines activate lymphocytes and upregulate adhesion molecules of the endothelial cells, which facilitates adhesion and influx of inflammatory cells, including macrophages, neutrophils, and lymphocytes, into the lung interstitium via the endothelium (Sleijfer 2001). Damage of the endothelial cells, along with infiltration of inflammatory cells into the interstitium, subsequently activates fibroblasts to deposit collagen, which causes pulmonary fibrosis (Sleijfer 2001).

2.2.1.2 Busulfan

Incidence

Busulfan is an alkylating agent with myelosuppressive properties, and is commonly used in the myeloablative conditioning regimen of bone marrow transplantation for hematologic malignancies (Limper 2004; Bilgrami et al. 2001) and idiopathic pneumonia syndrome (IPS) has been described in this population (Bilgrami et al. 2001). The incidence of busulfan pulmonary toxicity is approximately 6 %, with a range of 2.5–43 % (Limper 2004). The average time from initiation of therapy to onset of pulmonary symptoms is approximately 3.5 years, with some patients developing symptoms up to 10 years after treatment (Limper 2004). Dyspnea, cough, and fever are common clinical manifestations and occur in a more insidious nature than with other chemotherapy-related lung disease (Limper 2004). While some patients improve after discontinuation of busulfan and administration of corticosteroids, many develop progressive lung impairment that may ultimately lead to death (Limper 2004). Unlike bleomycin, it is uncertain if busulfan-related lung injury occurs in a dose-dependent fashion (Limper 2004). However, concomitant radiation and cytotoxic agents, such as cyclophosphamide, thiotepa, and melphalan, appear to increase pulmonary toxicities (Limper 2004; Bilgrami et al. 2001).

Pathophysiology

The exact mechanism for busulfan-induced lung injury is unknown, but cell-mediated immune reactions and release of cytokines are thought to be involved (Bilgrami et al. 2001). Atypical oval or elongated cells, intra-alveolar rather than interstitial fibrosis, and multinucleated giant cell containing eosinophilic nuclear inclusions are common histological features with busulfan-induced lung toxicity (Bilgrami et al. 2001). Furthermore, the number of type I pneumocytes decreases while type II pneumocytes proliferate, delamellate, and migrate into alveolar sacs (Bilgrami et al. 2001). Consequently, this may lead to extensive accumulation of alveolar debris that yields a pattern similar to alveolar proteinosis (Limper 2004).

2.2.2 Pulmonary Function Monitoring

Historically, pulmonary function test (PFT), which includes measurement of lung volumes and oxygen diffusion capacity, has been used to monitor for BIP (Fung and Vaughn 2011). Bleomycin was traditionally withheld if the diffusion capacity of carbon monoxide (DLCO) fell below 40–60 % of the pretreatment value (Comis 1990). Sleijfer et al. (1995) examined the validity of using DLCO to detect onset of BIP in testicular cancer patients and showed that DLCO declined in both groups of patients receiving bleomycin, etoposide, and cisplatin (BEP) and etoposide and cisplatin (EP). However, the decrease in DLCO of the BEP group became significant only at 12 weeks after completion of treatment ($P < 0.01$) when compared to the EP group. Therefore, the authors concluded that a decline in DLCO during active treatment should not be used as the basis for discontinuation of bleomycin therapy. In long-term survivors of Hodgkin's disease, PFT monitoring has been reported in several clinical trials and they showed that early decline in PFT is followed by subsequent improvement over time in most patients (Carver et al. 2007).

Aside from DLCO, Haugnes et al. (2009) have studied the validity of using other PFT measures to monitor for pulmonary damage in 1,049 long-term testicular survivors after chemotherapy. They reported a decline in both the predicted forced vital capacity (FVC) and forced expiratory volume in one second (FEV_1) in this cohort of patients. However, the onset of the decrease in these parameters is unclear and therefore, routine use of FVC and FEV_1 to monitor for chemotherapy-induced pulmonary damage is not currently recommended during chemotherapy for testicular cancer patients.

2.2.3 Management of Chemotherapy-Induced Pulmonary Toxicities

Withholding bleomycin at the earliest clinical signs or symptoms of pulmonary toxicities is the most effective treatment for BIP (Fung and Vaughn 2011). Although data regarding role of corticosteroids in management of BIP from prospective randomized trials is lacking, corticosteroids (for example, prednisone 60–100 mg/day) are the mainstay of treatment currently (Sleijfer 2001). For BIP that are refractory to standard-dose corticosteroids, azathioprine (150 mg/day) and high-dose corticosteroids have been used successfully (Fung and Vaughn 2011; Maher and Daly 1993). Similarly, early treatment with corticosteroids is common for busulfan-induced pulmonary toxicities (Bilgrami et al. 2001).

2.3 Nephrotoxicity

Nephrotoxicity is an inherent adverse effect of several chemotherapeutic agents (Kintzel 2001) as shown in Table 7. Mechanism of chemotherapy-induced renal dysfunction usually involves vasculature or tubular damage of the kidneys along with inadequate renal perfusion (Kintzel 2001; Skinner 2011). Hypertension, proteinuria, and varying degrees of renal insufficiency are common clinical manifestations of chemotherapy-induced nephrotoxicity (Jones et al. 2008). While these symptoms may be transient, chronic renal insufficiency may develop insidiously in a minority of patients (Skinner 2011). Long-term renal dysfunction associated with cisplatin and ifosfamide (Fung and Vaughn 2011; Jones et al. 2008) have been described and will be the main focus of this section.

2.3.1 Types of Chemotherapeutic Agents

2.3.1.1 Cisplatin

Cisplatin has broad antineoplastic activity, and plays an indispensible role in the curative treatment regimens for testicular cancer. It has activity against ovarian cancer as well as cancers of the head and neck, lung, bladder, and esophagus, and is used as adjuvant therapy in many of these cancers.

Incidence

Clinical manifestations of cisplatin nephrotoxicity include acute and/or chronic renal insufficiency, hypokalemia, and hypomagnesemia, which many cause paresthesia, tremor, tetany, and convulsions (Fung and Vaughn 2011; Skinner 2011). Among long-term testicular cancer survivors treated with cisplatin, approximately 20–30 % of them developed a long-term deterioration in renal function, with an average decline of 20–30 % in glomerular filtration rate (GFR) (Fung and Vaughn 2011). A recent study by Skinner et al. (2009) examined the incidence of long-term nephrotoxicity in 27 children who received cisplatin. At 10-year follow-up, they reported that there was no recovery of cisplatin-induced renal toxicity, as measured by GFR and serum

Table 7 Chemotherapy agents associated with nephrotoxicity (van Dalen et al. 2010)

Class of chemotherapy	Agents
Antibiotics	Mitomycin
Alkylating agents	Ifosfamide
Antimetabolites	Azacitidine
	Gemcitabine
	Methotrexate
	Pentostatin
Nitrosamines	Carmustine
	Semustine
Platinum agents	Carboplatin
	Cisplatin
Vascular endothelial growth inhibitors	Bevacizumab
	Sorafenib
	Sunitinib
Others	Interferon-α

Adapted from Kintzel and colleagues (van Dalen et al. 2010) with permission

magnesium. GFR was <60 ml/min/1.73 m^2 in 11 % of them at both completion and 10 years after chemotherapy.

Risk factors for development of cisplatin nephrotoxicity include high cumulative cisplatin dose (≥500 mg/m^2), increased rate of infusion, older age, pre-existing renal disease, renal radiation (≥15 Gy), and concomitant treatment with other nephrotoxins, such as aminoglycosides, amphotericin, immunosuppressants, and methotrexate (Fung and Vaughn 2011; Skinner 2011; Jones et al. 2008). In adults, renal toxicity is less common with low-dose cisplatin (20 mg/m^2/day) than high-dose (40 mg/m^2/day) (Skinner 2011) while children who received >40 mg/m^2/day developed significantly more nephrotoxicity than those at a lower dose (Skinner 2011).

Pathophysiology

Cisplatin exerts direct toxic effects on both the renal tubules and collecting ducts (Fung and Vaughn 2011). Filtration of unbound cisplatin at the glomerulus leads to its uptake into the renal tubular cells (Yao et al. 2007) where it is partially metabolized to nephrotoxic molecules, which subsequently cause cell injury (Yao et al. 2007). Cisplatin also has other intracellular effects that cause tubular damage and dysfunction which may explain sodium, potassium, and magnesium wasting in patients (Yao et al. 2007). These mechanisms include direct cytotoxicity with reactive oxygen species, activation of mitogen-activated protein kinases, induction of apoptosis, and stimulation of inflammation and fibrinogenesis (Yao et al. 2007). Furthermore, cisplatin may also induce renal vasculature damage, resulting in decreased blood flow and ischemic insult to the kidneys (Pabla and Dong 2008).

2.3.1.2 Ifosfamide

Incidence

Ifosfamide has a critical role in the treatment of many solid pediatric malignancies, including bone and soft-tissue sarcoma, Wilm's tumor, neuroblastoma, and germ cell tumors (Lawson et al. 2008). Proximal tubular dysfunction and decline in GFR, are the most common clinical manifestation of ifosfamide-induced nephrotoxicity (Jones et al. 2008), causing rise in serum creatinine and blood urea nitrogen levels, oliguria, and proximal tubular wasting of electrolytes, glucose, and amino acids (Kintzel 2001). Although most acute renal tubular dysfunction resolves, a minority of kidney damage is permanent and potentially progressive (Jones et al. 2008).

In a study of 16 pediatric osteosarcoma patients after high-dose ifosfamide (14 g/m^2 per course), 25 % of them experienced a reduction in GFR, as defined by ≥3 times increase in normal serum creatinine level (Berrak et al. 2005). Skinner et al. (2000) also reported that 17–50 % of pediatric sarcoma patients treated with conventional doses of ifosfamide subsequently developed progressive renal insufficiency. Furthermore, Suarez et al. (1991) reported that among 74 children with malignant mesenchymal tumors who received ifosfamide, 5 % of them developed persistent renal tubulopathy that resulted in Fanconi syndrome.

Risk factors that may predispose patients to ifosfamide-induced nephrotoxicity include younger age at treatment (<5 years at time of treatment), higher cumulative dose (≥60 g/m^2), renal radiation (≥15 Gy), and concurrent administration of other nephrotoxins, including cisplatin, amphotericin, immunosuppressants, and methotrexate (Skinner 2011; Jones et al. 2008; Skinner et al. 2000). While most published reports of ifosfamide-induced renal damage were in infants and young children, the significance of age as a risk factor remains unclear (Skinner 2011). Although several studies suggest that young age is a significant risk factor (Skinner 2011), this does not appear to predict long-term nephrotoxicity at 10 years (Skinner et al. 2010). Instead, Oberlin and colleagues recently reported that older age at treatment is associated with decreased GFR at 10 years among 183 pediatric patients who received a median dose of 54 g/m^2 of ifosfamide (RR = 1.08; 95 % CI 1.01–1.15). Concurrent cisplatin predisposes patients to higher risk of renal toxicity (Fung and Vaughn 2011). Loebstein et al. (1999) reported that the incidence of nephrotoxicity increased from 33.5 to 41.4 % when cisplatin was included in the chemotherapy of pediatric testicular cancer patients after a cumulative ifosfamide dose of 45 mg/m^2.

Pathophysiology

The underlying pathogenesis of ifosfamide-induced nephrotoxicity is currently poorly understood but direct cytotoxicity by ifosfamide or its metabolites is most likely implicated (Skinner 2011), which may involve production of reactive oxygen species that causes disruption in tubular cell energy pathways and membrane function (Skinner 2011). Chloroacetaldehyde (CAA), a metabolite of ifosfamide, is thought to be the primary causative agent for ifosfamide-induced renal damage (Skinner 2011). In a renal tubular cell culture model, CAA causes an experimental Fanconi syndrome possibly by blocking active transport and increasing the permeability of tubular cell membranes (Skinner 2011).

2.3.2 Renal Protective Interventions

Aggressive hydration is the best strategy to reduce the risk of cisplatin nephrotoxicity (Fung and Vaughn 2011). However, evidence for forced diuresis using mannitol or furosemide is controversial (Launay-Vacher et al. 2008). While several experimental reports (Cvitkovic et al. 1977; Pera et al. 1979) have suggested that these diuretics decreased cisplatin nephrotoxicity in animals, two randomized studies in humans (Al-Sarraf et al. 1982; Santoso et al. 2003) showed no such effect. At the same time, concomitant administration of nephrotoxic agents, such as aminoglycosides, non-steroidal anti-inflammatory drugs, and iodinated contrast media, should be avoided in patients receiving cisplatin (Fung and Vaughn 2011). In 2008, the European Society of Clinical Pharmacy Special Interest Group on Cancer Care published their recommendations on the prevention of cisplatin nephrotoxicity (Launay-Vacher et al. 2008) as shown in Table 8.

The most important measure to reduce the risk of ifosfamide nephrotoxicity is hydration (Fung and Vaughn 2011). While sodium 2-mercaptoethanesulfonate (Mesna) is effective in preventing hemorrhagic cystitis (Lawson et al. 2008), its renal protective effects are uncertain (Lawson et al. 2008). Electrolyte supplementation for patients with persistent electrolyte wasting is also critical after ifosfamide administration (Jones et al. 2008).

2.3.3 Surveillance of Nephrotoxicity

Due to risks of long-term nephrotoxicity from chemotherapy, patients should be monitored regularly using a defined surveillance protocol (Skinner 2011). According to the Children's Oncology Group of the United States (2008), pediatric oncology patients should have medical check-up at least yearly that includes blood pressure monitoring and urinalysis. At the first long-term follow-up visit (≥2 years after completion of chemotherapy), a basic metabolic panel should be obtained to monitor electrolytes, blood urea nitrogen, and creatinine levels. In addition, these patients should use over-the-counter non-steroidal anti-inflammatory drugs with caution.

Table 8 ESCP SIG Cancer Care recommendations on the prevention of cisplatin nephrotoxicity (van Dalen et al. 2009)

Before administration
1. Estimate GFR or CrCL using MDRD or Cockcroft-Gault formula, respectively
2. Ensure euvolemia is present
Dosage
Adjust cisplatin dosage according to the patient's renal function
Administration
Administer the platinum slowly
Hydration
1. Use a saline solution infusion that produces a brisk diuresis
2. Urine flow should be maintained at 3–4 1/24 h the preceding day and for the next 2–3 days
3. Do not use diuretics, neither mannitol nor furosemide
4. There are no data for patients who already are on diuretics, for another concomitant disease such as hypertension
After administration
1. When feasible, determine serum creatinine 3–5 days after completion of the course
2. Monitor magnesium levels routinely and supplement when necessary
3. Avoid co-adminstration of nephrotoxic drugs (aminoglycosides, non-steroidal anti-inflammatory drugs, iodinated contrast media, zoledronate, etc.)
4. Re-evaluate renal function before the next course

CrCL Creatinine clearance, *MDRD* Modification of Diet in Renal Disease

Adapted from Launay-Vacher (van Dalen et al. 2009) and colleagues with permission

2.4 Peripheral Neuropathy

Chemotherapy-induced peripheral neuropathy (CIPN) is a common, potentially severe side effect that can affect the quality of life in long-term cancer survivors (Cavaletti and Marmiroli 2010; Manji 2011). Sensory neuropathies, including paresthesias and pain, are the most common symptoms of CIPN (Pachman et al. 2011), and they usually begin from the fingers and toes and spread proximally in a "glove and stocking" distribution (Pachman et al. 2011). Onset of CIPN usually begins weeks to months after initial treatment with complete resolution of symptoms (Cavaletti and Marmiroli 2010; Manji 2011; Pachman et al. 2011). However, in some cases, CIPN is only partially reversible and can become permanent (Pachman et al. 2011). Table 9 lists the cytotoxic agents commonly associated with CIPN. In this section, we will focus on antimicrotubule agents, platinum analogs, and proteasome inhibitors.

Table 9 Chemotherapy agents associated with peripheral neuropathy (Giantris et al. 1998)

Class of chemotherapy	Agents
Antimicrotubules agents	Docetaxel
	Ixabepilone
	Paclitaxel
	Vincristine
Platinum agents	Carboplatin
	Cisplatin
	Oxaliplatin
Proteasome inhibitor	Bortezomib
Others	Thalidomide

Adpated from Cavaletti (Giantris et al. 1998) and colleagues with permission

2.4.1 Type of Chemotherapeutic Agents

2.4.1.1 Antimicrotubule Agents

Paclitaxel, ixabepilone, and vincristine are microtubule inhibitors commonly associated with CIPN (Cavaletti and Marmiroli 2010; Manji 2011). While paclitaxel and ixabepilone both induce polymerization and stabilization of tubulin dimers, vincristine prevents tubulin polymerization from soluble dimers into microtubules (Cavaletti and Marmiroli 2010).

Incidence

The incidence of paclitaxel-induced grade 3 and 4 sensory neuropathy ranges from 2 to 32 % depending on the dose and schedule of its administration (Carlson and Ocean 2011), with its clinical manifestations including paresthesias, numbness, and/or pain in a stocking-glove distribution; decreased proprioception and vibration; sensory ataxia; gait disturbance; and impaired deep tendon reflexes (Cavaletti and Marmiroli 2010; Carlson and Ocean 2011). In some patients, myopathy accompanied by muscle weakness in foot, finger, and ankle extensor muscles also develop (Cavaletti and Marmiroli 2010; Carlson and Ocean 2011). Onset of peripheral neuropathy usually occurs after cumulative doses of 100–300 mg/m^2 of paclitaxel (Carlson and Ocean 2011). Dose-dense administration of paclitaxel, albumin-bound paclitaxel, and concomitant administration of platinum agents are other risk factors for paclitaxel-induced CIPN (Manji 2011; Carlson and Ocean 2011).

Approximately 1–24 % of patients experienced grade 3 and 4 sensory neuropathy after ixabepilone, depending of its dose and administration schedule (Carlson and Ocean 2011). Onset of CIPN usually occurs after cumulative doses of 40–120 mg/m^2 of ixabepilone (Carlson and Ocean 2011). Compared to peripheral neuropathy associated with paclitaxel, peripheral neuropathy induced by ixabepilone is very similar in nature but its recovery appears to be considerably faster (Cavaletti and Marmiroli 2010; Carlson and Ocean 2011). Examining a dataset of 1,540 patients who received ixabepilone as a monotherapy or in combination with capecitabine, Vahdat et al. (2012) reported pre-existing neuropathy as the only risk factor for ixabepilone-associated peripheral neuropathy.

Vinca alkaloids, including vincristine, vinorelbine, and vinflunine, are all associated with CIPN (Cavaletti and Marmiroli 2010; Carlson and Ocean 2011). After discontinuation of vincristine, up to 30 % of patients may continue to experience peripheral neuropathy (Carlson and Ocean 2011). Aside from sensory neuropathy, moderate to severe autonomic dysfunction is also common after vincrisitine (Cavaletti and Marmiroli 2010; Carlson and Ocean 2011), with colicky abdominal pain and constipation being its symptoms (Cavaletti and Marmiroli 2010; Carlson and Ocean 2011). Furthermore, few cases of paralytic ileus and megacolon have also been reported (Carlson and Ocean 2011). With the newer generation of vinca alkaloids, such as vinorelbine and vinflunine, patients usually develop a primarily sensory neuropathy that is reversible after discontinuation of agents (Carlson and Ocean 2011).

Pathophysiology

The mechanisms for microtubules inhibitors-induced peripheral neuropathy have not been elucidated (Cavaletti and Marmiroli 2010; Carlson and Ocean 2011). Disruption of the active transport of proteins and other compounds within the neuron has been proposed as the main mechanism since intact function of the microtubules is critical for anterograde and retrograde axonal transport and the survival of neurons (Carlson and Ocean 2011). There are evidence that taxanes, such as paclitaxel and docetaxel, target both the axons and the soma of the sensory neurons (Cavaletti et al. 1995, 1997; Persohn et al. 2005) with dorsal root ganglions as the initial site of injury (Carlson and Ocean 2011; Cavaletti et al. 2000). Through signal transduction-mediated pathways, microglial activation within the spinal cord and macrophage activation within the dorsal root ganglion and peripheral nerves appear to be the key pathways in the pathogenesis of taxane-induced peripheral neuropathy (Cavaletti and Marmiroli 2010). The pathophysiology for ixabepilone-induced peripheral neuropathy is hypothesized to be similar to that of the taxanes due to their similar mechanism of action (Carlson and Ocean 2011). Unlike ixabepilone and the taxanes, however, vinca alkaloids induce depolymerization of microtubules (Cavaletti and Marmiroli 2010). This effect on tubulin dimers causes alteration in the length, arrangement, and orientation of axonal microtubules (Cavaletti and Marmiroli 2010), which may explain axonal transport dysfunction and Wallerian-like axonal degeneration (Cavaletti and Marmiroli 2010) observed in patients after treatment with vinca alkaloids.

2.4.1.2 Platinum Agents

Platinum compounds form DNA intrastrand adducts and interstrand crosslinks that disrupt the structure and function of DNA (Cavaletti and Marmiroli 2010) with peripheral neuropathy being a significant side effect of both cisplatin and oxaliplatin (Fung and Vaughn 2011; Cavaletti and Marmiroli 2010; Manji 2011).

Incidence

Approximately 7–31 % of testicular cancer patients undergoing cisplatin-based chemotherapy develop acute peripheral neuropathy (Bajorin et al. 1993; de Wit et al. 2001; Nichols et al. 1998). After a median follow-up of 10 years, persistent symptomatic peripheral neuropathy occurred in up to 30 % of testicular cancer patients after 3–4 cycles of cisplatin-based chemotherapy (Brydoy et al. 2009; Glendenning et al. 2010). Numbness, tingling, decreased proprioception, and impaired vibratory and temperature sensation are common clinical manifestations of cisplatin-induced peripheral neuropathy (Fung and Vaughn 2011; Cavaletti and Marmiroli 2010; Amptoulach and Tsavaris 2011). Onset of peripheral neuropathy usually occurs after a cumulative cisplatin dose of >300 mg/m^2 with 50–90 % of patients experiencing neuropathy after a cumulative dose of >500 mg/m^2 (Fung and Vaughn 2011; Amptoulach and Tsavaris 2011). Cumulative dose of cisplatin is the most significant risk factor for cisplatin-induced neuropathy (Fung and Vaughn 2011; Brydoy et al. 2009; Amptoulach and Tsavaris 2011).

The incidence of acute oxaliplatin-induced peripheral neuropathy ranges from 65 to 85 % depending on the dose and schedule of its administration (Argyriou et al. 2008), with its clinical symptoms including paresthesias and dysesthesias in the extremities and perioral region that are exacerbated by cold exposure (Amptoulach and Tsavaris 2011). In 1–2 % of patients, transient laryngopharyngeal dysesthesia that manifests as shortness of breath and swallowing difficulty may develop (Amptoulach and Tsavaris 2011; Argyriou et al. 2008). Although these acute toxicities are reversible in approximately 80 % of patients and usually resolve completely in about 40 % of patients 6–8 months after discontinuation of oxaliplatin (Amptoulach and Tsavaris 2011), chronic neuropathy has been reported (Amptoulach and Tsavaris 2011; Argyriou et al. 2008). Its incidence is related to various risk factors, including single dose per course, cumulative dose, administration schedule, and pre-existing peripheral neuropathy (Amptoulach and Tsavaris 2011; Argyriou et al. 2008). Table 10 compares the clinical characteristics of cisplatin and oxaliplatin-induced neurotoxicity.

Table 10 Comparison of cisplatin- and oxaliplatin-induced neuropathy (Nousiainen et al. 2002)

	Cisplatin	Oxaliplatin
Dose-limiting toxicity	Peripheral neuropathy	Peripheral neuropathy
Symptoms	Paresthesia	Paresthesia, sensory ataxia, and dysesthesia
Location	Extremities	Extremities, perioral area
Time-course onset	Delayed	Acute and delayed
After treatment	Deterioration	Usually recovery
Accompanying toxicities	Ototoxicity	Laryngospasms
Precipitating factors	None	Exposure to cold

Adapted from Amtoulach and colleagues (Nousiainen et al. 2002) with permission

Pathophysiology

Cisplatin causes damage to the dorsal root ganglion, which subsequently leads to anterograde axonal degeneration via several mechanisms (Fung and Vaughn 2011). By altering structures of neuronal DNA, it causes changes in the cell-cycle kinetics that promote apoptosis, oxidative stress, and mitochondrial dysfunction (Cavaletti and Marmiroli 2010; Manji 2011). The mechanisms of action for acute and chronic oxaliplatin-induced peripheral neuropathy are different and have not been fully elucidated (Argyriou et al. 2008). Evidence suggests that oxalate, a metabolite of oxaliplatin, interferes with the voltage-gated sodium channels that are critical for calcium transport of the neurons in acute oxaliplatin-induced neuropathy (Cavaletti and Marmiroli 2010; Argyriou et al. 2008). On the contrary, chronic oxaliplatin-induced neuropathy results from accumulation of oxaliplatin in the cells of dorsal root ganglia due to decreased cellular metabolism and axonal transport, which ultimately lead to direct cytotoxicity to the neurons (Argyriou et al. 2008). Furthermore, injury to the mitochondria by oxaliplatin has also been proposed as another potential mechanism (Argyriou et al. 2008).

2.4.1.3 Proteasome Inhibitors

Peripheral neuropathy is an important dose-limiting toxicity of bortezomib, which is a proteasome inhibitor approved for the treatment of multiple myeloma (Cavaletti and Marmiroli 2010; Cavaletti and Jakubowiak 2010). More importantly, up to 20 % of patients with multiple myeloma experience baseline sensory peripheral neuropathy from the disease itself, which further renders them susceptible to CIPN (Manji 2011).

Incidence

Approximately 37–44 % of patients developed bortezomib-induced peripheral neuropathy with painful distal sensory symptoms as the hallmark of its clinical manifestation (Cavaletti and Marmiroli 2010; Cavaletti and Jakubowiak 2010). This neuropathic pain can be severe and some patients also develop distal sensory loss, reduced deep tender reflexes, and impaired proprioception (Cavaletti and Marmiroli 2010). Onset of bortezomib-induced peripheral neuropathy usually occurs within 3 months of treatment initiation (Cavaletti and Jakubowiak 2010) with its recovery taking as long as 1.7 years in some patients (Cavaletti and Jakubowiak 2010). Furthermore, a minority of patients will experience persistent neuropathy after its discontinuation (Cavaletti and Jakubowiak 2010). Cumulative treatment dose appears as the most significant predictor for this risk (Cavaletti and Jakubowiak 2010).

Pathophysiology

The exact pathogenesis of bortezomib-induced neuropathy remains unknown. However, by targeting dorsal root ganglion, bortezomib may interfere with transcription, nuclear processing and transport, and cytoplasmic translation of messenger RNAs in these neurons (Cavaletti and Marmiroli 2010), which ultimately leads to extensive damage of both myelinated and unmyelinated axons (Cavaletti and Marmiroli 2010). Other mechanisms, including disruption of the neurotrophin network and dysregulation of the mitochondrial and endoplasmic reticulum-medicated calcium transport, may also be involved in bortezomib-induced neuropathy (Cavaletti and Marmiroli 2010).

2.4.2 Prevention and Treatment of CIPN

There are currently no pharmacological agents that are commonly used to prevent CIPN. However, the use of calcium and magnesium (Ca/Mg) infusion has shown promising results. A recent randomized, placebo-controlled, double-blind study by Grothey et al. (2011) investigated its efficacy in prevention of oxaliplatin-induced neuropathy in 102 patients undergoing adjuvant chemotherapy with 5-fluorouracil, leucovorin, and oxaliplatin (FOLFOX) for colon cancer. Ca/Mg reduced the incidence of chronic, cumulative $\geq$ grade 2 sensory neurotoxicity as measured by the National Cancer Institute Common Terminology Criteria for Adverse Events (NCI CTCAE) ($P = 0.038$) and by an oxaliplatin-specific sensory neurotoxicity scale ($P = 0.018$). On the contrary, a recent meta-analysis by Albers et al. (2011) examined eight purported neuroprotective agents for cisplatin-induced neuropathy, including acetylcysteine, amifostine, Ca/Mg, diethyldithiocarbamate, glutathione, Org2766, oxcarbazepine, and vitamin E, and concluded that there is insufficient data to show that any of them prevent or limit CIPN due to cisplatin.

There are currently no proven pharmacologic treatments for CIPN (Cavaletti and Marmiroli 2010; Pachman et al. 2011). Although the use of anticonvulsant or antidepressant drugs, including carbamazepine, lamotrigine, gabapentin, pregabalin, and venlafaxine, are common (Fung and Vaughn 2011; Cavaletti and Marmiroli 2010) and have shown efficacy in treatment of neuropathy from other causes (Pachman et al. 2011), such as diabetes, their data in CIPN are limited (Fung and Vaughn 2011; Pachman et al. 2011). As a result, modification or withdrawal of the insulting chemotherapeutic agent is usually the only option available for oncologists (Pachman et al. 2011). To assess severity of CIPN, several instruments (Pachman et al. 2011) are commonly used and they include the NCI CTCAE, the European Organization for Research and Treatment of Cancer Quality of Life CINP-20 questionnaire, the Total Neuropathy Score, the Functional Assessment of Cancer Therapy (FACT)/Gynecologic Oncology Group-Neurotoxicity questionnaire, the FACT-taxane tool, the Oxaliplatin-associated Neuropathy Questionnaire, Patient Neurotoxicity Questionnaire, and the Peripheral Neuropathy Scale.

2.5 Ototoxicity

Ototoxicity is a serious side effect among long-term cancer survivors after platinum-based chemotherapy (Fung and Vaughn 2011). This impairment has a particularly significant impact in the pediatric population since it can affect their learning, communication, school performance, social interaction, and overall health-related quality of life (Grewal et al. 2010). Ototoxicity is a dose-limiting adverse effect for both cisplatin and carboplatin (Fung and Vaughn 2011; Grewal et al. 2010) and will be discussed in this section.

2.5.1 Type of Chemotherapeutic Agents

2.5.1.1 Cisplatin

Incidence

Cisplatin causes high frequency hearing loss (4–8 kHz) and tinnitus (Fung and Vaughn 2011; Rybak et al. 2009) and these symptoms may occur within hours to days after treatment (Rybak et al. 2009). Young age at initial treatment (<5 years), high cumulative dose of cisplatin, impaired baseline renal and hearing function, and concurrent cochlear radiation (dose >48 Gy) are the most significant risk factors for ototoxicity (Fung and Vaughn 2011; Grewal et al. 2010; Rybak et al. 2009). Approximately 7–31 % of patients undergoing treatment with cisplatin-based chemotherapy develop transient tinnitus (Fung and Vaughn 2011). In a Pediatric Intergroup Study for children and adolescents with high-risk germ cell tumors (Cushing et al. 2004), 14 % of patients developed grade 3–4 hearing loss after high-dose cisplatin (800 mg/m^2) compared to 0 % of those with low-dose administration (400 mg/m^2). Similarly, Bokemeyer et al. (1998) reported that approximately 20 % of testicular cancer patients treated with ≤400 mg/m^2 experienced self-reported tinnitus and hearing loss chronically as compared to 50 % of those treated with >400 mg/m^2. In another study that compared the risks of ototoxicity in testicular cancer survivors who underwent dose-intensive chemotherapy (>100 mg/m^2 of cisplatin per cycle) to those without chemotherapy, Brydøy et al. (2009) found that patients in the dose-intensive group had 5.3 and 7.1 times higher risks of subjective hearing loss and tinnitus respectively.

Pathophysiology

Cisplatin causes damage to several areas of the cochlea, including the outer hair cells in the basal turn, spiral ganglion cells, and stria vascularis (Rybak et al. 2007, 2009). The underlying mechanism appears to involve generation of reactive oxygen species that triggers apoptosis in the inner ear (Rybak et al. 2007, 2009). Cisplatin has been shown to activate an enzyme known as a NOX-3, leading to an increase in superoxide production in both cochlear cell lines and cochlea of rates (Rybak et al. 2007). This superoxide production would subsequently activate a cascade of events resulting in oxidation of lipids and cell death (Rybak et al. 2007).

2.5.1.2 Carboplatin

Incidence

Although carboplatin is less ototoxic than cisplatin, approximately 0–38 % of patients still experience hearing impairment after treatment with carboplatin (Musial-Bright et al. 2011). Musial-Bright et al. (2011) recently examined the incidence of ototoxicity in 19 medulloblastoma patients who underwent treatment according to HIT protocols with carboplatin substitution and had adequate baseline and post-treatment audiological data. They reported that 10.5 % of patients developed hearing loss >20 dB. Younger age at diagnosis and higher cumulative carboplatin dose were both significant risk factors ($P < 0.05$) for hearing loss in this study cohort. Similarly, Qaddoumi et al. (2012) reported that twelve of sixty patients (20 %) with retinoblastoma who received front-line treatment with systemic carboplatin and vincristine developed ototoxicity. Furthermore, ten of these patients (17 %) had sustained hearing loss after a median follow-up of 6.1 years. Young age at the start of chemotherapy was again found to be associated with increased incidence of hearing loss. However, in three other studies (Friedman et al. 2000; Lambert et al. 2008; Smits et al. 2006) that examined carboplatin-induced ototoxicity in patients with retinoblastoma, no ototoxicity was reported.

Pathophysiology

The pathogenesis of carboplatin-induced ototoxicity is not well described in the current literature but it may resemble that of cisplatin due to their similar mechanisms of action.

2.5.2 Prevention and Treatment of Ototoxicity

The Food and Drug Administration in the United States has not approved any drugs as protective agents for cisplatin ototoxicity (Rybak et al. 2007). Several agents, including thiols, adenosine A1 receptor agonists, pifithrin or capase inhibitors, combination of ebselen and allopurinol, sodium butyrate, and salicylates, show potential promise for prevention of cisplatin ototoxicity (Fung and Vaughn 2011) and will require further studies in humans. To reduce the risk of ototoxicity, patients undergoing platinum-based chemotherapy should be encouraged to avoid loud noise and ototoxins, such as gentamicin, tobramycin, or furosemide (Fung and Vaughn 2011). Protective ear defenders or ear plugs should also be considered for those who work or live in a noisy environment (Fung and Vaughn 2011). Although there are no current effective treatment for cisplatin ototoxicity, gene therapy with antiapoptotic genes and intratympanic application of adenosine agonists both showed promising results in this regard (Rybak et al. 2007).

Since hearing impairment may adversely impact quality of life, socio-emotional development, and academic performance in children (Grewal et al. 2010), all childhood cancer survivors after ototoxic chemotherapy should undergo annual audiological evaluation and physical examination (Grewal et al. 2010). For children with progressive hearing loss, speech and language therapy, and other educational support, such as preferential classroom sitting and FM amplification system, should be considered (Grewal et al. 2010).

2.6 Reproductive Toxicity

In the United States, 1.4 million people are diagnosed with cancer every year with approximately 10 % of them <45 years of age (Jemal et al. 2009). As the number of young cancer survivors increases due to medical advancement, infertility due to chemotherapy, as defined by the inability to conceive after 1 year of intercourse without contraception (Lee et al. 2006), has become an important issue in this population. This section will review effects of various chemotherapy regimens on reproductive health including fertility, and describe different fertility preservation options that are available for adolescents and young adults with cancer.

2.6.1 Effects of Chemotherapy on Fertility

Cytotoxic damage to the rapidly differentiating spermatogonia is common during chemotherapy in males (Levine

Table 11 Effects of various chemotherapeutic regimen on sperm production in men (Kremer et al. 2001)

Degree of risk	Chemotherapy regimen	Common usage
High risk: prolonged azoospermia after treatment	Protocols containing procarbazine: COPP, MOPP, MVPP, ChIVPP, ChIVPP/EVA, MOPP/ABVD, COPP/ABVD	Hodgkin's lymphoma
	Alkylating chemotherapy for transplantation conditioning (cyclophosphamide, busulfan, melphalan)	BMT/SCT
	Any alkylating agent (e.g., procarbazine, nitrogen mustard, cyclophosphamide) + TBI, pelvic radiation, or testicular radiation	Testicular cancer, BMT/SCT, ALL, NHL, sarcoma, neuroblastoma, Hodgkin's lymphoma
	Cyclophosphamide >7.5 g/m^2	Sarcoma, NHL, neuroblastoma, ALL
Intermediate risk: prolonged azoospermia not common at standard dose	BEP × 2–4 cycles	Testicular cancer
	Cumulative cisplatin dose <400 mg/m^2	Testicular cancer
	Cumulative carboplatin dose ≤ 2 g/m^2	Testicular cancer
Low risk: temporary azoospermia after treatment	Nonalkylating chemotherapy: ABVD, OEPA, NOVP, CHOP, COP	Hodgkin's lymphoma, NHL
Very low/no risk: no effects on sperm production	Interferon alfa	Multiple cancers
Unknown risk	Irinotecan	Colon cancer
	Bevacizumab	Colon, non-small cell lung cancer
	Cetuximab	Colon, head and neck cancer
	Erlotinib	Non-small cell lung, pancreatic cancer
	Imatinib	Chronic myeloid leukemia, GI stromal tumor

TBI total-body irradiation, *BMT* bone marrow transplantation, *SCT* stem-cell transplantation, *ALL* acute lymphoblastic leukemia, *NHL* non-Hodgkin's lymphoma, *COPP* cyclophosphamide, vincristine, procarbazine, and prednisone, *MOPP* mechlorethamine, vincristine, procarbazine, and prednisone, *MVPP* mechlorethamine, vinblastine, procarbazine, and prednisone, *ChIVPP* chlorambucil, vinblastine, procarbazine, and prednisone, *EVA* etoposide, vinblastine, and doxorubicin, *ABVD* doxorubicin, bleomycin, vinblastine, and dacarbazine, *BEP* bleomycin etoposide, and cisplatin, *OEPA* vincristine, etoposide, prednisolone, and doxorubicin, *NOVP* mitoxantrone, vincristine, vinblastine, and prednisone, *CHOP* cyclophosphamide, doxorubicin, vincristine, and prednisone, *COP* cyclophosphamide, vincristine, and prednisone
Adapted from Levine and colleagues (Kremer et al. 2001) with permission

et al. 2010). Sperm count usually nadir at 6 months after completion of chemotherapy and may remain impaired for up to 2 years (Levine et al. 2010). For those with quantitative or qualitative injury to spermatogenic stem cells, infertility may become permanent (Levine et al. 2010). The risk of infertility depends on age of patient and the type, dose and schedule of cytotoxic treatments (Levine et al. 2010), with high dose alkylating agents and cisplatin predisposing patients to highest risk of prolonged or permanent infertility (Levine et al. 2010). Several other risk factors (Levine et al. 2010) include radiation to the testes (>1.2 Gy), total-body irradiation used as conditioning regimen for stem cell transplant, cranial radiation (>35–40 Gy) that results in deficiency of gonadotropin-releasing hormone, and baseline azoospermia preceding treatment as seen in patients with Hodgkin's lymphoma and testicular cancer. Table 11 describes the effect of various chemotherapy on sperm production in males (Levine et al. 2010).

On the contrary, females have a relatively finite number of ovarian primordial follicles and their reproductive potential declines when this population of follicles drops below a threshold number through normal atresia and maturation (Levine et al. 2010). Chemotherapy predisposes women to infertility by reducing this fixed number of primordial follicles as well as the number of larger maturing follicles (Levine et al. 2010) with the type, dose, and administration schedule of chemotherapy affecting the extent of injury to these follicles (Knopman et al. 2010). Other risk factors for infertility include older age at treatment, use of alkylating agents, pelvic irradiation, and cranial radiation (>35–40 Gy) (Levine et al. 2010). Table 12 describes the effect of various chemotherapy on development of amenorrhea (Levine et al. 2010).

2.6.2 Chemotherapy and Risks of Congenital Anomalies in Offspring

Due to the effects of chemotherapy on processes critical for embryogenesis, including DNA replication, cell division, and cellular metabolism, many patients who survived cancer reported fear of congenital anomalies in their offspring as the primary reason for not pursuing pregnancy (Knopman et al. 2010). Although this is a valid theoretical concern, several studies of the offspring of cancer reported no increased incidence of congenital or chromosomal anomalies in children

Table 12 Effects of various chemotherapeutic regimen on development of amenorrhea (Kremer et al. 2001)

Degree of risk	Chemotherapy regimen	Common usage
High risk: >80 % of women develop amenorrhea after treatment	CMF, CEF, or CAF × 6 cycles in women age 40+	Breast cancer
	Cyclophosphamide 5 g/m^2 in women 40+	Multiple cancers
	Cyclophosphamide 7.5 g/m^2 in female age <20	NHL, neuroblastoma, ALL, sarcoma
	Alkylating chemotherapy (e.g., cyclophosphamide, busulfan, melphalan) conditioning for transplantation	BMT/SCT
	Any alkylating agent (e.g., cyclophosphamide, ifosfamide, busulfan, CNU, CCNU) + TBI or pelvic radiation	BMT/SCT, ovarian cancer, sarcoma, neuroblastoma, Hodgkin's lymphoma
	Protocols containing procarbazine: MOPP, MVPP, COPP, ChIVPP, ChIVPP/EVA, BEACOPP, MOPP/ABVD, COPP/ABVD	Hodgkin's lymphoma
Intermediate risk: approximately 30–70 % of women develop amenorrhea after treatment	CMF, CEF, or CAF × 6 cycles in women age 30–39	Breast cancer
	AC in women age 40+	Breast cancer
Low risk: <20 % of women develop amenorrhea	AC in women age 30–39	Breast cancer
	CMF, CEF, or CAF × 6 cycles in women age <30	Breast cancer
	Nonalkylating chemotherapy: ABVD, CHOP, COP	Hodgkin's lymphoma, NHL
	Anthracycline + cytarabine	AML
	Multiagent therapies	ALL
Very low/no risk: negligible effect on menses	Methotrexate + fluorouracil	Breast cancer
	Vincristine (used in multiagent therapies)	Leukemia, Hodgkin's lymphoma, NHL, neuroblastoma, rhabdomyosarcoma, Wilms tumor, Kaposi's sarcoma
	Radioactive iodine	Thyroid cancer
Unknown risk	Paclitaxel, docetaxel (taxanes used in AC protocols)	Breast cancer
	Oxaliplatin	Ovarian cancer
	Irinotecan	Colon cancer
	Bevacizumab	Colon, non-small cell lung cancer
	Cetuximab	Colon, head and neck cancer
	Trastuzumab	Breast cancer
	Erlotinib	Non-small cell lung, pancreatic cancer
	Imatinib	Chronic myeloid leukemia, GI stromal tumor

TBI total-body irradiation, *CMF* cyclophosphamide, methotrexate, and fluorouracil, *CEF* cyclophosphamide, epirubicin, and fluorouracil, *CAF* cyclophosphamide, doxorubicin, and fluorouracil, *BMT* bone marrow transplantation, *SCT* stem-cell transplantation, *NHL* non-Hodgkin's lymphoma, *AML* acute myeloid leukemia, *ALL* acute lymphoblastic leukemia, *BCNU* carmustine, *CCNU* lomustine, *MOPP* mechlorethamine, vincristine, procarbazine, and prednisone, *MVPP* mechlorethamine, vinblastine, procarbazine, and prednisone, *COPP* cyclophosphamide, vincristine, procarbazine, and prednisone, *ChlVPP* chlorambucil, vinblastine, procarbazine, and prednisone, *EVA* etoposide, vinblastine, and doxorubicin, *BEACOPP* bleomycin, etoposide, doxorubicin, cyclophosphamide, vincristine, procarbazine, and prednisone, *ABVD* doxorubicin, bleomycin, vinblastine, and dacarbazine, *AC* doxorubicin and cyclophosphamide, *CHOP* cyclophosphamide, doxorubicin, vincristine, and prednisone, *COP* cyclophosphamide, vincristine, and prednisone

Adapted from Levine and colleagues (Kremer et al. 2001) with permission

(Byrne et al. 1998; Li et al. 1979). Boice et al. (2003) also reported that there was no difference in the incidence of genetic or chromosomal anomalies in 6,000 children of 25,000 survivors of childhood cancer when compared to their sibling controls in an international study. Finally, aside from malignancy arising from an inherited syndrome, there does not appear to be an increased risk of childhood cancer in the offspring of long-term cancer survivors (Knopman et al. 2010).

2.6.3 Fertility Preservation Options for Cancer Patients Undergoing Chemotherapy

For patients undergoing chemotherapy during their reproductive years, American Society of Clinical Oncology recommends assessment of their infertility risk as an integral part of the chemotherapy informed consent process (Lee et al. 2006). Furthermore, oncologists should be prepared to discuss fertility preservation options and refer

Table 13 Fertility preservation options for men (Kremer et al. 2001)

	Option						
Characteristics	Sperm banking (Masturbation)	Sperm banking (alternative collection methods)	Radiation shielding of gonads	Testicular tissue freezing	Testicular sperm extraction	Donor sperm	Adoption
Medical status	Standard	Experimental	Standard	Experimental	Standard	Standard	Standard
Definition	Sperm obtained through masturbation and then frozen	Sperm obtained through testicular extraction or electro-ejaculation under sedation	Use of shielding to reduce the dose of radiation delivered to the testes	Tissue obtained through biopsy and frozen for future use	Use of biopsy to obtain individual sperm from testicular tissue	Sperm donated by a man for artificial insemination or IVF	Process that creates a legal parent–child relationship
Pubertal status	After puberty	After puberty	Before or after puberty	Before or after puberty	After puberty	After puberty	After puberty
Time requirement	Outpatient procedure	Outpatient procedure	In conjunction with radiation treatments	Outpatient procedure	Outpatient procedure	Readily available for purchase	Varies depending on type of adoption
Success rates	Generally high; the most established technique for men	If sperm is obtained, similar to standard sperm banking	Possible with select radiation fields and anatomy	No available human success rates	30–70 % in postpubescent patients	50–80 %	NA
Cost	Approx. $1,500 for 3 samples; storage fees average $500/year	Varies greatly based on collection method	Generally included in the cost of radiation treatments	$500–$2,500 for surgery; $300–$1,000 for freezing; $500/year for storage	$4,000–$16,000 (in addition to costs to IVF)	$200–$500 per vial (in addition to costs for IUI or IVF)	$2,500–$35,000
Timing	Before treatment	Before treatment	During treatment	Before treatment	Before or after treatment	After treatment	After treatment
Special considerations	Deposits can be made every 24 h	Can be considered if male cannot ejaculate	Expertise required; does not protect against effects of chemotherapy	May be only cryopreservation option for prepubescent boys	Center should be able to freeze sperm found at time of biopsy	Can choose donor based on wide range of characteristics	Medical history often a factor

IVF in vitro fertilization, *NA* not applicable, *IUI* intrauterine insemination
Adapted from Levine and colleagues (Kremer et al. 2001) with permission

those interested to reproductive specialists (Lee et al. 2006). Sperm and embryo cryopreservation should be considered standard practice and be widely available for patients at significant risk of infertility (Lee et al. 2006; Wallace 2011) while other available fertility preservation methods should be considered experimental and only be conducted in institutions with the necessary expertise (Lee et al. 2006). Tables 13 and 14 summarize preservation option for men and women respectively (Levine et al. 2010).

2.7 Cognitive Impairment

There is growing evidence that a subset of long-term cancer survivors experience permanent cognitive impairment after completion of chemotherapy (Fardell et al. 2011; Tannock et al. 2004), which is particularly well documented in breast cancer survivors after adjuvant chemotherapy (Fardell et al. 2011; Tannock et al. 2004). Unfortunately, there is a lack of acknowledgment or education about this disabling adverse

Table 14 Fertility preservations options for women (Kremer et al. 2001)

	Option				
Characteristics	Embryo freezing	Egg freezing	Ovarian tissue freezing	Radiation shielding of gonads	Ovarian transplantation
Medical status	Standard	Experimental	Experimental	Standard	Standard
Definition	Harvesting eggs, IVF, and freezing of embryos for later implantation	Harvesting and freezing of unfertilized eggs	Freezing of ovarian tissue and reimplantation after cancer treatment	Use of shielding to reduce scatter radiation to the reproductive organs	Surgical repositioning of ovaries away from the radiation field
Pubertal status	After puberty	After puberty	Before or after puberty	Before or after puberty	Before or after puberty
Time requirement	10–14 days from menses; outpatient surgical procedure	10–14 days from menses; outpatient surgical procedure	Outpatient surgical procedure	In conjunction with radiation treatments	Outpatient procedure
Success rates	Approximately 40 % per transfer; varies by age and center; thousands of babies born	Approximately 21.6 % per embryo transfer; 900 live births	Case reports of seven live births	Only possible with selected radiation fields and anatomy	Approximately 50 % as a result of altered blood flow and scatter radiation
Cost	Approximately $12,000/cycle; storage fees and pregnancy costs additional	Approximately $12,000/cycle; storage fees and pregnancy costs additional	$12,000 for procedure; storage fees and reimplantation costs additional	Generally included in cost of radiation	Unknown; may be covered by insurance
Timing	Before or after treatment	Before or after treatment	Before or after treatment	During treatment	Before treatment
Special considerations	Need partner or donor sperm	May be attractive to single women or those opposed to embryo creation	Not suitable if high risk of ovarian metastases; only cryopreservation option for prepubescent girls	Expertise required; does not protect against effects of chemotherapy	Expertise required

	Option					
Characteristics	Radical trachelectomy	Ovarian suppression	Donor embryos	Donor eggs	Gestational surrogacy	Adoption
Medical status	Standard	Experimental	Standard	Standard	Standard	Standard
Definition	Surgical removal of the cervix with preservation of the uterus	GnRH analogs used to suppress ovaries	Embryos donated by a couple	Eggs donated by a woman	Woman carries a pregnancy for another woman or couple	Process that creates a legal parent–child relationship
Pubertal status	After puberty	After puberty	After puberty	After puberty	After puberty	After puberty
Time requirement	Inpatient surgical procedure	In conjunction with chemotherapy	Varies; is done in conjunction with IVF	Varies, is done in conjunction with IVF	Varies; time is required to find surrogate and implant embryos	Varies depending on types of adoption

(continued)

Table 14 (continued)

	Option					
Success rates	No evidence of high cancer recurrence rates in appropriate candidates	Unknown; conflicting results reported; larger randomized trials in progress	Unknown; high than that of frozen embryo IVF transfers	40–50 %	Similar to IVF; approximately 30 %	NA
Cost	Generally included in the cost of cancer treatment	$500/month	$5,000–$7,000 (in addition to cost for IVF)	$5,000–$15,000 (in addition to costs for IVF)	$10,000–$100,000	$2,500–$35,000
Timing	During treatment	During treatment	After treatment	After treatment	After treatment	After treatment
Special considerations	Limited to early-stage cervical cancer offered at a limited number of centers	Does not protect from radiation effects	Donor embryo available though IVF clinics or private agencies	Patient can choose donor based on various characteristics	Legal status varies by state	Medical history often a factor

IVF in vitro fertilization, *GnRH* gonadotroponin-releasing hormone, *NA* not applicable
Adapted from Levine and colleagues (Kremer et al. 2001) with permission

effect by healthcare providers to cancer survivors (Myers 2012). Long-term cognitive impairment in this increasing population of survivors has significant impact on their interpersonal relationships, their ability to perform at previous levels of competence, and their work performance (Fardell et al. 2011; Myers 2012). This section will discuss the incidence, mechanism, treatment, and prevention of this poorly understood yet serious side effect.

2.7.1 Effects of Chemotherapy on Cognitive Function

While up to 70 % of patients self-report persistent cognitive difficulties after completion of chemotherapy (Fardell et al. 2011), only 15–50 % of cancer survivors were found to have mild to moderate cognitive dysfunction using standardized neuropsychological assessment (Fardell et al. 2011). While two longitudinal studies (Ahles et al. 2010; Schagen et al. 2006) reported that this impairment can persist between 1 and 2 years after completion of chemotherapy, two cross-sectional studies (de Ruiter et al. 2011; Kreukels et al. 2006) suggested that this effect might last longer for up to 10 years after chemotherapy. Several domain of cognitive function may be affected by chemotherapy, including attention/concentration, verbal memory, visual memory, and speed of information processing (Fardell et al. 2011; Tannock et al. 2004).

Although the evidence at this juncture is not conclusive, several treatment-related factors may predispose patients to higher risk of long-term cognitive impairment, including high-dose chemotherapy, adjuvant hormonal therapy after chemotherapy, and the regimen of cyclophosphamide, methotrexate, and 5-fluorouracil (Fardell et al. 2011; Vardy and Tannock 2007). Furthermore, individual characteristics also affect this risk (Fardell et al. 2011). The presence of the APOE e4 allele (The epsilon4 allele of the apolipoprotein E gene which is associated with Alzheimer's disease), impaired baseline cognitive reserve before treatment, and increased age at diagnosis all seem to predispose patients to increased likelihood of chemotherapy-induced cognitive impairment (Fardell et al. 2011). Finally, in an overwhelming majority of studies to date, no association was found between cognitive impairment and psychological well being of patients (Fardell et al. 2011).

2.7.2 Mechanism of Chemotherapy-Induced Cognitive Impairment

Although the underlying neurobiological mechanisms linking chemotherapy with cognitive impairment is not fully elucidated in humans, it has been well studied in animal models. In healthy rodents, chemotherapy causes cell death of central nervous system, increase in oxidative stress and microglia activity, suppression of hippocampal neurogenesis, and decrease in levels of both neurotrophic factors and hippocampal catecholamines (Fardell et al. 2011).

Recently, neuroimaging has identified several structural and functional changes in brain region that are hypothesized to be involved in the cognitive deficits experienced by breast cancer survivors after chemotherapy. Silverman et al. (2007) used positron emission tomography scanning to examine metabolic activity of the brain in breast cancer patients who completed adjuvant chemotherapy 5–10 years ago. During performance of a short-term recall task, they identified significant altercation of cerebral blood flow to the frontal cortex and cerebellum in chemotherapy-treated patients. In particular, cerebral activation of the inferior frontal gyrus of patients with chemotherapy differed most from those without chemotherapy. Similarly, de Ruiter et al. (2011) used functional magnetic resonance imaging to compare cognitive function of those who completed high-dose adjuvant chemotherapy 10 years ago to those who are chemotherapy naïve. They reported hyporesponsiveness in both the prefrontal cortex and parahippocampal gyrus during executive functioning and episodic memory tasks in those with chemotherapy. Interestingly, by using diffusion tensor imaging, Abramham et al. (2008) reported that adjuvant chemotherapy for breast cancer affects normal-appearing white matter in the genu of the corpus callous, which may explain the cognitive deficits experienced by patients.

2.7.3 Prevention and Treatment of Chemotherapy-Induced Cognitive Impairment

There are currently no pharmacological interventions approved for prevention or treatment of chemotherapy-induced cognitive dysfunction. However, the following agents may have potential benefits for this indication (Fardell et al. 2011; Tannock et al. 2004), including erythropoietin, methylphenidate, modafinil, donepezil, fluoxetine, and antioxidants. Cognitive rehabilitation programs (Fardell et al. 2011; Tannock et al. 2004) may also be efficacious in cancer patients with cognitive deficits after chemotherapy. These programs usually retrain cancer patients to recover part of their lost cognitive functions; teach them compensatory methods of using their residual abilities to develop alternative methods of performing cognitive tasks, and address their social, emotional, and functional issues related to their cognitive dysfunction using a holistic approach (Fardell et al. 2011). Finally, regular exercises (Fardell et al. 2011), which have been shown to decrease inflammation, increase levels of neurotrophic factors, and promote neuronal cell proliferation and survival, may decrease the risk of cognitive decline after chemotherapy.

2.8 Second Malignant Neoplasms

Second malignant neoplasms (SMNs) are a potentially life-threatening late effect of chemotherapy. While both alkylating agents and topoisomerase II inhibitors are known causes of therapy-related myeloid neoplasms in cancer survivors (Fung and Vaughn 2011; Czader and Orazi 2009; Sill et al. 2011), risks of second solid cancer due to chemotherapy alone are less defined. In this section, we will review the risks of both second solid and hematological malignancies in cancer survivors after chemotherapy and discuss management options for this serious late effect.

2.8.1 Second Malignant Neoplasms After Chemotherapy

2.8.1.1 Hematological Malignancies

Therapy-related myeloid neoplasms represent 10–20 % of acute leukemias, myelodysplastic syndrome (MDS), and myelodysplastic/myeloproliferative neoplasms (Czader and Orazi 2009) and numerous cytotoxic agents are implicated in their development (Table 15). In this section, we will focus on alkylating agents and topoisomerase II inhibitors, which are known to increase risks of two distinct types of acute leukemias (Fung and Vaughn 2011; Czader and Orazi 2009; Sill et al. 2011). Leukemia due to alkylating agents usually has a latency period of 5–10 years after treatment and is frequently preceded by MDS (Fung and Vaughn 2011; Czader and Orazi 2009). Loss of part or all of chromosomes 5 or 7 are implicated in the development of this leukemia (Fung and Vaughn 2011; Czader and Orazi 2009). By contrast, acute leukemia after topoisomerase II inhibitors occurs within 2–3 years after therapy (Fung and Vaughn 2011), is not preceded by MDS (Fung and Vaughn 2011; Czader and Orazi 2009), and involves rearrangement of the MLL gene with 11q23 chromosomal translocations or shows recurrent cytogenetic abnormalities such as t(8;21), t(15;17), and inv(16) (Czader and Orazi 2009).

Cumulative doses of cisplatin (alkeylating agent) and etoposide (topoisomerase II inhibitor) directly correlate with risks of therapy-related myeloid neoplasms (Kollmannsberger et al. 1999; Travis et al. 1999, 2000). The cumulative incidence of leukemia at 5 years after etoposide increased from 0.5 % for testicular cancer patients with a cumulative dose of $<2{,}000$ mg/m^2 to 2.0 % for those with $\geq 2{,}000$ mg/m^2 (Kollmannsberger et al. 1999). Regarding risk of leukemia after cisplatin, Travis et al. (2000) reported that this risk has a highly significant relationship with cumulative dose of cisplatin in testicular cancer patients (P-trend = 0.001). They estimated that there is a 3.2-fold increased risk of leukemia after a cumulate dose of >650 mg of cisplatin although the excess risk is small (a total of 16 excess cases among 10,000 patients followed up for 15 years). Similarly, Travis et al. (1999) reported that a highly significant relationship exists between leukemia risk and cumulative cisplatin dose in patients with ovarian cancer (P-trend < 0.001). After a cumulative dose of 500–1,000 mg, they estimated that there is a total of 21 excess leukemia among 10,000 women followed up for 15 years.

2.8.1.2 Solid Malignancies

The risks of second solid cancer due to chemotherapy are less defined than those of hematological malignancies but

Table 15 Chemotherapy implicated in the development of therapy-related myeloid neoplasms (Krischer et al. 1997)

Class	Agent
Alkylating agents	Bulsulfan
	Carboplatin
	Carmustine
	Chlorambucil
	Cisplatin
	Cyclophosphamide
	Dacarbazine
	Dihydroxybusulfan
	Lomustine
	Mechlorethamine
	Melphalan
	Mitomycin C
	Procarbazine
	Semustine
	Thiotepa
Topoisomerase II inhibitors	Bimolane
	Dactinomycin
	Daunorubicin
	Doxorubicin
	4-Epi-doxorubicin
	Etoposide
	Mitoxantrone
	Razoxane
	Teniposide
Antimetabolites	Fludarabine
	6-Mercaptopurine
	Methotrexate
Antimicrotubule agents	Docetaxel
	Paclitaxel
	Vinblastine
	Vincristine

Adapted from Czader and colleagues (Krischer et al. 1997) with permission

were best studied in testicular cancer and Hodgkin's lymphoma patients. Travis et al. (2005) reported that the relative risk of second solid tumors was significantly increased after chemotherapy alone (RR = 1.8) in an international series of more than 40,000 patients. However, data on specific chemotherapeutic agents were not available. Another study (van den Belt-Dusebout et al. 2007) showed that the risk of solid tumors doubled in testicular cancer survivors after cisplatin-based regimens when compared with surgery alone, confirming findings of two other reports (Bokemeyer and Schmoll 1993; Wanderas et al. 1997). However, risk of solid cancer arising from modern era cisplatin-based chemotherapy remains to be elucidated in this population since these epidemiologic studies were conducted before current cisplatin-based chemotherapy became widely accepted. Furthermore, tobacco use increases risk of solid cancer to a similar extent as chemotherapy in testicular cancer patients (RR = 1.8) (van den Belt-Dusebout et al. 2007).

In a cohort of 5,798 patients with Hodgkin's lymphoma, Swerdlow et al. (2011) reported significantly increased lung cancer risk for those who received chemotherapy alone (RR = 2.9) and this was observed for both alkylating and non-alkylating regimens, whereas two earlier reports (Kaldor et al. 1992; Swerdlow et al. 1992) showed association with alkylating chemotherapy only. In particular, significant associations with lung cancer were identified for three chemotherapy regimens, mechlorethamine, vincristine, procarbazine, prednisone (MOPP), mechlorethamine, vinblastine, procarbazine, prednisone (MVPP), and chlorambucil, vinblastine, procarbazine, prednisone (ChIVPP), with each having relative risks of 3.1, 2.9, and 4.3, respectively. Furthermore, the authors suggested a dose-response effect for cycles of alkylating treatments in relation to lung cancer risk in their analyses. In particular, this increased lung cancer risk does not appear to be a consequence of confounding by smoking (Travis et al. 2002).

2.8.2 Management Considerations for Second Malignant Neoplasms

Currently, no consensus exists regarding interventions to minimize the risks of SMNs after chemotherapy. In general, all cancer survivors should adopt practices that are consistent with a healthy lifestyle, including routine exercise regimen, dietary modification, and smoking cessation (Fung and Vaughn 2011). Furthermore, adoption of age-appropriate cancer screening is important (Fung and Vaughn 2011). There are currently no evidence to suggest that frequent cancer screening with blood tests or radiographic studies is beneficial. Buchler et al. (2011) reported that only 27 % of second cancers were found on frequent oncology follow-up in their recent retrospective study.

3 Chemotherapy-Induced Late Effects in the Era of Pharmacogenomics

Genetic polymorphisms are inherited germline DNA sequence variations that may cause minor disruption in one or more biological pathways, and less commonly, complete loss of function when there is a deletion polymorphism. Elucidation of the molecular basis of germline genetic susceptibility to late effects of chemotherapy does not only provide invaluable insights and inform the development of therapeutic agents to target the underlying molecular pathways of these adverse effects, but it may also allow development of a risk-classification system that incorporates germline genetic markers to predict risks of chemotherapy-related side effects. In this section, we will review the current literatures regarding this rapidly emerging field within cancer survivorship.

3.1 Genes and Chemotherapy-Related Peripheral Neuropathy

Associations of CIPN with germline genetic variations of several genes have been identified, including *GSTP*1, *GSTM*1/*GSTM*3, *ERCC*1, *AGXT*, *ABCB*1, *CYP2C8*/*CYP3A5*, and *ITGB*3 genes (Cavaletti et al. 2011). *GSTP*1 encodes an enzyme of the glutathione S-transferases family that detoxifies chemotherapeutic agents by conjugating reactive electrophiles to glutathione (Mannervik et al. 1985). A single nucleotide polymorphism (SNP) of *GSTP*1 that causes substitution of isoleucine for valine (rs1695; Ile105Val) diminishes the activity of this enzyme and is associated with increased severity of CIPN in ten of twenty-three studies examining patients after platinum-based chemotherapy (Boige et al. 2010; Booton et al. 2006; Chen et al. 2010; Cho et al. 2010; Gamelin et al. 2007; Goekkurt et al. 2009; Hong et al. 2011; Inada et al. 2010; Kanai et al. 2010; Keam et al. 2008; Khrunin et al. 2010; Kim et al. 2009; Lecomte et al. 2006; Li et al. 2010; Marsh et al. 2007; McLeod et al. 2010; Mir et al. 2009; Oldenburg et al. 2007; Pare et al. 2008; Ruzzo et al. 2007; Seo et al. 2009; Stoehlmacher et al. 2002; Zarate et al. 2010).

Both *GSTM*1 and *GSTM*3 genes encode the μ class of glutathione S-transferases that are critical for detoxification of carcinogens, drugs, and environmental toxin through glutathione conjugation of electrophilic compounds (Cavaletti et al. 2011). Khrunin et al. (2010) reported recently that *GSTM*1 deletion and the AGG/AGG genotype in *GSTM*3 (rs1799735) were both associated with decreased risk of CIPN after treatment with platinum drugs. However, this association was not confirmed in other independent studies (Boige et al. 2010; Cho et al. 2010; Goekkurt et al. 2009; Kim et al. 2009; Lecomte et al. 2006; Mir et al. 2009; Oldenburg et al. 2007; Ruzzo et al. 2007; Seo et al. 2009; Zarate et al. 2010).

Excision repair cross-complementing group 1 (ERCC1), which is involved in the nucleotide excision-repair pathway and critical for DNA repair (Cavaletti et al. 2011), has also been studied for its role in development of CIPN. Two SNPs of *ERCC1*, rs11615 (542T → C) (Inada et al. 2010) and rs3212986 (809C → A) (Kim et al. 2009) were reported to predispose patients to higher risks of CIPN after oxaliplatin for colorectal cancer and after combination chemotherapy using taxanes and platinum drugs for ovarian cancer respectively. However, this association was not identified in other studies for patients treated with cisplatin or oxaliplatin (Boige et al. 2010; Chen et al. 2010; Goekkurt et al. 2009; Hong et al. 2011; Keam et al. 2008; Khrunin et al. 2010; Marsh et al. 2007; Seo et al. 2009; Zarate et al. 2010; Caponigro et al. 2009; Sissung et al. 2008).

Alanine-glyoxylate aminotransferase (AGXT) converts glyoxylate to glycolate, which is subsequently metabolized into oxalate by lactate dehydrogenase (Cavaletti et al. 2011). Gamelin et al. (2007) have examined if germline genetic variations of *AGXT* are associated with CIPN in colorectal cancer patients treated with oxaliplatin due to its critical role in oxalate metabolism. They identified two SNPs that predispose patients with more severe CIPN, rs4426527 (1141A → G) and rs34116584 (153C → T). However, this association was not identified by Kanai et al. (2010) in a cohort of 82 Japanese patients treated with oxaliplatin.

ATP-binding cassette proteins subfamily B member 1 (ABCB1) is involved in the transport of various molecules across extracellular and intracellular membranes (Cavaletti et al. 2011). In particular, ABCB 1 is known to mediate efflux of paclitaxel and docetaxel from cancer cells (Cavaletti et al. 2011). Sissung et al. (2008) reported that patients with SNP rs2032582 (2677G → T) had more rapid onset of CIPN after receiving docetaxel and thalidomide for prostate cancer. However, several other studies failed to detect this association (Marsh et al. 2007; Bergmann et al. 2011; Chang et al. 2009; Green et al. 2009; Leskela et al. 2011a; Rizzo et al. 2010; Sissung et al. 2006).

The enzymes CYP2C8 and CYP3A5 belong to the cytochrome P450 superfamily and are involved in the metabolism of taxanes through successive hydroxylation reactions (Cavaletti et al. 2011). Two studies (Green et al. 2009; Leskela et al. 2011a, b) have identified patients heterozygous for the CYP2C8*3 allele (rs11572080) were at increased risk of CIPN after chemotherapy regimens that include carboplatin and taxanes for various solid tumors. However, this result was not confirmed by two other studies; a study that examined white European women treated with paclitaxel or docetaxel for breast cancer (Rizzo et al. 2010) and a retrospective analysis that examined ovarian cancer patients (Bergmann et al. 2011). Regarding association of genetic variation of CYP3A5 gene with CIPN, Green et al. (2009) reported that the CYP3A5*3 polymorphism (rs776746) is associated with reduced risk of CIPN. However, this association is not confirmed by a retrospective study of ovarian cancer patients as previously mentioned (Bergmann et al. 2011). Finally, integrin B3 (ITGB3), which are cell surface proteins involved in cell adhesion and cell surface-mediated signaling, may be integral in the development of CIPN (Cavaletti et al. 2011). In a cohort of 55 colorectal cancer patients treated with oxaliplatin, Antonacopoulou et al. (2010) reported that patients with SNP rs5918 (196T → C) had increased risk of CIPN.

Fanconi anemia group D2 protein (FANCD2) is critical for assembly of DNA repair machinery (Sucheston et al. 2011) and variation in its expression has been linked to chemotherapy resistance in patients with glioma, ovarian cancer, and multiple myeloma (Sucheston et al. 2011). Recently, Sucheston et al. (2011) identified associations of 4 SNPs (rs7648104, rs7637888, rs6786638, and rs6442150) of the *FANCD2* gene with taxane-induced neurotoxicity in breast cancer patients. All these SNPs lie within the intronic region of the gene with three of them, including rs7648104, rs7637888, and rs6786638, directly correlating with gene expression levels of *FANCD2* (Sucheston et al. 2011).

Table 16 Summary of major research recommendations: late effects of testicular cancer and treatment (Travis et al. 2010)

Overall recommendations
1. Institution of lifelong follow-up of testicular cancer survivors with a large cohort setting to ascertain risks of emerging toxicities and the evolution of known late sequelae
2. Development of comprehensive risk prediction models that include treatment factors and genetic modifiers of late sequelae
3. Elucidation of the effect(s) of decades-long exposure of low serum level of platinum
4. Assessment of the overall burden of medical and psychosocial morbidity
5. The eventual formulation of evidence-based long-term follow-up guidelines and interventions

Adapted from Travis and colleagues (Travis et al. 2010) with permission

3.2 Genes and Cisplatin-Induced Ototoxicity

Associations of cisplatin-induced ototoxicity have been reported for several genes, including those encoding for glutathione-S-transferases (*GSTP1*, *GSTM1*, *GSTM3*) (Oldenburg et al. 2007a, b; Peters et al. 2000), thiopurine S-methyltransferase (*TPMT*) (Ross et al. 2009), catechol-O-methyltransferase (*COMT*) (Ross et al. 2009), and megalin. As mentioned previously, glutathione-S-transferases are important in detoxifying chemotherapeutic agents by conjugating reactive electrophiles to glutathione (Mannervik et al. 1985). Oldenburg and colleagues reported that patients with both SNP rs1695 of *GSTP1* (Ile105Val) (Oldenburg et al. 2007a, b) and homozygous deletion in *GSTM1* (Oldenburg et al. 2007) had decreased risk of developing cisplatin-induced ototoxicity. Furthermore, GSTM3*B allele was found to be protective of ototoxic effect of cisplatin (Peters et al. 2000).

TPMT transcribes an enzyme that metabolizes thiopurine drugs (Weinshilboum 2006) while *COMT* encodes an enzyme that metabolizes catecholamine-containing chemical via methylation (Weinshilboum 2006). Ross et al. (2009) reported that the risk alleles of SNP rs12201199 of *TPMT* and rs9332377 of *COMT* predisposed children who received cisplatin chemotherapy to 17.0 times and 5.5 times higher odds of cisplatin-induced hearing impairment respectively.

Megalin appears to play a critical role in hearing as it is strongly expressed within the marginal cells of the stria vascularis of the cochlea (Mukherjea and Rybak 2011). In a cohort of 74 patients with osteosarcoma, germ cell tumors, testicular cancers, hepatoblastoma, teratoma, neuroblastomas, and brain tumors, who received cisplatin-based chemotherapy, the A allele of rs2075252 of the megalin gene is found to be associated with the development of hearing impairment (Riedemann et al. 2008).

3.3 Genes and Therapy-Related Myeloid Leukemia

Three SNPs were recently reported to be associated with therapy-related myeloid leukemia in a genome-wide association study (Knight et al. 2009); rs1394384 of the *ACCN1* gene, rs1199098 that is in linkage disequilibrium with the *IPMK* gene, and rs1381392 that is not in proximity with any known genes, miRNAs, or regulatory elements but is in a genetic region frequently deleted in lung cancer. Functionally, *ACCN1* encodes an amiloride-sensitive cation channel. Genetic expression of *ACCN1* is not only observed in bone marrow and hematopoietic cells but is also associated with risks of both autism and multiple sclerosis (Knight et al. 2009). *IPMK* encodes a multikinase that upregulates the AKT kinase and may also alter Wnt/beta-catenin signaling (Knight et al. 2009).

3.4 Future Survivorship Research Directions in the Era of Pharmacogenomics

Currently, there is limited knowledge and understanding regarding how germline genetic variation may predispose cancer survivors to chemotherapy-related complications (Travis et al. 2006). Identification of such genetic markers is a prerequisite to understanding the molecular basis of the late effects and rational development of therapeutic agents. It will also be vital in the development of a risk classification system that will allow appropriate screening and early intervention with the goal of decreasing morbidity and mortality due to late effects of curative therapy of many cancers (Travis et al. 2006). An international meeting devoted to testicular cancer survivorship that was held in 2009 at the Wilmot P. Cancer Center in Rochester, New York by Travis et al. (2010) has summarized the major research recommendations in this area as shown in Table 16 and should be considered for cancer survivorship research in other malignancies.

References

Abraham J, Haut MW, Moran MT, Filburn S, Lemiuex S, Kuwabara H (2008) Adjuvant chemotherapy for breast cancer: effects on cerebral white matter seen in diffusion tensor imaging. Clin Breast Cancer 8:88–91

Ahles TA, Saykin AJ, McDonald BC et al (2010) Longitudinal assessment of cognitive changes associated with adjuvant treatment for breast cancer: impact of age and cognitive reserve. J Clin Oncol 28:4434–4440

Albers JW, Chaudhry V, Cavaletti G, Donehower RC (2011) Interventions for preventing neuropathy caused by cisplatin and related compounds. Cochrane Database Syst Rev 2011:CD005228

Al-Sarraf M, Fletcher W, Oishi N et al (1982) Cisplatin hydration with and without mannitol diuresis in refractory disseminated malignant melanoma: a southwest oncology group study. Cancer Treat Rep 66:31–35

Amptoulach S, Tsavaris N (2011) Neurotoxicity caused by the treatment with platinum analogues. Chemother Res Pract 2011:843019

Antonacopoulou AG, Argyriou AA, Scopa CD et al (2010) Integrin beta-3 L33P: a new insight into the pathogenesis of chronic oxaliplatin-induced peripheral neuropathy? Eur J Neurol 17:963–968

Argyriou AA, Polychronopoulos P, Iconomou G, Chroni E, Kalofonos HP (2008) A review on oxaliplatin-induced peripheral nerve damage. Cancer Treat Rev 34:368–377

Bajorin DF, Sarosdy MF, Pfister DG et al (1993) Randomized trial of etoposide and cisplatin versus etoposide and carboplatin in patients with good-risk germ cell tumors: a multiinstitutional study. J Clin Oncol 11:598–606

Bergmann TK, Green H, Brasch-Andersen C et al (2011) Retrospective study of the impact of pharmacogenetic variants on paclitaxel toxicity and survival in patients with ovarian cancer. Eur J Clin Pharmacol 67:693–700

Berrak SG, Pearson M, Berberoglu S, Ilhan IE, Jaffe N (2005) High-dose ifosfamide in relapsed pediatric osteosarcoma: therapeutic effects and renal toxicity. Pediatr Blood Cancer 44:215–219

Bilgrami SF, Metersky ML, McNally D et al (2001) Idiopathic pneumonia syndrome following myeloablative chemotherapy and autologous transplantation. Ann Pharmacother 35:196–201

Boice JD Jr, Tawn EJ, Winther JF et al (2003) Genetic effects of radiotherapy for childhood cancer. Health Phys 85:65–80

Boige V, Mendiboure J, Pignon JP et al (2010) Pharmacogenetic assessment of toxicity and outcome in patients with metastatic colorectal cancer treated with LV5FU2, FOLFOX, and FOLFIRI: FFCD 2000–05. J Clin Oncol 28:2556–2564

Bokemeyer C, Schmoll HJ (1993) Secondary neoplasms following treatment of malignant germ cell tumors. J Clin Oncol 11:1703–1709

Bokemeyer C, Berger CC, Hartmann JT et al (1998) Analysis of risk factors for cisplatin-induced ototoxicity in patients with testicular cancer. Br J Cancer 77:1355–1362

Booton R, Ward T, Heighway J, Ashcroft L, Morris J, Thatcher N (2006) Glutathione-S-transferase P1 isoenzyme polymorphisms, platinum-based chemotherapy, and non-small cell lung cancer. J Thorac Oncol 1:679–683

Brydoy M, Oldenburg J, Klepp O et al (2009) Observational study of prevalence of long-term Raynaud-like phenomena and neurological side effects in testicular cancer survivors. J Natl Cancer Inst 101:1682–1695

Buchler T, Kubankova P, Boublikova L et al (2011) Detection of second malignancies during long-term follow-up of testicular cancer survivors. Cancer 117:4212–4218

Byrne J, Rasmussen SA, Steinhorn SC et al (1998) Genetic disease in offspring of long-term survivors of childhood and adolescent cancer. Am J Hum Genet 62:45–52

Caponigro F, Lacombe D, Twelves C et al (2009) An EORTC phase I study of Bortezomib in combination with oxaliplatin, leucovorin and 5-fluorouracil in patients with advanced colorectal cancer. Eur J Cancer 45:48–55

Cardinale D, Sandri MT, Martinoni A et al (2002) Myocardial injury revealed by plasma troponin I in breast cancer treated with high-dose chemotherapy. Ann Oncol 13:710–715

Cardinale D, Sandri MT, Colombo A et al (2004) Prognostic value of troponin I in cardiac risk stratification of cancer patients undergoing high-dose chemotherapy. Circulation 109:2749–2754

Carlson K, Ocean AJ (2011) Peripheral neuropathy with microtubule-targeting agents: occurrence and management approach. Clin Breast Cancer 11:73–81

Carver JR, Shapiro CL, Ng A et al (2007) American Society of Clinical Oncology clinical evidence review on the ongoing care of adult cancer survivors: cardiac and pulmonary late effects. J Clin Oncol 25:3991–4008

Cavaletti G, Jakubowiak AJ (2010) Peripheral neuropathy during bortezomib treatment of multiple myeloma: a review of recent studies. Leuk Lymphoma 51:1178–1187

Cavaletti G, Marmiroli P (2010) Chemotherapy-induced peripheral neurotoxicity. Nat Rev Neurol 6:657–666

Cavaletti G, Tredici G, Braga M, Tazzari S (1995) Experimental peripheral neuropathy induced in adult rats by repeated intraperitoneal administration of taxol. Exp Neurol 133:64–72

Cavaletti G, Cavalletti E, Montaguti P, Oggioni N, De Negri O, Tredici G (1997) Effect on the peripheral nervous system of the short-term intravenous administration of paclitaxel in the rat. Neurotoxicology 18:137–145

Cavaletti G, Cavalletti E, Oggioni N et al (2000) Distribution of paclitaxel within the nervous system of the rat after repeated intravenous administration. Neurotoxicology 21:389–393

Cavaletti G, Alberti P, Marmiroli P (2011) Chemotherapy-induced peripheral neurotoxicity in the era of pharmacogenomics. Lancet Oncol 12:1151–1161

Chang H, Rha SY, Jeung HC et al (2009) Association of the ABCB1 gene polymorphisms 2677G>T/A and 3435C>T with clinical outcomes of paclitaxel monotherapy in metastatic breast cancer patients. Ann Oncol 20:272–277

Chen YC, Tzeng CH, Chen PM et al (2010) Influence of GSTP1 I105 V polymorphism on cumulative neuropathy and outcome of FOLFOX-4 treatment in Asian patients with colorectal carcinoma. Cancer Sci 101:530–535

Chia S, Clemons M, Martin LA et al (2006) Pegylated liposomal doxorubicin and trastuzumab in HER-2 overexpressing metastatic breast cancer: a multicenter phase II trial. J Clin Oncol 24:2773–2778

Kidney Health after Childhood Cancer. Children's Oncology Group (2008) (Accessed at http://www.survivorshipguidelines.org/pdf/KidneyHealth.pdf)

Cho HJ, Eom HS, Kim HJ, Kim IS, Lee GW, Kong SY (2010) Glutathione-S-transferase genotypes influence the risk of chemotherapy-related toxicities and prognosis in Korean patients with diffuse large B-cell lymphoma. Cancer Genet Cytogenet 198:40–46

Comis RL (1990) Detecting bleomycin pulmonary toxicity: a continued conundrum. J Clin Oncol 8:765–767

Cooper JA Jr, Zitnik RJ, Matthay RA (1988) Mechanisms of drug-induced pulmonary disease. Annu Rev Med 39:395–404

Cushing B, Giller R, Cullen JW et al (2004) Randomized comparison of combination chemotherapy with etoposide, bleomycin, and either high-dose or standard-dose cisplatin in children and adolescents with high-risk malignant germ cell tumors: a pediatric intergroup study—Pediatric Oncology Group 9049 and Children's Cancer Group 8882. J Clin Oncol 22:2691–2700

Cvitkovic E, Spaulding J, Bethune V, Martin J, Whitmore WF (1977) Improvement of cis-dichlorodiammineplatinum (NSC 119875): therapeutic index in an animal model. Cancer 39:1357–1361

Czader M, Orazi A (2009) Therapy-related myeloid neoplasms. Am J Clin Pathol 132:410–425

de Ruiter MB, Reneman L, Boogerd W et al (2011) Cerebral hyporesponsiveness and cognitive impairment 10 years after chemotherapy for breast cancer. Hum Brain Mapp 32:1206–1219

de Wit R, Roberts JT, Wilkinson PM et al (2001) Equivalence of three or four cycles of bleomycin, etoposide, and cisplatin chemotherapy and of a 3- or 5-day schedule in good-prognosis germ cell cancer: a randomized study of the European Organization for Research and Treatment of Cancer Genitourinary Tract Cancer Cooperative Group and the Medical Research Council. J Clin Oncol 19:1629–1640

Fardell JE, Vardy J, Johnston IN, Winocur G (2011) Chemotherapy and cognitive impairment: treatment options. Clin Pharmacol Ther 90:366–376

Floyd JD, Nguyen DT, Lobins RL, Bashir Q, Doll DC, Perry MC (2005) Cardiotoxicity of cancer therapy. J Clin Oncol 23:7685–7696

Friedman DL, Himelstein B, Shields CL et al (2000) Chemoreduction and local ophthalmic therapy for intraocular retinoblastoma. J Clin Oncol 18:12–17

Fung C, Vaughn DJ (2011) Complications associated with chemotherapy in testicular cancer management. Nat Rev Urol 8:213–222

Gamelin L, Capitain O, Morel A et al (2007) Predictive factors of oxaliplatin neurotoxicity: the involvement of the oxalate outcome pathway. Clin Cancer Res 13:6359–6368

Geiger S, Lange V, Suhl P, Heinemann V, Stemmler HJ (2010) Anticancer therapy induced cardiotoxicity: review of the literature. Anticancer Drugs 21:578–590

Giantris A, Abdurrahman L, Hinkle A, Asselin B, Lipshultz SE (1998) Anthracycline-induced cardiotoxicity in children and young adults. Crit Rev Oncol Hematol 27:53–68

Glendenning JL, Barbachano Y, Norman AR, Dearnaley DP, Horwich A, Huddart RA (2010) Long-term neurologic and peripheral vascular toxicity after chemotherapy treatment of testicular cancer. Cancer 116:2322–2331

Goekkurt E, Al-Batran SE, Hartmann JT et al (2009) Pharmacogenetic analyses of a phase III trial in metastatic gastroesophageal adenocarcinoma with fluorouracil and leucovorin plus either oxaliplatin or cisplatin: a study of the arbeitsgemeinschaft internistische onkologie. J Clin Oncol 27:2863–2873

Green H, Soderkvist P, Rosenberg P et al (2009) Pharmacogenetic studies of Paclitaxel in the treatment of ovarian cancer. Basic Clin Pharmacol Toxicol 104:130–137

Grewal S, Merchant T, Reymond R, McInerney M, Hodge C, Shearer P (2010) Auditory late effects of childhood cancer therapy: a report from the Children's Oncology Group. Pediatrics 125:e938–e950

Grothey A, Nikcevich DA, Sloan JA et al (2011) Intravenous calcium and magnesium for oxaliplatin-induced sensory neurotoxicity in adjuvant colon cancer: NCCTG N04C7. J Clin Oncol 29:421–427

Haugnes HS, Aass N, Fossa SD et al (2009) Pulmonary function in long-term survivors of testicular cancer. J Clin Oncol 27:2779–2786

Hayes DF, Picard MH (2006) Heart of darkness: the downside of trastuzumab. J Clin Oncol 24:4056–4058

Hensley ML, Hagerty KL, Kewalramani T et al (2009) American Society of Clinical Oncology 2008 clinical practice guideline update: use of chemotherapy and radiation therapy protectants. J Clin Oncol 27:127–145

Hong J, Han SW, Ham HS et al (2011) Phase II study of biweekly S-1 and oxaliplatin combination chemotherapy in metastatic colorectal cancer and pharmacogenetic analysis. Cancer Chemother Pharmacol 67:1323–1331

Huang TT, Hudson MM, Stokes DC, Krasin MJ, Spunt SL, Ness KK (2011) Pulmonary outcomes in survivors of childhood cancer: a systematic review. Chest 140:881–901

Inada M, Sato M, Morita S et al (2010) Associations between oxaliplatin-induced peripheral neuropathy and polymorphisms of the ERCC1 and GSTP1 genes. Int J Clin Pharmacol Ther 48:729–734

Isla D, Sarries C, Rosell R et al (2004) Single nucleotide polymorphisms and outcome in docetaxel-cisplatin-treated advanced non-small-cell lung cancer. Ann Oncol 15:1194–1203

Jemal A, Siegel R, Ward E, Hao Y, Xu J, Thun MJ (2009) Cancer statistics, 2009. CA Cancer J Clin 59:225–249

Jones DP, Spunt SL, Green D, Springate JE (2008) Renal late effects in patients treated for cancer in childhood: a report from the Children's Oncology Group. Pediatr Blood Cancer 51:724–731

Kaldor JM, Day NE, Bell J et al (1992) Lung cancer following Hodgkin's disease: a case-control study. Int J Cancer 52:677–681

Kanai M, Yoshioka A, Tanaka S et al (2010) Associations between glutathione S-transferase pi Ile105Val and glyoxylate aminotransferase Pro11Leu and Ile340Met polymorphisms and early-onset oxaliplatin-induced neuropathy. Cancer Epidemiol 34:189–193

Keam B, Im SA, Han SW et al (2008) Modified FOLFOX-6 chemotherapy in advanced gastric cancer: results of phase II study and comprehensive analysis of polymorphisms as a predictive and prognostic marker. BMC Cancer 8:148

Keefe DL (2002) Trastuzumab-associated cardiotoxicity. Cancer 95:1592–1600

Khrunin AV, Moisseev A, Gorbunova V, Limborska S (2010) Genetic polymorphisms and the efficacy and toxicity of cisplatin-based chemotherapy in ovarian cancer patients. Pharmacogenomics J 10:54–61

Kim HS, Kim MK, Chung HH et al (2009) Genetic polymorphisms affecting clinical outcomes in epithelial ovarian cancer patients treated with taxanes and platinum compounds: a Korean population-based study. Gynecol Oncol 113:264–269

Kintzel PE (2001) Anticancer drug-induced kidney disorders. Drug Saf 24:19–38

Knight JA, Skol AD, Shinde A et al (2009) Genome-wide association study to identify novel loci associated with therapy-related myeloid leukemia susceptibility. Blood 113:5575–5582

Knopman JM, Papadopoulos EB, Grifo JA, Fino ME, Noyes N (2010) Surviving childhood and reproductive-age malignancy: effects on fertility and future parenthood. Lancet Oncol 11:490–498

Kollmannsberger C, Hartmann JT, Kanz L, Bokemeyer C (1999) Therapy-related malignancies following treatment of germ cell cancer. Int J Cancer 83:860–863

Kremer LC, van Dalen EC, Offringa M, Ottenkamp J, Voute PA (2001) Anthracycline-induced clinical heart failure in a cohort of 607 children: long-term follow-up study. J Clin Oncol 19:191–196

Kreukels BP, Schagen SB, Ridderinkhof KR et al (2006) Effects of high-dose and conventional-dose adjuvant chemotherapy on long-term cognitive sequelae in patients with breast cancer: an electrophysiologic study. Clin Breast Cancer 7:67–78

Krischer JP, Epstein S, Cuthbertson DD, Goorin AM, Epstein ML, Lipshultz SE (1997) Clinical cardiotoxicity following anthracycline treatment for childhood cancer: the Pediatric Oncology Group experience. J Clin Oncol 15:1544–1552

Lambert MP, Shields C, Meadows AT (2008) A retrospective review of hearing in children with retinoblastoma treated with carboplatin-based chemotherapy. Pediatr Blood Cancer 50:223–226

Launay-Vacher V, Rey JB, Isnard-Bagnis C, Deray G, Daouphars M (2008) Prevention of cisplatin nephrotoxicity: state of the art and recommendations from the European Society of Clinical Pharmacy Special Interest Group on Cancer Care. Cancer Chemother Pharmacol 61:903–909

Lawson M, Vasilaras A, De Vries A, Mactaggart P, Nicol D (2008) Urological implications of cyclophosphamide and ifosfamide. Scand J Urol Nephrol 42:309–317

Lecomte T, Landi B, Beaune P, Laurent-Puig P, Loriot MA (2006) Glutathione S-transferase P1 polymorphism (Ile105Val) predicts cumulative neuropathy in patients receiving oxaliplatin-based chemotherapy. Clin Cancer Res 12:3050–3056

Lee SJ, Schover LR, Partridge AH et al (2006) American Society of Clinical Oncology recommendations on fertility preservation in cancer patients. J Clin Oncol 24:2917–2931

Leskela S, Jara C, Leandro-Garcia LJ et al (2011a) Polymorphisms in cytochromes P450 2C8 and 3A5 are associated with paclitaxel neurotoxicity. Pharmacogenomics J 11:121–129

Leskela S, Leandro-Garcia LJ, Mendiola M et al (2011b) The miR-200 family controls beta-tubulin III expression and is associated with paclitaxel-based treatment response and progression-free survival in ovarian cancer patients. Endocr Relat Cancer 18:85–95

Levine J, Canada A, Stern CJ (2010) Fertility preservation in adolescents and young adults with cancer. J Clin Oncol 28:4831–4841

Li FP, Fine W, Jaffe N, Holmes GE, Holmes FF (1979) Offspring of patients treated for cancer in childhood. J Natl Cancer Inst 62:1193–1197

Li QF, Yao RY, Liu KW, Lv HY, Jiang T, Liang J (2010) Genetic polymorphism of GSTP1: prediction of clinical outcome to oxaliplatin/5-FU-based chemotherapy in advanced gastric cancer. J Korean Med Sci 25:846–852

Limper AH (2004) Chemotherapy-induced lung disease. Clin Chest Med 25:53–64

Loebstein R, Atanackovic G, Bishai R et al (1999) Risk factors for long-term outcome of ifosfamide-induced nephrotoxicity in children. J Clin Pharmacol 39:454–461

Lyu YL, Kerrigan JE, Lin CP et al (2007) Topoisomerase IIbeta mediated DNA double-strand breaks: implications in doxorubicin cardiotoxicity and prevention by dexrazoxane. Cancer Res 67:8839–8846

Maher J, Daly PA (1993) Severe bleomycin lung toxicity: reversal with high dose corticosteroids. Thorax 48:92–94

Manji H (2011) Toxic neuropathy. Curr Opin Neurol 24:484–490

Mannervik B, Alin P, Guthenberg C et al (1985) Identification of three classes of cytosolic glutathione transferase common to several mammalian species: correlation between structural data and enzymatic properties. Proc Natl Acad Sci U S A 82:7202–7206

Marsh S, Paul J, King CR, Gifford G, McLeod HL, Brown R (2007) Pharmacogenetic assessment of toxicity and outcome after platinum plus taxane chemotherapy in ovarian cancer: the Scottish Randomised Trial in Ovarian Cancer. J Clin Oncol 25:4528–4535

McLeod HL, Sargent DJ, Marsh S et al (2010) Pharmacogenetic predictors of adverse events and response to chemotherapy in metastatic colorectal cancer: results from North American Gastrointestinal Intergroup Trial N9741. J Clin Oncol 28:3227–3233

Meinardi MT, Van Der Graaf WT, Gietema JA et al (2002) Evaluation of long term cardiotoxicity after epirubicin containing adjuvant chemotherapy and locoregional radiotherapy for breast cancer using various detection techniques. Heart 88:81–82

Mir O, Alexandre J, Tran A et al (2009) Relationship between GSTP1 Ile(105)Val polymorphism and docetaxel-induced peripheral neuropathy: clinical evidence of a role of oxidative stress in taxane toxicity. Ann Oncol 20:736–740

Mukherjea D, Rybak LP (2011) Pharmacogenomics of cisplatin-induced ototoxicity. Pharmacogenomics 12:1039–1050

Musial-Bright L, Fengler R, Henze G, Hernaiz Driever P (2011) Carboplatin and ototoxicity: hearing loss rates among survivors of childhood medulloblastoma. Childs Nerv Syst 27:407–413

Myers JS (2012) Chemotherapy-related cognitive impairment: the breast cancer experience. Oncol Nurs Forum 39:E31–E40

Nichols CR, Catalano PJ, Crawford ED, Vogelzang NJ, Einhorn LH, Loehrer PJ (1998) Randomized comparison of cisplatin and etoposide and either bleomycin or ifosfamide in treatment of advanced disseminated germ cell tumors: an Eastern Cooperative Oncology Group, Southwest Oncology Group, and Cancer and Leukemia Group B Study. J Clin Oncol 16:1287–1293

Nousiainen T, Jantunen E, Vanninen E, Hartikainen J (2002a) Early decline in left ventricular ejection fraction predicts doxorubicin cardiotoxicity in lymphoma patients. Br J Cancer 86:1697–1700

Nousiainen T, Vanninen E, Jantunen E et al (2002b) Natriuretic peptides during the development of doxorubicin-induced left ventricular diastolic dysfunction. J Intern Med 251:228–234

Oldenburg J, Kraggerud SM, Brydoy M, Cvancarova M, Lothe RA, Fossa SD (2007a) Association between long-term neuro-toxicities in testicular cancer survivors and polymorphisms in glutathione-s-transferase-P1 and -M1, a retrospective cross sectional study. J Transl Med 5:70

Oldenburg J, Kraggerud SM, Cvancarova M, Lothe RA, Fossa SD (2007b) Cisplatin-induced long-term hearing impairment is associated with specific glutathione s-transferase genotypes in testicular cancer survivors. J Clin Oncol 25:708–714

Pabla N, Dong Z (2008) Cisplatin nephrotoxicity: mechanisms and renoprotective strategies. Kidney Int 73:994–1007

Pachman DR, Barton DL, Watson JC, Loprinzi CL (2011) Chemotherapy-induced peripheral neuropathy: prevention and treatment. Clin Pharmacol Ther 90:377–387

Pare L, Marcuello E, Altes A et al (2008) Pharmacogenetic prediction of clinical outcome in advanced colorectal cancer patients receiving oxaliplatin/5-fluorouracil as first-line chemotherapy. Br J Cancer 99:1050–1055

Pera MF Jr, Zook BC, Harder HC (1979) Effects of mannitol or furosemide diuresis on the nephrotoxicity and physiological disposition of cis-dichlorodiammineplatinum-(II) in rats. Cancer Res 39:1269–1278

Persohn E, Canta A, Schoepfer S et al (2005) Morphological and morphometric analysis of paclitaxel and docetaxel-induced peripheral neuropathy in rats. Eur J Cancer 41:1460–1466

Peters U, Preisler-Adams S, Hebeisen A et al (2000) Glutathione S-transferase genetic polymorphisms and individual sensitivity to the ototoxic effect of cisplatin. Anticancer Drugs 11:639–643

Qaddoumi I, Bass JK, Wu J et al (2012) Carboplatin-associated ototoxicity in children with retinoblastoma. J Clin Oncol 30(10):1034

Rayson D, Suter TM, Jackisch C et al (2011) Cardiac safety of adjuvant pegylated liposomal doxorubicin with concurrent trastuzumab: a randomized phase II trial. Ann Oncol 18(1):48–59

Riedemann L, Lanvers C, Deuster D et al (2008) Megalin genetic polymorphisms and individual sensitivity to the ototoxic effect of cisplatin. Pharmacogenomics J 8:23–28

Rizzo R, Spaggiari F, Indelli M et al (2010) Association of CYP1B1 with hypersensitivity induced by taxane therapy in breast cancer patients. Breast Cancer Res Treat 124:593–598

Ross CJ, Katzov-Eckert H, Dube MP et al (2009) Genetic variants in TPMT and COMT are associated with hearing loss in children receiving cisplatin chemotherapy. Nat Genet 41:1345–1349

Ruzzo A, Graziano F, Loupakis F et al (2007) Pharmacogenetic profiling in patients with advanced colorectal cancer treated with first-line FOLFOX-4 chemotherapy. J Clin Oncol 25:1247–1254

Rybak LP, Whitworth CA, Mukherjea D, Ramkumar V (2007) Mechanisms of cisplatin-induced ototoxicity and prevention. Hear Res 226:157–167

Rybak LP, Mukherjea D, Jajoo S, Ramkumar V (2009) Cisplatin ototoxicity and protection: clinical and experimental studies. Tohoku J Exp Med 219:177–186

Santoso JT, Lucci JA 3rd, Coleman RL, Schafer I, Hannigan EV (2003) Saline, mannitol, and furosemide hydration in acute cisplatin nephrotoxicity: a randomized trial. Cancer Chemother Pharmacol 52:13–18

Schagen SB, Muller MJ, Boogerd W, Mellenbergh GJ, van Dam FS (2006) Change in cognitive function after chemotherapy: a prospective longitudinal study in breast cancer patients. J Natl Cancer Inst 98:1742–1745

Schwartz RG, McKenzie WB, Alexander J et al (1987) Congestive heart failure and left ventricular dysfunction complicating doxorubicin therapy. Seven-year experience using serial radionuclide angiocardiography. Am J Med 82:1109–1118

Senkus E, Jassem J (2011) Cardiovascular effects of systemic cancer treatment. Cancer Treat Rev 37:300–311

Seo BG, Kwon HC, Oh SY et al (2009) Comprehensive analysis of excision repair complementation group 1, glutathione S-transferase, thymidylate synthase and uridine diphosphate glucuronosyl transferase 1A1 polymorphisms predictive for treatment outcome in patients with advanced gastric cancer treated with FOLFOX or FOLFIRI. Oncol Rep 22:127–136

Sill H, Olipitz W, Zebisch A, Schulz E, Wolfler A (2011) Therapy-related myeloid neoplasms: pathobiology and clinical characteristics. Br J Pharmacol 162:792–805

Silverman DH, Dy CJ, Castellon SA et al (2007) Altered frontocortical, cerebellar, and basal ganglia activity in adjuvant-treated breast cancer survivors 5–10 years after chemotherapy. Breast Cancer Res Treat 103:303–311

Sissung TM, Mross K, Steinberg SM et al (2006) Association of ABCB1 genotypes with paclitaxel-mediated peripheral neuropathy and neutropenia. Eur J Cancer 42:2893–2896

Sissung TM, Baum CE, Deeken J et al (2008) ABCB1 genetic variation influences the toxicity and clinical outcome of patients with androgen-independent prostate cancer treated with docetaxel. Clin Cancer Res 14:4543–4549

Skinner R (2011) Nephrotoxicity—what do we know and what don't we know? J Pediatr Hematol Oncol 33:128–134

Skinner R, Cotterill SJ, Stevens MC (2000) Risk factors for nephrotoxicity after ifosfamide treatment in children: a UKCCSG Late Effects Group study. United Kingdom Children's Cancer Study Group. Br J Cancer 82:1636–1645

Skinner R, Parry A, Price L, Cole M, Craft AW, Pearson AD (2009) Persistent nephrotoxicity during 10-year follow-up after cisplatin or carboplatin treatment in childhood: relevance of age and dose as risk factors. Eur J Cancer 45:3213–3219

Skinner R, Parry A, Price L, Cole M, Craft AW, Pearson AD (2010) Glomerular toxicity persists 10 years after ifosfamide treatment in childhood and is not predictable by age or dose. Pediatr Blood Cancer 54:983–989

Slamon DJ, Leyland-Jones B, Shak S et al (2001) Use of chemotherapy plus a monoclonal antibody against HER2 for metastatic breast cancer that overexpresses HER2. N Engl J Med 344:783–792

Sleijfer S (2001) Bleomycin-induced pneumonitis. Chest 120:617–624

Sleijfer S, van der Mark TW, Schraffordt Koops H, Mulder NH (1995) Decrease in pulmonary function during bleomycin-containing combination chemotherapy for testicular cancer: not only a bleomycin effect. Br J Cancer 71:120–123

Smith LA, Cornelius VR, Plummer CJ et al (2010) Cardiotoxicity of anthracycline agents for the treatment of cancer: systematic review and meta-analysis of randomised controlled trials. BMC Cancer 10:337

Smits C, Swen SJ, Theo Goverts S, Moll AC, Imhof SM, Schouten-van Meeteren AY (2006) Assessment of hearing in very young children receiving carboplatin for retinoblastoma. Eur J Cancer 42:492–500

Stoehlmacher J, Park DJ, Zhang W et al (2002) Association between glutathione S-transferase P1, T1, and M1 genetic polymorphism and survival of patients with metastatic colorectal cancer. J Natl Cancer Inst 94:936–942

Suarez A, McDowell H, Niaudet P, Comoy E, Flamant F (1991) Long-term follow-up of ifosfamide renal toxicity in children treated for malignant mesenchymal tumors: an international society of pediatric oncology report. J Clin Oncol 9:2177–2182

Sucheston LE, Zhao H, Yao S et al (2011) Genetic predictors of taxane-induced neurotoxicity in a SWOG phase III intergroup adjuvant breast cancer treatment trial (S0221). Breast Cancer Res Treat 130:993–1002

Swain SM, Whaley FS, Gerber MC et al (1997) Cardioprotection with dexrazoxane for doxorubicin-containing therapy in advanced breast cancer. J Clin Oncol 15:1318–1332

Swerdlow AJ, Douglas AJ, Hudson GV, Hudson BV, Bennett MH, MacLennan KA (1992) Risk of second primary cancers after Hodgkin's disease by type of treatment: analysis of 2846 patients in the British National Lymphoma Investigation. BMJ 304:1137–1143

Swerdlow AJ, Higgins CD, Smith P et al (2011) Second cancer risk after chemotherapy for Hodgkin's lymphoma: a collaborative British cohort study. J Clin Oncol 29:4096–4104

Tannock IF, Ahles TA, Ganz PA, Van Dam FS (2004) Cognitive impairment associated with chemotherapy for cancer: report of a workshop. J Clin Oncol 22:2233–2239

Trachtenberg BH, Landy DC, Franco VI et al (2011) Anthracycline-associated cardiotoxicity in survivors of childhood cancer. Pediatr Cardiol 32:342–353

Travis LB, Holowaty EJ, Bergfeldt K et al (1999) Risk of leukemia after platinum-based chemotherapy for ovarian cancer. N Engl J Med 340:351–357

Travis LB, Andersson M, Gospodarowicz M et al (2000) Treatment-associated leukemia following testicular cancer. J Natl Cancer Inst 92:1165–1171

Travis LB, Gospodarowicz M, Curtis RE et al (2002) Lung cancer following chemotherapy and radiotherapy for Hodgkin's disease. J Natl Cancer Inst 94:182–192

Travis LB, Fossa SD, Schonfeld SJ et al (2005) Second cancers among 40,576 testicular cancer patients: focus on long-term survivors. J Natl Cancer Inst 97:1354–1365

Travis LB, Rabkin CS, Brown LM et al (2006) Cancer survivorship—genetic susceptibility and second primary cancers: research strategies and recommendations. J Natl Cancer Inst 98:15–25

Travis LB, Beard C, Allan JM et al (2010) Testicular cancer survivorship: research strategies and recommendations. J Natl Cancer Inst 102:1114–1130

Vahdat LT, Thomas ES, Roche HH et al (2012) Ixabepilone-associated peripheral neuropathy: data from across the phase II and III clinical trials. Support Care Cancer 20:2661

van Dalen EC, van der Pal HJ, Caron HN, Kremer LC (2009) Different dosage schedules for reducing cardiotoxicity in cancer patients receiving anthracycline chemotherapy. Cochrane Database Syst Rev 2009:CD005008

van Dalen EC, Michiels EM, Caron HN, Kremer LC (2010) Different anthracycline derivates for reducing cardiotoxicity in cancer patients. Cochrane Database Syst Rev 2010:CD005006 van Dalen EC, Caron HN, Dickinson HO, Kremer LC (2011) Cardioprotective interventions for cancer patients receiving anthracyclines. Cochrane Database Syst Rev 2011:CD003917

van den Belt-Dusebout AW, de Wit R, Gietema JA et al (2007) Treatment-specific risks of second malignancies and cardiovascular disease in 5-year survivors of testicular cancer. J Clin Oncol 25:4370–4378

Vardy J, Tannock I (2007) Cognitive function after chemotherapy in adults with solid tumours. Crit Rev Oncol Hematol 63:183–202

Von Hoff DD, Layard MW, Basa P et al (1979) Risk factors for doxorubicin-induced congestive heart failure. Ann Intern Med 91:710–717

Wallace WH (2011) Oncofertility and preservation of reproductive capacity in children and young adults. Cancer 117:2301–2310

Wanderas EH, Fossa SD, Tretli S (1997) Risk of subsequent non-germ cell cancer after treatment of germ cell cancer in 2006 Norwegian male patients. Eur J Cancer 33:253–262

Weinshilboum RM (2006) Pharmacogenomics: catechol O-methyltransferase to thiopurine S-methyltransferase. Cell Mol Neurobiol 26:539–561

Wouters KA, Kremer LC, Miller TL, Herman EH, Lipshultz SE (2005) Protecting against anthracycline-induced myocardial damage: a review of the most promising strategies. Br J Haematol 131:561–578

Yao X, Panichpisal K, Kurtzman N, Nugent K (2007) Cisplatin nephrotoxicity: a review. Am J Med Sci 334:115–124

Yeh ET, Bickford CL (2009) Cardiovascular complications of cancer therapy: incidence, pathogenesis, diagnosis, and management. J Am Coll Cardiol 53:2231–2247

Yousem SA, Lifson JD, Colby TV (1985) Chemotherapy-induced eosinophilic pneumonia. Rclation to bleomycin. Chest 88:103–106

Zarate R, Rodriguez J, Bandres E et al (2010) Oxaliplatin, irinotecan and capecitabine as first-line therapy in metastatic colorectal cancer (mCRC): a dose-finding study and pharmacogenomic analysis. Br J Cancer 102:987–994

Zhu X, Wu S, Dahut WL, Parikh CR (2007) Risks of proteinuria and hypertension with bevacizumab, an antibody against vascular endothelial growth factor: systematic review and meta-analysis. Am J Kidney Dis 49:186–193

Zuppinger C, Suter TM (2010) Cancer therapy-associated cardiotoxicity and signaling in the myocardium. J Cardiovasc Pharmacol 56:1 41–146

General References

Band P (2010) The birth of the subspecialty of medical oncology and examples of its early scientific foundations. J Clin Oncol 28:3653–3658

Goodman and Gilman's The Pharmacologic Basis of Therapeutics, 12th edition. New York, McGraw-Hill 2012, Brunton LL, Chabner BA, Knollmann BC, eds. Editors of the online editon: Editor-in-Chief: Brunton LL. Assoc eds: Blumenthal DK, Murri N, Hilal-Dandan R. Consulting ed: Knollmann BC. Chapter 60, Chabner BA. General Principles of Cancer Chemotherapy. Chapter 61, Chabner BA, Bertino J, Cleary J et al. Cytotoxic Agents. Chapter 62, Chabner BA, Barnes J, Neal J et al. Targeted Therapies: Tyrosine Kinase Inhibitors, Monoclonal Antibodies, and Cytokines

Perry MC (ed) (2008) The chemotherapy source book, 4th edn. Lippincott, Williams and Wilkins, Philadelphia

BioSurveillance and Longitudinal Lifelong Guidelines

Andrea K. Ng and Melissa M. Hudson

Contents

A. K. Ng (✉)
Radiation Oncology, Dana-Farber/Harvard Cancer Center,
75 Francis St ASB1-L2, Boston, MA 02115, USA
e-mail: ang@lroc.harvard.edu

M. M. Hudson
Cancer Survivorship Division, St. Jude Children's
Research Hospital, MS 735, Room S-6014,
262 Danny Thomas Place, Memphis, TN 38105-3678, USA

Abstract

- Given the increased risk of a wide range of late effects faced by cancer survivors, lifelong follow-up of these patients are essential.
- Existing guidelines are largely based on the known types of late effects, their temporal trend and modifying risk factors after specific treatments for various primary malignancies.
- Well-established follow-up guidelines exist for survivors of pediatric malignancies, most of which are based on prior treatment exposures.
- Less data are available on the optimal follow-up strategies for survivors of adult-onset cancer.
- Additional efforts are needed to prospectively evaluate the feasibility and efficacy of the follow-up recommendations including screening and prevention strategies.
- Need to initiate transition from multidisciplinary oncology to medical community care through *individualized survivorship care plan* (p 5, paragraph 1).
- Community health care providers are unfamiliar with health risks associated with cancer survivors and need to be *supplemented by patient education and self advocacy* (p 5, paragraph 2, 3).
- Currently, deficiencies include lack of standard definitions of toxicity, *use of variable testing strategies*, inconsistency as to evaluation time in relation to therapeutic exposures (p 6, paragraph 1).
- *Early identification leads to early intervention* for late onset therapy-related complications (p 6, paragraph 4).
- NCCN guidelines provide follow-up *algorithms for cancer relapse* rather than late effects of treatment (p 8, paragraph 1).
- Long-term surveillance guidelines beyond 5 years are available for 15 different cancers and again are designed for detecting cancer recurrence (p 9, paragraph 2).
- *Second malignant neoplasms* (SMN) have been most actively pursued in Hodgkin's lymphoma survivors

P. Rubin et al. (eds.), *ALERT – Adverse Late Effects of Cancer Treatment*, Medical Radiology. Radiation Oncology,
DOI: 10.1007/978-3-540-72314-1_10, © Springer-Verlag Berlin Heidelberg 2014

(breast cancer and lung cancer) (p 10, paragraph 3, p 11, paragraph 1, p 12).

- *SMN skin cancers* are increased in Hodgkin's lymphoma and TBI/BMT survivors (p 13).
- *SMN uterine cancer* is increased in breast cancer survivors on estrogen therapy by 50 % in high-risk women (p 19).
- *Cardiovascular disease* complications are seen after radiation in breast cancer and Hodgkin's lymphoma survivors, with varied guidelines for annual blood pressure, serum glucose and lipid screening, and utility of baseline stress test/echocardiogram (p 16).
- *Endocrine deficiencies* after head and neck radiation leads to 30–40 % risk of hypothyroidism (p 18).
- *Osteopenia* can occur due to increased bone turnover in treatment-induced ovarian ablation and prostate cancer treated with gonadotrophin-releasing hormone agonists (p 18).
- *Osteonecrosis and bone fracture* can occur after radiation doses of 60 Gy and have been shown in survivors of cervix cancer (p 18).
- *Psychosocial distress issues* include fear, anxiety, suicidal ideation, depression, highlighting importance of implementing routine psychological screening and access to mental health professionals (p 20).

Future Directions

- Recognize need for *adult guidelines in follow-up* of cancer survivors, especially those treated by radiation ± chemotherapy and surgery (p 20).
- Need information on feasibility, level of compliance efficacy, *cost-effectiveness for surveillance strategies* (p 20).
- Optimal types of testing and interventions, *their timing and frequency* needs to be better defined and assessed in *prospective cohorts* of cancer survivors (p 20).
- Develop *internet contact and resources* that may provide optimal means to maintain contact for long-term follow-up of cancer survivors in our highly mobile society (p 20).

1 Introduction

Improvement in cancer screening, advances in cancer therapy and supportive care, along with the aging population have led to an increasing number of cancer survivors. After successful cancer therapy, a substantial proportion of patients face a wide range of late effects, including medical and psychosocial sequelae. According to the American Society of Clinical Oncology (ASCO), late effects are defined as a side effect that occurs more than 5 years after a diagnosis of cancer because of the related treatments, such as chemotherapy, radiation therapy, and surgery. It should be noted, however, that survivors are also at risk for other events unrelated to their prior therapy, but that may be due to shared etiologic risk factors with the initial cancer, such as genetic predisposition, health habits, environmental exposures, immune dysfunction, or infectious causes.

While ample data exist describing the increased risk of various late effects after cancer therapy, especially for selected subtypes of cancers which are characterized by young age at diagnosis, high cure rate and/or a long natural history, relatively little information are available on how to cope with the known increased risk. Potential approaches include early detection of late effects through surveillance and screening, allowing early intervention and treatment, as well as risk reduction and prevention strategies. Raising the awareness of patients and health care providers of the increased risks of late effects, and education on risk reduction through health habit modification and adherence to screening recommendations are also key to the success of a survivorship program.

Currently, concrete guidelines and recommendations for the follow-up of long-term cancer survivors are lacking. The key exception is with pediatric oncology, a group in which historically significant effort is dedicated to the lifelong care of childhood cancer survivors (Landier et al. 1999; Bhatia et al. 2005; Robison 2005; Hudson 2008). In addition to careful documentation and reporting of late effects, well-established guidelines, based on existing evidence and/or expert consensus, have been specifically developed to provide recommendations on the follow-up of long-term childhood cancer survivors (Landier et al. 2004). Although follow-up guidelines for survivors of adult-onset cancer exist, these often focused on detection of cancer recurrences, rather than management of late effects. In this chapter, we will review and discuss available follow-up guidelines designed to screen for, reduce the risk of, and provide intervention for late effects in long-term cancer survivors.

2 Follow-up Guidelines for Survivors of Pediatric Malignancies

Therapeutic success has made long-term survival a reality for the vast majority of children, adolescents, and young adults diagnosed with cancer. Following contemporary therapy, over 80 % of children and adolescents will survive 5 or more years from their cancer diagnosis and most are effectively cured of the disease (Ries et al. 2007). Investigations of long-term health outcomes in the growing population of childhood cancer survivors have identified morbidity predisposed by specific therapeutic exposures, as well host-, cancer-, and behavioral-related factors influencing risk of future disease (Oeffinger et al. 2004). These cancer-related sequelae, known as late effects, encompass a spectrum of health problems that may adversely affect quality of life and predispose to early mortality (Oeffinger et al. 2004; Mertens 2007). Moreover, late effects are commonly experienced by adults surviving childhood cancer and become more prevalent with increasing time from cancer diagnosis (Oeffinger et al. 2006; Geenen et al. 2007).

The substantial knowledge about cancer-related effects gained through health outcomes research has established a foundation for risk-based survivor care and the currently available health screening guidelines proposed for childhood cancer survivors (Skinner et al. 2005). Optimal risk-based care involves as a systematic plan for lifelong screening, surveillance, and prevention that incorporates risks based on the previous cancer, cancer therapy, genetic predispositions, lifestyle behaviors, and comorbid health conditions (Oeffinger 2003; Oeffinger et al. 2004). Information that is essential to the coordination of risk-based care includes age at cancer diagnosis, cancer histology, organs/tissues involved by cancer, and therapeutic interventions undertaken such as surgery, chemotherapy administration, radiation treatment (fields and doses), hematopoietic cell transplantation, and blood product transfusion. Knowledge of cumulative dosages or dose intensity of chemotherapeutic agents like anthracyclines is also important in estimating risk and determining screening frequency. Ideally, this information is outlined in a treatment summary organized by staff at the pediatric cancer center. Figure 1 provides an example of a treatment summary detailing therapeutic exposures and health screening recommended by the Children's Oncology Group.

It is anticipated that early detection of health problems, institution of preventive or remedial therapy, and modification of maladaptive health behaviors will provide aging childhood cancer survivors with opportunities to maintain or improve health. Implementation of risk-based care requires a working knowledge about health risks predisposed by treatment for childhood cancer, an expertise that is likely to be available only at a long-term follow-up program in a pediatric cancer center (Aziz et al. 2006). An essential service of these multidisciplinary programs is to facilitate the transition from oncology to community care by organizing an individualized survivorship care plan that includes details about therapeutic interventions undertaken for childhood cancer and their potential health risks, personalized health screening recommendations, and information about lifestyle factors that modify risks. The survivorship prescription is extremely important because the survivor's contact with the cancer center becomes less frequent with increasing passage of time from diagnosis and therapy (Oeffinger et al. 2004).

Coordination of risk-based care becomes more challenging as survivors age out of pediatric long-term follow-up programs and return to community providers for both their primary and cancer-related care. Research has demonstrated that community providers are largely unfamiliar with the health risks associated with childhood cancer, which includes a heterogeneous group of relatively rare diseases managed with diverse therapeutic approaches that have evolved over the years (Landier et al. 2006). Access to preventive care may also be hindered by survivors who are uninformed about their cancer history and its associated health risks (Kadan-Lottick et al. 2002).

Because most survivors do not have access to late effects experts in their community to coordinate health care after cancer, patient education and self-advocacy have been promoted as a means of disseminating awareness about cancer-related health risks to community providers (Landier et al. 2006). Resources that provide busy clinicians with accurate and succinct information about cancer-related late effects can help survivors gain access to appropriate health screening. To address this need, several groups have developed guidelines aiming to facilitate and standardize risk-based care of childhood cancer survivors (Skinner et al. 2005). Limitations in high quality health outcomes investigations posed challenges in efforts to organize an evidence-base to support specific screening recommendations. Deficiencies encountered included the lack of standard definitions of toxicity, use of variable testing strategies, and inconsistency in evaluation time in relation to therapeutic exposure, and bias related to incomplete participation of at-risk cohorts. Since childhood cancer comprises a relatively small proportion of cancer diagnoses, establishing through randomized clinical trials that screening of asymptomatic survivors can reduce morbidity and mortality is not feasible. Consequently, studies evaluating utility and cost-effectiveness of screening asymptomatic survivors are unlikely to be undertaken.

Despite the considerable limitations in the evidence currently available to guide health screening recommendations for childhood cancer survivors, compelling evidence does exist linking adverse outcomes to specific therapeutic exposures. These data prompted the use of a hybrid-model for the development of health screening recommendations to address the medically vulnerable and growing population of childhood cancer survivors. Group methods have varied in the magnitude and scope of the assessment of the evidence-base of adverse outcomes. However, all proposed screening recommendations based on the collective clinical experience of late effects experts that matched the magnitude of the risk with the intensity of the screening recommendation. A brief description of the guideline development methodology and content used by the Children's Oncology Group (COG), the Scottish Intercollegiate Guideline Network (SIGN) and the Late Effects Group of the United Kingdom Children's Cancer Study Group (UKCCSG) is summarized in Table 1.

The COG and SIGN Guidelines and UKCCSG Practice Statement represent important educational resources for survivors of childhood cancer and providers who supervise

SUMMARY OF CANCER TREATMENT

Date Prepared: 06/30/2008

Survivor Name:		**Date of Birth:**	
Treatment Center: St. Jude Children's Research Hospital			
Cancer Diagnosis: Acute lymphoblastic leukemia			
Date of Diagnosis: 02/18/1972		**Age at Diagnosis:** 4.9 years	**Date of Completion of Therapy**: 09/18/1974
Cancer Treatment			
Radiation Therapy			
Date start	**Date Stop**	**Field**	**Dose (cGy)**
03/20/1972	04/05/1972	Cranium	2400
Chemotherapy			
Drug Name		**Dose (units or mg/m^2)**	
L-asparaginase		Yes	
Daunorubicin		Yes – 50 mg/m^2	
Mercaptopurine		Yes	
Methotrexate		Yes	
Prednisone		Yes	
Vincristine		Yes	
Cancer Treatment	**Late Effects Risks**	**Screening Recommendations****	**Health Behavior Recommendations**
Any cancer history	Difficulty with healthcare and insurance access	Complete physical exam every year	Have regular screening exams appropriate for cancer treatment exposures
Hypothalamic-pituitary axis radiation	Hypothyroidism Metabolic syndrome Hypertension Dyslipidemia Overweight/Obesity Hyperinsulinism/Insulin resistance	Body mass index Free T4, TSH Fasting glucose, insulin and lipid profile	Get regular exercise (≥ 20-30 3 times weekly). Eat a variety of healthy foods with an emphasis on plant sources and calcium rich foods. Limit fat in diet to ≤ 30%. Maintain a healthy weight.
Daunorubicin	Cardiomyopathy	Baseline EKG at 2 or more years after completion of therapy Echocardiogram every 5 years	Do not smoke. Get regular exercise (≥ 20-30 minutes 3 times weekly). Eat a variety of healthy foods with an emphasis on plant sources and calcium rich foods. Limit fat in diet to ≤ 30%. Maintain a healthy weight.
Methotrexate/Corticosteroids	Osteopenia/Osteoporosis	Bone density test	Do not smoke. Get regular weight-bearing exercise (≥ 20-30 minutes 3 times weekly). Eat a variety of healthy foods with an emphasis on plant sources and calcium rich foods. Limit your intake of alcohol (≤ 1 drink/day for women; ≤ 2 drinks/day for men)

**Screening recommendations from the CureSearch Children's Oncology Group Long-Term Follow-Up Guidelines at http://www.survivorshipguidelines.org.

Fig. 1 After completion of therapy clinical summary for an adult survivor of childhood acute lymphoblastic leukemia detailing therapeutic exposures and health screening recommended by the Children's Oncology Group

their care. It is anticipated that increased awareness about adverse outcomes after childhood cancer offer the potential benefits of early identification of and intervention for late onset therapy-related complications. However, survivors may also experience potential harms including anxiety about health risks and false-positive screening evaluations. In addition, the costs of long-term follow-up care may be prohibitive for some patients. These issues are particularly relevant since the evidence supporting optimal screening methods for most outcomes and the benefits of treating

Table 1 Guidelines for follow-up care after childhood cancer

Organization	Search methods	Scoring of evidence	Content/Features
Children's Oncology Group *Long-Term Follow-Up Guidelines for Survivors of Childhood, Adolescent and Young Adult Cancers* Version 1.0 released March 2003 Version 2.0 released March 2006	Systematic literature review via MEDLINE (National Library of Medicine, Bethesda, MD) using key search words comprised "childhood cancer therapy," "complications," "late effects", and specific toxicities	Scoring by multidisciplinary panel of late effects experts according to a modified version of the National Comprehensive Cancer Network "Categories of Consensus" system (high to lower level of evidence)	136 sections of exposure-based potential late effects with periodic health screening recommendations, and supporting references. Delineation of "At Risk" and "Highest Risk" groups
Available at: http://www.survivorshipguidelines.org	References from the bibliographies of selected articles were used to broaden the search" Multidisciplinary system-based (e.g., cardiovascular, neurocognitive, reproductive, etc.) task forces monitor the literature and provide recommendations for guideline revision as new information becomes available	Each score reflects expert panel's assessment of strength of evidence from the literature linking specific adverse outcomes to specific therapeutic exposures Assessment of appropriateness of screening recommendation based on expert panel's collective clinical experience	Health counseling and further considerations complemented by patient education materials handouts called "Health Links" Adult cancer screening recommendations for standard and high-risk groups
Scottish Intercollegiate Guidelines Network *Long-Term Follow-Up of Survivors of Childhood Cancer—SIGN 76: A National Clinical Guideline* Release date January 2004 Updated March 2005 Available at: http://www.sign.ac.uk/guidelines/fulltext/76.	Systematic review and critical appraisal of literature using SIGN methodology	Rating of methodological quality (low to high risk of bias) of eligible studies by two independent reviewers. Recommendation for evidence's use in guiding management decisions graded (A to D) based on multidisciplinary team's collective clinical experience and knowledge of evidence Recommendation of "best practices" based on clinical experience of guideline development group	Detailed analysis of 5 key survivor outcomes: (1) growth (2) puberty and fertility (3) cardiac abnormalities (4) thyroid function (5) neurodevelopment and psychological health Recommendations for levels of long-term follow-up care based on intensity of treatment received
United Kingdom Children's Cancer Study Group Late Effects Group *Practice Statement: Therapy Based Long Term Follow Up.* 1st Edition released 1995 2nd Edition released April 2005 2nd Edition updated June 2006 Available at: http://www.ukccsg.org/public/followup/PracticeStatement	Formal literature searches of key topics	Assessment of data from literature review complemented by expert committee reports and opinions and clinical experience and practice of respected authorities Formal critical appraisal undertaken in specific contributions cross-referenced to the SIGN 76 Guidelines	Brief summary of exposure-based outcomes by any treatment, chemotherapy, radiation, and surgery 25 key content sections highlighting potential adverse outcomes, risk factors, screening recommendations, further management, and supporting references Appendices offering expanded detail about health outcomes in high risk groups (CNS tumors, transplant recipients), other general topics (puberty, fertility, immunization), and template of treatment summary

asymptomatic survivors with subclinical dysfunction have not been established. Prospective and scientifically rigorous research is required to identify accurate and cost-effective screening modalities and appropriate screening frequency and to establish the impact of screening on long-term survivor health outcomes.

3 Follow-up Guidelines for Survivors of Adult-Onset Malignancies

In contrast to follow-up guidelines for survivors of pediatric malignancies, which are based on treatment exposures, guidelines for survivors of adult-onset malignancies are largely based on cancer types, in part because of the wider range of malignancies and the greater patient and clinical scenario heterogeneity in the adult population. In addition, follow-up recommendations for the adult-onset cancer survivors tend to be less comprehensive and specific, and are available only for a restricted number of primary cancer diagnosis.

One of the most well-recognized and widely-used guidelines in adult oncology is the National Comprehensive Cancer Network (NCCN) Clinical Practice Guidelines in Oncology, developed through review of the evidence in conjunction with expert judgment by multidisciplinary panels from NCCN Member Institutions (2008). For each disease entity, guidelines for diagnosis and staging, primary intervention, adjuvant treatment, surveillance, management of recurrent, or disseminated disease, as well as guidelines for symptom management/supportive care are provided and continually updated. Table 2 summarizes the NCCN follow-up recommendations for each of the cancer sites. The algorithms for all disease entities included surveillance recommendations. However, many were intended solely for detection of relapses rather than for late effects. For several cancer sites, references were made for the follow-up and/or management of treatment-related late effects, most notably for survivors of breast cancer, head and neck cancer and Hodgkin lymphoma. For some cancer sites, the recommendations were based on anticipated adverse events related to their original cancer diagnosis rather than cancer therapy exposures. These include survivors of breast cancers who were also BRCA-1 and/or -2 carriers, survivors of patients with hereditary nonpolyposis colorectal cancer (HNPCC), survivors of melanoma or non-melanoma skin cancers whose first skin malignancy were likely related to sun exposures, and survivors of lung cancer in whom the first lung malignancy may be related to tobacco use. For these survivors the NCCN provide recommendations regarding more intensive cancer screening, prevention and health habit modifications.

The American College of Radiology Appropriateness Criteria also provide evidence-based guidelines for management of a selected number of primary cancer sites, including breast cancer, Hodgkin lymphoma, lung cancer, prostate cancer, and rectal-anal cancer (www.acr.org). The guidelines were developed by expert panels that consisted of oncologists as well as other specialists depending on the disease site. Of these disease sites, a separate topic dedicated to follow-up of patients were only available for lung cancer and Hodgkin lymphoma. For post-therapy follow-up for lung cancer, in addition to recommendations regarding follow-up for recurrences, discussions were made on the role of life-long chest computed tomography (CT) screening due to the increased risk of second lung cancer in these patients, although the frequency of the screening CT was considered controversial. For follow-up after Hodgkin lymphoma therapy, more detailed discussions were available on the follow-up of a number of late effects, including hypothyroidism, second malignancy, in particular breast cancer and lung cancer, and cardiovascular complications. Recommendations were also made regarding areas of patient counseling and education, both for raising patient awareness as well as for promoting life style changes.

Increasingly, information specific to cancer survivors are available on websites of major cancer centers as well as cancer organizations including the American Society of Clinical Oncology and the American Cancer Society (www.cancer.net; www.cancer.org). Most of these sites describe the key late effects in cancer survivors and provide additional links to other relevant sites and resources. At MD Anderson Cancer Center, follow-up guidelines, entitled "Long-Term Surveillance Guidelines Beyond 5 Years" for 15 different disease sites were listed (www.mdanderson.org). These included acute myelogenous leukemia, bladder cancer, bone cancer, breast cancer, cervical cancer, colorectal cancer, endometrial, head and neck, kidney, lung, lymphoma, melanoma, ovarian cancer, prostate cancer, and soft tissue sarcoma. Although most of these guidelines were again designed for detection of recurrence, some of the recommendations were related to the screening for second malignancy, thyroid dysfunction, and bone loss associated prior cancer therapy.

4 Specific Areas for Surveillance/ Interventions

There are several well-documented late effects in long-term cancer survivors, some of which may be life-threatening, while others may have considerable impact on patients' quality of life, that deserve special attention. Early detection at a treatable stage, and increased efforts toward risk

Table 2 NCCN surveillance guidelines for individual cancer types

Disease site	Surveillance guidelines
Acute myeloid leukemia	Surveillance for relapse only
Bladder cancer	Surveillance for relapse only
Bone cancer	Surveillance for relapse
	Surveillance/intervention for late effects
	Survivorship prescription to schedule follow-up with multidisciplinary team
	Extended therapy and surveillance may be necessary to address potential late effects of surgery, radiation and chemotherapy for long-term survivors
Breast cancer	Surveillance for relapse
	Surveillance/intervention for late effects
	After tamoxifen, annual gynecological examination if uterus present and rapid assessment of any vaginal spotting
	After aromatase inhibitor or ovarian failure, monitoring of bone health
	Consider breast MRI in women at high risk of bilateral disease, e.g. BRCA-1 or -2 carriers[a]
	Cardiac monitoring at baseline, 3 , 6 and 9 months after Trastuzumab therapy
Central nervous system cancer	Surveillance for relapse only
Cervical cancer	Surveillance for relapse
	Surveillance/intervention for late effects
	Use of vaginal dilator after radiation therapy in women who wish to remain sexually active
Chronic myelogenous leukemia	Surveillance for relapse only
Colorectal cancer	Surveillance for relapse
	Surveillance/intervention for late effects
	Surveillance post-treatment colonoscopy aimed at identifying and removing metachronous polyps given the increased risk of developing second cancers[a]
	More frequent (annual) surveillance colonoscopy for patients with HNPCC[a]
Anal cancer	Surveillance for relapse only
Esophageal cancer	Surveillance/intervention for relapse Surveillance for late effects Some patients may require dilatation of an anastamotic or a chemoradiation-induced stricture Nutritional counseling may be extremely valuable
Gastric cancer	Surveillance for relapse
	Surveillance/intervention for late effects
	Vitamin B12 levels should be monitored for patients who have had proximal/total gastrectomy
Head and neck cancer	Surveillance for relapse
	Surveillance/intervention for late effects
	TSH q 6–12 months if neck irradiated.
	Speech/hearing and swallowing evaluation and rehabilitation as indicated
	Smoking cessation counseling[a]
	Dental follow-up
Hepatobiliary cancer	Surveillance for relapse only

(continued)

Table 2 (continued)

Disease site	Surveillance guidelines
Hodgkin lymphoma	Surveillance for relapse
	Surveillance/intervention for late effects after > 5 years
	Annual blood pressure, serum glucose, lipids screening
	Consider baseline echo/stress echo after 10 years
	Pneumococcal revaccination q 5–7 years in patients who had splenectomy or splenic irradiation
	Meningococcal/H. flu vaccination in selected patients
	Consider annual influenza vaccine in high-risk patients
	Annual TSH if neck irradiated
	Annual chest imaging for patients at increased risk for lung cancer
	Mammogram/Breast MRI screening 8–10 years after irradiation or by age 40
	Counseling on reproduction, health habits, psychosocial, cardiovascular, breast self-exam, skin cancer risk
Kidney cancer	Surveillance for relapse only
Melanoma	Surveillance for relapse
	Surveillance/intervention for late effects
	Patient education on skin self-exam, protection, and subsequent skin cancer risks[a]
	Structured follow-up program to detect subsequent second primary melanoma and non-melanoma primary skin malignances; at least annual skin examination for life[a]
Multiple myeloma	Surveillance for relapse only
Myelodysplastic syndrome	Surveillance for relapse only
Neuroendocrine tumor	Surveillance for relapse only
Non-Hodgkin's lymphoma	Surveillance for relapse only
Non-melanoma skin cancer	Surveillance for relapse
	Surveillance/intervention for late effects:
Basal cell and squamous cell	Complete skin examination q 6–12 months, annually for life after 3 years[a]
Dermatofibrosarcoma protuberans	Patient education on sun exposure and self examination[a]
Merkel cell cancer	Prevention with oral retinoids in high-risk patients to reduce risk of subsequent skin cancers[a] Aggressive treatment of precancers can prevent development of subsequent invasive tumors[a]
	Surveillance for relapse only
	Surveillance for relapse only
Non-small cell lung cancer	Surveillance for relapse only
Occult primary	Surveillance for relapse only
Ovarian cancer	Surveillance for relapse only
Pancreatic adenocarcinoma	Surveillance for relapse only
Prostate cancer	Surveillance for relapse
	Surveillance/intervention for late effects:
	Increased risk of osteoporosis after either medical or surgical castration; recommended baseline bone density test and supplementation with calcium and vitamin D
	If osteopenia or osteoporosis, strongly consider bisphosphonate therapy
Small cell lung cancer	Surveillance for relapse
	Surveillance/intervention for late effects:
	Smoking cessation intervention after recovery from primary therapy[a]
	New pulmonary nodules after 2 years follow-up should initiate work-up for potential new primary[a]

(continued)

Table 2 (continued)

Disease site	Surveillance guidelines
Soft tissue sarcoma	Surveillance for relapse only
Testicular cancer	Surveillance for relapse only
Thymic cancer	Surveillance for relapse only
Thyroid cancer	Surveillance for relapse only
Uterine cancer	Surveillance for relapse only

[a] Surveillance/intervention recommendations for late events unrelated to cancer treatment exposures but related to other underlying risk factors

reduction and prevention of these late effects may play an important role in improving the well-being of long-term cancer survivors.

4.1 Second Malignancy

Second malignancy is one of the most serious late effects in patients who had survived their first cancer. There is a large body of literature describing the increased risk of second malignancy among survivors of childhood cancers (Cardous-Ubbink et al. 2007; Davies 2007; MacArthur et al. 2007), as well as survivors of several adult-onset cancers, with most information available in survivors of Hodgkin lymphoma (Biti et al. 1994; Doria et al. 1995; Donaldson et al. 1999; Swerdlow et al. 2000; van Leeuwen et al. 2000; Dores et al. 2002; Ng et al. 2002; Franklin et al. 2006; Hodgson et al. 2007). Increasing data are also available on second malignancy risk after treatment for testicular cancer (Kollmannsberger et al. 1999; Travis et al. 2000, 2005), breast cancer (Boice et al. 1992; Fisher et al. 1994; Neugut et al. 1994; Roychoudhuri et al. 2004; Kirova et al. 2007), prostate cancer (Brenner et al. 2000; Pickles et al. 2002; Chrouser et al. 2005; Moon et al. 2006), cervical cancer (Boice et al. 1987; Kleinerman et al. 1995; Chaturvedi et al. 2007), and non-Hodgkin's lymphoma (Travis et al. 1995; Mudie et al. 2006; Tward et al. 2006). The following lists a number of second malignancies that have been shown to have an increased incidence among specific cancer survivors, and in which screening and/or prevention may be warranted.

4.1.1 Breast Cancer as a Second Malignancy

An increased risk of breast cancer is clearly shown in survivors of a number of childhood malignancies and Hodgkin lymphoma, largely as a result of prior chest irradiation (Travis et al. 2003; van Leeuwen et al. 2003; Kenney et al. 2004). An excess risk of contralateral breast cancer related to radiation therapy has also been demonstrated in women treated with breast or chest wall irradiation (Boice et al. 1992; Gao et al. 2003; Hemminki et al. 2007). In addition to young age at treatment, hormonal exposures as well as other traditional breast cancer risk factors may further modify the risk (Travis et al. 2003; van Leeuwen et al. 2003). Mammography screening is a widely accepted screening modality that has been shown to significantly reduce breast cancer mortality in the general population (Frisell et al. 1997; Tabar et al. 2000; Duffy et al. 2005). Although its efficacy has not been specifically assessed in cancer survivors with breast cancer mortality as an endpoint, given the known significantly increased risk, mammography screening 8–10 years after chest irradiation is recommended in most follow-up guidelines for survivors. Breast MRI has been shown to be more sensitive than mammogram in high-risk women based on their genetic predisposition, although its role in detecting treatment-related breast cancer has not been assessed. Nevertheless, the ACS currently recommends yearly breast MRI imaging as an adjunct to mammography in women who received chest radiation between the age of 10 and 30 years (Saslow et al. 2007).

Chemoprevention with selective estrogen-receptor modulators (SERMS) have been evaluated in high-risk populations, mostly based on genetic predisposition but also including survivors of breast cancers, for breast cancer risk reduction (Cuzick 2008). Although it has not been assessed in other cancer survivors, in women at high risk due to their treatment history and other risk factors, tamoxifen for women who have completed child-bearing, and raloxifene in post-menopausal women can be considered on a case-by-case basis.

4.1.2 Lung Cancer as a Second Malignancy

An increased risk for lung cancer have been shown in survivors of Hodgkin lymphoma (Swerdlow et al. 2000; van Leeuwen et al. 2000; Dores et al. 2002; Ng et al. 2002; Travis et al. 2002; Hodgson et al. 2007), non-Hodgkin's lymphoma (Andre et al. 2004; Mudie et al. 2006; Tward et al. 2006), breast cancer (Neugut et al. 1994; Kaufman et al. 2008), lung cancer (Rubin et al. 2007), testicular cancer (Argiris et al. 2004), and cervical cancer (Boice et al. 1987; Kleinerman et al. 1995; Chaturvedi et al. 2007). Radiation therapy and alkylating chemotherapy both contribute to the risk, as has been demonstrated in survivors of

Hodgkin and non-Hodgkin's lymphoma (Swerdlow et al. 2001; Travis et al. 2002; Andre et al. 2004). The increased risk seen in survivors of cancers of the head and neck, lungs, and cervix is more likely to be related to tobacco history being a common etiologic factor for both the primary malignancy and the subsequent lung cancer.

The role of low-dose chest CT screening in other high-risk populations has been studied and reported in nonrandomized studies, and the results are conflicting and controversial (Bach 2008; Henschke et al. 2008; Midthun et al. 2008). The National Lung Screening Trial, a randomized study comparing chest X-ray versus chest CT screening in the noncancer population showed a 20 % reduction in lung cancer-specific mortality with chest CT screening (Aberle et al. 2011). The role of chest CT screening in cancer survivors has not been studied. However, for selected survivors who are deemed at high risk based on the their treatment and smoking history, and in whom further radiation therapy is not feasible because of their prior chest irradiation, they may particularly benefit from early detection through a more sensitive screening modality such as CT scan, with the goal of detecting lung cancers at an early, operable, and presumably more curable stage.

Given the known contribution of smoking to lung cancer risk, and the multiplicative effect of smoking on lung cancer risk after cancer therapy (Travis et al. 2002; Kaufman et al. 2008), survivors who continue to be smokers would greatly benefit from smoking cessation counseling and referral to smoking cessation programs.

4.1.3 Skin Cancer as a Second Malignancy

An increased risk of non-melanomatous skin cancer, in particular basal cell carcinoma, within prior radiation treatment fields have been demonstrated (Colman et al. 1988; Levi et al. 2006a). Synchronous or metachronous skin malignancies are also commonly seen in patients who already have a skin cancer diagnosis (Karagas et al. 1996; Goggins et al. 2003; Revenga et al. 2004; Levi et al. 2006b; Titus-Ernstoff et al. 2006; Cardous-Ubbink et al. 2007), as well as in patients with history of non-Hodgkin's lymphoma (Goggins et al. 2001; Hemminki et al. 2003; Loriot et al. 2006), chronic leukemia (Travis et al. 1992), and in patients status bone marrow or stem cell transplantation (Hasegawa et al. 2005; Cavalier et al. 2006). The increased risk of skin cancer in these patients are likely related to sun exposure and compromised immune status, rather than from prior cancer therapy. In cancer survivors at high risk of developing a skin malignancy, risk-reduction through sun-safety practice, and early-detection through regular self-examination and at least annual skin examination by a dermatologist are essential.

4.1.4 Endometrial Cancer as a Second Malignancy

Tamoxifen is commonly used as adjuvant therapy in women with estrogen-receptor positive breast cancer, and has been shown to reduce the risk of contralateral breast cancer by 30–40 % (Swerdlow et al. 2001). It is also an effective chemoprevention agent, reducing the risk of breast cancer by 50 % in high-risk women (Fisher et al. 1998). However, several large studies have shown that tamoxifen therapy is associated with a 2- to 4-fold significantly increased risk of endometrial caner (Magriples et al. 1993; Fisher et al. 1994; Bergman et al. 2000). In most cases, the endometrial cancers are detected an early, resectable stage. Although there are no proven effective screening tests for endometrial cancer, survivors of breast cancer who have received tamoxifen should be made aware of the increased risk, encouraged to undergo regular gynecological examinations, and have prompt evaluation of any vaginal spotting or abdominal/pelvic pain.

4.1.5 Colorectal Cancer as a Second Malignancy

An increased risk of colorectal cancer is seen among childhood cancer survivors who had received prior abdominal/pelvic irradiation, most notably in survivors of Wilms' tumor (Densmore et al. 1996; Metayer et al. 2000; Bhatia et al. 2003). In addition, the risk of colorectal cancer has been shown to be significantly elevated among survivors of Hodgkin lymphoma, testicular cancer, cervical cancer and prostate cancer (Brenner et al. 2000; Travis et al. 2005; Chaturvedi et al. 2007; Hodgson et al. 2007). Currently, the COG guidelines recommend colonoscopy screening in patients who have received radiation therapy to the abdominal/pelvic region for childhood malignancies, to be performed every 5 years beginning at 10 years after radiation or by age 35. Although recommendations for colorectal cancer screening prior to age 50 in survivors of adult-onset malignancies are not available, the COG recommendations may apply to selected young adult cancer survivors based on their primary cancer diagnosis, radiation therapy history, time since treatment and other risk factors such as family history.

4.2 Cardiovascular Disease

A broad spectrum of cardiovascular complications after cancer therapy can be seen after exposure to chest radiation therapy, specific chemotherapeutic agents and targeted therapy, and hormonal therapy. An increased risk of cardiovascular disease has been demonstrated in survivors of childhood malignancies (Krischer et al. 1997; Pein et al.

2004; Guldner et al. 2006), Hodgkin lymphoma (Heidenreich et al. 2003, 2005, 2007; Hull et al. 2003; Aleman et al. 2007), non-Hodgkin's lymphoma (Moser et al. 2006), breast cancer (Jones et al. 1989; Seidman et al. 2002; Ewer et al. 2005) and more recently prostate cancer (Smith 2004; Smith 2007; Tsai et al. 2007) and testicular cancer (Huddart et al. 2003; van den Belt-Dusebout et al. 2006, 2007). In general, prior chest irradiation is associated with an increased risk of coronary vessel disease, pericardial disease, valvular dysfunction, cardiomyopathy, conduction defects (Benoff et al. 1995; Adams et al. 2003), while exposure to anthracyclines is associated with ventricular dysfunction in a dose-related fashion (Shan et al. 1996; Keefe 2001; Steingart 2005). Among breast cancer survivors, earlier data had shown that patients treated with left-sided breast or chest wall irradiation had an increased risk for ischemic heart disease and cardiac deaths, although for patients treated in recent years with modern techniques and conformal therapy, an increased risk was no longer seen (Cuzick et al. 1994; Nixon et al. 1998; Patt et al. 2005). Trastuzumab (Herceptin) has been shown to significantly improve disease-free and overall survival in women with HER-2/neu positive breast cancer in both metastatic and adjuvant therapy settings. However, it is also associated with an increased risk of congestive heart failure and ventricular dysfunction (Seidman et al. 2002; Tan-Chiu et al. 2005). Unlike anthracycline-related cardiac dysfunction, however, the long-term cardiac risk Herceptin use is not clear. For survivors of testicular cancer, an increased risk of small and large artery disease has been demonstrated after cisplatin-based chemotherapy, which may be related to direct endothelial damage (van den Belt-Dusebout et al. 2006). For patients with prostate cancer, treatment with gonadotropin-releasing hormone agonists increases subcutaneous fat mass, decreases insulin sensitivity, increases serum lipoproteins, leading to greater risk of diabetes, cardiovascular disease, and cardiac deaths (Smith 2007).

The COG guidelines recommend baseline and periodic screening with echocardiogram and MUGA scans after exposure to anthracyclines, and for patients treated with chest irradiation, fasting blood glucose, lipid profile every 3–5 years, as well as baseline and periodic echocardiogram (2006).

The NCCN guidelines provide some cardiac-related follow-up recommendations after treatment for breast cancer and Hodgkin lymphoma (2008). Specifically, for breast cancer patients treated with trastuzumab-containing regimens, cardiac monitoring at baseline, 3 , 6 , and 9 months was recommended, although the type of cardiac monitoring was not specified. For survivors of Hodgkin lymphoma, the NCCN recommended annual blood pressure, serum glucose and lipid screening, and that baseline stress test/echocardiogram at 10 years should be considered (2008). The ACR appropriateness criteria recommended routine exercise tolerance testing and echocardiography in symptomatic patients and periodic screening in patients depending on the mediastinal radiation dose, cumulative anthracycline dose, and presence of other cardiac risk factors.

ASCO recently reviewed the clinical evidence for ongoing care related to cardiac and pulmonary late effects (Carver et al. 2007). Potential strategies for monitoring of chemotherapy-related cardiac complications, including serial endocardial biopsy, serial B-type natriuretic peptide (BNP) and troponin level testing, radionucleotide MUGA or radionucleotide angiography, exercise testing, and echocardiogram were discussed, although it was concluded that at the present time evidence supporting the use of any of these screening tools as standard monitoring for long-term survivors of cancer is lacking. In addition, it was determined that the value of any treatment, including combinations of beta blockers, angiotensin-converting enzyme (ACE) inhibitors, angiotensin receptor blockers, spironolactone, diuretics, nitrates, and hydralazine in altering the natural history of cardiac disease in the asymptomatic survivor remains to be clarified.

4.3 Endocrine Function

Reproductive health is often affected by cancer therapy, and this is especially relevant for survivors of cancers diagnosed during childhood or young adulthood. Both alkylating-agent based chemotherapy and radiation therapy to the pelvic region increase the risk of early ovarian failure in women and permanent azospermia in men. In addition, history of cranial irradiation, particularly in childhood cancer survivors, can lead to growth hormone deficiencies and hypogonadism. The COG guidelines recommend baseline screening follicle-stimulating hormone (FSH), luteinizing hormone (LH), testosterone or estradiol levels at age 14 or as clinically indicated in patients with delayed puberty or clinical signs and symptoms of hormone deficiency (2006).

A number of adult-onset cancers can occur in patients in their reproductive age, and in whom treatment can affect their reproductive function. Examples include patients with breast cancer (Partridge et al. 2008), gynecological cancers (Carter et al. 2007), testicular cancer (Taksey et al. 2003) and lymphoma (Howell et al. 2002; Franchi-Rezgui et al. 2003; Sieniawski et al. 2008). These patients would benefit from baseline evaluation by reproductive endocrinology to discuss options of preserving fertility prior to treatment initiation, and in their follow-up, referral to specialists, as applicable, for counseling and to review reproductive options (Demeestere et al. 2006).

Several primary cancer sites involve radiation therapy that included treatment to the neck region. In these patients, there is a 30–40 % risk of developing hypothyroidism over time (Chin et al. 1997). Screening thyroid stimulating hormone (TSH) levels should be obtained in all patients with prior radiation exposure to the neck as part of their follow-up for detection and treatment of subclinical hypothyroidism.

4.4 Bone Health

Bone health can be compromised through different mechanisms after cancer therapy. In the COG guidelines, screening bone density evaluation is recommended as part of long-term follow-up in patients who had received antimetabolites or corticosteroids (2006).

This recommendation may also apply to survivors of adult-onset cancer including women with treatment-induced ovarian failure, and men with prostate cancer treated with gonadotropin-releasing hormone agonists, which can increase bone turnover, decrease bone mineral density, and increase fracture risk. The role of preventative treatment against osteopenia, including bisphosphonates and selective estrogen receptor modulators in high risk cancer survivors remain to be determined. In the NCCN Task Force Report on Bone Health and Cancer Care, the role of imaging techniques to assess bone health and potential therapeutic strategies to maintain bone health in high-risk cancer survivors were discussed (Theriault et al. 2006).

History of exposure to radiation doses of 60 Gy or higher region places patients at increased risk of osteoradionecrosis (Ramli et al. 2006; Goldwaser et al. 2007). Similar doses of radiation to weight-bearing bones have been associated with an increased risk of bone fractures. This has been demonstrated in survivors of gynecological cancers who have received pelvic irradiation (Ikushima et al. 2006), and survivors of soft tissue sarcoma treated with radiation therapy (Holt et al. 2005), who typically receive doses of 60 Gy or higher to at least part of the bone. Survivors with this treatment history should be made aware of the increased fracture risk and should have prompt attention to and evaluation of any bone pain or swelling, or non-healing wounds.

4.5 Psychosocial Issues

Cancer survivors face a broad range of psychosocial challenges related to their prior cancer diagnosis and treatment. Survivors can be distressed by fear of recurrence, adverse health consequences related to cancer treatment, disruption or alteration of social support, difficulties at the workplace, and barriers in obtaining health and life insurance. Considerable data are available describing psychological distress in childhood cancer survivors. In one study on pediatric cancer survivors, alarmingly, suicidal ideation was found in 18 % of patients (Recklitis et al. 2006). Data on psychosocial function of long-term survivors of several individual adult-onset cancers are also available, most notably for survivors of breast cancer, Hodgkin lymphoma and testicular cancer (Fobair et al. 1986; Rieker et al. 1989; Bloom et al. 1993; Arai et al. 1996; Loge et al. 1997; Dorval et al. 1998; Ozen et al. 1998; Ganz et al. 2002, 2003; Wettergren et al. 2004; Helgeson et al. 2005; Thorsen et al. 2005). The influence of the time from treatment on the level of distress appears to vary, with some studies showing improvement in psychosocial function over time (Bloom et al. 2004), while others showing persistent distress beyond 7–10 years after treatment (Loge et al. 1997; Mehanna et al. 2006). In a study examining the risk of significant depressive symptoms over an 8-year period among 8,387 adults after a diagnosis of cancer, diabetes, hypertension, heart disease, arthritis, chronic lung disease, or stroke, only patients with an initial diagnosis of cancer or heart disease continued to have significant depressive symptoms beyond 4– 8 years (Polsky et al. 2005). These findings highlight the importance of implementing routine psychological screening and access to mental health professionals for long-term cancer survivors.

5 Conclusions

Successful cancer therapy often comes at the price of increased risk of adverse late events. In addition to lifelong follow-up of cancer survivors with reducing the risks of, monitoring for, and prompt treatment of late effects, early education of newly diagnosed patients regarding potential future events are essential. Survivors may also benefit from being regularly evaluated at dedicated survivorship clinics where pertinent experts for addressing specific late effects and from the most up-to-date information on management of cancer survivors are available. In addition, follow-up at survivorship clinics may facilitate patient participation in survivorship research, allowing further improvement in the care of long-term cancer survivors.

6 Future Directions

It is important to recognize that currently available guidelines in the follow-up of cancer survivors are largely based on the known late effects after specific treatment exposures. Little are available on the feasibility, level of compliance, efficacy, and cost-effectiveness of the recommended surveillance strategies. The optimal types of testing and intervention, as well as their timing and frequency also need to be better defined. Prospective evaluation of these strategies represents an important component of survivorship research.

To optimize care for cancer survivors and for successful conduction of survivorship research, the ability to reach out to long-term cancer survivors is crucial. It can be logistically difficult for survivors who no longer live locally to return to their oncology center for regular follow up visits. Long-term survivors, especially for those who are young and asymptomatic, may also be less motivated in maintaining contact with their health care providers. An innovative approach is to utilize the Internet, which has the potential to stay in contact with a large number of patients and provide individualized and interactive information at considerably lower costs than in-person contact. Researchers at Texas Children's Cancer Center and Baylor College, in conjunction with COG, are developing an interactive internet resource for childhood cancer survivors, entitled "Passport for Care" (2006). Data are also beginning to become available on the use Internet-based survivorship care plans for survivors of adult-onset malignancies (Hill-Kayser et al. 2008). The role of the Internet to provide follow-up and preventative care for cancer survivors need to be further investigated.

Finally, as cancer therapy evolve, it is imperative to continue the long-term follow-up of survivors with careful documentation of types of late effects associated with new treatments, their temporal trend, and modifying effect of other existing risk factors, efforts which will allow advances in the care of future cancer survivors.

References

Aberle DR, Adams AM, Berg CD, Black WC, Clapp JD, Fagerstrom RM, Gareen IF, Gatsonis C, Marcus PM, Sicks JD (2011) Reduced lung-cancer mortality with low-dose computed tomographic screening. N Engl J Med 365(5):395–409

Adams MJ, Hardenbergh PH, Constine LS, Lipshultz SE (2003) Radiation-associated cardiovascular disease. Crit Rev Oncol Hematol 45(1):55–75

Aleman BM, van den Belt-Dusebout AW, De Bruin ML, van 't Veer MB, Baaijens MH, de Boer JP, Hart AA, Klokman WJ, Kuenen MA, Ouwens GM, Bartelink H, van Leeuwen FE (2007) Late cardiotoxicity after treatment for Hodgkin lymphoma. Blood 109(5): 1878–1886

Andre M, Mounier N, Leleu X, Sonet A, Brice P, Henry-Amar M, Tilly H, Coiffier B, Bosly A, Morel P, Haioun C, Gaulard P, Reyes F, Gisselbrecht C (2004) Second cancers and late toxicities after treatment of aggressive non-Hodgkin lymphoma with the ACVBP regimen: a GELA cohort study on 2837 patients. Blood 103(4):1222–1228

Arai Y, Kawakita M, Hida S, Terachi T, Okada Y, Yoshida O (1996) Psychosocial aspects in long-term survivors of testicular cancer. J Urol 155(2):574–578

Argiris A, Brockstein BE, Haraf DJ, Stenson KM, Mittal BB, Kies MS, Rosen FR, Jovanovic B, Vokes EE (2004) Competing causes of death and second primary tumors in patients with locoregionally advanced head and neck cancer treated with chemoradiotherapy. Clin Cancer Res 10(6):1956–1962

Aziz NM, Oeffinger KC, Brooks S, Turoff AJ (2006) Comprehensive long-term follow-up programs for pediatric cancer survivors. Cancer 107(4):841–848

Bach PB (2008) Lung cancer screening. J Natl Compr Cancer Netw 6(3):271–275

Benoff LJ, Schweitzer P (1995) Radiation therapy-induced cardiac injury. Am Heart J 129(6):1193–1196

Bergman L, Beelen ML, Gallee MP, Hollema H, Benraadt J, van Leeuwen FE (2000) Risk and prognosis of endometrial cancer after tamoxifen for breast cancer. Comprehensive Cancer Centres' ALERT Group. Assessment of liver and endometrial cancer risk following tamoxifen. Lancet 356(9233):881–887

Bhatia S, Landier W (2005) Evaluating survivors of pediatric cancer. Cancer J 11(4):340–354

Bhatia S, Yasui Y, Robison LL, Birch JM, Bogue MK, Diller L, DeLaat C, Fossati-Bellani F, Morgan E, Oberlin O, Reaman G, Ruymann FB, Tersak J, Meadows AT (2003) High risk of subsequent neoplasms continues with extended follow-up of childhood Hodgkin's disease: report from the late effects study Group. J Clin Oncol 21(23):4386–4394

Biti G, Cellai E, Magrini SM, Papi MG, Ponticelli P, Boddi V (1994) Second solid tumors and leukemia after treatment for Hodgkin's disease: an analysis of 1121 patients from a single institution. Int J Radiat Oncol Biol Phys 29(1):25–31

Bloom JR, Fobair P, Gritz E, Wellisch D, Spiegel D, Varghese A, Hoppe R (1993) Psychosocial outcomes of cancer: a comparative analysis of Hodgkin's disease and testicular cancer. J Clin Oncol 11(5):979–988

Bloom JR, Stewart SL, Chang S, Banks PJ (2004) Then and now: quality of life of young breast cancer survivors. Psycho oncol 13(3):147–160

Boice JD Jr, Blettner M, Kleinerman RA, Stovall M, Moloney WC, Engholm G, Austin DF, Bosch A, Cookfair DL, Krementz ET et al (1987) Radiation dose and leukemia risk in patients treated for cancer of the cervix. J Natl Cancer Inst 79(6):1295–1311

Boice JD Jr, Harvey EB, Blettner M, Stovall M, Flannery JT (1992) Cancer in the contralateral breast after radiotherapy for breast cancer. N Engl J Med 326(12):781–785

Brenner DJ, Curtis RE, Hall EJ, Ron E (2000) Second malignancies in prostate carcinoma patients after radiotherapy compared with surgery. Cancer 88(2):398–406

Cardous-Ubbink MC, Heinen RC, Bakker PJ, van den Berg H, Oldenburger F, Caron HN, Voute PA, van Leeuwen FE (2007) Risk of second malignancies in long-term survivors of childhood cancer. Eur J Cancer 43(2):351–362

Carter J, Lewin S, Abu-Rustum N, Sonoda Y (2007) Reproductive issues in the gynecologic cancer patient. Oncology (Williston Park) 21(5): 598–606; discussion 606–609

Carver JR, Shapiro CL, Ng A, Jacobs L, Schwartz C, Virgo KS, Hagerty KL, Somerfield MR, Vaughn DJ (2007) American society of clinical oncology clinical evidence review on the ongoing care of adult cancer survivors: cardiac and pulmonary late effects. J Clin Oncol 25(25):3991–4008

Cavalier M, Shmalo JA, Yu M, Billings SD, Abonour R, Nelson RP Jr (2006) Skin cancer after nonmyeloablative hematopoietic cell transplantation. Bone Marrow Transpl 37(12):1103–1108

Chaturvedi AK, Engels EA, Gilbert ES, Chen BE, Storm H, Lynch CF, Hall P, Langmark F, Pukkala E, Kaijser M, Andersson M, Fossa SD, Joensuu H, Boice JD, Kleinerman RA, Travis LB (2007) Second cancers among 104,760 survivors of cervical cancer: evaluation of long-term risk. J Natl Cancer Inst 99(21):1634–1643

Chin D, Sklar C, Donahue B, Uli N, Geneiser N, Allen J, Nirenberg A, David R, Kohn B, Oberfield SE (1997) Thyroid dysfunction as a late effect in survivors of pediatric medulloblastoma/primitive neuroectodermal tumors: a comparison of hyperfractionated versus conventional radiotherapy. Cancer 80(4):798–804

Chrouser K, Leibovich B, Bergstralh E, Zincke H, Blute M (2005) Bladder cancer risk following primary and adjuvant external beam radiation for prostate cancer. J Urol 174(1): 107–110; discussion 110–111

Colman M, Easton DF, Horwich A, Peckham MJ (1988) Second malignancies and Hodgkin's disease–the Royal Marsden Hospital experience. Radiother Oncol 11(3):229–238

Cuzick J (2008) Chemoprevention of breast cancer. Breast Cancer 15(1):10–16

Cuzick J, Stewart H, Rutqvist L, Houghton J, Edwards R, Redmond C, Peto R, Baum M, Fisher B, Host H et al (1994) Cause-specific mortality in long-term survivors of breast cancer who participated in trials of radiotherapy. J Clin Oncol 12(3):447–453

Davies SM (2007) Subsequent malignant neoplasms in survivors of childhood cancer: childhood cancer survivor study (CCSS) studies. Pediatr Blood Cancer 48(7):727–730

Demeestere I, Simon P, Emiliani S, Delbaere A, Englert Y (2006) Options to preserve fertility before oncological treatment: cryopreservation of ovarian tissue and its clinical application. Acta Clin Belg 61(5):259–263

Densmore TL, Langer JC, Molleston JP, Dehner LP, Coffin CM (1996) Colorectal adenocarcinoma as a second malignant neoplasm following Wilms' tumor and rhabdomyosarcoma. Med Pediatr Oncol 27(6):556–560

Donaldson SS, Hancock SL, Hoppe RT (1999) The Janeway lecture. Hodgkin's disease–finding the balance between cure and late effects. Cancer J Sci Am 5(6):325–333

Dores GM, Metayer C, Curtis RE, Lynch CF, Clarke EA, Glimelius B, Storm H, Pukkala E, van Leeuwen FE, Holowaty EJ, Andersson M, Wiklund T, Joensuu T, van't Veer MB, Stovall M, Gospodarowicz M, Travis LB (2002) Second malignant neoplasms among long-term survivors of Hodgkin's disease: a population-based evaluation over 25 years. J Clin Oncol 20(16): 3484–3494

Doria R, Holford T, Farber LR, Prosnitz LR, Cooper DL (1995) Second solid malignancies after combined modality therapy for Hodgkin's disease. J Clin Oncol 13(8):2016–2022

Dorval M, Maunsell E, Deschenes L, Brisson J, Masse B (1998) Long-term quality of life after breast cancer: comparison of 8-year survivors with population controls. J Clin Oncol 16(2):487–494

Duffy SW, Smith RA, Gabe R, Tabar L, Yen AM, Chen TH (2005) Screening for breast cancer. Surg Oncol Clin N Am 14(4):671–697

Ewer MS, Vooletich MT, Durand JB, Woods ML, Davis JR, Valero V, Lenihan DJ (2005) Reversibility of trastuzumab-related cardiotoxicity: new insights based on clinical course and response to medical treatment. J Clin Oncol 23(31):7820–7826

Fisher B, Costantino JP, Redmond CK, Fisher ER, Wickerham DL, Cronin WM (1994) Endometrial cancer in tamoxifen-treated breast cancer patients: findings from the National Surgical Adjuvant Breast and Bowel Project (NSABP) B-14. J Natl Cancer Inst 86(7):527–537

Fisher B, Costantino JP, Wickerham DL, Redmond CK, Kavanah M, Cronin WM, Vogel V, Robidoux A, Dimitrov N, Atkins J, Daly M, Wieand S, Tan-Chiu E, Ford L, Wolmark N (1998) Tamoxifen for prevention of breast cancer: report of the National Surgical Adjuvant Breast and Bowel Project P-1 Study. J Natl Cancer Inst 90(18):1371–1388

Fobair P, Hoppe RT, Bloom J, Cox R, Varghese A, Spiegel D (1986) Psychosocial problems among survivors of Hodgkin's disease. J Clin Oncol 4(5):805–814

Franchi-Rezgui P, Rousselot P, Espie M, Briere J, Pierre Marolleau J, Gisselbrecht C, Brice P (2003) Fertility in young women after chemotherapy with alkylating agents for Hodgkin and non-Hodgkin lymphomas. Hematol J 4(2):116–120

Franklin J, Pluetschow A, Paus M, Specht L, Anselmo AP, Aviles A, Biti G, Bogatyreva T, Bonadonna G, Brillant C, Cavalieri E, Diehl V, Eghbali H, Ferme C, Henry-Amar M, Hoppe R, Howard S, Meyer R, Niedzwiecki D, Pavlovsky S, Radford J, Raemaekers J, Ryder D, Schiller P, Shakhtarina S, Valagussa P, Wilimas J, Yahalom J (2006) Second malignancy risk associated with treatment of Hodgkin's lymphoma: meta-analysis of the randomised trials. Ann Oncol 17(12):1749–1760

Frisell J, Lidbrink E, Hellstrom L, Rutqvist LE (1997) Followup after 11 years–update of mortality results in the Stockholm mammographic screening trial. Breast Cancer Res Treat 45(3):263–270

Ganz PA, Desmond KA, Leedham B, Rowland JH, Meyerowitz BE, Belin TR (2002) Quality of life in long-term, disease-free survivors of breast cancer: a follow-up study. J Natl Cancer Inst 94(1):39–49

Ganz PA, Greendale GA, Petersen L, Kahn B, Bower JE (2003) Breast cancer in younger women: reproductive and late health effects of treatment. J Clin Oncol 21(22):4184–4193

Gao X, Fisher SG, Emami B (2003) Risk of second primary cancer in the contralateral breast in women treated for early-stage breast cancer: a population-based study. Int J Radiat Oncol Biol Phys 56(4):1038–1045

Geenen MM, Cardous-Ubbink MC, Kremer LC, van den Bos C, van der Pal HJ, Heinen RC, Jaspers MW, Koning CC, Oldenburger F, Langeveld NE, Hart AA, Bakker PJ, Caron HN, van Leeuwen FE (2007) Medical assessment of adverse health outcomes in long-term survivors of childhood cancer. JAMA 297(24):2705–2715

Goggins WB, Finkelstein DM, Tsao H (2001) Evidence for an association between cutaneous melanoma and non-Hodgkin lymphoma. Cancer 91(4):874–880

Goggins WB, Tsao H (2003) A population-based analysis of risk factors for a second primary cutaneous melanoma among melanoma survivors. Cancer 97(3):639–643

Goldwaser BR, Chuang SK, Kaban LB, August M (2007) Risk factor assessment for the development of osteoradionecrosis. J Oral Maxillofac Surg 65(11):2311–2316

Guldner L, Haddy N, Pein F, Diallo I, Shamsaldin A, Dahan M, Lebidois J, Merlet P, Villain E, Sidi D, Sakiroglu O, Hartmann O, Leftakopoulos D, de Vathaire F (2006) Radiation dose and long term risk of cardiac pathology following radiotherapy and anthracyclin for a childhood cancer. Radiother Oncol 81(1):47–56

Hasegawa W, Pond GR, Rifkind JT, Messner HA, Lau A, Daly AS, Kiss TL, Kotchetkova N, Galal A, Lipton JH (2005) Long-term follow-up of secondary malignancies in adults after allogeneic bone marrow transplantation. Bone Marrow Transpl 35(1):51–55

Heidenreich PA, Hancock SL, Lee BK, Mariscal CS, Schnittger I (2003) Asymptomatic cardiac disease following mediastinal irradiation. J Am Coll Cardiol 42(4):743–749

Heidenreich PA, Hancock SL, Vagelos RH, Lee BK, Schnittger I (2005) Diastolic dysfunction after mediastinal irradiation. Am Heart J 150(5):977–982

Heidenreich PA, Schnittger I, Strauss HW, Vagelos RH, Lee BK, Mariscal CS, Tate DJ, Horning SJ, Hoppe RT, Hancock SL (2007) Screening for coronary artery disease after mediastinal irradiation for Hodgkin's disease. J Clin Oncol 25(1):43–49

Helgeson VS, Tomich PL (2005) Surviving cancer: a comparison of 5-year disease-free breast cancer survivors with healthy women. Psycho Oncol 14(4):307–317

Hemminki K, Ji J, Forsti A (2007) Risks for familial and contralateral breast cancer interact multiplicatively and cause a high risk. Cancer Res 67(3):868–870

Hemminki K, Jiang Y, Steineck G (2003) Skin cancer and non-Hodgkin's lymphoma as second malignancies. markers of impaired immune function? Eur J Cancer 39(2):223–229

Henschke CI, Yankelevitz DF (2008) CT screening for lung cancer: update 2007. Oncologist 13(1):65–78

Hill-Kayser C, Vachani C, Hampshire MK, Jacobs LA, Metz J (2008) First report of internet-based survivorship care plans and utilization by colorectal cancer (CRC) survivors. Gastrointest Cancers Symp Abstract No. 398

Hodgson DC, Gilbert ES, Dores GM, Schonfeld SJ, Lynch CF, Storm H, Hall P, Langmark F, Pukkala E, Andersson M, Kaijser M, Joensuu H, Fossa SD, Travis LB (2007) Long-term solid cancer risk among 5-year survivors of Hodgkin's lymphoma. J Clin Oncol 25(12):1489–1497

Holt GE, Griffin AM, Pintilie M, Wunder JS, Catton C, O'Sullivan B, Bell RS (2005) Fractures following radiotherapy and limb-salvage surgery for lower extremity soft-tissue sarcomas. a comparison of high-dose and low-dose radiotherapy. J Bone Joint Surg Am 87(2):315–319

Howell SJ, Shalet SM (2002) Fertility preservation and management of gonadal failure associated with lymphoma therapy. Curr Oncol Rep 4(5):443–452

Huddart RA, Norman A, Shahidi M, Horwich A, Coward D, Nicholls J, Dearnaley DP (2003) Cardiovascular disease as a long-term complication of treatment for testicular cancer. J Clin Oncol 21(8):1513–1523

Hudson MM (2008) Survivors of childhood cancer: coming of age. Hematol Oncol Clin North Am 22(2): 211–231, v–vi

Hull MC, Morris CG, Pepine CJ, Mendenhall NP (2003) Valvular dysfunction and carotid, subclavian, and coronary artery disease in survivors of hodgkin lymphoma treated with radiation therapy. JAMA 290(21):2831–2837

Ikushima H, Osaki K, Furutani S, Yamashita K, Kishida Y, Kudoh T, Nishitani H (2006) Pelvic bone complications following radiation therapy of gynecologic malignancies: clinical evaluation of radiation-induced pelvic insufficiency fractures. Gynecol Oncol 103(3):1100–1104

Jones JM, Ribeiro GG (1989) Mortality patterns over 34 years of breast cancer patients in a clinical trial of post-operative radiotherapy. Clin Radiol 40(2):204–208

Kadan-Lottick NS, Robison LL, Gurney JG, Neglia JP, Yasui Y, Hayashi R, Hudson M, Greenberg M, Mertens AC (2002) Childhood cancer survivors' knowledge about their past diagnosis and treatment: childhood cancer survivor study. JAMA 287(14):1832–1839

Karagas MR, McDonald JA, Greenberg ER, Stukel TA, Weiss JE, Baron JA, Stevens MM (1996) Risk of basal cell and squamous cell skin cancers after ionizing radiation therapy. for the skin cancer prevention study group. J Natl Cancer Inst 88(24):1848–1853

Kaufman EL, Jacobson JS, Hershman DL, Desai M, Neugut AI (2008) Effect of breast cancer radiotherapy and cigarette smoking on risk of second primary lung cancer. J Clin Oncol 26(3):392–398

Keefe DL (2001) Anthracycline-induced cardiomyopathy. Semin Oncol 28(4 Suppl 12):2–7

Kenney LB, Yasui Y, Inskip PD, Hammond S, Neglia JP, Mertens AC, Meadows AT, Friedman D, Robison LL, Diller L (2004) Breast cancer after childhood cancer: a report from the childhood cancer survivor study. Ann Intern Med 141(8):590–597

Kirova YM, Gambotti L, De Rycke Y, Vilcoq JR, Asselain B, Fourquet A (2007) Risk of second malignancies after adjuvant radiotherapy for breast cancer: a large-scale, single-institution review. Int J Radiat Oncol Biol Phys 68(2):359–363

Kleinerman RA, Boice JD Jr, Storm HH, Sparen P, Andersen A, Pukkala E, Lynch CF, Hankey BF, Flannery JT (1995) Second primary cancer after treatment for cervical cancer. an international cancer registries study. Cancer 76(3):442–452

Kollmannsberger C, Hartmann JT, Kanz L, Bokemeyer C (1999) Therapy-related malignancies following treatment of germ cell cancer. Int J Cancer 83(6):860–863

Krischer JP, Epstein S, Cuthbertson DD, Goorin AM, Epstein ML, Lipshultz SE (1997) Clinical cardiotoxicity following anthracycline treatment for childhood cancer: the pediatric oncology group experience. J Clin Oncol 15(4):1544–1552

Landier W, Bhatia S (1999) Long-term complications following childhood cancer. Indian Pediatr 36(10):975–980

Landier W, Bhatia S, Eshelman DA, Forte KJ, Sweeney T, Hester AL, Darling J, Armstrong FD, Blatt J, Constine LS, Freeman CR, Friedman DL, Green DM, Marina N, Meadows AT, Neglia JP, Oeffinger KC, Robison LL, Ruccione KS, Sklar CA, Hudson MM (2004) Development of risk-based guidelines for pediatric cancer survivors: the Children's Oncology Group Long-Term Follow-Up Guidelines from the Children's Oncology Group Late Effects Committee and Nursing Discipline. J Clin Oncol 22(24):4979–4990

Landier W, Wallace WH, Hudson MM (2006) Long-term follow-up of pediatric cancer survivors: education, surveillance, and screening. Pediatr Blood Cancer 46(2):149–158

Levi F, Moeckli R, Randimbison L, Te VC, Maspoli M, La Vecchia C (2006a) Skin cancer in survivors of childhood and adolescent cancer. Eur J Cancer 42(5):656–659

Levi F, Randimbison L, Maspoli M, Te VC, La Vecchia C (2006b) High incidence of second basal cell skin cancers. Int J Cancer 119(6):1505–1507

Loge JH, Abrahamsen AF, Ekeberg O, Hannisdal E, Kaasa S (1997) Psychological distress after cancer cure: a survey of 459 Hodgkin's disease survivors. Br J Cancer 76(6):791–796

Loriot Y, Chaoui D, Dorval T, Vincent-Salomon A, Lumbroso-Le Rouic L, Dendale R, Desjardins L, Levy C, Decaudin D (2006) Association between lymphoma and melanoma: report of a single-center series of eight patients and a review of the literature. Leuk Lymphoma 47(6):1023–1028

MacArthur AC, Spinelli JJ, Rogers PC, Goddard KJ, Phillips N, McBride ML (2007) Risk of a second malignant neoplasm among 5-year survivors of cancer in childhood and adolescence in British Columbia, Canada. Pediatr Blood Cancer 48(4):453–459

Magriples U, Naftolin F, Schwartz PE, Carcangiu ML (1993) High-grade endometrial carcinoma in tamoxifen-treated breast cancer patients. J Clin Oncol 11(3):485–490

Mehanna HM, Morton RP (2006) Deterioration in quality-of-life of late (10-year) survivors of head and neck cancer. Clin Otolaryngol 31(3):204–211

Mertens AC (2007) Cause of mortality in 5-year survivors of childhood cancer. Pediatr Blood Cancer 48(7):723–726

Metayer C, Lynch CF, Clarke EA, Glimelius B, Storm H, Pukkala E, Joensuu T, van Leeuwen FE, van't Veer MB, Curtis RE, Holowaty EJ, Andersson M, Wiklund T, Gospodarowicz M, Travis LB (2000) Second cancers among long-term survivors of Hodgkin's disease diagnosed in childhood and adolescence. J Clin Oncol 18(12): 2435–2443

Midthun DE, Jett JR (2008) Update on screening for lung cancer. Semin Respir Crit Care Med 29(3):233–240

Moon K, Stukenborg GJ, Keim J, Theodorescu D (2006) Cancer incidence after localized therapy for prostate cancer. Cancer 107(5):991–998

Moser EC, Noordijk EM, van Leeuwen FE, le Cessie S, Baars JW, Thomas J, Carde P, Meerwaldt JH, van Glabbeke M, Kluin-Nelemans HC (2006) Long-term risk of cardiovascular disease after treatment for aggressive non-Hodgkin lymphoma. Blood 107(7):2912–2919

Mudie NY, Swerdlow AJ, Higgins CD, Smith P, Qiao Z, Hancock BW, Hoskin PJ, Linch DC (2006) Risk of second malignancy after non-Hodgkin's lymphoma: a British cohort study. J Clin Oncol 24(10):1568–1574

NCCN clinical practice guidelines in oncology (2008) www.nccn.org

Neugut AI, Murray T, Santos J, Amols H, Hayes MK, Flannery JT, Robinson E (1994) Increased risk of lung cancer after breast cancer radiation therapy in cigarette smokers. Cancer 73(6): 1615–1620

Ng AK, Bernardo MV, Weller E, Backstrand K, Silver B, Marcus KC, Tarbell NJ, Stevenson MA, Friedberg JW, Mauch PM (2002) Second malignancy after Hodgkin disease treated with radiation therapy with or without chemotherapy: long-term risks and risk factors. Blood 100(6):1989–1996

Nixon AJ, Manola J, Gelman R, Bornstein B, Abner A, Hetelekidis S, Recht A, Harris JR (1998) No long-term increase in cardiac-related mortality after breast-conserving surgery and radiation therapy using modern techniques. J Clin Oncol 16(4):1374–1379

Oeffinger KC (2003) Longitudinal risk-based health care for adult survivors of childhood cancer. Curr Probl Cancer 27(3):143–167

Oeffinger KC, Hudson MM (2004) Long-term complications following childhood and adolescent cancer: foundations for providing risk-based health care for survivors. CA Cancer J Clin 54(4): 208–236

Oeffinger KC, Mertens AC, Hudson MM, Gurney JG, Casillas J, Chen H, Whitton J, Yeazel M, Yasui Y, Robison LL (2004) Health care of young adult survivors of childhood cancer: a report from the childhood cancer survivor study. Ann Fam Med 2(1):61–70

Oeffinger KC, Mertens AC, Sklar CA, Kawashima T, Hudson MM, Meadows AT, Friedman DL, Marina N, Hobbie W, Kadan-Lottick NS, Schwartz CL, Leisenring W, Robison LL (2006) Chronic health conditions in adult survivors of childhood cancer. N Engl J Med 355(15):1572–1582

Ozen H, Sahin A, Toklu C, Rastadoskouee M, Kilic C, Gogus A, Kendi S (1998) Psychosocial adjustment after testicular cancer treatment. J Urol 159(6):1947–1950

Partridge AH, Gelber S, Peppercorn J, Gunsburg E, Sampson E, Rosenberg R, Przypyszny M, Winer EP (2008) Fertility and menopausal outcomes in young breast cancer survivors. Clin Breast Cancer 8(1):65–69

Passport for care: an internet-based survivorship care plan (2006) http://www.cancer.gov/ncicancerbulletin/NCI_Cancer_Bulletin_06 0606/page9.

Patt DA, Goodwin JS, Kuo YF, Freeman JL, Zhang DD, Buchholz TA, Hortobagyi GN, Giordano SH (2005) Cardiac morbidity of adjuvant radiotherapy for breast cancer. J Clin Oncol 23(30):7475–7482

Pein F, Sakiroglu O, Dahan M, Lebidois J, Merlet P, Shamsaldin A, Villain E, de Vathaire F, Sidi D, Hartmann O (2004) Cardiac abnormalities 15 years and more after adriamycin therapy in 229 childhood survivors of a solid tumour at the Institut Gustave Roussy. Br J Cancer 91(1):37–44

Pickles T, Phillips N (2002) The risk of second malignancy in men with prostate cancer treated with or without radiation in British Columbia, 1984–2000. Radiother Oncol 65(3):145–151

Polsky D, Doshi JA, Marcus S, Oslin D, Rothbard A, Thomas N, Thompson CL (2005) Long-term risk for depressive symptoms after a medical diagnosis. Arch Intern Med 165(11):1260–1266

Ramli R, Ngeow WC, Rahman RA, Chai WL (2006) Managing complications of radiation therapy in head and neck cancer patients: part IV. Management of osteoradionecrosis. Singap Dent J 28(1):11–15

Recklitis CJ, Lockwood RA, Rothwell MA, Diller LR (2006) Suicidal ideation and attempts in adult survivors of childhood cancer. J Clin Oncol 24(24):3852–3857

Revenga F, Paricio JF, Vazquez MM, Del Villar V (2004) Risk of subsequent non-melanoma skin cancer in a cohort of patients with primary basal cell carcinoma. J Eur Acad Dermatol Venereol 18(4):514–515

Rieker PP, Fitzgerald EM, Kalish LA, Richie JP, Lederman GS, Edbril SD, Garnick MB (1989) Psychosocial factors, curative therapies, and behavioral outcomes. A comparison of testis cancer survivors and a control group of healthy men. Cancer 64(11):2399–2407

Ries L, Melbert D, Krapcho M, al E (2007) SEER Cancer Statistics Review, 1975–2004. National Cancer Institute, Bethesda

Robison LL (2005) The Childhood Cancer Survivor Study: a resource for research of long-term outcomes among adult survivors of childhood cancer. Minn Med 88(4):45–49

Roychoudhuri R, Evans H, Robinson D, Moller H (2004) Radiation-induced malignancies following radiotherapy for breast cancer. Br J Cancer 91(5):868–872

Rubins J, Unger M, Colice GL (2007) Follow-up and surveillance of the lung cancer patient following curative intent therapy: ACCP evidence-based clinical practice guideline (2nd edition). Chest 132(3 Suppl):355S–367S

Saslow D, Boetes C, Burke W, Harms S, Leach MO, Lehman CD, Morris E, Pisano E, Schnall M, Sener S, Smith RA, Warner E, Yaffe M, Andrews KS, Russell CA (2007) American Cancer Society guidelines for breast screening with MRI as an adjunct to mammography. CA Cancer J Clin 57(2):75–89

Seidman A, Hudis C, Pierri MK, Shak S, Paton V, Ashby M, Murphy M, Stewart SJ, Keefe D (2002) Cardiac dysfunction in the trastuzumab clinical trials experience. J Clin Oncol 20(5): 1215–1221

Shan K, Lincoff AM, Young JB (1996) Anthracycline-induced cardiotoxicity. Ann Intern Med 125(1):47–58

Sieniawski M, Reineke T, Josting A, Nogova L, Behringer K, Halbsguth T, Fuchs M, Diehl V, Engert A (2008) Assessment of male fertility in patients with Hodgkin's lymphoma treated in the German Hodgkin Study Group (GHSG) clinical trials. Ann Oncol 19(10):1751–1801

Skinner R, Wallace WH, Levitt GA (2005) Therapy based long-term follow-up practice statement. http://www.ukccsg.org/public/follow up/PracticeStatement/index.html **(2nd edn)**

Smith MR (2004) Changes in fat and lean body mass during androgen-deprivation therapy for prostate cancer. Urology 63(4):742–745

Smith MR (2007) Androgen deprivation therapy for prostate cancer: new concepts and concerns. Curr Opin Endocrinol Diabetes Obes 14(3):247–254

Steingart R (2005) Mechanisms of late cardiovascular toxicity from cancer chemotherapy. J Clin Oncol 23(36):9051–9052

Swerdlow AJ, Barber JA, Hudson GV, Cunningham D, Gupta RK, Hancock BW, Horwich A, Lister TA, Linch DC (2000) Risk of second malignancy after Hodgkin's disease in a collaborative British cohort: the relation to age at treatment. J Clin Oncol 18(3):498–509

Swerdlow AJ, Schoemaker MJ, Allerton R, Horwich A, Barber JA, Cunningham D, Lister TA, Rohatiner AZ, Vaughan Hudson G, Williams MV, Linch DC (2001) Lung cancer after Hodgkin's disease: a nested case-control study of the relation to treatment. J Clin Oncol 19(6):1610–1618

Tabar L, Vitak B, Chen HH, Duffy SW, Yen MF, Chiang CF, Krusemo UB, Tot T, Smith RA (2000) The Swedish two-county trial twenty years later. Updated mortality results and new insights from long-term follow-up. Radiol Clin North Am 38(4):625–651

Taksey J, Bissada NK, Chaudhary UB (2003) Fertility after chemotherapy for testicular cancer. Arch Androl 49(5):389–395

Tan-Chiu E, Yothers G, Romond E, Geyer CE Jr, Ewer M, Keefe D, Shannon RP, Swain SM, Brown A, Fehrenbacher L, Vogel VG, Seay TE, Rastogi P, Mamounas EP, Wolmark N, Bryant J (2005) Assessment of cardiac dysfunction in a randomized trial comparing doxorubicin and cyclophosphamide followed by paclitaxel, with or without trastuzumab as adjuvant therapy in node-positive, human epidermal growth factor receptor 2-overexpressing breast cancer: NSABP B-31. J Clin Oncol 23(31):7811–7819

Theriault RL, Biermann JS, Brown E, Brufsky A, Demers L, Grewal RK, Guise T, Jackson R, McEnery K, Podoloff D, Ravdin P, Shapiro CL, Smith M, Van Poznak CH (2006) NCCN Task Force Report: Bone Health and Cancer Care. J Natl Compr Canc Netw 4 Suppl 2: S1–20

Thorsen L, Nystad W, Stigum H, Dahl O, Klepp O, Bremnes RM, Wist E, Fossa SD (2005) The association between self-reported physical activity and prevalence of depression and anxiety disorder in long-term survivors of testicular cancer and men in a general population sample. Support Care Cancer 13(8):637–646

Titus-Ernstoff L, Perry AE, Spencer SK, Gibson J, Ding J, Cole B, Ernstoff MS (2006) Multiple primary melanoma: two-year results from a population-based study. Arch Dermatol 142(4):433–438

Travis LB, Andersson M, Gospodarowicz M, van Leeuwen FE, Bergfeldt K, Lynch CF, Curtis RE, Kohler BA, Wiklund T, Storm H, Holowaty E, Hall P, Pukkala E, Sleijfer DT, Clarke EA, Boice JD Jr, Stovall M, Gilbert E (2000) Treatment-associated leukemia following testicular cancer. J Natl Cancer Inst 92(14):1165–1171

Travis LB, Curtis RE, Glimelius B, Holowaty EJ, Van Leeuwen FE, Lynch CF, Hagenbeek A, Stovall M, Banks PM, Adami J et al (1995) Bladder and kidney cancer following cyclophosphamide therapy for non-Hodgkin's lymphoma. J Natl Cancer Inst 87(7):524–530

Travis LB, Curtis RE, Hankey BF, Fraumeni JF Jr (1992) Second cancers in patients with chronic lymphocytic leukemia. J Natl Cancer Inst 84(18):1422–1427

Travis LB, Fossa SD, Schonfeld SJ, McMaster ML, Lynch CF, Storm H, Hall P, Holowaty E, Andersen A, Pukkala E, Andersson M, Kaijser M, Gospodarowicz M, Joensuu T, Cohen RJ, Boice JD Jr, Dores GM, Gilbert ES (2005) Second cancers among 40,576 testicular cancer patients: focus on long-term survivors. J Natl Cancer Inst 97(18):1354–1365

Travis LB, Gospodarowicz M, Curtis RE, Clarke EA, Andersson M, Glimelius B, Joensuu T, Lynch CF, van Leeuwen FE, Holowaty E, Storm H, Glimelius I, Pukkala E, Stovall M, Fraumeni JF Jr, Boice JD Jr, Gilbert E (2002) Lung cancer following chemotherapy and radiotherapy for Hodgkin's disease. J Natl Cancer Inst 94(3):182–192

Travis LB, Hill DA, Dores GM, Gospodarowicz M, van Leeuwen FE, Holowaty E, Glimelius B, Andersson M, Wiklund T, Lynch CF, Van't Veer MB, Glimelius I, Storm H, Pukkala E, Stovall M, Curtis R, Boice JD Jr, Gilbert E (2003) Breast cancer following radiotherapy and chemotherapy among young women with Hodgkin disease. JAMA 290(4):465–475

Tsai HK, D'Amico AV, Sadetsky N, Chen MH, Carroll PR (2007) Androgen deprivation therapy for localized prostate cancer and the risk of cardiovascular mortality. J Natl Cancer Inst 99(20):1516–1524

Tward JD, Wendland MM, Shrieve DC, Szabo A, Gaffney DK (2006) The risk of secondary malignancies over 30 years after the treatment of non-Hodgkin lymphoma. Cancer 107(1):108–115

van den Belt-Dusebout AW, de Wit R, Gietema JA, Horenblas S, Louwman MW, Ribot JG, Hoekstra HJ, Ouwens GM, Aleman BM, van Leeuwen FE (2007) Treatment-specific risks of second malignancies and cardiovascular disease in 5-year survivors of testicular cancer. J Clin Oncol 25(28):4370–4378

van den Belt-Dusebout AW, Nuver J, de Wit R, Gietema JA, ten Bokkel Huinink WW, Rodrigus PT, Schimmel EC, Aleman BM, van Leeuwen FE (2006) Long-term risk of cardiovascular disease in 5-year survivors of testicular cancer. J Clin Oncol 24(3):467–475

van Leeuwen FE, Klokman WJ, Stovall M, Dahler EC, van't Veer MB, Noordijk EM, Crommelin MA, Aleman BM, Broeks A, Gospodarowicz M, Travis LB, Russell NS (2003) Roles of radiation dose, chemotherapy, and hormonal factors in breast cancer following Hodgkin's disease. J Natl Cancer Inst 95(13): 971–980

van Leeuwen FE, Klokman WJ, Veer MB, Hagenbeek A, Krol AD, Vetter UA, Schaapveld M, van Heerde P, Burgers JM, Somers R, Aleman BM (2000) Long-term risk of second malignancy in survivors of Hodgkin's disease treated during adolescence or young adulthood. J Clin Oncol 18(3):487–497

Wettergren L, Bjorkholm M, Axdorph U, Langius-Eklof A (2004) Determinants of health-related quality of life in long-term survivors of Hodgkin's lymphoma. Qual Life Res 13(8):1369–1379

BioPediatric Complexities of Growth and Development

Arnold C. Paulino, Sughosh Dhakal, and Louis S. Constine

Contents

L. S. Constine (✉)
Department of Radiation Oncology, James P. Wilmot Cancer Center, University of Rochester Medical Center, 647, Rochester, NY 14642, USA
e-mail: Louis_constine@urmc.rochester.edu

A. C. Paulino
Radiation Oncology, Department of Radiation Oncology, The Methodist Hospital, 6565 Fannin St, 77030 Houston, TX, USA

S. Dhakal
Radiation Oncology, Department of Radiation Oncology, University of Rochester School of Medicine and Dentistry, 601 Elmwood Ave, Box 647, Rochester, NY 14642, USA

Abstract

Although increased survival and ultimately cure of cancer remains the primary goal of treatment, the quality of survival is largely dependent on the toxicities of treatment. In particular, the late effects of treatment, which may manifest months to years or even decades after therapy, have been a driving force in the evolution of the treatment of many curable cancers. Advances in radiation oncology and diagnostic radiology have led to more conformal treatments that spare adjacent normal structures, and chemotherapy regimens have likewise evolved. In addition, in many cancers, perhaps most notably Hodgkin lymphoma, favorable subsets of patients are now treated with decreased doses of chemotherapy and radiation while maintaining overall efficacy.

1 Introduction

Although increased survival and ultimately cure of cancer remains the primary goal of treatment, the quality of survival is largely dependent on the toxicities of treatment. In particular, the late effects of treatment, which may manifest months to years or even decades after therapy, have been a driving force in the evolution of the treatment of many curable cancers. Advances in radiation oncology and diagnostic radiology have led to more conformal treatments that spare adjacent normal structures, and chemotherapy regimens have likewise evolved. In addition, in many cancers, perhaps most notably Hodgkin lymphoma, favorable subsets of patients are now treated with decreased doses of chemotherapy and radiation while maintaining overall efficacy.

The development and manifestation of late effects in children differ greatly when compared to adults. The late effects in adults are primarily a result of inflammatory and fibrogenic processes. While these processes can also occur

P. Rubin et al. (eds.), *ALERT – Adverse Late Effects of Cancer Treatment*, Medical Radiology. Radiation Oncology,
DOI: 10.1007/978-3-540-72314-1_11, © Springer-Verlag Berlin Heidelberg 2014

in children, the inability of an organ to grow and mature properly is a late complication which is unique to children. Differences in tissue and organ development explain many of the susceptibilities to and manifestations of radiation-induced injury when delivered throughout the early years of life, whereas a differential ability to repair injury is the primary determinant of chronic tissue injury in the mature and senescing adult. Furthermore, comorbid illness and prolonged environmental and lifestyle factors are much more likely to affect the development of treatment related injury in adults.

Many of these principles are illustrated by the example of chest wall irradiation. Both the adult and child will be prone to pulmonary consequences, such as inflammation and fibrosis; however, the child also will be susceptible to a direct restriction of lung compliance from bone hypoplasia and malformation in the developing ribs and spine, as well as indirect effects of compliance due to greater levels of atelectasis and air trapping. Such is not the case in the adult, where the bones are fully grown and hypoplasia and malformation are not an issue. However, comedical factors generally absent in children but oftentimes present in adults, such as smoking or other environment exposures, will affect the risk of treatment-related pneumonitis. In addition, the capacity for tissue repair may be relatively limited in the elderly.

This chapter will review organogenesis in the developing human, from the embryo to adulthood, and the complexities involved in manifestation of late effects from radiation therapy according to stage of development. It will review the four classic growth curves for normal tissues in children and briefly discuss a selected number of confounding factors that may influence the degree of late effects in the pediatric and adult population. Secondary malignant neoplasms will not be covered in this chapter as they are discussed extensively elsewhere.

2 Organogenesis: Sensitivity to Late Effects According to Stage of Development

2.1 Embryo and Fetus

Growth starts after fertilization of the egg by the sperm. Radiotherapy to the developing embryo or fetus may affect growth depending on its stage of development. There are three recognized phases of the developmental period in utero: (1) preimplantation, (2) prenatal organogenesis, and (3) fetal period (Russell and Russell 1954).

Preimplantation starts from the time of fertilization to the time when the embryo attaches to the uterine wall (implantation). It is the most sensitive phase to the lethal effects of radiation and occurs within the first 2 weeks postconception. In some mammals, this can be manifested by a decrease in litter size secondary to prenatal death of the accompanying progeny. The irradiated preimplanted embryo that survives until term grows normally in the prepartum and postpartum periods. Growth is not affected by irradiation at this period as only a few cells are present; if substantial numbers of cells die, the embryo is resorbed. In those that have survived, cells usually divide to "make-up" what cells were destroyed. Data regarding the effects of radiation therapy during this phase of development are largely derived from animal models and in vitro experiments, utilizing mouse embryos grown in tissue culture (Streffer and Molls 1987). Doses as low as 5–15 cGy can kill fertilized eggs in mice and rats (Rugh 1962; Brent and Ghorson 1972).

The second phase of development in utero is prenatal organogenesis, which occurs immediately after implantation and extends through the first 60 days after conception. It is a period of marked radiosensitivity as this corresponds to differentiation of body structures. Irradiation during this period has resulted in malformations secondary to disruption of morphogenesis of different organ systems. Most of the clinical information regarding malformations occurring in this period come from atomic bomb survivors in Hiroshima. Reported anomalies have largely affected a few organ systems including the central nervous system, skeletal system and dentition, eye and genitalia. The gastrointestinal, cardiovascular, and renal systems, which are common sites of anomalies, are not particularly involved in those receiving radiation (Metler and Upton 1995). This may be related to the length and time of organ development. If death occurs as a result of irradiation during organogenesis, it is likely to manifest as neonatal death or death occurring at time of or around birth, in contrast to death during irradiation at time of preimplantation or implantation, in which case the embryo is resorbed.

The fetal period occurs from 60 days after conception through parturition. Body and organ growth predominates as differentiation becomes more complete; hence, structural malformations gradually decrease while disturbances of growth are more prominent. Much higher doses are required to cause death during this phase compared to earlier periods of development. Irradiation of an early fetus results in the largest degree of permanent growth retardation, in contrast to an irradiated early embryo, which will exhibit greater growth retardation at birth but largely recover later in life. As can be expected, tissues undergoing the most rapid cell division at the time of exposure are the most susceptible to growth disturbances. For example, the highest incidence of mental retardation in atomic bomb survivors are seen in those exposed at 8–15 weeks of intrauterine life, with a relative risk four times higher than those exposed at

16 weeks or greater. Mental retardation was not seen in subjects irradiated at <8 weeks in utero (Otake et al. 1991). Irradiation of the fetus between 16 and 20 weeks of gestation may also lead to microcephaly and stunting of growth. Irradiation after 30 weeks of gestation is not likely to produce gross structural abnormalities leading to serious problems in early life.

2.2 Postnatal Period and Childhood

Unlike the prenatal stage, postnatal development after radiation exposure has been less studied, both in animal models and humans. The majority of our information comes from descriptive studies of children irradiated for cancer with adjacent normal tissue incidentally receiving dose. The postnatal period and childhood span years where organs and functional subunits continue to proliferate and develop. This period is divided into three growth phases: neogenesis, genesis, and pubogenesis. This period covers the time from birth to the beginning of adulthood which, for simplicity, is arbitrarily set at 18 years of age in this chapter.

Neogenesis refers to the time between birth and approximately 5 years of age, when most normal tissues are newly formed and their development consists of rapid growth of their functional subunits. Brain tissue is rapidly developing during this phase and is hence more susceptible to radiation injury. Musculoskeletal growth, likewise, is more vulnerable when bone growth is most rapid, during neogenesis and pubogenesis; however, mitotic potential is greater for neogenesis rather than pubogenesis. Therefore, it is not surprising that the neonatal bone would be more susceptible to growth retardation than adolescent bone given the same dose of radiation.

Genesis refers to the time between 5 years of age and just prior to the onset of puberty. Growth is more stable during this period, and the organs have full complement of functional subunits. Irradiation at this time would in general be less detrimental to different organ systems compared to neogenesis as mitotic potential decreases.

Pubogenesis refers to the time from the onset of puberty to the beginning of adulthood. It is the phase when sexual organs grow as well as the second growth spurt in the musculoskeletal system. As will be discussed later, genitalia and breast tissues undergo rapid change. Certain organs such as the brain have less growth during pubogenesis, and irradiation at this time has less potential detrimental effects on neurocognitive function.

2.3 Adulthood

Adulthood can be defined as a time of normal tissue regeneration to maintain homeostasis rather than true growth in size and content of an organ system. Three phases have been described: (1) maturation, (2) renewal, and (3) senescence. Radiotherapy during these adult phases will lead to reactions that are primarily both inflammatory and fibrogenic.

Maturation occurs from approximately 18–40 years of age. It is a time when the normal tissues are fully regenerative and functional units are replaced. Repair recovery is usually rapid. This phase can also be defined as a balance of regenesis. Losses of molecular fidelity that occur during this phase are maintained by a repair and turnover system that is capable of achieving a homeostatic state until reproductive maturation is totally achieved (Hayflick 2007). This assures that the species would be able to survive.

The renewal phase refers to the period from 40–60 years of age in which some cellular senescence starts occurring and normal tissue regeneration loses its capacity to restore cells. As a result, some parenchymal atrophy occurs as senescence sets in. Cellular senescence is the phenomenon where normal diploid differentiated cells lose the ability to divide, generally after about 50 cell divisions in vitro (Hayflick 1965). In response to deoxyribonucleic acid (DNA) damage, cells either age or self-destruct through apoptosis if the damage cannot be repaired. It is believed that the death of a fraction of the cells may benefit the tissue and ultimately the organism as a whole. The renewal phase is also the time after the female has achieved reproductive maturation. The imbalance that occurs in youth where repair and maintenance of molecules exceeds any loss of fidelity slowly shifts after reproductive maturation to a state where the loss of molecular fidelity begins to exceed repair capacity (Hayflick 2007).

The senescence phase refers to the period from 60–80 years of age and beyond, during which time cellular senescence exceeds the normal tissue capacity to regenerate. Thus, normal tissue atrophy or compensatory hypertrophy or hyperplasia occurs in order to compensate for loss of functional subunits. Table 1 lists some of the bodily changes which occur during the senescence phase.

3 Growth Patterns of Normal Tissues: Influence on Manifestations of Normal Tissue Effects

The growth period for the human body is unusually long among mammalian species, extending for more than a quarter of the normal life span. This long growth period is associated with a delay in most aspects of bodily development, especially skeletal and endocrine maturation. Total body mass continues to increase after maturity, but the rate of increase is slowed considerably after about age 18 years in males and about age 16 years in females.

Table 1 Bodily changes during the senescence phase

Cessation of organ growth
Wrinkling of skin
Loss of teeth
Graying of hair
Atrophy of gonads
Weakening of muscles
Bent posture
Slowed reaction time
Presbyopia
Reduction in rapid eye movement (REM) sleep
Diminution of sense of smell
Loss of fine coordination
Decline of memory and mental efficiency
Loss of hearing, particularly for higher frequencies
Decline in ability to taste, particularly salt and bitter
Diminution of vibratory sense in toes and feet

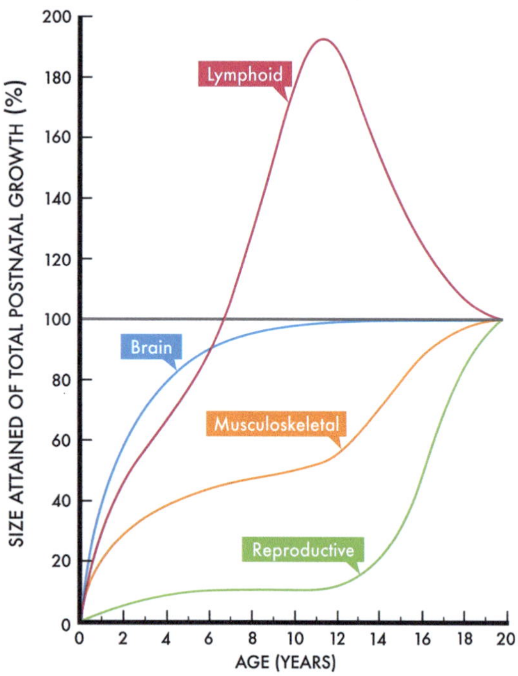

Fig. 1 Four classic growth curves according to age and organ size. Modified with permission from Tanner (1962)

The growth of specific tissues from birth to adulthood has been categorized by four classic patterns: (1) lymphoid, with accelerated growth followed by involution at the time of puberty; (2) brain, with rapid postnatal growth that slows and essentially completes by early adolescence; (3) gonadal, with little change during early life but rapid development just before and coincident with puberty; and (4) a more general pattern characterized by two major periods of rapid growth during the postnatal period and puberty. Figure 1 shows the growth relationships according to time and type of organ in the neonatal period and childhood (Tanner 1962), while Table 2 provides specific data for a broader number of organs and systems.

In general, one can expect the timing of radiation therapy along the curve to influence the type and severity of possible late effects, with more pronounced and severe complications occurring if radiation is administered during the periods of increased mitotic activity. These growth curves provide a context in which to explore and discuss the incidence and differential responses of children with respect to the normal tissue effects.

3.1 Lymphoid Growth Pattern

This type of growth pattern is characterized by gradual evolution and involution to the time of puberty. An example of an organ that follows this pattern is the thymus. It reaches its greatest relative weight at birth, but its absolute weight continues to increase until the onset of puberty. In fact in the renewal phase of adulthood, it is estimated that the thymus gland is only about 5–10 % of its original size. No significant late effects from RT occur in the lymphoid system. In particular, there are no age-specific effects, perhaps because the inherent radiation sensitivity of lymphoid tissues outweighs any differential that could be observed due to age.

3.2 Brain Growth Pattern

This type of growth pattern is characterized by rapid postnatal growth which slows down and is almost complete in adolescence. Naturally, the head and neck also follow this pattern of growth.

The brain is most sensitive to ionizing radiation in the early fetal period, but postnatally during the first few years of life. Brain growth during the first 3 years of life is not secondary to increase in number of neurons but due to axonal growth, dendritic arborization, and synaptogenesis. Myelinization, though well developed at about the second year of life, is not complete until the second to third decade of life (Dobbing and Sands 1963). By 6 years of age, the child's brain has reached adult size. Several studies have shown greater cognitive impairment in younger children compared to older children receiving cranial irradiation (Ris et al. 2001; Conklin et al. 2008). It is for this reason that for many years prior to the era of conformal radiotherapy, in an effort to avoid the deleterious effects of radiotherapy, chemotherapy after surgery was the treatment for children <3 years of age with medulloblastoma, ependymoma,

Table 2 Anatomy and physiology: relative rate of development

	Age 0–5 years	Age 5–10 years	Age 10–15 years	Age 15–Adult
Brain	4	1	1	1
Thyroid	2	3	3	4
GI	4	3	3	2
Gonadal	1	1	4	4
Lung	3	2	3	4
Urinary system	4	3	3	2
Skin	3	2	4	4
Lymphoid tissues	4	4	hypoplasia	hypoplasia
Liver	4	2	3	2
Musculoskeletal	3	2	4	2
Head and neck	4	2	2	1
Circulatory	3	2	4	2

1 static, *2* mild, *3* moderate, *4* significant

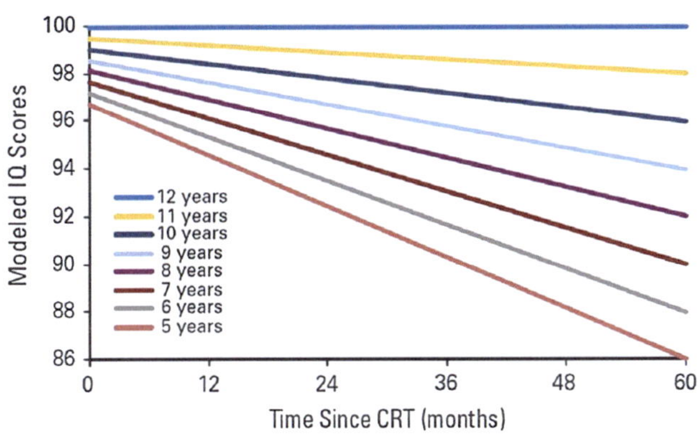

Fig. 2 Intelligence quotient (IQ) scores after conformal radiotherapy in children with low grade glioma. Reprinted with permission from Merchant et al. (2009)

and high-grade gliomas (Duffner et al. 1993). A report from St. Jude Children's Research Hospital showed cognitive decline after conformal radiotherapy for children under 12 years of age with low-grade glioma (Fig. 2). In fact, age at time of irradiation was more important than radiation dose in predicting cognitive decline. Children <5 years old show the most cognitive decline (Merchant et al. 2009). Consistent with this, most children who are affected with radiation-induced Moyamoya syndrome were irradiated when they were <5 years of age, a time when brain growth is rapid (Desai et al. 2006).

One study attributed a greater degree of deficient development with loss of white matter, and this was presumptively correlated with the impaired cognitive outcome of younger children (Mulhern et al. 2001). This description of white matter changes is consistent with the classic finding after radiation insult of the normal brain of a focal or diffuse area of white matter necrosis (Martins et al. 1977). It is also consistent with the premise that radiotherapy would have more effect during the time when there is greater growth of the brain. Table 3 shows the growth and development of the brain according to time of irradiation.

In adulthood, late effects of RT to the brain involve neurocognitive dysfunction which is discussed in greater detail elsewhere in this textbook.

3.3 Gonadal Growth Pattern

This type of growth pattern is characterized by little change during early life but rapid development just before and coincident with puberty. Examples of organs with this growth pattern are the testicle, ovary, and breast.

This unique growth pattern explains why, unlike in other sites where children are more vulnerable to the late effects of radiotherapy compared with their adult counterparts, the ovary is different with respect to sterility. The ovary contains a fixed pool of primordial oocytes, maximal at 5 months of gestational age, declining with increasing age in an exponential fashion, culminating at menopause (Wallace and Kelsey 2010) (Fig. 3). In contrast to other organs that are able to maintain homeostasis, the ovary does not replenish oocytes, similar to other organs in cellular senescence during the past years.

A classic study showed that the effective sterilizing dose to the ovary after fractionated radiotherapy decreased at increasing age of irradiation: 20.3 Gy at birth, 18.4 Gy at 10 years, 16.5 Gy at 20 years, and 14.3 Gy at 30 years of age (Wallace et al. 2005). The study authors estimated the sterilizing dose of radiotherapy at any given age by integrating known data on the radiosensitivity of human oocytes with their model for natural oocyte decline (Fig. 4).

This finding is also supported by the Childhood Cancer Survivor Study, which showed that cyclophosphamide

Table 3 Growth and development of brain with respect to time of irradiation

Phase	Time	Manifestation after radiation therapy
Preimplantation	First 2 weeks post-conception	Death of pre-implanted embryo
Prenatal organogenesis and fetal period	2 weeks to parturition	Microcephaly, mental retardation (greatest risk at 8–15 weeks post-conception)
Neogenesis	Birth to 6 years	Mental retardation, severe cognitive deficits especially in children <3 years of age when myelin formation is still not nearly complete. Hypoplasia of portion of skull and soft tissues which receive radiation therapy
Genesis	6 years to puberty	Mild to moderate cognitive deficits. Mild or no hypoplasia of skull as brain reaches its adult size at 6 years of age
Pubogenesis	Puberty to 18 years	Mild cognitive deficits. No hypoplasia of skull
Maturation	18–40 years	Mild cognitive deficits. No hypoplasia of skull
Renewal and senescence phase	40 years +	Brain atrophy, cognitive deficits seen but a combination of senescence and radiotherapy effect

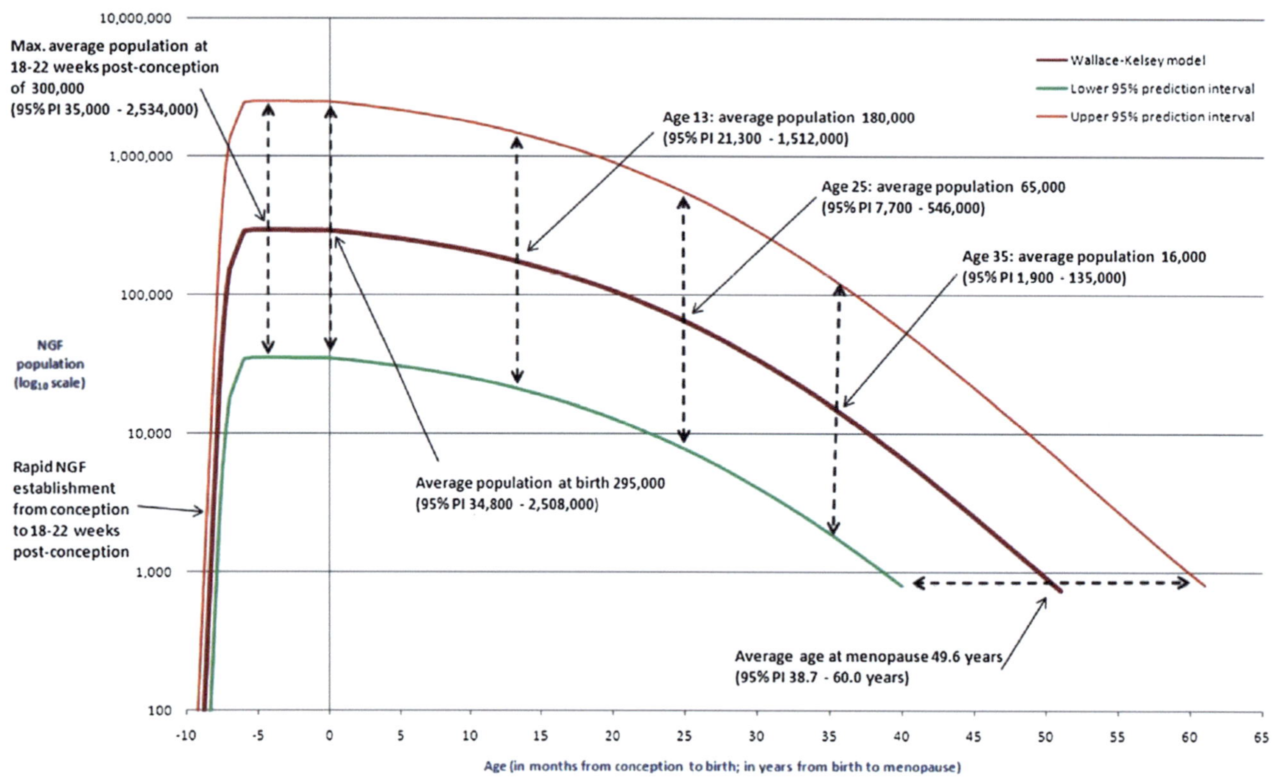

Fig. 3 The average non-growing follicles population at ages 20 weeks after conception, birth, 13, 25, and 35 years is given, along with predicted average age of menopause at 49.6 years, together with the respective 95 % PI. Max, maximum. Reprinted from Wallace and Kelsey (2010)

exposure was a risk factor for sterility in older (13–20 years), but not younger (<13 years) children (Chemaitilly et al. 2006). Finally, data exist showing that ovarian dysfunction may be less in children receiving total body irradiation at an age before menarche, compared with those who were older and received radiotherapy after menarche (Ogilvy-Stuart et al. 1992), although this difference is temporary as longer follow-up of patients reveals the same incidence of permanent ovarian dysfunction.

Similarly, children and adults have different manifestations of late radiation injury in the breast, with breast hypoplasia being the most common type of late toxicity in children. In 129 children, <4 years of age receiving a mean dose of 2.3 Gy for hemangioma, breast hypoplasia was observed in 53 % (Furst et al. 1989). Others have also observed breast hypoplasia after relatively low doses of radiation, such as for pulmonary metastases from Wilms' tumor where children receive bilateral lung irradiation to

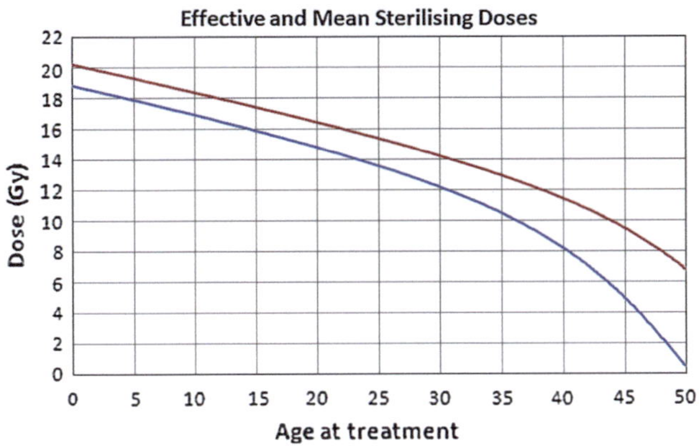

Fig. 4 Effective (*red line*) and mean (*blue line*) estimates of the dose required to sterilize a patient at a known age of treatment. Gy, gray. Reprinted with permission from Wallace et al. (2005)

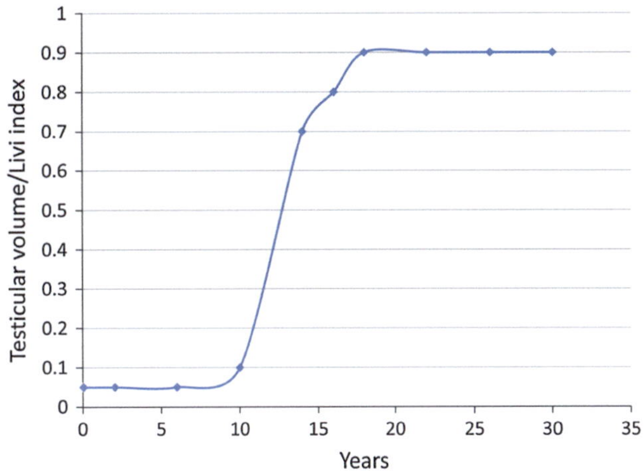

Fig. 5 Testicular volume/Livi index curve as the function of age in a non-gypsy sample. Modified from Beres (1989)

doses of 10–12 Gy (Macklis et al. 1991). Although the dose was quite low, the breast in the young has not fully developed, with hyperplasia of the breast not occurring till puberty. The development of secondary breast malignancies is discussed in great detail elsewhere in this text.

With regard to the testes, it is important to note that unlike in the ovary, where fertility and hormone production are closely related because of their dependence on the ova and primary follicle, these functions differ in the testes because of the differing sensitivity of the spermatogonia and Leydig cells to cytotoxic therapy. Because the spermatogonia are exquisitely sensitive to radiation, even small dosages can produce measurable damage. Depression of sperm counts is discernible at dosages as low as 15 cGy. This decrease in sperm counts may evolve 3–6 weeks after irradiation, and, depending on the dosage, recovery may take 1–3 years. The germinal epithelium is damaged by much lower dosages (less than 1 Gy) of RT than Leydig cells (20–30 Gy) (Sklar et al. 1990). Complete sterilization may occur with fractionated irradiation to a dosage of 1–2 Gy. Spermatocytes generally fail to complete maturation division at dosages of 2–3 Gy and are visibly damaged after 4–6 Gy with resulting azoospermia. Higher dosages are necessary to damage spermatids than will damage the more sensitive spermatocytes. At the highest dosages, permanent sterility is common. At lower dosages, this reduced sperm count is seen 60–80 days after exposure, which is the time at which maturation would otherwise be complete (Shalet et al. 1976).

The growth of the testicle reflects its functional evolution. While at the ages of 0–9 the volume does not significantly change, there is a rapid (about tenfold) increase between 10 and 15 years. The maximum size is attained at 17–22 years depending on race (Beres 1989) (Fig. 5).

3.4 General Growth Pattern

This type of growth pattern is characterized by peak growth rates in the early postnatal period and during puberty. It is perhaps best exemplified by the musculoskeletal system; however, the liver and gastrointestinal tract, kidneys, and urinary system, and skin also follow this pattern.

Bone growth is not a uniform process and does not grow at a gradual rate. There is accelerated growth from birth to about 5 years old, steady slow growth from 5 to 10, and accelerated growth during the pubertal years, which of course generally occurs a few years earlier for females compared to males. Radiation damage to bone is expressed in the epiphysis by arrested chondrogenesis, in the metaphysis by deficient absorptive processes in the calcified bone and cartilage, and in the diaphysis by an alteration in periosteal activity causing abnormal bone modeling (Probert and Parkers 1975). Doses >20 Gy are usually necessary to arrest endochondral bone formation. In a classic study of spinal growth after radiotherapy, the greatest retardation of growth was seen during the periods of most active growth in children < 6 years of age and those undergoing puberty (Probert and Parker 1975). In another study of slipped epiphysis secondary to radiation therapy, doses of >2500 cGy and young age at time of irradiation were the main risk factors for this complication (Silverman et al. 1981), which occurred in 50 % of children <4 years and 5 % of children 5–15 years of age. In contrast to children and adolescents, adult bone is much more tolerant to radiation damage; doses of 6000 cGy or more are needed to cause osteoradionecrosis.

Muscular growth parallels bone growth, and is bimodal, again occurring during the early postnatal and pubertal periods. Muscular hypoplasia and atrophy have been reported in young children receiving radiotherapy to the spine and extremities.

Another example of the general growth pattern is the urinary system, although its radiosensitivity varies widely, with the ureter being the most resistant, the bladder having intermediate sensitivity, and the kidney the most sensitive. The tolerance of dose for the adult kidney appears to be approximately 23 Gy in 5 weeks to the parenchyma of both kidneys, with 28 Gy to both kidneys in 5 weeks carrying a high risk of severe radiation nephritis (Luxton and Kunkler 1964). It is not clear whether renal injury is more severe in children than adults or during varying points of the growth curve, with the possible perhaps exception of irradiation during neogenesis (Cassady 1995; Peschel et al. 1981). This comparison is greatly confounded by the fact that much of the data in regards to the effect of radiation therapy on the pediatric kidney has been collected from survivors of pediatric Wilms tumor, who undergo resection and/or irradiated for their primary renal malignancy (and also sometimes present with bilateral disease), as opposed to adults whose kidneys are often only tangentially or incidentally irradiated during the treatment of a range of abdominal/pelvic malignancies.

4 Growth Patterns in Adults

Hayflick's studies with human fibroblasts in cell culture have demonstrated that the capacity to divide becomes less as a person gets older; an infant's cells divide about 50 times, those of a 20-year old about 30 times and those of an 80-year old about 20 times (Hayflick 1974). This decline in the ability to repair damage, together with cell attrition and the effects of comorbid illness are particularly important in the manifestation of late effects in the elderly.

4.1 Maintenance of Homeostasis

Achieving homeostasis is a delicate balance between cell proliferation and attrition. When stem cells move beyond the pleuripotent stage, under the influence of intrinsic and extrinsic factors they follow one of two paths: (1) self renewal or multipotency or (2) differentiation, giving rise to more specialized cells. In the final stages of life, differentiated or nondividing cells play a greater role in injury response as cells within the proliferative compartment move toward a quiescent or senescent state.

Hypertrophy and hyperplasia can occur in response to injury. Hypertrophy, which refers to the increase in the size of cells and ultimately the tissue and organ in response to function demand or hormonal stimulation, becomes relatively more important in the maintenance of normal tissues of adults than hyperplasia, which refers to the increase in the number of cells due to division when stressed or stimulated to increase activity. The skin and intestinal epithelium, hepatocytes, fibroblasts, and bone marrow cells can undergo hyperplasia whereas nerve cells and cardiac and skeletal muscle have relatively no capacity for hyperplastic growth.

Atrophy of an organ is a result of impaired repair process. Atrophy refers to the shrinkage of a cell by loss of cell substance, or shrinkage of tissue or an organ from cell atrophy or death. Several factors can contribute to atrophic organs or tissues such as decreased workload, loss of innervation, diminished blood supply, inadequate nutrition, or loss of endocrine stimulation (Robbins et al. 1984).

4.2 Confounding Factors in Adults

Many changes occur in various organ systems during the aging process. For example, in the musculoskeletal system, collagen undergoes stiffening and loss of elasticity, resulting in decreased integrity and function. Both men and women lose bone mass, starting at around the renewal phase of adulthood. Physical inactivity and malnutrition (especially for calcium and Vitamin D) of the elderly can also result in bone loss. In postmenopausal women, decrease in estrogen production can lead to osteoporosis. By the time an adult has reached the peak of the senescence phase, it is not unusual to see a decrease in height of 1–3 inches, with women having more loss.

For many organs in the body, specific disease states associated with aging are of more significance than generalized deterioration. Generalized reduction in blood flow due to atherosclerosis, accelerated by hypertension and diabetes, has an adverse effect on most organ systems. For example, after radiation treatment to the extremity in a child bone and muscle growth are the primary late toxicities whereas in an adult, soft tissue or bone necrosis, atrophy of the extremity and fracture may be the concern because of change of cellular composition and diminished blood flow to the irradiated area. A recent study from Florence showed that seven of 214 patients treated for extremity soft tissue sarcoma and postoperative radiotherapy developed a fracture. The fractures were all in older patients >55 years of age. Interestingly these seven fractures were seen only in postmenopausal women, indicative of the interaction between age and coexisting hormonal changes on bone density and late radiotherapy complications (Livi et al. 2006).

Other organs can also be more susceptible in older adults because of comorbidities and the aging process where the inability to repair normal tissues and maintain homeostasis is problematic. In the kidney, chronic renal failure is more common in older patients (>30 years) after total body irradiation (Delgado et al. 2006). In the radiotherapeutic management of brain tumors, cognitive function is severely affected in young children while in the older adult, cognitive loss can occur but not necessarily from the treatment but because of other disease states affecting the brain as well as part of normal aging process when a small amount of neurons are lost. Both age and educational level, for example, are included in the determination of cognitive impairment after whole brain radiotherapy for brain metastases using the Folstein Mini-Mental status examination (Corn et al. 2008).

5 Summary

The developing human organism is complex with multiple organ systems developing at different times and rates. Late effects of radiotherapy are influenced not only by total dose, volume, and fractionation but also the stage of normal tissue development, comorbid disease, and various host factors, both intrinsic and extrinsic. While late effects in adults are primarily inflammatory and fibrogenic, in children a major and unique contributor to late toxicity is impairment of maturation of the organ. Confounding factors such as comorbid disease, physiologic changes, and environmental factors play a big part in the determination of late toxicity in the adult patient. Knowledge of the growth and development of various organ systems will help the radiation oncologist to understand potential degree of late effects both in children and adults.

References

Beres J (1989) Testicular volume variations from 0 to 28 years of age. Int Urol Nephrol 21:159–167

Brent RL, Ghorson RO (1972) Radiation exposure in pregnancy. Curr Probl Radiol 2:1–48

Cassady JR (1995) Clinical radiation nephropathy. Int J Radiat Oncol Biol Phys 31:1249–1256

Chemaitilly W, Mertens AC, Mitby P (2006) Acute ovarian failure in the Childhood Cancer Survivor Study. J Clin Endo Metab 91:1723–1728

Conklin HM, Li C, Xiong X, Ogg RJ, Merchant TE (2008) Predicting change in academic abilities after conformal radiation therapy for localized ependymoma. J Clin Oncol 26:3965–3970

Corn BW, Moughan J, Knisely JPS, Fox SW, Chakravarti A, Yung WKA, Curran WJ, Robins HI, Brachman DG, Henderson RH, Mehta MP, Movsas B (2008) Prospective evaluation of quality of life and neurocognitive effects in patients with multiple brain metastases receiving whole-brain radiotherapy with or without thalidomide on Radiation Therapy Oncology Group (RTOG) Trial 0118. Int J Radiat Oncol Biol Phys 71:71–78

Delgado J, Cooper N, Thomson K, Duarte R, Jarmulowicz M, Cassoni A, Kottaridis P, Peggs K, Mackinnon S (2006) The importance of age, fludarabine and total body irradiation in the incidence and severity of chronic renal failure after allogeneic hematopoietic cell transplantation. Biol Blood Marrow Transplant 12:75–83

Desai SS, Paulino AC, Mai WY, Teh BS (2006) Radiation-induced Moyamoya syndrome. Int J Radiat Oncol Biol Phys 65:1222–1227

Dobbing J, Sands J (1963) The quantitative growth and development of the human brain. Arch Dis Child 48:757–767

Duffner PK, Horowitz ME, Krischer JP, Friedman HS, Burger PC, Cohen ME, Sanford RA, Mulhern RK, James HE, Freeman CR, Seidel FG, Kun LE (1993) Postoperative chemotherapy and delayed radiation in children less than three years of age with malignant brain tumors. N Engl J Med 328:1725–1731

Furst CJ, Lundell M, Ahlback SO, Holm LE (1989) Breast hypoplasia following irradiation of the female breast in infancy and early childhood. Acta Oncol 28:519–523

Hayflick L (1965) The limited in vitro lifetime of human diploid cell strains. Exp Cell Res 37:614–636

Hayflick L (1974) The longevity of human cultured cells. J Am Geriatr Soc 22:1–12

Hayflick L (2007) Biological aging is no longer an unsolved problem. Ann N Y Acad Sci 1100:1–13

Livi L, Santoni R, Paiar F, Bastiani P, Beltrami G, Caldora P, Capanna R, De Biase P, Detti B, Fondelli S, Meldolesi E, Pertici M, Polli C, Simontacchi G, Biti G (2006) Late treatment-related complications in 214 patients with extremity soft-tissue sarcoma treated by surgery and postoperative radiation therapy. Am J Surg 191:230–234

Luxton RW, Kunkler PB (1964) Radiation nephritis. Acta Radiol Ther Phys Biol 66:169–178

Macklis RM, Oltikar A, Sallan SE (1991) Wilms' tumor patients with pulmonary metastases. Int J Rad Onc Biol Phys 21:1187–1193

Martins AN, Johnston JS, Henry MJ, Stoffel TJ, Dichiro G (1977) Delayed radiation necrosis of the brain. J Neurosurg 47:336–345

Merchant TE, Conklin HM, Wu S, Lustig RH, Xiong X (2009) Late effects of conformal radiotherapy for pediatric patients with low-grade glioma: prospective evaluation of cognitive, endocrine and hearing deficits. J Clin Oncol 27:3691–3697

Metler FA, Upton AC (1995) Medical effects of ionizing radiation, 2nd edn. WB Saunders Co, Philadelphia

Mulhern RK, Palmer SL, Reddick WE, Glass JO, Kun LE, Taylor J, Langston J, Gajjar A (2001) Risks of young age for selected neurocognitive deficits in medulloblastoma are associated with white matter loss. J Clin Oncol 19:472–479

Ogilvy-Stuart AL, Clark DJ, Wallace WH, Gibson BE, Stevens RF, Shalet SM, Donaldson MD (1992) Endocrine deficit after fractionated total body irradiation. Arch Dis Child 67:1107–1110

Otake M, Schull WJ, Yoshimura H (1991) Brain damage among the prenatally exposed. J Radiat Res (Suppl) 32:249–264

Peschel RE, Chen M, Seashore J (1981) The treatment of massive hepatomegaly in stage IV-S neuroblastoma. Int J Radiat Oncol Biol Phys 7:549–553

Probert JC, Parker BP (1975) The effects of radiation therapy on bone growth. Radiology 114:155–162

Ris MD, Packer R, Goldwein J, Jones-Wallace D, Boyett JM (2001) Intellectual outcome after reduced-dose radiation therapy plus adjuvant chemotherapy for medulloblastoma: a Children's Cancer Group study. J Clin Oncol 19:3470–3476

Robbins SL, Cotran RS, Kumar V (1984) Pathologic basis of disease, 3rd edn. WB Saunders, Philadelphia

Rugh R (1962) The impact of ionizing radiation on the embryo and fetus. Am J Roentgenol 87:559–566

Russell LB, Russell WL (1954) An analysis of the changing radiation response of the developing mouse embryo. J Cell Physiol (Suppl 1) 43:103–149

Shalet SM, Beardwell CG, Pearson D, Jones PH (1976) The effects of varying doses of cerebral irradiation on growth hormone production in childhood. Clin Endocrinol (Oxf) 5:287–290

Silverman CL, Thomas PRM, McAlister WH, Walker S, Whiteside LA (1981) Slipped capital femoral epiphysis in irradiated children: dose volume and age relationships. Int J Radiat Oncol Biol Phys 7:1357–1363

Sklar CA, Robison LL, Nesbit ME, Sather HN, Meadows AT, Ortega JA, Kim TH, Hammond GD (1990) Effects of radiation on testicular function in long-term survivors of childhood acute lymphoblastic leukemia: a report from the Children's Cancer Study Group. J Clin Oncol 8:1981–1987

Streffer C, Molls M (1987) Cultures of preimplantation mouse embryos: a model for radiobiological studies. Adv Radiat Biol 13:169–213

Tanner JM (1962) Growth at adolescence. Blackwell Scientific Publications, Oxford

Valentin J (2002) Basic anatomical and physiological data for use in radiological protection: reference values. ICRP Publication 89. Ann ICRP 32:5–265

Wallace WH, Kelsey TM (2010) Human ovarian reserve from conception to menopause. PLoS ONE 5:e8772

Wallace WH, Thomson AB, Saran F, Kelsey TW (2005) Predicting age of ovarian failure after radiation to a field that includes the ovaries. Int J Radiat Oncol Biol Phys 62:738–744

BioGenetic and Host Implications

Barry S. Rosenstein

Contents

Abstract

It has been of substantial interest to identify the inherent factors that individuals may possess which could render them more likely to suffer adverse effects resulting from a standard radiation therapy treatment for cancer. Case reports have been published suggesting that patients with certain diseases, including collagen vascular diseases, diabetes, and inflammatory bowel disease, are at greater risk for developing normal tissue toxicities following radiation therapy. However, retrospective studies have generally not found substantial increases in the susceptibility of these patients for the development of normal tissue toxicities following radiotherapy. The focus of many research studies has been to develop cell-based assays to identify radiosensitive patients, but the only approach that appears promising in this regard is the lymphocyte apoptosis assay. On the genomic level, expression studies have suggested that altered expression of certain genes may correlate with adverse radiation effects. A major focus of the effort to identify markers for potential radiosensitivity, is the identification of genetic alterations, primarily single nucleotide polymorphisms (SNPs) that are associated with the development of radiation-induced toxicities. A series of candidate gene SNP studies has been performed whose results are supportive of the role for genetic factors conferring an increased risk for the development of radiation injuries. The current emphasis in this area of research is to perform genome wide association studies involving simultaneous screening of a broad range of genes for each patient using high density microarrays to identify SNPs that have the strongest associations with adverse effects arising from radiotherapy. Identification of such genetic markers may be of clinical significance as it could lead to the development of a predictive assay that will permit identification of potential radiotherapy patients that are at greatest risk for the development of radiation injuries. In addition, the discovery of genes

B. S. Rosenstein (✉)
Radiation Oncology, Dermatology and Community and Preventive Medicine, Mount Sinai School of Medicine, NYU School of Medicine, 1 Gustave L. Levy Place, New York, NY 10029, USA
e-mail: barry.rosenstein@mssm.edu

P. Rubin et al. (eds.), *ALERT – Adverse Late Effects of Cancer Treatment*, Medical Radiology. Radiation Oncology, DOI: 10.1007/978-3-540-72314-1_12,
© Springer-Verlag Berlin Heidelberg 2014

whose products alter the susceptibility of patients for the development of normal tissue toxicities may provide valuable information as to the molecular pathways through which these radiation effects arise.

1 Introduction

A substantial degree of variability among patients in the response to a standard course of radiotherapy has long been observed. When a patient exhibits an unusual reaction to a conventional protocol, generally the first approach is to examine whether any tissues received an excessively high dose due to overlapping fields or a dosimetric error was made in treatment planning. However, more often than not, there is not a clear explanation for an excessive normal tissue response. Therefore, it has generally been assumed when treating patients to a dose which represents tolerance for a normal tissue, that by chance, some patients will develop a radiation injury. This has often been ascribed to the random nature of cell killing and the stochastic nature of the pathways leading to the expression of radiation injury. However, a number of studies have suggested that often the explanation for the development of an adverse response is not simply random, but may be more a reflection of some genetic attribute of the patient that confers a susceptibility for the development of an adverse response (Safwat et al. 2002). Thus, if it were possible to identify the "host" factors that render certain patients more likely to develop complications from a radiation treatment, it could then be feasible to adjust the treatment protocols for these patients. Thus, depending upon the cancer being treated, it may be prudent to use a lower total dose or attempt a more conformal treatment. Alternatively, for those patients who could be reasonably treated with surgery alone, it may be best to avoid the use of radiotherapy. The purpose of this chapter is to review the evidence that certain inherent genetic patient factors may play a role in the response of normal tissues and organs to radiotherapy.

2 Diseases Associated with Adverse Responses to Radiotherapy

Patients with certain underlying conditions or diseases may be more susceptible for the development of adverse responses to a standard course of radiotherapy. The main groups of patients that have been investigated are radiotherapy patients who had been diagnosed with either collagen vascular diseases, diabetes/hypertension, or inflammatory bowel disease.

2.1 Collagen Vascular Disease

Collagen vascular disease (CVD) represents a spectrum of disorders characterized by abnormalities in immunoregulatory processes resulting in the production of autoantibodies and anomalies in cell-medicated immunity (Hamilton 2005). The autoantibodies are typically formed against components of the extracellular matrix, including collagen and elastin. Patients with CVDs may exhibit skin rash, fibrosis, arthritis, and in more severe cases, organ damage. A series of case reports, often of pronounced and even dramatic radiation reactions and toxicity, initially suggested that patients diagnosed with CVDs were at an increased risk for radiation injuries resulting from radiotherapy (Nilsen et al. 1967; Glasenapp 1968; Urtasun 1971; Ransom and Cameron 1987; Olivotto et al. 1989; Robertson et al. 1991; Varga et al. 1991; Rathmell and Taylor 1992; Abu-Shakra and Lee 1993; Hareyama et al. 1995; Bliss et al. 1996; Mayr and Riggs 1997; Rakfal and Deutsch 1998; Khoo et al. 2004; Wo and Taghian 2007). In response to these case reports, radiation oncologists have been cautious in treating patients with CVDs. In addition, based upon these findings, the American College of Radiology stated in their guidelines concerning breast cancer (Winchester and Cox 1998) that "a history of collagen vascular disease is a relative contraindication to breast conservation treatment because published reports indicate that such patients tolerate irradiation poorly".

To examine the question as to whether patients with CVD are at increased risk for radiation injuries following radiotherapy, several retrospective studies were performed (Ross et al. 1993; Morris and Powell 1997; Chen and Obedian 2001; Phan et al. 2003; Gold et al. 2007, 2008; Pinn et al. 2008). The patients studied primarily included those affected with rheumatoid arthritis (RA), systemic lupus erythematosus (SLE), dermatomyositis, polymyositis, and systemic sclerosis (scleroderma). In addition, some of these patients exhibited overlapping syndromes, referred to as mixed connective tissue disorders. In a study of 20 patients specifically diagnosed with scleroderma, Gold et al. (2007) reported that only 15 % of the subjects developed late radiation toxicities, which is similar to the rates of historical controls. In addition, only a small percentage of patients displayed grade 3 or worse acute toxicities, comparable to the rates in historic control populations. However, in a subsequent publication, Gold et al. (2008) reported in a study of 41 patients with either scleroderma or SLE, that patients who were diagnosed with high severity CVD were at greater risk to develop radiation-induced toxicities resulting from radiotherapy compared with patients with low-severity CVD. In addition, the manifestations of radiation injury appeared earlier in the high-severity CVD group. In a study of 21 patients with SLE, Pinn et al. (2008) reported that patients with SLE renal involvement were at a greater risk for the development of chronic radiation toxicity resulting from radiotherapy. These authors concluded that both acute and chronic toxicities resulting from radiotherapy were moderate among patients with SLE and therefore the use of RT should not be avoided in these patients, although patients with more advanced SLE may be at an increased risk for the development of adverse effects resulting from RT.

In order to reach a more definitive conclusion as to whether CVDs predispose patients to complications from RT, the results of three matched case–control studies (Ross et al. 1993; Chen and Obedian 2001; Phan et al. 2003) and one large retrospective study (Morris and Powell 1997) have been published. Ross et al. (1993) reported the results for 61 patients with CVDs (39 RA, 13 SLE, 4 scleroderma, 4 dermatomyositis, and 1 polymyositis) treated with radiotherapy. No significant difference was found between the group of patients with CVDs and matched controls in terms of either acute or late effects of radiation. Phan (2003) performed a case–control study of 38 patients with CVDs (21 SLE, two scleroderma, four Raynaud's phenomena, three fibromyalgia, three polymyalgia, three Sjogren's syndrome, two polymyositis-dermatomyositis) and reported no significant differences in the incidence of either early or late complications between the case and control groups, although the patients with scleroderma exhibited an increase in both acute and late effects. Chen et al. (2001) performed a case control study of patients diagnosed with CVDs who received breast conserving therapy. Similar to previous studies, no significant differences were found in the incidence of acute effects between the cases and controls. However, this study found an increased risk of late radiation toxicity in the CVD patients compared with controls. This was primarily due to the development of late morbidity in 75 % of the scleroderma patients, although this group consisted of only four subjects. A retrospective report from Morris and Powell (1997) of 209 patients diagnosed with CVDs (136 RA, 28 SLE, 17 polymyositis-dermatomyositis, 16 scleroderma, 8 ankylosing spondylitis, 4 mixed tissue disorders) reported a similar rate of acute reactions to the Ross et al. study (1993). However, this study found that severe late radiation toxicity was significantly associated with non-RA CVDs. Thus, these authors concluded that aside from RA, CVD may be associated with an enhanced risk of late effects following standard radiotherapy. Holscher et al. (2006) performed a review of the literature and calculated a pooled relative risk of 2.0 (95 % confidence interval, 0.99–4.1) for the development of late effects in patients diagnosed with CVDs following radiotherapy compared with RT patients without a history of CVD.

Thus, although some studies have suggested an increased risk of late effects in certain patients, particularly those people diagnosed with scleroderma, none of the retrospective series has confirmed the substantial increase in the susceptibility of patients with CVDs to radiation-induced normal tissue toxicities that were reported in earlier case reports.

2.2 Diabetes and Hypertension

Diabetes and hypertension often have similar vascular pathologies to patients with CVDs, although without an autoimmune etiology. Herold et al. (1999); Chon and Loeffler (2002) reported upon radiation toxicities in a population of 944 patients treated with EBRT for prostate cancer, 121 of whom had diabetes. They found that the rates of gastrointestinal and genitourinary morbidity were somewhat higher in the diabetic patients compared with men not exhibiting evidence of diabetes. Maruyama et al. (1974) reviewed the records of 271 patients treated with RT for cervical cancer and concluded that patients with diabetes were more likely to develop small bowel obstructions following RT. VanNagell et al. (1974) also reported on cervical cancer RT patients with the finding of a correlation between diabetes with the development of radiation-induced bladder and rectal injuries.

2.3 Inflammatory Bowel Disease

Inflammatory bowel diseases (IBD) comprise patients with ulcerative colitis and Crohn's disease. IBD has been considered a relative contraindication for pelvic or abdominal RT since this disease is characterized by an inflammatory reaction in the mucosa and it has been thought that radiation would exacerbate this condition. Willet et al. (2000) reported on 28 patients with IBD (10 Crohn's disease and 18 ulcerative colitis). A higher rate of radiation toxicities was observed in IBD patients who underwent abdominal or pelvic RT compared with morbidity rates of non-IBD patients who received similar treatments. Thus, these authors suggested that RT should be used judiciously in these patients. Green et al. (1999) reported on the outcomes for 47 IBD patients (35 ulcerative colitis and 12 Crohn's disease) treated with RT for rectal cancer. The rates of acute and late complications were similar in this group to those reported in randomized trials of RT for rectal cancer. In addition, two studies (Grann and Wallner 1998; Peters et al. 2006) of patients with IBD who received brachytherapy for prostate cancer reported that these patients tolerated this treatment and exhibited similar rates of rectal complications to non-IBD patients.

In summary, a series of case reports have described radiotherapy-related injuries in patients with CVDs, diabetes, hypertension, and IBD, thereby raising concerns about patients diagnosed with these types of diseases as to their suitability for radiotherapy. However, retrospective series, with several exceptions, have generally reported a tolerable incidence of complications among these patients. In addition, publication bias may have prevented some negative studies from being reported. Thus, the avoidance of radiotherapy for patients diagnosed with these diseases based upon case reports may have resulted in overly cautious treatment recommendations. However, it must be recognized that some people, in particular patients with active CVD, IBD, or a combination of uncontrolled hypertension with diabetes, may be at a greater risk for the development of normal tissue injuries resulting from a standard course of radiotherapy and should be treated with particular care.

3 Genetic Factors

It has long been speculated that genetic factors could play an important role influencing the susceptibility of a patient for the development of a radiation injury (Andreassen et al. 2002, 2005; Baumann et al. 2003; Fernet and Hall 2004; Bourguignon et al. 2005; Jones et al. 2005). To examine the role of potential genetic influences, the incidence and time to development of radiation-induced telangiectasia in breast cancer patients treated with radiotherapy was examined (Safwat et al. 2002). A large range in the severity and latent times prior to the manifestation of telangiectasia was observed in this population despite a uniform radiotherapy treatment. Consistent with previous results (Tucker et al. 1992, 1996; Turesson and Joiner 1996), it was estimated that 80–90 % of the variability among patients could be attributed to deterministic effects, associated possibly with individual genetic differences. By comparison, it was calculated that only about 10–20 % of the variation resulted from stochastic events associated with the random variations in dosimetry and dose delivery.

3.1 Skin Fibroblast Radiosensitivity

As a manifestation of an inherent genetic susceptibility to radiation toxicity, studies were performed in which the in vitro radiosensitivity of skin fibroblasts was measured. It should be noted that although it could be expected that cell killing by radiation may play a central role in the etiology of early effects, late radiation effects in the skin are more likely a manifestation of a cytokine cascade induced by radiation resulting in an inflammatory response leading to a fibrotic reaction (Bentzen 2006). Thus, a correlation between killing of skin fibroblasts with late effects would be unlikely. Nevertheless, several initial studies reported an association between dermal fibroblast radiation sensitivity with the severity for both early and late effects (Loeffler et al. 1990; Oppitz et al. 2001). However, replication studies generally were not able to validate these initial findings as there was a lack of correlation between fibroblast radiosensitivity with late effects and only a weak association with early skin responses (Begg et al. 1993).

3.2 Lymphocyte Assays

The initial results examining lymphocyte radiosensitivity did not suggest a correlation with adverse radiotherapy effects. In addition, because lymphocytes display differential radiation sensitivity, the changes in the levels of different lymphocyte cell-types resulted in large experimental variation (Stewart et al. 1988; Crompton and Ozsahin 1997). However, in more recent work that takes into account the cell-type specific radiosensitivities, it has been reported that the response of CD4 and CD8 T-lymphocytes to irradiation correlates with radiation-induced morbidity in a breast cancer patient population treated with radiotherapy (Crompton et al. 1999, 2001; Ozsahin et al. 1997; Azria et al. 2004; Ozsahin et al. 2005). In particular, an inverse correlation has been reported between radiation-induced T-lymphocyte apoptosis, especially in CD8 cells, with the development of late effects in patients from whom the lymphocytes were derived.

3.3 Gene Expression Profiling

With the development of gene expression microarrays that provide the ability to measure the expression of a large number of genes following irradiation, it is now possible to examine whether differential expression of certain genes following irradiation correlates with the development of radiation-induced injuries resulting from radiotherapy. Expression was studied in fibroblast cell lines derived from breast cancer patients exhibiting a range of subcutaneous fibrotic reactions following post-mastectomy radiotherapy (Alsner et al. 2007; Rodningen et al. 2008). RNA was isolated 2 h following irradiation of fibroblasts and analyzed using a 15 K cDNA microarray. The results were compared with gene expression in unirradiated fibroblasts. A minimum set of 18 genes was identified that could differentiate patients who were at low risk for fibrosis compared with patients at high risk based upon the differential expression of these genes in the two populations. Using quantitative real time PCR, it was found that the relative magnitude of the increase in irradiated compared with unirradiated fibroblasts provided even greater discrimination between patients who were either sensitive or resistant to the development of subcutaneous fibrosis following radiotherapy. The results of this study indicated that differential gene expression of specific genes could distinguish between patients at low risk from those at high risk for a fibrotic response.

3.4 Identification of Single Nucleotide Polymorphisms

The most direct way to identify the genetic factors associated with susceptibility for the development of radiation-induced adverse effects is to identify the genetic variants that correlate with the manifestation of different forms of radiation-induced injuries resulting from radiotherapy. Putting aside copy number variants, humans are 99.9 % identical in their genetic makeup. Thus, about once every 1,000 nucleotides at least 1 % of the population exhibits a change in the DNA sequence that is the result of an ancestral mutation which has spread throughout the population resulting in substitution of a variant base pair at a specific nucleotide in the human genome for the one observed in the majority of the population (Frazer et al. 2007). These are referred to as single nucleotide polymorphisms or SNPs. Therefore, each individual is either homozygous for the major allele (the more common base pair), homozygous for the minor allele (less common pair base) or heterozygous for the allele (possessing the more common base pair in one copy of the chromosome and the less common base pair in the other chromosome of the pair). Although many of the SNPs in the human genome have little or no functional consequence, it is thought that some number of these genetic variants are associated with a susceptibility to the development of a diversity of biological end-points including physical attributes such height, weight and intelligence, an increased risk for a particular disease, and variation in the response to drugs and radiotherapy. This forms the basis of personalized medicine, which is the use of a person's genotype to select a medical treatment for a certain disease or a preventative measure against the development of a specific disorder that is most appropriate for that particular person.

In order to identify the SNPs associated with adverse radiation effects, a series of case–control studies has been performed over the past 10 years in which SNPs in specific candidate genes have been screened in radiotherapy patients who developed complications from radiotherapy and control subjects who received similar treatments, but did not develop adverse responses. Although associations of certain SNPs with normal tissue toxicities resulting from radiotherapy have been detected, it should be noted that few of these studies have been validated. Another important limitation of these findings is that generally corrections were not made for multiple testing, even though routinely multiple SNPs were screened. Thus, it is likely that some SNPs reported as being significantly associated with a particular form of radiation injury were actually false positives. It should be noted that when reference is made to possession of a SNP in the following discussion, this indicates that the patients were either heterozygous or homozygous for the minor SNP allele.

3.4.1 Prostate Cancer

Hall et al. (1998) first reported an association between the possession of "significant mutations" in *ATM* with proctitis and cystitis in prostate cancer patients treated with radiotherapy. This was followed by two studies by Cesaretti et al. (2005, 2006) in which they discovered an association between missense SNPs (causes substitution of the encoded amino acid) in *ATM* with rectal bleeding and erectile dysfunction and that the impact of the SNPs upon proctitis was radiation dose dependent. In contrast to these positive findings, Meyer et al. (2007) found no association between the codon 1054 SNP in *ATM* with either urinary morbidity or erectile dysfunction. Damaraju et al. (2006) screened for SNPs in multiple genes and identified an association between SNPs in *LIG4*, *ERCC2* and *CP2D6*4* with bladder and rectal toxicity. Peters et al. (2007) detected a correlation between SNPs in *TGFB1* with both erectile dysfunction and rectal bleeding. Burri et al. (2008) reported that patients with a particular SNP in *XRCC1* were more likely to develop erectile dysfunction and that men who harbored either a specific SNP in *SOD2* or a combination of SNPs in *SOD2* and *XRCC3* displayed an increased incidence of rectal bleeding.

3.4.2 Breast Cancer

The first report of a positive association between possession of SNPs and radiation injury in breast cancer patients treated with radiotherapy was from Iannuzzi et al. (2002) followed later by Ho et al. (2007) who reported a correlation between missense SNPs in *ATM* with subcutaneous fibrosis and telangiectasias. In contrast, Bremer (2003) did not detect an association between SNPs in *ATM* with radiation effects. Edvardsen (2007) found a correlation between an *ATM* SNP with a reduced frequency of telangiectasia, indicating a protective effect associated with possession of this SNP. Andreassen (2003, 2005, 2006) reported an association between SNPs in *TGFB1*, *SOD2*, *XRCC3*, *XRCC1* and *ATM* with subcutaneous fibrosis. However, in a validation study in which a separate replication set of subjects was screened, this group was unable to confirm their initial findings (Andreassen et al. 2006). Angele et al. (2003), Moullan et al. (2003), Quarmby et al. (2003) and Giotopulos et al. (2007) found associations between adverse radiation responses with SNPs in either *ATM*, *XRCC1*, *TGFB1*, and *TGFB1/XRCC1*, respectively. In addition,

Edvardsen et al. (2007) reported that possession of a SNP in *GSTP1* was associated with pleural thickening.

3.4.3 Other Sites

De Ruyck et al. (2005, 2006) reported a correlation between SNPs in *XRCC3* and *TGFB1* with an increase risk of late radiation effects following treatment for either cervical or endometrial cancers whereas a SNP in *XRCC1* with associated with a reduced incidence of late effects. Severin et al. (2001) published an association between a SNP in *RAD21* with radiation effects following treatment at any one of multiple sites.

3.4.4 Multiple SNP Screening

In order to expand the number of SNPs being screened, Suga et al. (2007) have reported results performed as part of the Japanese RadGenomics Project in which breast cancer patients treated with radiotherapy were screened for 999 SNPs in a total of 137 candidate genes. It was discovered in this study that haplotypes in six loci were associated with the development of early skin reactions. In a separate study performed by this group (Suga et al. 2008), prostate cancer patients who had undergone carbon ion radiotherapy were screened for 450 SNPs in 118 genes and an association was found between SNPs in *SART1*, *ID3*, *EPDR1*, *PAI1*, and *XRCC6* with urinary morbidity.

3.4.5 Genome Wide Association Studies

In recent years, an effort has been made to expand the list of genes and SNPs that are being screened. The logical extension of this work is to perform genome wide association studies (GWAS). Thus, work has been initiated to conduct GWAS by the GENE-PARE (Ho et al. 2006), GENEPI (Baumann et al. 2003; West et al. 2005) and RadGenomics (Suga et al. 2007) consortia to identify SNPs associated with adverse radiotherapy responses. Each of these groups has developed a large biorepository and databank of radiotherapy patients. This area of research has only recently become feasible due to two major scientific and technical breakthroughs. The first is the HapMap project (Frazer et al. 2007) which has now identified roughly 3 million of the estimated 10 million SNPs that are thought to exist in the human population. In addition, HapMap has demonstrated that SNPs are inherited in "haplotype blocks" which represent groups of SNPs that are in linkage disequilibrium and are thus inherited together since they are rarely separated through recombination. Therefore, it is in fact not necessary to genotype all possible SNPs, but just a portion, since one SNP in a haplotype block can serve essentially as a "tag" SNP. Once this tag SNP has been identified, comprehensive sequencing in the area surrounding the SNP will identify the actual functional SNP whose presence confers susceptibility to the development of the end-point of interest. The other important event that has fueled the tremendous increase in GWAS during recent years has been the development of relatively low cost SNP genotyping arrays. These arrays permit the simultaneous genotyping of roughly one million SNPS in each person. Using this approach, the cost of SNP genotyping has fallen nearly 10,000-fold in the past decade. It is therefore now not necessary to limit screening to only a handful of genes and SNPs. Thus, there has been virtually an explosion of GWAS published over the past few years reporting associations between SNPs with a variety of traits and susceptibility to a range of diseases (Manolio et al. 2008). It must also be recognized that the technology for DNA re-sequencing is developing rapidly with a commensurate drop in price. Hence, the time is likely not very far into the future when it may be possible to determine the complete nucleotide sequence for an individual at a modest cost.

In addition to the identification of most SNPs and the ability to genotype at a relatively low cost, there are several other reasons why the preferred approach for SNP association studies is to perform this research on a genome-wide basis. The first is recognition of the relative ignorance as to genes involved in the pathways leading to normal tissue effects. A candidate gene approach permits examination of only a limited number of genes whose proteins play known roles in the development of radiation injuries. In contrast, GWAS will facilitate the discovery of new genes and proteins involved in etiology of radiation effects and help to elucidate novel pathways for the development of radiation responses. In addition, it has been found in some GWAS that the critical SNPs were not located within coding regions of genes, but in non-coding portions of the genome. Presumably, in these instances, the changes in DNA sequence exert some type of regulatory control over a particular gene. These SNPs clearly would not have been identified using a candidate gene approach. Also, it must be appreciated that it is not adequate for a certain protein to play an important role in a radiation-response pathway, but the gene that encodes that protein must also possess a SNP(s) that exerts an important functional impact for there to be a genetic basis associated with clinical radiosensitivity related to that particular gene.

In addition to SNPs, the other major source of genetic variation between people is copy number variants. These represent relatively long nucleotide stretches in which more than one copy for that portion of the genome may be present in an individual. If a copy number variant is present in greater than 1 % of a population, it is referred to as a copy number polymorphism. Although there are relatively few studies which have correlated specific effects with CNPs, it is possible to use SNP microarrays to also analyze CNPs. Thus, most GWAS are also screening for association between CNPs and the particular end-point of interest since this source of genetic variation may prove to be of importance.

In summary, there is evidence to support the hypothesis that much of the individual variation in susceptibility for the development of radiation-induced normal tissue toxicities is the result of inherent host or genetic susceptibilities, which each patient brings into radiotherapy. Thus, the development of complications resulting from a treatment with radiation does not necessarily arise from random chance, but may be a manifestation of predisposing factors that render certain patients more likely to suffer injuries from radiotherapy. It is anticipated that identification of the genetic and host factors that predispose individuals to the development of adverse effects from radiotherapy will greatly facilitate the ability to optimize cancer treatment for each patient on an individual basis.

References

Abu-Shakra M, Lee P (1993) Exaggerated fibrosis in patients with systemic sclerosis (scleroderma) following radiation therapy. J Rheumatol 20(9):1601–1603

Alsner J, Rodningen OK, Overgaard J (2007) Differential gene expression before and after ionizing radiation of subcutaneous fibroblasts identifies breast cancer patients resistant to radiation-induced fibrosis. Radiother Oncol 83(3):261–266

Andreassen CN (2005) Can risk of radiotherapy-induced normal tissue complications be predicted from genetic profiles? Acta Oncol 44(8):801–815

Andreassen CN, Alsner J, Overgaard J (2002) Does variability in normal tissue reactions after radiotherapy have a genetic basis–where and how to look for it? Radiother Oncol 64(2):131–140

Andreassen CN, Alsner J, Overgaard M, Overgaard J (2003) Prediction of normal tissue radiosensitivity from polymorphisms in candidate genes. Radiother Oncol 69(2):127–135

Andreassen CN, Alsner J, Overgaard J et al (2005) TGFB1 polymorphisms are associated with risk of late normal tissue complications in the breast after radiotherapy for early breast cancer. Radiother Oncol 75(1):18–21

Andreassen CN, Overgaard J, Alsner J et al (2006a) ATM sequence variants and risk of radiation-induced subcutaneous fibrosis after postmastectomy radiotherapy. Int J Radiat Oncol Biol Phys 64(3):776–783

Andreassen CN, Alsner J, Overgaard M, Sorensen FB, Overgaard J (2006b) Risk of radiation-induced subcutaneous fibrosis in relation to single nucleotide polymorphisms in TGFB1, SOD2, XRCC1, XRCC3, APEX and ATM–a study based on DNA from formalin fixed paraffin embedded tissue samples. Int J Radiat Biol 82(8):577–586

Angele S, Romestaing P, Moullan N et al (2003) ATM haplotypes and cellular response to DNA damage: association with breast cancer risk and clinical radiosensitivity. Cancer Res 63(24):8717–8725

Azria D, Gourgou S, Sozzi WJ et al (2004) Concomitant use of tamoxifen with radiotherapy enhances subcutaneous breast fibrosis in hypersensitive patients. Br J Cancer 91(7):1251–1260

Baumann M, Holscher T, Begg AC (2003) Towards genetic prediction of radiation responses: ESTRO's GENEPI project. Radiother Oncol 69(2):121–125

Begg AC, Russell NS, Knaken H, Lebesque JV (1993) Lack of correlation of human fibroblast radiosensitivity in vitro with early skin reactions in patients undergoing radiotherapy. Int J Radiat Biol 64(4):393–405

Bentzen SM (2006) Preventing or reducing late side effects of radiation therapy: radiobiology meets molecular pathology. Nat Rev Cancer 6(9):702–713

Bliss P, Parsons CA, Blake PR (1996) Incidence and possible aetiological factors in the development of pelvic insufficiency fractures following radical radiotherapy. Br J Radiol 69(822):548–554

Bourguignon MH, Gisone PA, Perez MR et al (2005) Genetic and epigenetic features in radiation sensitivity. Part II: implications for clinical practice and radiation protection. Eur J Nucl Med Mol Imaging 32(3):351–368

Bremer M, Klopper K, Yamini P, Bendix-Waltes R, Dork T, Karstens JH (2003) Clinical radiosensitivity in breast cancer patients carrying pathogenic ATM gene mutations: no observation of increased radiation-induced acute or late effects. Radiother Oncol 69(2):155–160

Burri RJ, Stock RG, Cesaretti JA et al (2008) Association of single nucleotide polymorphisms in SOD2, XRCC1 and XRCC3 with susceptibility for the development of adverse effects resulting from radiotherapy for prostate cancer. Radiat Res 170(1):49–59

Cesaretti JA, Stock RG, Lehrer S et al (2005) ATM sequence variants are predictive of adverse radiotherapy response among patients treated for prostate cancer. Int J Radiat Oncol Biol Phys 61(1):196–202

Cesaretti J, Stock R, Atencio D et al (2006) A genetically determined dose volume histogram predicts for rectal bleeding among patients treated with prostate brachytherapy. Int J Radiat Oncol Biol Phys 66(3):S37–S50

Chen AM, Obedian E, Haffty BG (2001) Breast-conserving therapy in the setting of collagen vascular disease. Cancer J 7(6):480–491

Chon BH and Loeffler JS (2002) The effect of nonmalignant systemic disease on tolerance to radiation therapy. Oncologist 7(2):136–143

Crompton NE and Ozsahin M (1997) A versatile and rapid assay of radiosensitivity of peripheral blood leukocytes based on DNA and surface-marker assessment of cytotoxicity. Radiat Res 147(1):55–60

Crompton NE, Miralbell R, Rutz HP et al (1999) Altered apoptotic profiles in irradiated patients with increased toxicity. Int J Radiat Oncol Biol Phys 45(3):707–714

Crompton NE, Shi YQ, Emery GC et al (2001) Sources of variation in patient response to radiation treatment. Int J Radiat Oncol Biol Phys 49(2):547–554

Damaraju S, Murray D, Dufour J et al (2006) Association of DNA repair and steroid metabolism gene polymorphisms with clinical late toxicity in patients treated with conformal radiotherapy for prostate cancer. Clin Cancer Res 12(8):2545–2554

De Ruyck K, Van Eijkeren M, Claes K et al (2005) Radiation-induced damage to normal tissues after radiotherapy in patients treated for gynecologic tumors: association with single nucleotide polymorphisms in XRCC1, XRCC3, and OGG1 genes and in vitro chromosomal radiosensitivity in lymphocytes. Int J Radiat Oncol Biol Phys 62(4):1140–1149

De Ruyck K, Van Eijkeren M, Claes K et al (2006) TGFbeta1 polymorphisms and late clinical radiosensitivity in patients treated for gynecologic tumors. Int J Radiat Oncol Biol Phys 65(4): 1240–1248

Edvardsen H, Kristensen VN, Grenaker Alnaes GI et al (2007) Germline glutathione S-transferase variants in breast cancer: relation to diagnosis and cutaneous long-term adverse effects after two fractionation patterns of radiotherapy. Int J Radiat Oncol Biol Phys 67(4):1163–1171

Edvardsen H, Tefre T, Jansen L et al (2007) Linkage disequilibrium pattern of the ATM gene in breast cancer patients and controls; association of SNPs and haplotypes to radio-sensitivity and post-lumpectomy local recurrence. Radiat Oncol 2:25

Fernet M, Hall J (2004) Genetic biomarkers of therapeutic radiation sensitivity. DNA Repair (Amst) 3(8–9):1237–1243

Frazer KA, Ballinger DG, Cox DR et al (2007) A second generation human haplotype map of over 3.1 million SNPs. Nature 449(7164):851–861

Giotopoulos G, Symonds RP, Foweraker K et al (2007) The late radiotherapy normal tissue injury phenotypes of telangiectasia, fibrosis and atrophy in breast cancer patients have distinct genotype-dependent causes. Br J Cancer 96(6):1001–1007

Glasenapp GB (1968) Osteomyelitis of the maxilla following radiotherapy for facial lupus. HNO, 16(2):46–49

Gold DG, Miller RC, Petersen IA, Osborn TG (2007) Radiotherapy for malignancy in patients with scleroderma: the mayo clinic experience. Int J Radiat Oncol Biol Phys 67(2):559–567

Gold DG, Miller RC, Pinn ME, Osborn TG, Petersen IA, Brown PD (2008) Chronic toxicity risk after radiotherapy for patients with systemic sclerosis (systemic scleroderma) or systemic lupus erythematosus: association with connective tissue disorder severity. Radiother Oncol 87(1):127–131

Grann A and Wallner K (1998) Prostate brachytherapy in patients with inflammatory bowel disease. Int J Radiat Oncol Biol Phys 40(1):135–138

Green S, Stock RG, Greenstein AJ (1999) Rectal cancer and inflammatory bowel disease: natural history and implications for radiation therapy. Int J Radiat Oncol Biol Phys 44(4):835–840

Hall EJ, Schiff PB, Hanks GE et al (1998) A preliminary report: frequency of A-T heterozygotes among prostate cancer patients with severe late responses to radiation therapy. Cancer J Sci Am 4(6):385–389

Hamilton CD (2005) Immunosuppression related to collagen-vascular disease or its treatment. Proc Am Thorac Soc 2(5):456–460

Hareyama M, Nagakura H, Tamakawa M et al (1995) Severe reaction after chemoradiotherapy of nasopharyngeal carcinoma with collagen disease. Int J Radiat Oncol Biol Phys 33(4):971

Herold DM, Hanlon AL, Hanks GE (1999) Diabetes mellitus: a predictor for late radiation morbidity. Int J Radiat Oncol Biol Phys 43(3):475–479

Ho AY, Atencio DP, Peters S et al (2006) Genetic predictors of adverse radiotherapy effects: the Gene-PARE project. Int J Radiat Oncol Biol Phys 65(3):646–655

Ho AY, Fan G, Atencio DP et al (2007) Possession of ATM sequence variants as predictor for late normal tissue responses in breast cancer patients treated with radiotherapy. Int J Radiat Oncol Biol Phys 69:677–684

Holscher T, Bentzen SM, Baumann M (2006) Influence of connective tissue diseases on the expression of radiation side effects: a systematic review. Radiother Oncol 78(2):123–130

Iannuzzi CM, Atencio DP, Green S, Stock RG, Rosenstein BS (2002) ATM mutations in female breast cancer patients predict for an increase in radiation-induced late effects. Int J Radiat Oncol Biol Phys 52(3):606–613

Jones IM, Thomas CB, Xi T, Nelson DO, Mohrenweiser HW (2005) The genetic basis for variation in radiation sensitivity in the general population. Radiat Res 163(6):700–701

Khoo VS, Saunders MP, Gowda R, Price P, Cummings BJ (2004) Anal canal cancer and chemoradiation treatment in two patients with systemic lupus erythematosus treated by chronic therapeutic immunosuppression. Clin Oncol (R Coll Radiol) 16(1):1–5

Loeffler JS, Harris JR, Dahlberg WK, Little JB (1990) In vitro radiosensitivity of human diploid fibroblasts derived from women with unusually sensitive clinical responses to definitive radiation therapy for breast cancer. Radiat Res 121(2):227–231

Manolio TA, Brooks LD, Collins FS (2008) A HapMap harvest of insights into the genetics of common disease. J Clin Invest 118(5):1590–1605

Maruyama Y, Van Nagell JR, Utley J, Vider ML, Parker JC (1974) Radiation and small bowel complications in cervical carcinoma therapy. Radiology 112(3):699–703

Mayr NA, Riggs CE Jr., Saag KG, Wen BC, Pennington EC, Hussey DH (1997) Mixed connective tissue disease and radiation toxicity. a case report. Cancer 79(3):612–618

Meyer A, Wilhelm B, Dork T et al (2007) ATM missense variant P1054R predisposes to prostate cancer. Radiother Oncol 83(3):283–288

Morris MM and Powell SN (1997) Irradiation in the setting of collagen vascular disease: acute and late complications. J Clin Oncol 15(7):2728–2735

Moullan N, Cox DG, Angele S, Romestaing P, Gerard JP, Hall J (2003) Polymorphisms in the DNA repair gene XRCC1, breast cancer risk, and response to radiotherapy. Cancer Epidemiol Biomarkers Prev 12(11 Pt 1):1168–1174

Nilsen LB, Missal ME, Condemi JJ (1967) Appearance of Hodgkin's disease in a patient with systemic lupus erythematosus. Cancer 20(11):1930–1933

Olivotto IA, Fairey RN, Gillies JH, Stein H (1989) Fatal outcome of pelvic radiotherapy for carcinoma of the cervix in a patient with systemic lupus erythematosis. Clin Radiol 40(1):83–84

Oppitz U, Baier K, Wulf J, Schakowski R, Flentje M (2001) The in vitro colony assay: a predictor of clinical outcome. Int J Radiat Biol 77(1):105–110

Ozsahin M, Ozsahin H, Shi Y, Larsson B, Wurgler FE, Crompton NE (1997) Rapid assay of intrinsic radiosensitivity based on apoptosis in human CD4 and CD8 T-lymphocytes. Int J Radiat Oncol Biol Phys 38(2):429–440

Ozsahin M, Crompton NE, Gourgou S et al (2005) CD4 and CD8 T-lymphocyte apoptosis can predict radiation-induced late toxicity: a prospective study in 399 patients. Clin Cancer Res 11(20):7426–7433

Peters CA, Cesaretti JA, Stone NN, Stock RG (2006) Low-dose rate prostate brachytherapy is well tolerated in patients with a history of inflammatory bowel disease. Int J Radiat Oncol Biol Phys 66(2):424–429

Peters CA, Stock RG, Cesaretti JA et al (2007) TGFB1 single nucleotide polymorphisms are associated with adverse quality of life in prostate cancer patients treated with radiotherapy. Int J Radiat Oncol Biol Phys 70:752–759

Phan C, Mindrum M, Silverman C, Paris K, Spanos W (2003) Matched-control retrospective study of the acute and late complications in patients with collagen vascular diseases treated with radiation therapy. Cancer J 9(6):461–466

Pinn ME, Gold DG, Petersen IA, Osborn TG, Brown PD, Miller RC (2008) Systemic lupus erythematosus, radiotherapy, and the risk of acute and chronic toxicity: the mayo clinic experience. Int J Radiat Oncol Biol Phys 71(2):498–506

Quarmby S, Fakhoury H, Levine E et al (2003) Association of transforming growth factor beta-1 single nucleotide polymorphisms with radiation-induced damage to normal tissues in breast cancer patients. Int J Radiat Biol 79(2):137–143

Rakfal SM, Deutsch M (1998) Radiotherapy for malignancies associated with lupus: case reports of acute and late reactions. Am J Clin Oncol 21(1):54–57

Ransom DT and Cameron FG (1987) Scleroderma–a possible contra-indication to lumpectomy and radiotherapy in breast carcinoma. Australas Radiol, 31(3):317–318

Rathmell AJ and Taylor RE (1992) Enhanced normal tissue response to radiation in a patient with discoid lupus erythematosus. Clin Oncol (R Coll Radiol) 4(5):331–332

Robertson JM, Clarke DH, Pevzner MM (1991) Breast conservation therapy. Severe breast fibrosis after radiation therapy in patients with collagen vascular disease. Cancer 68(3):502–508

Rodningen OK, Borresen-Dale AL, Alsner J, Hastie T, Overgaard J (2008) Radiation-induced gene expression in human subcutaneous fibroblasts is predictive of radiation-induced fibrosis. Radiother Oncol 86(3):314–320

Ross JG, Hussey DH, Mayr NA, Davis CS (1993) Acute and late reactions to radiation therapy in patients with collagen vascular diseases. Cancer 71(11):3744–3752

Safwat A, Bentzen SM, Turesson I, Hendry JH (2002) Deterministic rather than stochastic factors explain most of the variation in the expression of skin telangiectasia after radiotherapy. Int J Radiat Oncol Biol Phys 52(1):198–204

Severin DM, Leong T, Cassidy B et al (2001) Novel DNA sequence variants in the hHR21 DNA repair gene in radiosensitive cancer patients. Int J Radiat Oncol Biol Phys 50(5):1323–1331

Stewart CC, Stevenson AP, Habbersett RC (1988) The effect of low-dose irradiation on unstimulated and PHA-stimulated human lymphocyte subsets. Int J Radiat Biol Relat Stud Phys Chem Med 53(1):77–87

Suga T, Ishikawa A, Kohda M et al (2007) Haplotype-based analysis of genes associated with risk of adverse skin reactions after radiotherapy in breast cancer patients. Int J Radiat Oncol Biol Phys 69(3):685–693

Suga T, Iwakawa M, Tsuji H et al (2008) Influence of multiple genetic polymorphisms on genitourinary morbidity after carbon ion radiotherapy for prostate cancer. Int J Radiat Oncol Biol Phys 72(3):808–813

Tucker SL, Turesson I, Thames HD (1992) Evidence for individual differences in the radiosensitivity of human skin. Eur J Cancer 28A(11):1783–1791

Tucker SL, Geara FB, Peters LJ, Brock WA (1996) How much could the radiotherapy dose be altered for individual patients based on a predictive assay of normal-tissue radiosensitivity? Radiother Oncol 38(2):103–113

Turesson I and Joiner MC (1996) Clinical evidence of hypersensitivity to low doses in radiotherapy. Radiother Oncol 40(1):1–3

Urtasun RC (1971) A complication of the use of radiation for malignant neoplasia in chronic discoid lupus erythematosus. J Can Assoc Radiol, 22(2): 168–169

van Nagell JR, Parker JC, Maruyama Y, Utley J, Vider ML, Luckett P (1974) Bladder or rectal injury following radiation therapy for cervical cancer. Am J Obstet Gynecol 119(6):727–732

Varga J, Haustein UF, Creech RH, Dwyer JP (1991) and Jimenez, SA Exaggerated radiation-induced fibrosis in patients with systemic sclerosis. JAMA 265(24):3292–3295

West CM, McKay MJ, Holscher T et al (2005) Molecular markers predicting radiotherapy response: report and recommendations from an International Atomic Energy Agency technical meeting. Int J Radiat Oncol Biol Phys 62(5):1264–1273

Willett CG, Ooi CJ, Zietman AL et al (2000) Acute and late toxicity of patients with inflammatory bowel disease undergoing irradiation for abdominal and pelvic neoplasms. Int J Radiat Oncol Biol Phys 46(4):995–998

Winchester DP and Cox JD (1998) Standards for diagnosis and management of invasive breast carcinoma. American College of Radiology. American College of Surgeons. College of American Pathologists. Society of Surgical Oncology. CA Cancer J Clin 48(2): 83–107

Wo J and Taghian A (2007) Radiotherapy in setting of collagen vascular disease. Int J Radiat Oncol Biol Phys 69(5):1347–1353

Bioengineering of Irradiated Normal Tissues by Bone Marrow Stem Cells

Joel S. Greenberger and Michael W. Epperly

Contents

Supported by Research Grants: RO1CA11927 and RO1CA083876.

J. S. Greenberger (✉) · M. W. Epperly
Department of Radiation Oncology, University of Pittsburgh Cancer Institute, UPMC Cancer Pavilion, POB2, 5th Floor, Rm. 533, 5150, Centre Avenue, Pittsburgh, PA 15232, USA
e-mail: Greenbergerjs@umpc.edu

Abstract

Irradiation damage of normal tissue during radiation therapy is repaired by stem cells and differentiated progeny derived from both the irradiated tissue and from cells migrating through the blood from the bone marrow. The bone marrow contains both pluripotential hematopoietic stem cells and their committed progenitors, and bone marrow stromal cells (mesenchymal stem cells). Using defined conditions in vitro or in animal model systems in vivo, each of these marrow origin cell populations has been shown to differentiate into multiple cell lineages. Irradiation of epithelial organs stimulates migration of bone marrow cells to sites of injury where incorporation leads to either repair of acute injury or to formation of late fibrosis. The degree to which marrow origin stem and committed progenitor cells contribute to repair of irradiation damage is not known. This chapter discusses the roles of the different marrow origin cell populations in repair of irradiation-induced damage to epithelial organs.

1 Introduction

There has always been a fascination with tissue healing. Scientists and physicians have made tremendous discoveries over the past several decades with respect to the molecular and cellular mechanisms of wound repair and methods by which to optimize recovery of tissue function and minimize late fibrosis or scarring (Rubin and Cassarett 1968; Hall 1988; Epperly et al. 2003; Dileto and Travis 1996; Franko and Sharplin 1994). The fields of tissue engineering (Lanza and Atala 2002), bioengineering (Stripp and Reynolds 2005), and regenerative medicine (Lagasse et al. 2001) have evolved from the wealth of basic science, and clinical data obtained from a variety of disciplines including both medical and tissue physiology.

P. Rubin et al. (eds.), *ALERT – Adverse Late Effects of Cancer Treatment*, Medical Radiology. Radiation Oncology,
DOI: 10.1007/978-3-540-72314-1_13, © Springer-Verlag Berlin Heidelberg 2014

In the medical field, pioneering studies in plastic and reconstructive surgery (Stripp and Reynolds 2005), wound and burn management (Lagasse et al. 2001), ischemia and reperfusion damage (Kaminski et al. 2004), organ failure (Novakova-Jiresova et al. 2004), regeneration following functional organ reduction (Giangreco et al. 2009), and others have uncovered clear evidence of age-related changes in the biological repair process, the critical role of inflammatory cytokines in tissue regeneration, and the role of stem cells in the process of repair.

In the basic science disciplines of cellular physiology and stem cell biology, many revolutionary changes in the past decades have occurred most prominently. The discovery of the multilineage epithelial differentiating capacity of subsets of bone marrow stem cells that were previously thought to be restricted to the lymphohematopoietic lineage (Petersen et al. 1999; Krause et al. 2001). Fibroblasts of the bone marrow microenvironment (Friedenstein et al. 1982), renamed mesenchymal stem cells (Pittenger et al. 1999) were shown to have a capacity not only for multilineage differentiation to osteoblasts, chondrocytes, and adipocytes, but also to display migratory and homing capacity to different sites within the bone marrow and other organs (Erices et al. 2000; Anklesaria et al. 1989; Quesenberry et al. 2005; Werts et al. 1980). Both intrinsic genetic (Boggs et al. 1981) and microenvironmentally determinative (Tjwa et al. 2009; Hazen et al. 2009; Heissig et al. 2002) influences on stem cell differentiation have been established.

Tissue damage from ionizing irradiation parallels many features of injury from other insults including thermal burn, ultraviolet irradiation damage, and ischemia/reperfusion injury (Kaminski et al. 2004). Common to each form of tissue injury is the phenomenon of oxidative stress (Tyurina et al. 2008, Tyurin 2008; Kagan et al. 2009; Jiang et al. 2007; Greenberger and Epperly 2007). The antioxidant pool within cells, tissues, and organs has been shown to critically influence the capacity of the repair process following each form of injury (Epperly et al. 2004). However, ionizing irradiation injury is unique in several aspects. Ionizing irradiation-induced DNA strand breaks that initiate cellular death are highly localized within the nucleus (Olive and Banath 2004), and have been shown to activate a set of signal transduction events that lead to a unique form of injury (Bakkenist and Kastan 2003). The direct irradiation dose–response relationships of cellular, tissue, and organ injury are influenced by *radiation quality* (high-linear energy transfer particle damage compared to X-ray photon-induced damage (Ibanez et al. 2009)), direct and indirect *bystander effects* (Mothersill and Seymour 2004) (Unirradiated cells can facilitate and stimulate repair of irradiated cells, and conversely irradiated cells can release cytokines and/or communicate damage through cell contact to induce cell death in unirradiated cells, respectively (Prise and O'Sullivan 2009)), and *volume* effects. Tissue and organ volume effects of ionizing irradiation present a complex challenge in explaining the mechanism of total body irradiation damage from a specific dose of irradiation that is significantly more severe than the same dose delivered to hemibody or partial body volumes. For example, the length of spinal cord receiving a given irradiation dose determines tissue capacity for recovery (van der Kogel et al. 1982). However, the cellular and molecular mechanisms of the volume effect are poorly understood (Prise and O'Sullivan 2009).

It is now clear that damage to self-renewing cell populations that have a supportive role in the microenvironment can significantly limit recovery capacity not only by effects on other surviving cells within the irradiated volume, but also with respect to hosting reparative cells that migrate in from distant sites through the circulation (Greenberger 1991). This chapter will review both the state of knowledge and future challenges with respect to exploiting the potential effectiveness of bone marrow-derived stem cells to reconstitute irradiated tissues.

2 Bone Marrow Stem Cell Reconstitution of the Irradiated Bone Marrow

The role of bone marrow-derived stem cells in what is now called regenerative medicine in fact began in radiation biology. The pioneering studies of Till and McCulloch (1961) first demonstrated a direct cell dose response curve with respect to the capacity of bone marrow-derived cells to produce hematopoietic cell foci in the total body irradiated mouse spleen. This assay called the colony forming unit spleen was the first clear demonstration that bone marrow could quantitatively restore tissue and organ function (McCulloch and Till 1962). Over the next several decades, researchers established several basic principles of the biology of bone marrow transplantation, each of which serves as a focus for continuing research efforts:

1. There is a bone marrow toxic dose of total body ionizing irradiation, below which marrow transplantation can facilitate survival. Above that threshold total body irradiation dose, damage to other organs overrides the reconstitution capacity of bone marrow stem cells to rescue the animal/human from lethality. There remains great controversy as to the mechanism of the "dose threshold for survival by bone marrow transplantation".
2. A subset of cells in the bone marrow contains totipotential or pluripotential hematopoietic stem cells. Separation and concentration of this subset of cells, then injected intravenously after total body irradiation will promote survival as well as will whole bone marrow (Krause et al. 2001; Tsao et al. 2009; Zaibak et al. 2009;

Montini et al. 2009; Dickson et al. 2009; Carotta et al. 2004; Cerdan et al. 2004; Yoyooka et al. 2003; Torres et al. 2007). The other subsets of cells (usually those already displaying differentiation markers on the cell surface) may provide short-term protection, but do not result in donor cell origin mediated long-term reconstitution of hematopoiesis in the irradiated recipient. Non-stem cell subpopulations within the bone marrow are referred to as committed progenitors and sub-sets have been shown to be unilineage (granulocyte progenitors, macrophage progenitors), bilineage (granulocyte–macrophage progenitors), and multilineage hematopoietic or lymphohematopoietic progenitors. The genetic profile of the true totipotential, lymphohematopoietic reconstituting stem cell has been a subject of intense investigation (Terskikh et al. 2003). Gene-Array and proteomics studies have shown specific gene expression (Terskikh et al. 2003) and protein profiles (Unwin et al. 2006) with true stem cells; however, the precise identification of this cell subset is still unknown.

3. The irradiated microenvironment into which bone marrow stem cells migrate significantly influences the parameters of engraftment. Stem cell introduction through the circulation leads to the phenomena of migration and homing. Before the identification of bone marrow-derived stem cells, it was known that other differentiated nucleated committed cells within the peripheral circulation (polymorphonuclear leukocytes, monocytes, and lymphocytes) respond to inflammatory cytokines, peptide signals, and endothelial cell surface adhesion molecules which influence their attachment and stable residence within a particular tissue or organ. The past decades have identified other primitive cell types which also migrate through the circulation including bone marrow stromal cell progenitors (bone marrow fibroblasts, mesenchymal stem cells), committed hematopoietic progenitor cells, and true pluripotential hematopoietic stem cells. Factors which induce migration of cell populations from one site in the bone marrow to another site in marrow or other organs have clearly been shown to include several cytokines, the most prominent granulocyte-colony stimulating factor. Migration which has also been called "trafficking" leads to the enhanced availability of tissue regenerating cells in the circulation (Bonig et al. 2009; Schmitz et al. 1996; Switzer et al. 2001; Semerad et al. 2005; Kim et al. 2006; Carlo-Stella et al. 2000).

   Migration is not always followed by homing. Homing (stable residence and return to an integrated basal state) of bone marrow-derived stem cells to specific sites is dependent upon specific microenvironmental factors in the target site (Calvi et al. 2003; Matsuzaki et al. 2004; Cancelas et al. 2005; Adams et al. 2007; Zhang et al. 2003; Ara et al. 2003; Kiel et al. 2005; Wright et al. 2001). Controversy persists as to whether these homing signals are microenvironment cell type-specific (endothelial cell (Kiel et al. 2005), osteoblast progenitor cell (Calvi et al. 2003), and bone marrow fibroblast (Ara et al. 2003)) or common to all cells and are rather dependent on expression of adhesion molecules (Greenberger 1991). Homing can be transient, such as the known initial concentration of intravenously injected bone marrow-derived stem cells in the recipient lung (Albera et al. 2005). However, for stable engraftment to the marrow the trafficking or homing cell must arrive at a specific microenvironmental space or niche. Controversy also persists as to the physical site within the bone marrow space of this stem cell niche, whether it is periosteal, contained within the vascular space of reticular adventitial cells, or involves sites of osteoblast activity (Jones and Wagers 2008). Attentively, the site may be a region of relative hypoxia (Parmar et al. 2007).

4. Transplanted bone marrow stem cells must return to a state of quiescence to provide stable reconstitution (Zipori 2004; Roy and Verfaillie 1999). The mechanism by which engrafted cells return to a nondividing state (G_0, or quiescence) is unknown. Several observations suggest that this phenomenon is absolutely required for stable bone marrow transplantation (van Hennik et al. 1999). Manipulation of purified hematopoietic stem cells in tissue culture, in bioreactors, or by rapid in vitro serial transplantation, using tissue culture dishes or other materials produces cells that are altered and rendered insufficient to allow homing and return to quiescence, and results in loss of the stem cell phenotype and often inability to stably engraft.

   Another proof of the need for quiescence of stem cells is that those hematopoietic cells surviving chemotherapy using drugs that target cycling or dividing cells, leave a residual population that is still capable of in vivo transplantation (Rice et al. 1993).

5. Toxicity to the engraftment site (hematopoietic microenvironment) can prevent engraftment of healthy stem cells. Radiation dose dependent toxicity has been shown to limit healthy stem cell engraftment to a high dose irradiated marrow site compared to a lower dose irradiated site (Werts et al. 1980). The recovery capacity of a high dose irradiated site can be observed over time, or a late toxic effect to the irradiated microenvironment can permanently prevent the return of hematopoiesis at this site. The late toxic effect involves fibrosis and replacement of functioning tissue with proliferating fibroblasts. Fibrosis is a common phenomenon to many irradiated organs and prevents both recovery of resident in situ stem populations as well as engraftment of circulating progenitors derived from bone marrow (Dileto and

Travis 1996; Franko and Sharplin 1994; Werts et al. 1980).

There are bone marrow stem cell and microenvironmental niche cell specific genetic determinants of tissue repair (Boggs et al. 1981; Tjwa et al. 2009; Hazen et al. 2009; Heissig et al. 2002). Mouse genotype specific factors can determine total body radiosensitivity of the hematopoietic system. Specific genes have been shown to modulate transplantation capacity (Christopherson II et al. 2004; Boggs et al. 1973), but also genetic factors of the hematopoietic microenvironment or niche can be specific modulators of engraftment (Anklesaria et al. 1989).

The genetic factors influencing both stem cell and microenvironment specific components of stem cell transplantation appear to be independent of the intrinsic radiosensitivity of each of those cell types (Anklesaria et al. 1989).

3 Endothelial Progenitor Cell Involvement in Tissue Regeneration and Bioengineering

There continues to be controversy over the distinct phenotype of the circulating endothelial progenitor cell of bone marrow origin. Initial studies suggested that the hematopoietic stem cell was capable of differentiation to endothelial cells (Takakura et al. 2000; Sakai et al. 2009). A subset of circulating, bone marrow-derived hematopoietic cells containing FLT1 receptors was shown to be specific for endothelial differentiation capacity (Shimonaka et al. 2003). The ability of these cells to migrate through the circulation and reconstitute blood vessels at a distant site was documented (Bompais et al. 2004). However, the unique cells surface phenotype of the endothelial progenitor remains controversial.

Bone marrow-derived cells are known to contribute to the vasculature within tumors (Murayama et al. 2002). In several in vivo orthotopic tumor models, migration of bone marrow-derived cells into the tumor microenvironment has been shown (Murayama et al. 2002). Tumor-derived endothelial cells share many properties with endothelial cells from normal organs including liver and brain (Aird et al. 1995). However, organ-specific endothelial cells have been shown to be dependent in their response to specific transcriptional factors including Von Willebrand factor (Jahroudi et al. 1996). Fetal endothelial cells share microenvironmental properties with those endothelial cells of the adult brain (Aird et al. 1995). These observations suggest the potential capacity of bone marrow-derived endothelial progenitors to be involved in critical aspects of tissue repair, namely revascularization following injury (Murayama et al. 2002). The capacity of endothelial progenitors to revascularize the damaged cardiac vasculature and central nervous system vasculature has been shown (Young et al. 2007).

The role of endothelial progenitors in revascularization of irradiation damaged tissue remains controversial. A common factor limiting bone marrow-derived endothelial progenitor cell reconstitution of irradiation in damaged tissue is toxicity to the microenvironment. Revascularization has been shown to depend upon both vascular budding of intrinsic endothelial cells (Hirschi and Goodell 2002) as well as the involvement of migrating, circulation/bone marrow-derived endothelial cell progenitors (Takakura et al. 2000). Revascularization of cutaneous wounds has been shown to depend upon vascular bud recruitment into the repairing tissue (Hirschi and Goodell 2002). The reaction of neurons, fibroblast progenitor cells (mesenchymal stem cells), and budding endothelial cells within irradiation-damaged tissue influences whether vascular repair will occur or attentively whether deleterious fibrosis will limit vascular extension (Lei et al. 2006). Within the local tissue, cells migrating into the wound area through the circulation include not only endothelial progenitors, but those involved in the inflammatory response (Miyahara et al. 2006). In thermal, ultraviolet irradiation, and ischemia reperfusion injury (Link et al. 1996), dead and dying cells within the tissue recruit inflammatory cells through the circulation to serve a role in limiting tissue damage, but also in the clean-up process of removing dead and damaged cells (Jackson et al. 2001). A successful revascularization depends upon limitation of the fibrotic response, but also on rapid and efficient removal of dead cells (Lei et al. 2006). Tipping the balance away from successful revascularization and toward organ failure can result from continued inflammatory cytokine production by cells of the irradiated microenvironment (Greenberger 1991). A chronic inflammatory phenomenon may limit the capacity of both in situ surviving vascular progenitor cells that produce the budding phenomenon, as well as circulatory stem cells from providing tissue repair.

4 Epithelial Progenitor Cells Derived from the Bone Marrow

The studies of Peterson et al. (1999) first demonstrated that bone marrow cells could differentiate to regenerating liver. These studies were followed by those of Krauss et al. (2001) demonstrating that single bone marrow cell reconstituted, lethally irradiated recipient, mice had rare cells in multiple epithelial organs which were epithelial and had markers of the donor hematopoietic cell (Krause et al. 2001). Numerous studies followed demonstrating the evidence of non-hematopoietic organ reconstitution capacity of bone

Table 1 Published reports of donor bone marrow-derived progenitor/stem cell origin of normal tissues

Tissue	Reference	Methodology demonstration of differentiation self-renewal			
		In situ localization by donor cell marker	In situ localization by functional marker	In vitro explant	Demonstration in vivo
Hematopoietic stem cell	Till and McCulloch (1961), McCulloch and Till (1962)	+	+	+	+
Endothelial cell (blood vessel)	Bompais et al. (2004), Lombaert et al. (2008)	+	+	+	−
Liver (hepatocyte, oval cell, biliary duct cell)	Petersen et al. (1999), Krause et al. (2001), Spyridonidis et al. (2004), Korbling et al. (2002), Theise et al. (2000)	+	+	+	−
Esophagus	Epperly et al. (2004), Niu et al. (2008)	+	+	+	+
Lung	Albera et al. (2005), Engelhardt (2001), Kyung et al. (2004), Reynolds et al. (2004)	+	+	+	−
Skeletal muscle	Proksch et al. (2009), Mookerjee et al. (2009), Gussoni et al. (1999)	+	+	+	−
Cardiac muscle	Yoon et al. (2005)	+	+	+	−
Marrow stromal cell	Anklesaria et al. (1989)	+	+	+	+
Osteoblast	Sasportas et al. (2009), Gronthos et al. (1994), Prockop (1997)	+	+	+	−
Chondrocyte	Zhou et al. (2005)	+	+	+	−
Pancreas	Hess et al. (2003), Chen et al. (2004), Zeng et al. (2006)	+	+	+	−
Intestine	Ishikawa et al. (2004)	+	+	+	−
Skin (dermis)	Deng et al. (2005)	+	+	+	−
Central nervous system neurological cell	Barberi et al. (2003), Lim et al. (2009), Cheng et al. (2009), Brazelton et al. (2000), Mezey et al. (2000), Kamishina et al. (2008), Davoust et al. (2006), Munoz et al. (2005), Simard and Rivest (2004), Habich et al. (2006), Goolsby et al. (2003), Ohtaki et al. (2008)	+	+	+	−
Retina	Chadderton et al. (2009), Lamba et al. (2006)	+	+	+	−
Peripheral nervous system neurons, spinal cord	Sigurjonsson et al. (2005), Lin et al. (2008), Barnabe-Heider and Frisen (2008), Park et al. (2005)	+	+	+	−
Ear	Li et al. (2003)	+	+	+	−
Germ cell	Lue et al. (2007)	+	+	+	−
Breast	Li et al. (2009), Woodward et al. (2007)	+	+	+	−
Salivary gland	Lombaert et al. (2008)	+	−	+	−

marrow fibroblast or hematopoietic cells (Table 1). These reports document the capacity of bone marrow cells to differentiate to cells of the brain, spinal cord, skin, eye, lung, esophagus, oral cavity, salivary gland, osteoblast/bone, glandular tissues, and germ cells. A problem with many reports in this area has been the failure to properly apply the correct definition of "stem cell" when using a conclusion that stated evidence of bone marrow "stem cell" origin of organ-specific cells.

Bone marrow transplantation can result in epithelial organ recovery, but this need not be attributed to transplanted stem cells (Fig. 1). The stem cell is not the same as committed progenitor cells. Bone marrow committed progenitor cells can migrate into an irradiated tissue, proliferate, and assume characteristics of that tissue either through the inductive microenvironment causing differentiation, or through cell fusion (Ogle et al. 2005). However, stabilization of tissue damage and transient early appearance of

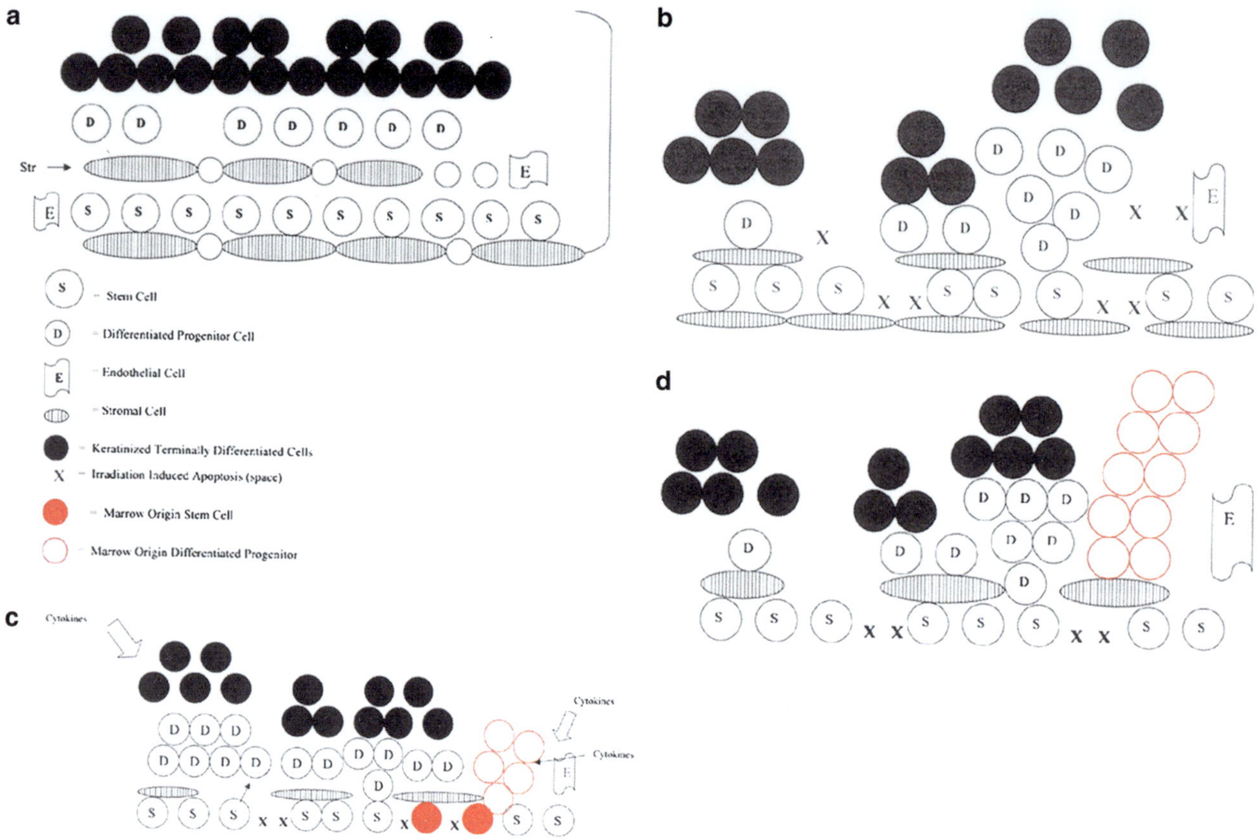

Fig. 1 Irradiation-induced bone marrow stem cell migration to epithelial tissues via the circulation serves as a restorative countermeasure to stimulate organ recovery. **a** Esophagus stem cells and stromal cells in a basal state. **b** Esophagus irradiation depletes basal stem cells causing proliferative response. **c** The effect of bone marrow stem cell regenerative migration (*red*) into the esophagus restoring the epithelial stem cell niche. **d** The effect of differentiated/committed bone marrow-derived cells (not true stem cells) moving into the irradiated esophagus restoring committed esophageal progenitor cells (*red*). True esophageal stem cells remain in their niche and repopulate the esophagus at a later time pushing out the marrow origin cells (Greenberger and Epperly 2009, reproduced with permission of the publisher (Elsevier, Inc.).)

donor cell-derived marked cells within tissue does not prove that bone marrow-derived stem cells were responsible.

The true definition of a stem cell is that it retains capacity for not only differentiation but self-renewal to generate other stem cells. Studies in which self-renewal has been documented represent a small subset of the total published studies reporting bone marrow stem cells derived regeneration of epithelial organs (Table 1). It is well established that damage to the microenvironment of the irradiated organ can limit bone marrow-derived stem cell or differentiated cell homing and proliferative capacity in that organ (Fig. 2) (Quesenberry et al. 2005; Epperly et al. 2004; Niu et al. 2008).

Damage to the irradiated tissue microenvironment can be decreased by treatment of that organ with agents that reduce oxidative stress and production of free radicals (Greenberger 1991; Demedts et al. 2005; Naparstek et al. 1985; Greenberger et al. 1988). The capacity of an irradiated tissue to favorably support the migration, homing, and stable functioning of bone marrow-derived cells, arriving from the circulation has been shown to be critically dependent on the functional status of the microenvironment of that target organ.

Irradiation damage to a specific organ includes both acute and chronic side effects (van Rongen et al. 1993). The eclipse or quiet phase between the disappearance of acute irradiation effects and appearance of late effects has been shown to be attributable to a second phase of cytokine production that is associated with the initiation of the late effects (Leask and Abraham 2004). It is generally accepted that for bone marrow-derived stem cells to have a functional role in tissue reconstitution of an epithelial organ, the deleterious effect of continuous free radical production by the microenvironment in that tissue must be ameliorated (Oberley and Buettner 1979). Research efforts have focused on development of techniques by which to supply stable antioxidant delivery to cells of the irradiated microenvironment to facilitate stem cell homing. At the present time, there still remain challenges for proof of the concept that bone marrow-derived cells can reconstitute an epithelial

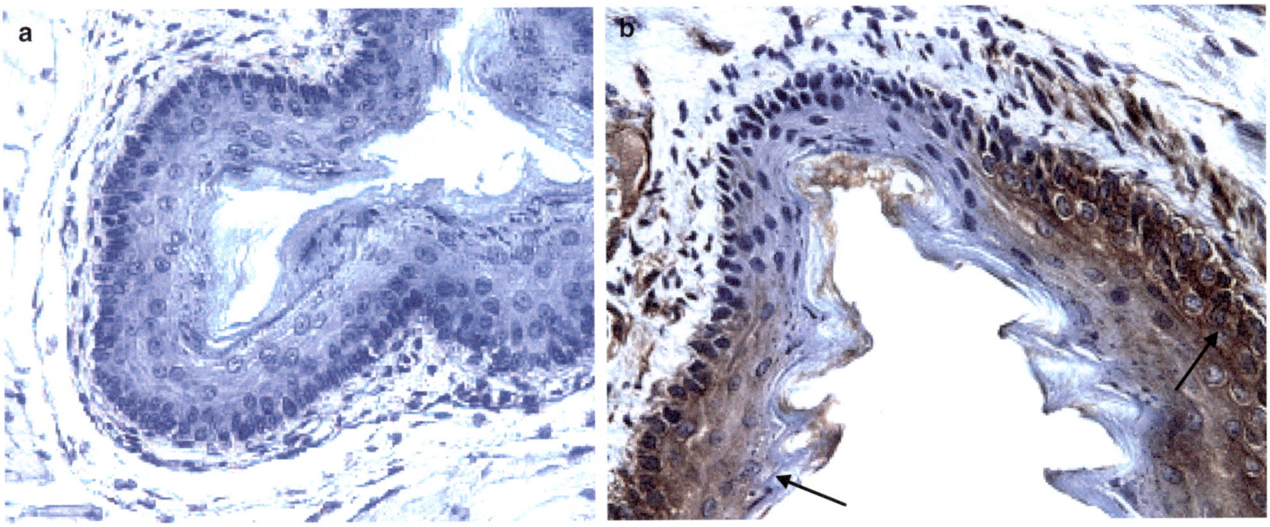

Fig. 2 ROSA positive male donor bone marrow-derived squamous epithelium in MnSOD-PL treated irradiated esophagus of C57BL/6HNsd female mouse. LacZ expression in ROSA positive cells (*brown color arrows*). Female C57BL/6NHsd mice were administered MnSOD-PL (100 μg plasmid DNA in 100 μl lipofectin) at the top of the esophagus and the mice were permitted to swallow. 24 h later mice were irradiated to 27 Gy to the upper body. Five days later mice were injected with 1×10^6 bone marrow cells from a ROSA (LacZ+) male mouse. Mice were sacrificed 14 days later, esophagus removed, fixed in 10 % formalin, sectioned, and stained for LacZ expression using goat anti-LacZ antibody followed by biotinylated labeled antigoat antibody and ExtrAvidin-Peroxidase reagent (Sigma Chemical Co., St. Louis, MO). Nuclei were stained with hematoxylin. **a** Esophagus section from an MnSOD-PL treated, irradiated control mouse. **b** Section from a mouse receiving MnSOD-PL before irradiation and injected ROSA bone marrow. LacZ positive foci of ROSA bone marrow (**arrows**) (**b**) (×40)

organ. These challenges include the demonstration that functional cellular physiologic units within the recipient's irradiated tissue are derived from donor bone marrow cells. Some representative challenges include:

1. Alveolar respiratory complexes in the lung must be shown to be of donor marrow cellular origin.
2. Functioning muscle bundles producing muscle contraction and contributing to muscle strength must be shown to be associated with skeletal myocytes derived from donor bone marrow origin cells.
3. Elements of glandular secretion/glandular buds and production of donor bone marrow genotype-derived secretary products must be shown to be derived from bone marrow genotype specific cells.

These criteria have been met in few situations including at present only the target recipient organs of liver and bone marrow itself (Wagers et al. 2002).

5 Bone Marrow-Derived Mesenchymal Stem Cells

Bone marrow fibroblasts were originally thought to be those cells supporting the homing and proliferation of hematopoietic cells (Friedenstein et al. 1982). Continuous bone marrow cultures provided a system by which to study cells of the hematopoietic microenvironment and their interaction with hematopoietic stem cells in vitro (Dexter et al. 1977). Hematopoietic stem cells derived from long-term bone marrow culture were shown to have the properties of freshly derived stem cells from donor mice (Dexter et al. 1977). Hematopoietic reconstitution of lethally irradiated mice by transplant of stem cells derived from long-term bone marrow cultures that had been in vitro for months, demonstrated the capacity of an in vitro culture system to contain persistent totipotential stem cells. Within the hematopoietic niche of these marrow cultures "cobblestone islands" were shown to contain quiescent cells that harbored true stem cells (Greenberger 1978; Mauch et al. 1980; Sakakeeny and Greenberger 1982). The aging of continuous bone marrow cultures was associated with decline in the number of stem cells and production of committed hematopoietic progenitors (Sakakeeny and Greenberger 1982). The long-term bone marrow culture system remains the only in vitro system for maintenance of true stem cells outside the body for long durations (Sakakeeny and Greenberger 1982).

Other organ explant systems have been shown to share some properties of the long-term bone marrow culture system (Kataoka et al. 2003; Kalabis et al. 2008; Engelhardt et al. 1993). The success of the long-term bone marrow culture system allowed focus on those cells of the microenvironment (nonhematopoietic) which were responsible for stable quiescence of hematopoietic stem cells (Mauch et al. 1980). Following explant to culture, long-term marrow cultures were shown to contain cells with endothelial markers, fibroblast markers, as well as macrophage markers (Sakakeeny and Greenberger 1982). The hematopoietic microenvironment was thought to be composed of these three cell types (Dexter et al. 1977). Accumulation of neutral fat/lipid in bone marrow stromal cell association of lipid containing droplets in stromal cells near hematopoietic niches, suggested that the adipocyte was the critical hemopoiesis supporting stromal cell (Greenberger 1978). Further information indicated that lipid accumulation was in fact the toxic response of bone marrow to the high concentrations of fat and corticosteroid in horse serum used to establish the cultures (Greenberger 1978). Cultures with limited fat accumulation led to longer duration of hematopoiesis (Sakakeeny and Greenberger 1982). This data was consistent with the clinical observation that accumulation of yellow fat occurs in bone marrow during aging, and the fatty repopulation of the marrow microenvironment was associated with hematopoietic failure (Sakakeeny and Greenberger 1982).

Ionizing irradiation effects on the hematopoietic microenvironment were shown to be similar to those in natural aging (Zhou et al. 2008). Irradiated cells accumulated fat more quickly (Greenberger 1991), irradiated cells in culture showed upregulation of p53 and p21, stress response elements also shown to be upregulated during aging of bone marrow stromal cells (Zhou et al. 2008). Factors which reversed fat accumulation and aging effects in bone marrow stromal cells were shown to enhance hematopoiesis (Lechpammer et al. 2005; Epperly et al. 2007).

There is evidence that the cells of bone marrow microenvironment can be repopulated/replenished by cells of donor bone marrow origin (Anklesaria et al. 1989; Werts et al. 1980). Replacement of the microenvironment was first demonstrated by Werts and Degowin (Werts et al. 1980) and confirmed by Anklesaria et al. (1989) who showed that bone marrow stromal cells engrafted less effectively to high dose irradiated sites compared to low dose irradiated sites. These cells were called bone marrow fibroblasts, but later were shown to be those cells capable of multilineage differentiation (Pittenger et al. 1999).

Bone marrow stromal cells can engraft into a fracture/bone wound healing defect in vivo (Gokhale et al. 2010) and they are involved in regeneration/osteogenesis in irradiation damage tissue. Higher irradiation doses limit the capacity of migratory cells to be involved in bone healing (Gokhale et al. 2010). Antioxidant administration facilitates improved mesenchymal stem cell engraftment. However, serious negative effect of bone marrow stromal cell engraftment is the role of these cells in late tissue irradiation damage. Bone marrow stromal cells have been shown to contribute significantly to the fibrosis in irradiated lung (Epperly et al. 2003). Bone marrow stromal cell involvement in fibrosis is also a factor in chemotherapeutic drug induced lung damage such as that by bleomycin injury (Ortiz et al. 2003). Under one set of conditions, bone marrow-derived cells can be involved in tissue repair and potentially organ reconstitution, and under another set of conditions a distinct mesenchymal stem cell subset can contribute to late fibrotic damage which limits organ recovery. The subtle dynamics of cell migration into an irradiated microenvironment can be either beneficial or deleterious depending on the cell population and the timing.

6 The Irradiated Tissue Microenvironment: Niche or Vascular Space?

It is clear that above a toxic threshold dose of irradiation (which may differ between tissues and organs) spontaneous tissue reconstitution may not follow. The protection or replacement by bone marrow cells of the irradiation damaged tissue microenvironment after such a toxic dose may lead to improved tissue recovery. There is controversy as to whether the microenvironment for stem cells is in fact a vascular space (Lombaert et al. 2008) or a specific cell type which functions as the niche (Anklesaria et al. 1989; Adams et al. 2007; Zhang et al. 2003). There is further controversy over whether the cells of the microenvironment as well as the stem cell population itself can be replaced by bone marrow.

Reconstitution of irradiated epithelial and nonepithelial tissues is dependent upon a subtle interplay between migratory beneficial cells (tissue reparative stem cells) and deleterious late damage inducing cells (fibrosis inducing mesenchymal stem cells). One approach toward tipping the balance toward repair may be to limit oxidative stress responses in the irradiated tissue microenvironment which change the makeup of cytokine production and release. Therefore, in addition to marrow-derived stem cell transplant, local delivery of antioxidants by stimulation of the in situ replenishment of antioxidant stores, by specific antioxidant diets, or by direct perfusion with antioxidants may facilitate tissue repair. Research is ongoing and important to achieve the goal of replacing irradiation-damaged tissue through donor stem cell transplantation.

References

Adams GB, Martin RP, Alley IR et al (2007) Therapeutic targeting of a stem cell niche. Nat Biotechnol 25:238–242

Aird WC, Jahroudi N, Weiler-Guettler H, Rayburn HB, Rosenberg RD (1995) Human von Willebrand factor gene sequences target expression to a subpopulation of endothelial cells in transgenic mice. Proc Natl Acad Sci U S A 92:4567

Albera C, Polak JM, Janes S, Griffiths MJD, Alison MR, Wright NA, Navaratnarasah S, Poulsom R, Jeffrey R, Fisher C, Burke M, Bishop AE (2005) Repopulation of human pulmonary epithelium by bone marrow cells: a potential means to promote repair. Tissue Eng 11:7–8

Anklesaria P, FitzGerald TJ, Kase K et al (1989) Improved hematopoiesis in anemic S1/S1d mice by therapeutic transplantation of a hematopoietic microenvironment. Blood 74:1144–1152

Ara T, Tokoyoda K, Sugiyama T, Egawa T, Kawabata K, Nagasawa T (2003) Long-term hematopoietic stem cells require stromal cell-derived factor-1 for colonizing bone marrow during ontogeny. Immunity 19:257–267

Bakkenist CJ, Kastan MB (2003) DNA damage activates ATM through intermolecular autophosphorylation and dimer association. Nature 30(421):499–506

Barberi T, Klivenyi P, Calingasan NY, Lee H, Kawamata H, Loonam K, Perrier AL, Bruses J, Rubio ME, Topf N, Tabar V, Harrison NL, Beal MF, Moore MAS, Studer L (2003) Neural subtype specification of fertilization and nuclear transfer embryonic stem cells and application in parkinsonian mice. Nat Biotechnol 21(10): 1200–1210

Barnabe-Heider F, Frisen J (2008) Stem cells for spinal cord repair. Cell Stem Cell 3:16–20

Boggs SS, Wilson SM, Smith WW (1973) Effects of endotoxin on hematopoiesis in irradiated and non-irradiated W/W^v mice. Rad Res 56:481

Boggs DR, Boggs SS, Ruscetti FW (1981) The W/W^v mouse as a model system for the study of aplastic anemia. In: Levine AS (ed) Proceedings of the conference on aplastic anemia: a stem cell disease, No. 81-1008. NIH Publication, San Francisco, p 197

Bompais H, Chagraoui J, Canron X, Crisan M, Liu XH, Anjo A, Tolla-Le Port C, Leboeuf M, Charbord P, Bikfalvi A, Uzan G (2004) Human endothelial cells derived from circulating progenitors display specific functional properties compared with mature vessel wall endothelial cells. Blood 103(7): 2577–2584

Bonig H, Chudziak D, Priestley G, Papayannopoulou T (2009) Insights into the biology of mobilized hematopoietic stem/progenitor cells through innovative treatment schedules of the CXCR4 antagonist AMD3100. Exp Hematol 37:402–415

Brazelton TR, Rossi FM, Keshet GI, Blau HM (2000) From marrow to brain: expression of neuronal phenotypes in adult mice. Science 290:1775–1779

Calvi LM, Adams GB, Weibrecht KW et al (2003) Osteoblastic cells regulate the haematopoietic stem cell niche. Nature 425:844–848

Cancelas JA, Lee AW, Prabhakar R et al (2005) GTPases differentially integrate signals regulating hematopoietic stem cell localization. Nat Med 11:886–894

Carlo-Stella C, Cesana C, Regazzi E et al (2000) Peripheral blood progenitor cell mobilization in healthy donors receiving recombinant human granulocyte colony-stimulating factor. Exp Hematol 28:216–224

Carotta S, Pilat S, Mairhofer A, Schmidt U, Dolznig H, Steinlein P, Beug H (2004) Directed differentiation and mass cultivation of pure erythroid progenitors from mouse embryonic stem cells. Blood 104:1873–1880

Cerdan C, Rouleau A, Bhatia M (2004) VEGF-A_{165} augments erythropoietic development form human embryonic stem cells. Blood 103:2504–2510

Chadderton N, Millington-Ward S, Palfi A, O'Reilly M, Tuohy G, Humphries MM, Li T, Humphries P, Kenna PF, Farrar GJ (2009) Improved retinal function in a mouse model of dominant retinitis pigmentosa following AAV-delivered gene therapy. Mol Ther 17(4):593–599

Chen LB, Jiang XB, Yang L (2004) Differentiation of rat marrow mesenchymal stem cells into pancreatic islet beta-cells. World J Gastroenterol 10:3016–3020

Cheng L-C, Pastrana E, Tavazoie M, Doetsch F (2009) miR-124 regulates adult neurogenesis in the subventricular zone stem cell niche. Nat Neurosci 12(4):399–405

Christopherson II KW, Hangoc G, Mantel CR, Broxmeyer HE (2004) Modulation of hematopoietic stem cell homing and engraftment by CD26. Science 305:1000–1004

Davoust N, Vuaillat C, Cavillon G, Domenget C, Hatterer E, Bernard A, Dumontel C, Jurdic P, Malcus C, Confavreux C, Belin MF, Nataf S (2006) Bone marrow CD34+/B220+ progenitors target the inflamed brain and display in vitro differentiation potential toward microglia. FASEB J 20:2081–2092

Demedts M, Behr J, Buhl R, Costabel U, Dekhuijzen R, Jansen HM, MacNee W, Thomeer M, Wallaert B, Laurent F, Nicholson AG, Verbeken EK, Verschakelen J, Flower CDR, Capron F, Petruzzelli S, DeVuyst P, van den Bosch JMM, Rodriguez-Becerra E, Corvasce G, Lankhorst I, Sardina M, Montanari M (2005) High-dose acetylcysteine in idiopathic pulmonary fibrosis. N Engl J Med 353:2229–2242

Deng W, Han Q, Liao L, Li C, Ge W, Zhao Z, You Sheng, Deng H, Murad F, Zhao RCH (2005) Engrafted bone marrow-derived Flk-1+ mesenchymal stem cells regenerate skin tissue. Tissue Eng 11:110–119

Dexter TM, Allen TD, Lajtha LG (1977) Conditions controlling the proliferation of hematopoietic stem cells in vitro. J Cell Physiol 91:335–344

Dickson GJ, Kwasniewska A, Mills KI, Lappin TRJ, Thompson A (2009) Hoxa6 potentiates short-term hematopoietic cell proliferation and extended self-renewal. Exp Hematol 37:322–333

Dileto C, Travis EL (1996) Fibroblast radiosensitivity in vitro and lung fibrosis in vivo: comparison between a fibrosis-prone and fibrosis-resistant mouse strain. Radiat Res 146:61–67

Engelhardt JF (2001) Stem cell niches in the mouse airway. Am J Respir Cell Mol Biol 24:649–652

Engelhardt JF, Yang Y, Stratford-Perricaudet LD, Allen ED, Kozarsky K, Perricaudet M, Yankaskas JR, Wilson JM (1993) Direct gene transfer of human CFTR into human bronchial epithelia of xenografts with E1-deleted adenoviruses. Nat Genet 4:27–34

Epperly MW, Sikora CA, Defilippi S, Gretton JE, Greenberger JS (2003) Bone marrow origin of myofibroblasts in irradiation pulmonary fibrosis. Am J Resp Mol Cell Biol 29:213–224

Epperly MW, Osipov AN, Martin I, Kawai K, Borisenko GG, Jefferson M, Bernarding M, Greenberger JS, Kagan VE (2004a) Ascorbate as a "redox-sensor" and protector against irradiation-induced oxidative stress in 32D cl 3 hematopoietic cells and subclones overexpressing human manganese Superoxide Dismutase. Int J Radiat Oncol Biol Phys 58(3):851–861

Epperly MW, Goff JP, Sikora CA, Shields DS, Greenberger JS (2004b) Bone marrow origin of cells with capacity for homing and differentiation to esophageal squamous epithelium. Radiat Res 162:233–240

Epperly MW, Cao S, Zhang X, Franicola D, Kanai AJ, Greenberger EE, Greenberger JS (2007) Increased longevity of hematopoiesis in continuous bone marrow cultures derived from mtNOS−/− homozygous recombinant negative mice correlates with increased radioresistance of hematopoietic and bone marrow stromal cells. Exp Hematol 35:137–145

Erices A, Conget P, Minguell JJ (2000) Mesenchymal progenitor cells in human umbilical cord blood. Br J Haematol 109:235–242

Franko AJ, Sharplin J (1994) Development of fibrosis after lung irradiation in relation to inflammation and lung function in a mouse strain prone to fibrosis. Radiat Res 140:347–355

Friedenstein AJ, Lat-Zink NW, Grosheva AG, Gorskaya VF (1982) Microenvironment transfer by heterotopic transplantation of freshly cultured cells in porous sponges. Exp Hematol 10:217–227

Giangreco A, Arwert EN, Rosewell IR, Snyder J, Watt FM, Stripp BR (2009) Stem cells are dispensable for lung homeostasis but restore airways after injury. PNAS 106(23):9286–9291

Gokhale AS, Epperly M, Glowacki J, Wang H, Wipf P, Pierce JG, Dixon T, Patrene K, Greenberger JS (2010) Small molecule GS-nitroxide ameliorate ionizing irradiation-induced delay in bone wound healing in a novel murine model. In vivo 24:377–384

Goolsby J, Marty MC, Heletz D, Chiappelli J, Tashko G, Yarnell D, Fishman PS, Dhib-Jalbut S, Bever CT, Pessac B, Trisler D (2003) Hematopoietic progenitors express neural genes. PNAS 100: 14926–14931

Greenberger JS (1978) Sensitivity of corticosteroid-dependent, insulin-resistant lipogenesis in marrow preadipocytes of mutation diabetic-obese mice. Nature 275:752–754

Greenberger JS (1991) Toxic effects on the hematopoietic microenvironment. Exp Hematol 19:1101–1109

Greenberger JS, Epperly MW (2007) Antioxidant therapeutic approaches toward amelioration of the pulmonary pathophysiological damaging effects of ionizing irradiation. Curr Respir Med Rev 3:29–37

Greenberger JS, Epperly MW (2009) Bioengineering in the repair of irradiated normal tissue by bone marrow derived stem cell populations. Semi Radiat Oncol (19(2):133–139

Greenberger JS, FitzGerald TJ, Kleason V, Anklesaria P, Bushnell D, Kase K, Sakakeeny MA (1988) Alteration in hematopoietic stem cell seeding and proliferation by low-dose-rate irradiation of bone marrow stromal cells in vitro. Int J Radiat Oncol Biol Phys 14:85–94

Gronthos S, Graves SE, Ohta S, Simmons PJ (1994) The STRO-1+ fraction of adult human bone marrow contains the osteogenic precursors. Blood 84:4164–4173

Gussoni E, Soneoka Y, Strickland CD et al (1999) Dystrophin expression in the mdx mouse restored by stem cell transplantation. Nature 401:390–394

Habich A, Jurga M, Markiewicz I, Lukomska B, Bany-Laszewicz U, Domanska-Janik K (2006) Early appearance of stem/progenitor cells with neural-like characteristics in human cord blood mononuclear fraction cultured in vitro. Exp Hematol 34:914–925

Hall EJ (ed) (1988) Radiobiology for the radiobiologist, 3rd edn. JB Lippincott Company, Philadelphia

Hazen AL, Smith MJ, Desponts C, Winter O, Moser K, Kerr WG (2009) SHIP is required for a functional hematopoietic stem cell niche. Blood 113:2924–2930

Heissig B, Hattori K, Dias S, Friedrich M, Ferris B, Hackett NR, Crystal RG, Besmer P, Lyden D, Moore MAS, Werb Z, Rafii S (2002) Recruitment of stem and progenitor cells from the bone marrow niche requires MMP-9 mediated release of Kit-Ligand. Cell 109:625–637

Hirschi KK, Goodell MA (2002) Hematopoietic, vascular, and cardiac fates of bone marrow-derived stem cells. Gene Ther 9:648–652

Ibanez IL, Bracalente C, Molinari BL, Palmieri MA, Policastro L, Kreiner AJ, Burlon AA, Valda A, Navalesi D, Davidson J, Davidson M, Vazquez M, Ozafran M, Duran H (2009) Induction and rejoining of DNA double strand breaks assessed by H2AX phosphorylation in melanoma cells irradiated with proton and lithium beams. Int J Radiat Oncol Biol Phys 74:1226–1235

Ishikawa F, Yasukawa M, Yoshida S, Nakamura KI, Nagatoshi Y, Kanemaru T, Shimoda K, Shimoda S, Miyamoto T, Okamura J, Shultz LD, Harada M (2004) Human cord blood- and bone marrow-derived CD34+ cells regenerate gastrointestinal epithelial cells. FASEBJ 18:1958–1960

Jackson KA, Majka SM, Wang H, Pocius J, Hartley CJ, Majesky MW, Entman ML, Michael LH, Hirschi KK, Goodell MA (2001) Regeneration of ischemic cardiac muscle and vascular endothelium by adult stem cells. J Clin Invest 107:1395–1402

Jahroudi N, Ardekani AM, Greenberger JS (1996) Ionizing irradiation increases transcription of the von Willebrand factor gene in endothelial cells. Blood 88:3801–3814

Jiang J, Kurnikov I, Belikova NA, Xiao J, Zhao Q, Vlasova IL, Amoscato AA, Braslau R, Studer A, Fink MP, Greenberger JS, Wipf Pe, Kagan VE (2007) Structural requirements for optimized delivery, inhibition of oxidative stress an anti-apoptotic activity of targeted nitroxides. J Pharmacol Exp Ther 320(5):1050–1060

Jones DL, Wagers J (2008) No place like home: anatomy and function of the stem cell niche. Mol Cell Biol 9:11–20

Kagan VE, Bayir A, Bayir H, Stoyanovsky D, Borisenko GG, Tyurina YY, Wipf P, Atkinson J, Greenberger JS, Chapkin RS, Belikova NA (2009) Mitochondria-targeted disruptors and inhibitors of cytochrome c/cardiolipin peroxidase complexes: a new strategy in anti-apoptotic drug discovery. Mol Nutr Food Res 53:104–114

Kalabis J, Oyama K, Okawa T, Nakagawa H, Michaylira CZ, Stairs DB, Figueiredo J-L, Mahmood U, Diehl JA, Rustgi AK (2008) A subpopulation of mouse esophageal basal cells has properties of stem cells with the capacity for self-renewal and lineage specification. J Clin Invest 118:3860–3868

Kaminski A, Pohl CB, Sponholz C, Ma N, Stamm C, Vollmar B, Steinhoff G (2004) Up-regulation of endothelial nitric oxide synthase inhibits pulmonary *leukocyte* migration following lung ischemia-reperfusion in mice. Am J Pathol 164(6):2241–2249

Kamishina H, Cheeseman JA, Clemmons RM (2008) Nestin-positive spheres derived from canine bone marrow stromal cells generate cells with early neuronal and glial phenotypic characteristics. In Vitro Cell Dev Biol Animal 44:140–144

Kataoka K, Medina RJ, Kageyama T, Miyazaki M, Yoshino T, Makino T, Huh Nam-ho (2003) Participation of adult mouse bone marrow cells in reconstitution of skin. Am J Pathol 163(4): 1227–1231

Kiel MJ, Yilmaz OH, Iwashita T, Yilmaz OH, Terhorst C, Morrison SJ (2005) SLAM family receptors distinguish hematopoietic stem and progenitor cells and reveal endothelial niches for stem cells. Cell 121:1109–1121

Kim HK, De La Luz Sierra M, Williams CK, Gulino AV, Tosato G (2006) G-CSF down-regulation of CXCR4 expression identified as a mechanism for mobilization of myeloid cells. Blood 108:812–820

Korbling M, Katz RL, Khanna A, Ruifrok AC, Rondon G, Albitar M, Champlin RE, Estrov Z (2002) Hepatocytes and epithelial cells of donor origin in recipients of peripheral-blood stem cells. N Engl J Med 346:738–746

Krause D, Theise N, Collector M et al (2001) Multi-organ, multi-lineage engraftment by a single bone marrow-derived stem cell. Cell 105:369–377

Kyung UH, Reynolds SD, Watkins S, Fuchs E, Stripp BR (2004) Basal cells are a multipotent progenitor capable of renewing the bronchial epithelium. Am J Pathol 164:577–588

Lagasse E, Shizuru JA, Uchida N, Tsukamoto A, Weissman IL (2001) Toward regenerative medicine. Immun 14:425–436

Lamba BA, Karl MO, Ware CB, Reh TA (2006) Efficient generation of retinal progenitor cells from human embryonic stem cells. PNAS 103:12769–12774

Lanza RP, Atala A (eds) (2002) Methods of tissue engineering. Academic Press, New York

Leask A, Abraham DJ (2004) TGF-B signaling and the fibrotic response. FASEB J 18:816–827

Lechpammer S, Epperly MW, Zhou S, Nie S, Glowacki J, Greenberger JS (2005) Antioxidant pool regulated adipocyte differentiation Sod2−/− bone marrow stromal cells. Exp Hematol 33:1201–1208

Lei Ye, Haider HKA, Sim EKW (2006) Adult stem cells for cardiac repair: a choice between skeletal myoblasts and bone marrow stem cells. Exp Biol Med 231:8–19

Li H, Liu H, Heller S (2003) Pluripotent stem cells from the adult mouse inner ear. Nat Med 9(10):1293–1299

Li W, Ferguson BJ, Khaled WT, Tevendale M, Stingl J, Poli V, Rich T, Salomoni P, Watson CJ (2009) DML depletion disrupts normal mammary gland development and skews the composition of the mammary luminal cell progenitor pool. PNAS 106:4725–4730

Lim DA, Huang Y-C, Swigut T, Mirick AL, Garcia-Verdugo JM, Wysocka J, Ernst P, Alvarez-Bo (2009) Chromatin remodeling factor Mll1 is essential for neurogenesis from postnatal neural stem cells. Nature 458:529–336

Lin W, Chen X, Wang X, Liu J, Gu X (2008) Adult rat bone marrow stromal cells differentiate into Schwann cell-like cells in vitro. In Vitro Cell Dev Biol Animal 44:31–40

Link CJ, Orren D, Muldoon R, Cook JA, Bohr VA (1996) Pentoxifylline inhibits gene-specific repair of UV-induced DNA damage in hamster cells. Rad Onc Invest 4:115–121

Lombaert IMA, Brunsting JF, Wierenga PK, Kampinga HH, de Haan G, Coppes RP (2008) Cytokine treatment improves parenchymal and vascular damage of salivary glands after irradiation. Clin Cancer Res 14(23):7741–7748

Lue Y, Erkkila K, Liu PY, Ma K, Wang C, Hikim AS, Swerdloff RS (2007) Fate of bone marrow stem cells transplanted into the testis: potential implication for men with testicular failure. Am J Pathol, 170(3):899–908

Matsuzaki Y, Kinjo K, Mulligan RC et al (2004) Unexpectedly efficient homing capacity of purified murine hematopoietic stem cells. Immunity 20:87–93

Mauch P, Greenberger JS, Botnick LE, Hannon EC, Hellman S (1980) Evidence for structured variation in self-renewal capacity within long-term bone marrow cultures. PNAS 77:2927–2930

McCulloch EA, Till JE (1962) The sensitivity of cells from normal mouse bone marrow to gamma radiation in vitro and in vivo. Radiat Res 16:822–832

Mezey E, Chandross KJ, Harta G, Maki RA, McKercher SR (2000) Turning blood into brain: cells bearing neuronal antigens generated in vivo from bone marrow. Science 290:1779–1783

Miyahara Y, Nagaya N, Kataoka M, Yanagawa B, Tanaka K, Hao H, Ishino K, Ishida H, Shimizu T, Kangawa K, Sano S, Okano T, Kitamura S, Mori H (2006) Monolayered mesenchymal stem cells repair scarred myocardium after myocardial infarction. Nat Med 12(4):459–468

Montini E, Cesana D, Schmidt M, Sanvito F, Bartholomae CC, Ranzani M, Benedicenti F, Sergi LS, Ambrosi A, Ponzoni M, Doglioni C, Di SC, von Kalle C, Naldini L (2009) The genotoxic potential of retroviral vectors is strongly modulated by vector design and integration site selection in a mouse model of HSC gene therapy. J Clin Invest 110:964–975

Mookerjee I, Hewitson TD, Halls ML, Summers RJ, Mathai ML, Bathgate RAD, Tregear GW, Samuel CS (2009) Relaxin inhibits renal myofibroblast differentiation via RXFP1, the nitric oxide pathway and Smad2. FASEBJ 23:1219–1229

Mothersill C, Seymour CB (2004) Radiation-induced bystander effects-implications for cancer. Nat Rev Cancer 4:158–164

Munoz JR, Stoutenger BR, Robinson AP, Spees JL, Prockop DJ (2005) Human stem/progenitor cells from bone marrow promote neurogenesis of endogenous neural stem cells in the hippocampus of mice. PNAS 102:18171–18176

Murayama T, Tepper OM, Silver M, Ma H, Losordo DW, Isner JM, Asahara T, Kalka C (2002) Determination of bone marrow-derived endothelial progenitor cell significance in angiogenic growth factor-induced neovascularization in vivo. Exp Hematol 30:967–972

Naparstek E, Donnelly T, Kase K, Greenberger JS (1985) Biologic effects of in vitro x-irradiation of murine long-term bone marrow cultures on the production of granulocyte-macrophage colony stimulating factors. Exp Hematol 13:701–708

Niu Y, Epperly MW, Shen H, Smith T, Lewis D, Gollin S, Greenberger JS (2008) Intraesophageal MnSOD-plasmid liposome administration enhances engraftment and self-renewal capacity of bone marrow derived progenitors of esophageal squamous epithelium. Gene Therapy 15:347–356

Novakova-Jiresova A, van Gameren MM, Coppes RP, Kampinga HH, Groen HJM (2004) Transforming growth factor-B plasma dynamics and post-irradiation lung injury in lung cancer patients. Radiother Oncol 71:183–189

Oberley LW, Buettner GR (1979) Role of superoxide dismutase in cancer: a review. Cancer Res 39:1141–1149

Ogle BM, Cascalho M, Platt JL (2005) Biological implications of cell fusion. Mol Cell Biol 6:567

Ohtaki H, Ylostalo JH, Foraker JE, Robinson AP, Reger RL, Shioda S, Prockop DJ (2008) Stem/progenitor cells from bone marrow decrease neuronal death in global ischemia by modulation of inflammatory/immune responses. PNAS 105:14638–14643

Olive PL, Banath JP (2004) Phosphorylation of histone H2AX as a measure of radiosensitivity. Int J Radiat Oncol Biol Phys 58:331–335

Ortiz LA, Gambelli F, McBride C, Gaupp D, Baddoo M, Kaminski N, Phinney DG (2003) Mesenchymal stem cell engraftment in lung is enhanced in response to bleomycin exposure and ameliorates its fibrotic effects. PNAS 100(14):8407–8411

Park HC, Shim YS, Ha Y, Yoon SH, Park SR, Choi BH, Park HS (2005) Treatment of complete spinal cord injury patients by autologous bone marrow cell transplantation and administration of granulocyte-macrophage colony stimulating factor. Tissue Eng 11:913–922

Parmar K, Mauch P, Vergilio Jo-A, Sackstein R, Down JD (2007) Distribution of hematopoietic stem cells in the bone marrow according to regional hypoxia. PNAS 104:5431–5436

Petersen BE, Bowen WC, Patrene KD, Mars WM, Sullivan AK, Boggs SS, Greenberger JS, Goff JP (1999) Bone marrow as a potential source of hepatic oval cells. Science 284:1168–1170

Pittenger MF, Mackay AM, Beck SC et al (1999) Multilineage potential of adult human mesenchymal stem cells. Science 284:143–147

Prise KM, O'Sullivan JM (2009) Radiation-induced bystander signaling in cancer therapy. Nat Rev Cancer 9:351–365

Prockop DJ (1997) Marrow stromal cells as stem cells for nonhematopoietic tissues. Science 276:71

Proksch S, Bel A, Puymirat E, Pidial L, Bellamy V, Peyrard S, Larghero J, Augereau-Vacher B, Menasche P (2009) Does the human skeletal muscle harbor the murine equivalents of cardiac precursor cells? Mol Ther 17(4):733–741

Quesenberry PJ, Colvin G, Abedi M (2005) Perspective fundamental and clinical concepts on stem cell homing and engraftment: a journey to niches and beyond. Exp Hematol 33:9–19

Reynolds SD, Giangreco A, Hong KU, McGrath KE, Ortiz LA, Stripp BR (2004) Airway injury in lung disease pathophysiology: selective depletion of airway stem and progenitor cell pools potentiates lung inflammation and alveolar dysfunction. Am J Physiol Lung Cell Mol Physiol 287:L1256–L1265

Rice A, Barbot C, Lacombe F, Dubosc-Marchenay N, Marit G, Hau F, Boiron JM, Reiffers J (1993) 5-fluorouracil permits access to a primitive subpopulation of peripheral blood stem cells. Stem Cells 11:326–335

Roy V, Verfaillie CM (1999) Expression and function of cell adhesion molecules on fetal liver, cord blood and bone marrow hematopoietic progenitors: implications for anatomical localization and developmental stage specific regulation of hematopoiesis. Exp Hematol 27:302–312

Rubin P, Cassarett GW (1968) Clinical radiation pathology, vol 1. WB Saunders, Philadelphia

Sakai E, Kitajima K, Sato A, Nakano T (2009) Increase of hematopoietic progenitor and suppression of endothelial gene expression by Runx1 expression during in vitro ES differentiation. Exp Hematol 37:334–345

Sakakeeny MA, Greenberger JS (1982) Granulopoiesis longevity in continuous bone marrow cultures and factor dependent cell line generation: significant variation among 28 inbred mouse strains and outbred stocks. J Nat Cancer Inst 68:305–317

Sasportas LS, Kasmieh R, Wakimoto H, Hingtgen S, van de Water Jeroen AJM, Mohapatra G, Figueiredo JL, Martuza RL, Weissleder R, Shah K (2009) Assessment of therapeutic efficacy and fate of engineered human mesenchymal stem cells for cancer therapy. Proc Natl Acad Sci U S A 106(12):4822–4827

Schmitz N, Linch DC, Dreger P et al (1996) Randomized trial of filgrastim-mobilized peripheral blood progenitor cell transplantation versus autologous bone-marrow transplantation in lymphoma patients. Lancet 347:353–357

Semerad CL, Christopher MJ, Liu F et al (2005) G-CSF potently inhibits osteoblast activity and CXCL12 mRNA expression in the bone marrow. Blood 106:3020–3027

Shimonaka M, Katagiri K, Nakayama T, Fujita N, Tsuruo T, Yoshie O, Kinashi T (2003) Rap1 translates chemokine signals to integrin activation, cell polarization, and motility across vascular endothelium under flow. J Cell Biol 161(2):417–427

Sigurjonsson OE, Perreault MC, Egeland T, Glover JC (2005) Adult human hematopoietic stem cells produce neurons efficiently in the regenerating chicken embryo spinal cord. PNAS 102:5227–5232

Simard AR, Rivest S (2004) Bone marrow stem cells have the ability to populate the entire central nervous system into fully differentiated parenchymal microglia. FASEB J 18:998–1000

Spyridonidis A, Schmitt-Graff A, Tomann T, Dwenger A, Follo M, Behringer D, Finke J (2004) Epithelial tissue chimerism after human hematopoietic cell transplantation is a real phenomenon. Am J Pathol 164:1147–1155

Stripp BR, Reynolds SD (2005) Bioengineered lung epithelium: implications for basic and applied studies in lung tissue regeneration. Am J Respir Cell Mol Biol 32:85–86

Switzer GE, Goycoolea JM, Dew MA, Graeff EC, Hegland J (2001) Donating stimulated peripheral blood stem cells vs. bone marrow: do donors experience the procedures differently? Bone Marrow Transplant 27:917–923

Takakura N, Watanabe T, Suenobu S, Yamada Y, Noda T, Ito Y, Satake M, Suda T (2000) A role for hematopoietic stem cells in promoting angiogenesis. Cell 102:199–209

Terskikh AV, Miyamoto T, Chang C, Diatchenko L, Weissman IL (2003) Gene expression analysis of purified hematopoietic stem cells and committed progenitors. Blood 102:94–102

Theise ND, Badve S, Saxena R, Henegariu O, Sell S, Crawford JM, Krause DS (2000) Derivation of hepatocytes from bone marrow cells in mice after radiation-induced myeloablation. Hepatology 31:235–240

Till JE, McCulloch EA (1961) Developmental aspects of the cell cycle, vol 971. Academic Press, New York, pp 297–313

Tjwa M, Sidenius N, Moura R, Jansen S, Theunissen K, Andolfo A, DeMol M, Dewerchin M, Moons L, Blasi F, Verfailie C, Carmeliet P (2009) Membrane-anchored uPAR regulates the proliferation, marrow pool size, engraftment, and mobilization of mouse hematopoietic stem/progenitor cells. J Clin Invest 119(4):1008–1018

Torres P, Maria E, Parfitt David E, Kouzarides T, Zernicka-Goetz M (2007) Histone arginine methylation regulates pluripotency in the early mouse embryo. Nature 445:214–220

Tsao GJ, Allen JA, Logronio KA, Lazzeroni LC, Shizuru JA (2009) Purified hematopoietic stem cell allografts reconstitute immunity superior to bone marrow. PNAS 106:3288–3293

Tyurin VA, Tyurina YY, Kochanek PM, Hamilton R, DeKosky ST, Greenberger JS, Bayir H, Kagan VE (2008) Oxidative lipidomics of programmed cell death. Methods Enzymol 442:375–393

Tyurina YY, Tyurin VA, Epperly MW, Greenberger JS, Kagan VE (2008) Oxidative lipidomics of γ-irradiation induced intestinal injury. Free Radic Biol Med 44:299–314

Unwin RD, Smith DL, Blinco D, Wilson CL, Miller CJ, Evans CA, Jaworska E, Baldwin SA, Barnes K, Pierce Andrew, Spooncer Elaine, Whetton Anthony D (2006) Quantitative proteomics reveals posttranslational control as a regulatory factor in primary hematopoietic stem cells. Blood 107:4687–4693

van der Kogel AJ, Sissingh HA, Zoetelief J (1982) Effect of x-rays and neutrons on repair and regeneration in the rat spinal cord. Int J Radiat Oncol Biol Phys 8:2095–2097

van Hennik PB, de Koning AE, Ploemacher RE (1999) Seeding efficiency of primitive human hematopoietic cells in nonobese diabetic/severe combined immune deficiency mice: implications for stem cell frequency assessment. Blood 94(9):3055–3061

van Rongen E, Thames HD, Travis EL (1993) Recovery from radiation damage in mouse lung: Interpretations in terms of two rates of repair. Radiat Res 133:225–233

Wagers AJ, Christensen JL, Weissman IL (2002) Cell fate determination from stem cells. Gene Ther 9:606–612

Werts ED, Gibson DP, Knapp SA et al (1980) Bone marrow fibroblasts circulate to replace damaged marrow sites. Radiat Res 81:20–30

Woodward WA, Chen MS, Behbod F, Alfaro MP, Buchholz TA, Rosen JM (2007) WNT/β-catenin mediates radiation resistance of mouse mammary progenitor cells. PNAS 104:618–623

Wright DE, Wagers AJ, Gulati AP, Johnson FL, Weissman IL (2001) Physiological migration of hematopoietic stem and progenitor cells. Science 294:1933–1936

Hess D, Li L, Martin M, Sakano S, Hill D, Strutt B, Thyssen S, Gray DA, Bhatia M (2003) Bone marrow-derived stem cells initiate pancreatic regeneration. Nat Biotechnol 21:763–770

Yoon Y, Wecker A, Heyd L, Park J, Tkebuchava T, Kusano K, Hanley A, Scadova H, Qin G, Cha D, Johnson KL, Aikawa R, Asahara T, Losordo DW (2005) Clonally expanded novel multipotent stem cells from human bone marrow regenerate myocardium after myocardial infarction. J Clin Invest 115:326–338

Young PP, Vaughan DE, Hatzopoulos AK (2007) Biologic properties of endothelial progenitor cells and their potential for cell therapy. Prog Cardiovasc Dis 49:421–429

Yoyooka Y, Tsunekawa N, Akasu R, Noce T (2003) Embryonic stem cells can form germ cells in vitro. PNAS 100:11457–11462

Zaibak F, Kozlovski J, Vadolas J, Sarsero JP, Williamson R, Howden SE (2009) Integration of functional bacterial artificial chromosomes into human cord blood-derived multipotent stem cells. Gene Ther 16:404–414

Zeng F, Chen M, Baldwin DA, Gong Z, Yan J, Qian H, Wang J, Jiang X, Ren Z, Sun Deming, Huang S (2006) Multiorgan engraftment and differentiation of human cord blood CD34+ Lin- cells in goats assessed by gene expression profiling. PNAS 103:7801–7806

Zhang J, Niu C, Ye L et al (2003) Identification of the haematopoietic stem cell niche and control of the niche size. Nature 425:836–841

Zhou S, Yates KE, Eid K, Glowacki J (2005) Demineralized bone promotes chondrocyte or osteoblast differentiation of human

marrow stromal cells cultured in collagen sponges. Cell Tissue Banking 6:33–44
Zhou S, Greenberger JS, Epperly MW, Goff JP, Adler C, LeBoff MS, Glowacki J (2008) Age-related intrinsic changes in human bone marrow-derived mesenchymal stem cells and their differentiation to osteoblasts. Aging Cell 7:335–343
Zipori D (2004) The nature of stem cells: state rather than entity. Nat Rev 5:873–883

Radiotherapy-Induced Carcinogenesis and Leukemogenesis: Mechanisms and Quantitative Modeling

David J. Brenner, Igor Shuryak, and Rainer K. Sachs

Contents

D. J. Brenner (✉) · I. Shuryak
Center for Radiological Research,
Columbia University Medical Center,
New York, NY, USA
e-mail: djb3@columbia.edu

R. K. Sachs
Departments of Mathematics and Physics,
University of California, Berkeley, CA, USA

Abstract

Biologically-based modeling of spontaneous and radiation-induced carcinogenesis has a history spanning several decades. Such models are important conceptual and quantitative tools, particularly useful whenever cancer risks must be estimated under exposure situations for which no data yet exist, e.g., for novel and prospective radiotherapy protocols. Direct extrapolation from existing data is often not possible due to complex differences between the data sets, but quantitative models can accommodate such extrapolation. Many carcinogenesis models can be characterized as short-term, in that they focus on those processes occurring during and shortly after irradiation. The main advantage of this class of models is that they provide a detailed initial dose response for short-term endpoints which are used as surrogates for carcinogenesis. The main disadvantage is that the possibly substantial modulations of the magnitude and shape of this initial dose response during the lengthy period between irradiation and manifestation of typical solid tumors are not considered. In contrast with the short-term models, another class of biologically-motivated models can be characterized as long-term, in the sense that they track carcinogenesis mechanisms throughout the entire human life span. The main advantages of long-term models are: (1) modulation of the radiation dose response during the long latency period between exposure and diagnosis of cancer is included; and (2) extensive data on spontaneous cancers can be used to help determine the adjustable parameters needed to estimate cancer risks. The main disadvantage is that the early radiation response is typically treated in a less-mechanistic manner than in the short-term models. Here we review some short- and long-term model examples and the carcinogenesis mechanisms which they incorporate. We also discuss an example of unification of both model classes, focusing on application of such formalisms for quantifying radiotherapy-induced second cancer risks.

P. Rubin et al. (eds.), *ALERT – Adverse Late Effects of Cancer Treatment*, Medical Radiology. Radiation Oncology,
DOI: 10.1007/978-3-540-72314-1_14, © Springer-Verlag Berlin Heidelberg 2014

1 Introduction

Ionizing radiation is a well-known cytotoxic and carcinogenic agent. As such, it is effective as a treatment for cancer, but can also induce secondary malignancies (Curtis et al. 2006) (see also the chapter titled "Understanding and Predicting Radiation-Associated Normal Tissue Injury: A Global and Historical Perspective"). As more patients undergo cancer radiotherapy, and live longer after treatment, the number of cancer survivors has tripled over the past three decades and continues to increase, reaching >10 million (Curtis et al. 2006; Anonymous 2004). The lifetime risk of radiation-induced second cancers in these individuals is not negligible (Brenner et al. 2007), and these second cancers can result in high mortality and morbidity—for example, breast cancer radiotherapy can cause lung cancer, and lung cancer has a poor prognosis. Consequently, second malignancies induced by radiotherapy are becoming a growing concern (Brenner et al. 2000; Ron 2006). This is the case particularly for patients irradiated in childhood, who have a long life expectancy during which second cancers can develop, and in whom the relative risk of some radiogenic second cancers is on the order of 10–100 (Ron 2006; Ronckers et al. 2006; Neglia et al. 2006).

It has recently become clearer (Lindsay et al. 2001; Sachs and Brenner 2005) that even at high radiation doses—tens of Gy—radiation-induced cancer risk remains substantial, presumably due to cellular repopulation, instead of dropping essentially to zero due to cell inactivation (killing), as was previously thought by many radiobiologists (Bennett et al. 2004; Dasu et al. 2005). Thus, tissues surrounding the tumor, which unavoidably receive doses not much smaller than the prescribed treatment dose, may be a source of much of the second cancer risk attributable to radiotherapy (Hodgson et al. 2007; Koh et al. 2007). The remaining portion of the radiation-induced risk is derived from large volumes of tissues more distant from the treatment target, which receive lower radiation doses. An example of the estimated relative contributions of high- and low-dose regions to overall radiogenic cancer risk is shown in Fig. 1.

A reasonable approach to minimizing radiation-induced second cancers would be to compare radiotherapy protocols of equal efficacy against the primary tumor, and identify the ones with the lowest second cancer risk. However, because the latency period for radiation-induced solid tumors is long (Curtis et al. 2006; Brenner et al. 2000; BEIR VII Report 2005; Ivanov et al. 2004), the carcinogenic effects of radiotherapy have been directly measured only for regimens used several decades ago. The risks which may be associated with newer treatment methods are for the most part not yet observable. Biologically motivated mathematical/computational models, calibrated using data from older protocols, can address this problem by predicting risks of current (and prospective) treatment regimens.

A systematic review of the epidemiological data on second cancers has been given in the chapter titled "Understanding and Predicting Radiation-Associated Normal Tissue Injury: A Global and Historical Perspective ". Here, we discuss some biologically based models of spontaneous and radiation-induced carcinogenesis in the literature, and analyze their potential for predicting second cancers due to modern treatment protocols. Most of the discussion focuses on solid tumors. Leukemias, which can be substantially different from solid tumors in terms of latency period and dose–response relationships, are treated separately. We also discuss an example of a potentially useful approach for improving biologically based second cancer modeling by unifying some current model concepts to produce a formalism which includes both short- and long-term mechanisms important for radiation carcinogenesis.

2 Short-Term Biologically Based Models

Biologically motivated mathematical modeling of spontaneous and ionizing radiation-induced carcinogenesis has a history spanning more than 50 years (Nordling 1953; Armitage and Doll 1954). Many biologically based models can be characterized as *short-term,* in that they focus on those processes occurring during and shortly (i.e., about 1 month or less) after irradiation (Sachs and Brenner 2005; Nilsson et al. 1990; Thames 1985; Dale 1986; Sontag 1997; Lange et al. 1997; Zaider and Wuu 1995; Stewart 2001; Curtis 1986; Tobias 1985; Radivoyevitch et al. 2001; Hahnfeldt and Hlatky 1996, 1998; Mebust et al. 2002; Schollnberger et al. 2002; Hofmann et al. 2006; Sachs et al. 2007; Shuryak et al. 2006; Little 2007; Schneider and Kaser-Hotz 2005; Schneider and Walsh 2008). These models typically analyze the induction of short-term endpoints which are used as surrogates for carcinogenesis, such as mutations or chromosome aberrations (Radivoyevitch et al. 2001; Ottolenghi et al. 1999). Different short-term models analyze DNA damage induction and DNA repair/misrepair (Nilsson et al. 1990; Sontag 1997; Stewart 2001; Curtis 1986; Tobias 1985). Short-term models take into account a variety of phenomena such as dose rate effects (Thames 1985; Rossi and Kellerer 1986; Brenner et al. 1996), induction and/or saturation of particular repair pathways (Schollnberger et al. 2002), and alterations of the cell cycle distribution during/after irradiation (Zaider and Wuu 1995; Hahnfeldt and Hlatky 1996, 1998). Many short-term models are motivated toward radiation-induced cancer risk estimation at low radiation doses (Bennett et al. 2004), but some have also been adapted to predict radiotherapy-induced second cancers

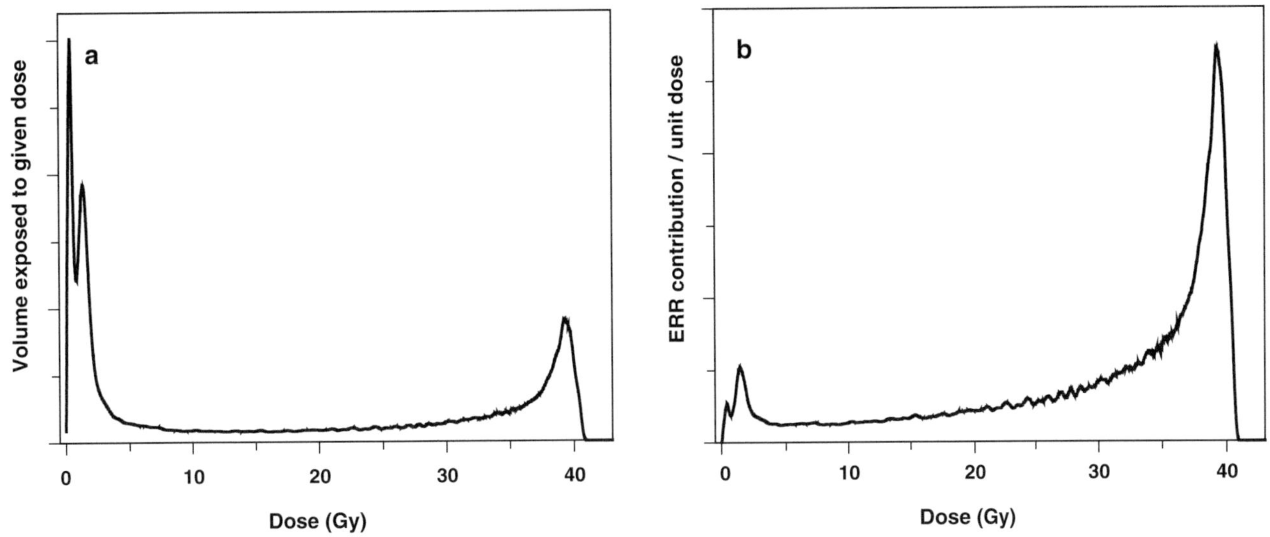

Fig. 1 Estimation of radiation-induced second-cancer risks based on a dose-volume histogram (DVH). The DVH (**a**) is for the left breast of a female treated for breast cancer by radiotherapy; the doses are in 0.5 cGy intervals. **b** The estimated contribution of different dose intervals within the irradiated breast to the overall excess relative risk (ERR), assuming the dose–response relationship for the ERR is approximately linear in dose

(Dasu et al. 2005; Dale 1986; Schneider and Kaser-Hotz 2005; Schneider and Walsh 2008). The common feature of these short-term models is that the long-term processes involved in carcinogenesis, which are dominant before radiation exposure and in the long latency period after initial tissue recovery from radiation damage, are typically treated indirectly, nonmechanistically, or not at all. Often a proportional hazards assumption is used to justify taking the shape of the cancer incidence dose–response curve as being the same, apart from an overall scaling factor, as the shape of the dose–response curve for some short-term surrogate endpoint (BEIR VII Report 2005; Upton 2003; NCRP Report 136 2001).

The main advantage of this class of models is that they provide a detailed initial dose response for short-term endpoints which are used as surrogates for carcinogenesis. The main disadvantage is that the possibly substantial modulations of the magnitude and shape of this initial dose response during the lengthy period (multiple years decades in humans) between irradiation and manifestation of typical solid tumors are not considered; a simple proportional hazards assumption, plausible at low doses, becomes questionable at the high doses responsible for some second cancers.

Among the great variety of mathematical formalisms which can be classified as short-term radiation carcinogenesis models, we here focus on those models designed specifically for analyzing radiotherapy-induced second cancers.

2.1 The Linear Quadratic Exponential Model

The assumption that radiation-induced carcinogenesis is primarily governed by a balance of cell mutation (also commonly referred to as initiation) and cell killing (often referred to as inactivation) has been used for many years (Gray 1957). It has generally been quantified by use of the so called linear-quadratic-exponential (LQE) equation. This equation uses the classic linear-quadratic form both for radiation induced initiation (i.e., $a\ D + b\ D^2$, where D is radiation dose and a and b are adjustable parameters) and for radiation-induced inactivation ($\exp[-\ \alpha\ D - \beta\ D^2]$, where α and β are adjustable parameters). It has been applied to data from Japanese atomic bomb survivors (Bennett et al. 2004), and to radiotherapy-treated cancer patients (Dasu et al. 2005).

At very low doses ($\ll$1 Gy), the quadratic terms for both initiation and inactivation in the LQE equation are negligible, given realistic parameter values. The dose response is, therefore, effectively linear. This qualitatively agrees with the linear-no-threshold (LNT) approach generally used for radiation protection estimates at low doses (BEIR VII Report 2005; NCRP Report 136 2001). At intermediate radiation doses (i.e., up to a few Gy), the equation predicts that the radiogenic cancer risk is an increasing function of dose. This is because at such doses the risk is dominated by initiation, and inactivation has a limited effect since the majority of cells can survive the exposure. At high doses

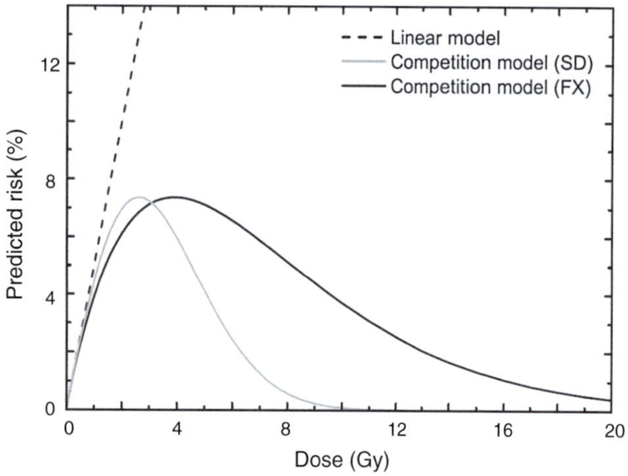

Fig. 2 Typical dose responses for radiogenic cancer risk predicted by the LQE model involving competition between cell mutation and killing for single radiation doses (SD) and fractionated doses (FX), using the same parameters. A strictly linear dose response that neglects cell killing is shown for comparison. The figure is reproduced from Dasu et al. (2005)

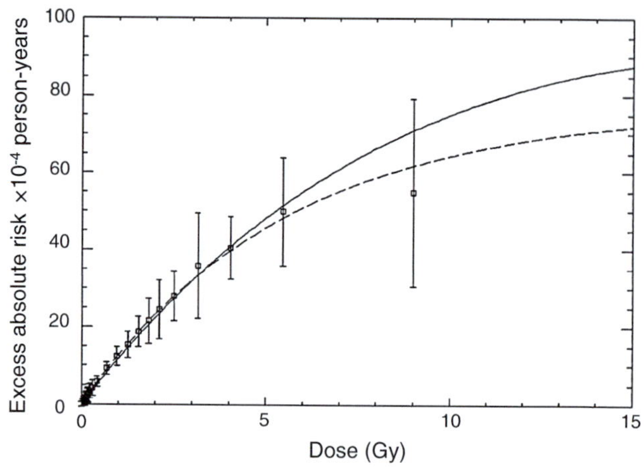

Fig. 3 Predicted cancer incidence as a function of organ absorbed dose of the atomic bomb survivors (*squares*). Shown are the fits to the combined dataset of A-bomb survivor data and Hodgkin's patients using a linear-exponential model (*solid line*) and a plateau-dose model (*dashed line*). The data and fits are presented for a neutron RBE of 10. The figure and caption are reproduced from Schneider and Walsh (2008)

(e.g. $\gg$5 Gy), however, the exponential inactivation term leads to a very small predicted radiogenic risk, because essentially all radiation-initiated cells would be inactivated by the radiation. These model behaviors are illustrated graphically in Fig. 2, for both single and for fractionated radiation doses.

2.2 Semi-Empirical Models with Cell Proliferation

The LQE model often underestimates the risks of high radiation doses (Sachs and Brenner 2005), presumably because it describes only the processes of cell initiation and inactivation. A biologically plausible explanation for the persistence of large risks at high fractionated doses delivered during cancer radiotherapy is that cell proliferation during the time intervals between dose fractions and shortly after treatment stops negates much of the effect of cell inactivation. The recent models by Schneider and Kaser-Hotz (2005), Schneider and Walsh (2008) address this issue by providing a semi-empirical or phenomenological treatment of cell proliferation (and possibly other relevant factors that alter the dose response at high doses) by means of the following alternative assumptions:

(1) A linear-exponential model, which assumes that the dose response consists of a linearly increasing term and an exponentially decreasing term. The linearly increasing term can be interpreted as a combination of all the factors leading to cell initiation, and the exponentially decreasing term can be interpreted as the combination of cell inactivation and proliferation, along with possible other contributing factors. At low doses, the predicted risk grows approximately linearly. At higher doses it turns over, and tends to zero at very high doses.
(2) A phenomenological plateau-dose model, which assumes that the dose response grows linearly at low doses and saturates at high doses by asymptotically approaching a plateau. The plateau can be interpreted as a balance of inactivation and proliferation, which tend to equilibrium by cancelling each other. The main difference from the linear-exponential model is that this formalism predicts a substantial radiogenic cancer risk even at very large doses.

One or other of these alternative models can potentially be applied to any dose distribution if the dose-volume histogram is available. They can also be used to calculate the organ equivalent dose (OED), which is defined as the integral of the dose-volume distribution weighted by the predicted cancer risk (Schneider and Kaser-Hotz 2005; Schneider and Walsh 2008). For a strictly linear dose response, OED is proportional to mean dose. For inhomogeneous dose distributions, it may differ considerably from the mean dose. Best fits of the two model versions to data on atomic bomb survivors and patients treated with radiotherapy for Hodgkin's disease are shown in Fig. 3. This approach describes the atomic bomb survivor and second cancer data adequately and is potentially useful for additional second cancer risk estimation.

2.3 Initiation, Inactivation, and Proliferation Models

In contrast to phenomenological models, the so called initiation, inactivation, and proliferation (*iip*) models (Lindsay et al. 2001; Sachs and Brenner 2005; Sachs et al. 2007; Shuryak et al. 2006; Little 2007; Wheldon et al. 2000) involve a relatively detailed mechanistic treatment of the three short-term processes that give the models their name throughout the course of a typical high-dose (tens of Gy) fractionated radiotherapy regimen, and during a subsequent tissue recovery period of a number of weeks.

The model developed by Wheldon and Lindsay (Lindsay et al. 2001; Wheldon et al. 2000) is based on familiar two-stage concepts: Normal stem cells can be mutated to a pre-malignant (initiated) state, either spontaneously or by radiation. These once-mutated cells can, with a certain probability, acquire the second mutation, which makes them fully malignant. In addition to elevating the initiation rate, radiation can inactivate (kill, i.e., reproductively sterilize) both normal and initiated cells.

A key concept in the model involves compensatory proliferation of both normal and initiated cells after some of these cells have been inactivated by radiation. This process is assumed to occur in response to intercellular signals, restoring the homeostatically controlled total number of stem cells in the organ which existed before irradiation. Partial or complete impairment of the homeostatic mechanism by radiation is allowed in the model: Under complete impairment, no proliferation occurs after cell killing, and under no impairment surviving cells repopulate to exactly the same number, as was present before exposure. Intermediate scenarios are easily accommodated. The proliferation rate of initiated cells relative to normal ones is also treated as an adjustable parameter. They can proliferate as fast as, faster than or slower than normal cells. The model is mainly deterministic, but an approximation for stochastic extinction of all initiated cells after high doses of radiation is made. If all initiated cells in the organ are killed, then only normal cells participate in repopulation.

Typical radiation dose responses generated by the Wheldon-Lindsay model are shown in Fig. 4. The figure demonstrates the following important consequence of detailed modeling of cell proliferation in addition to initiation and inactivation: If compensatory cell proliferation is not accounted for, cell inactivation by radiation begins to overpower cell initiation at relatively low radiation doses of a few Gy. At higher doses (e.g., 10 Gy), predicted radiogenic cancer incidence would therefore quickly decline. However, cell proliferation stimulated by homeostatic mechanisms can compensate for much of the cell killing. So when proliferation is taken into account, radiogenic cancer incidence remains high even at doses >10 Gy. The latter situation is supported by some recent epidemiological data on radiotherapy-induced second cancers (Travis, the chapter titled " Understanding and Predicting Radiation-Associated Normal Tissue Injury: A Global and Historical Perspective" this volume, and Curtis et al. 2006; Sachs and Brenner 2005; Travis et al. 2002, 2003). Therefore, modeling cell proliferation of normal and initiated cells appears to be an important component of reasonably predicting the risks of second malignancies caused by radiotherapy for existing tumors.

The *iip* modeling approach for solid tumors was further refined by Sachs and Brenner (2005). Here a typical fractionated dosing radiotherapy regimen was modeled, and the *iip* processes were tracked in detail throughout the radiotherapy and subsequent tissue recovery periods. In particular, cell proliferation of both normal and pre-malignant cells was calculated in the time gaps between dose fractions, as well as during a recovery period after radiotherapy ends. Eventual risk of cancer was assumed to be proportional to the number of pre-malignant (initiated) cells present after radiotherapy and recovery, by the time when homeostatic organ repopulation has been completed. The relevant proportionality constants were estimated by using data on atomic bomb survivors. The main adjustable parameter in the model was the relative proliferation rate of initiated cells compared with normal ones, there called r. The model was fitted to epidemiological data on lung and breast cancers in patients irradiated for Hodgkin's disease. The fits were adequate, as shown in Fig. 5.

The fits shown in Fig. 5 were produced using the relative proliferation rate of initiated cells compared with normal ones of $r \leq 1$, e.g., $r = 0.8$. If r was >1, the model generated cancer excess relative risk (ERR) curves that increase faster than linearly with radiation dose, which was contrary to the data. This means that the model successfully describes the data only if initiated cells have a growth disadvantage during the tissue recovery period, rather than an advantage, which contrasts with the more commonly made assumption of clonal expansion. One explanation could be that the growth disadvantage occurs only on the relatively short-term time scale of a few weeks-months during and after radiotherapy, for example because some initiated cells could be selectively eliminated during interactions with surrounding normal cells. On the long-term time scale of multiple years on the pathway towards cancer, this disadvantage could disappear and a small growth advantage for initiated cells could emerge.

An alternative explanation is that the slope of the cancer ERR dose–response relationship is reduced at high doses by stochastic effects, i.e. due to stochastic extinction of a substantial proportion of initiated cells during radiotherapy. This possibility was explored in a stochastic extension of

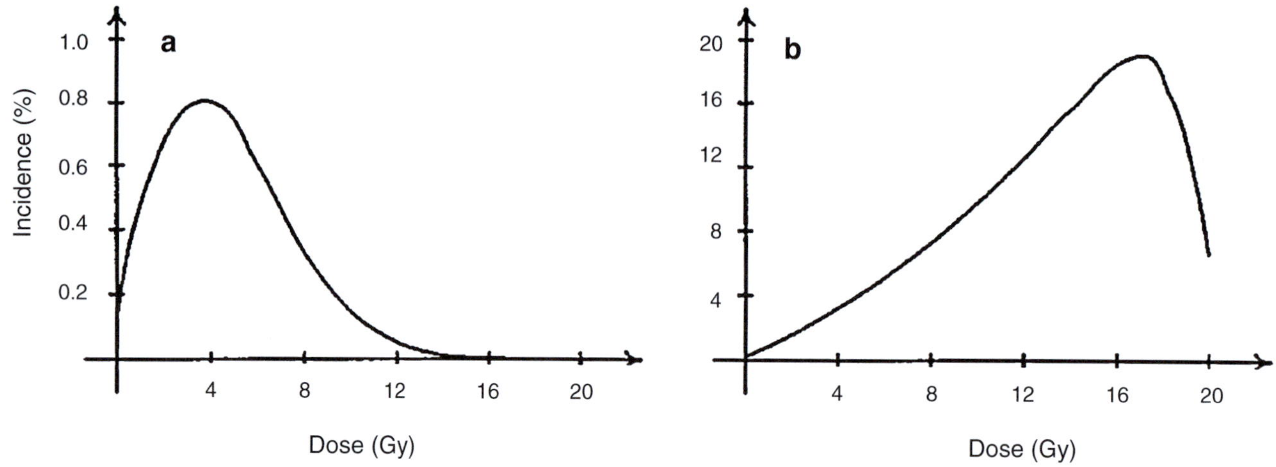

Fig. 4 The percentage incidence of carcinogenesis 20 years after irradiation is illustrated for **a** no cell repopulation and **b** full cell repopulation to 10^8 cells, using the Wheldon-Lindsay model. The figure and caption are reproduced from Wheldon et al. (2000)

the deterministic *iip* model (Sachs et al. 2007). Indeed, it was found that, with realistic parameter values, stochastic effects due to cell killing during radiotherapy could be substantial. The variance of the number of live initiated cells after the multifraction radiotherapy protocol was typically much larger than the mean, and the probability that the simulated organ contains zero such cells after repopulation has run its course was quite high. This stochastic model allowed the epidemiological second cancer data to be fitted well even if a growth advantage for initiated cells was present during the recovery period (i.e., $r > 1$). It showed that reducing the overall radiotherapy treatment time, e.g., by treating on weekends, can reduce the second cancer risk by increasing the probability of stochastic extinction of pre-malignant clones.

3 Long-Term Biologically Based Models

By contrast with the short-term models described so far, another class of biologically motivated quantitative models can be characterized as *long-term*, in the sense that they track carcinogenesis mechanisms throughout the entire human or animal life span, e.g., the Armitage-Doll model (Armitage and Doll 1954; Armitage 1985), the Moolgavkar-Venzon-Knudson two-stage clonal expansion (TSCE) model (Moolgavkar 1980; Moolgavkar 1978; Moolgavkar and Knudson 1981), the two-stage logistic (TSL) model (Sachs et al. 2005), and many others (Little and Li 2007; Little and Wright 2003; Pierce and Mendelsohn 1999; Pierce and Vaeth 2003; Ritter et al. 2003; Yakovlev and Polig 1996). The main advantages of long-term models are: (1) including the modulation of the radiation dose response during the long latency period between radiation exposure and diagnosis of cancer; and (2), the fact that radiation carcinogenesis is usually treated as just a perturbation of background carcinogenesis, so that extensive data on spontaneous cancers can be used to help determine the adjustable parameters needed to estimate cancer risks. The main disadvantage is that the early radiation response is typically treated in a less-mechanistic, more phenomenological, manner than in the short-term models, and similarly for the dose-rate response. This disadvantage can be partially alleviated by suitable semi-mechanistic assumptions about the short-term aspects of the dose response, e.g., the effects of cell repopulation which partially compensates for cell killing by radiation (Heidenreich and Hoogenveen 2001), cell–cell interactions which can accelerate the proliferation of pre-malignant cells causing radiogenic promotion, etc. Some examples of long-term models that are relevant or potentially relevant to second-cancer estimation are discussed below.

3.1 Multistage Models Without Clonal Expansion

This class includes the earliest of the commonly used mathematical models of carcinogenesis—the pioneering models of Nordling (1953) and Armitage and Doll (1954). They are based on the concept that cancer originates from an ancestral target somatic cell, whose lineage has accumulated several relevant alterations (i.e., changes that are passed on to daughter cells). In current applications of these models, the target cells are usually thought of as organ-specific stem cells; the relevant alterations are thought to be mutations occurring in oncogenes and tumor suppressor genes, though chromosome rearrangements such as balanced translocations or inversions, copy number changes, or epigenetic changes are also sometimes discussed. Once a

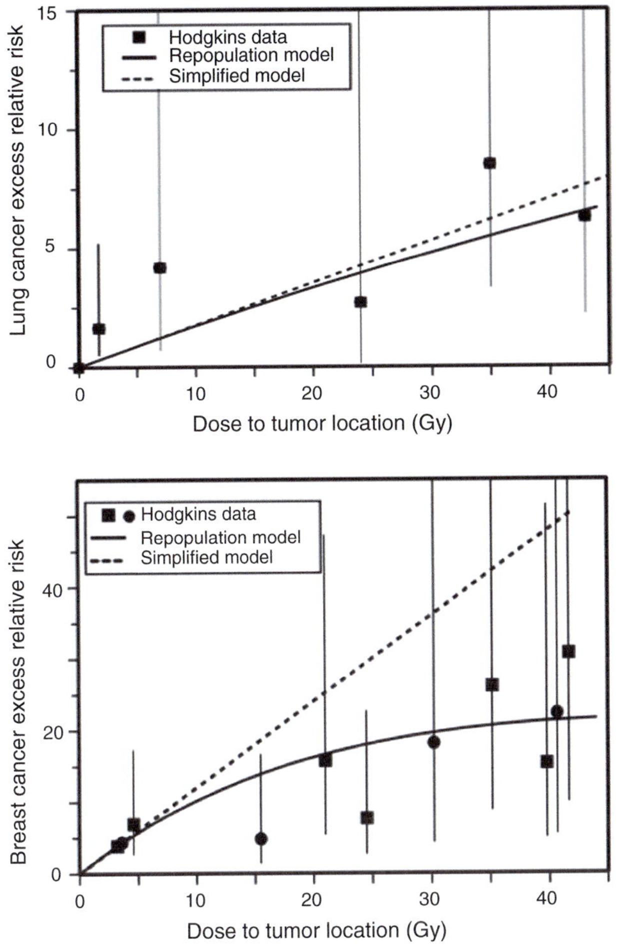

Fig. 5 Measured and predicted excess relative risks for lung cancer and female breast cancer induced by high doses of ionizing radiation, using the Sachs-Brenner *iip* model (*solid curves*). The data points are from studies of second cancers after radiotherapy of Hodgkin's disease patients. The *dashed lines* are the predictions of the simplified repopulation model based on the slope at low doses derived from the excess relative risks of the atomic bomb survivors. The figure and caption are reproduced from Sachs and Brenner (2005)

cell has accumulated all the necessary mutations, it becomes fully malignant, and can subsequently (after some lag period) develop into a clinical cancer. A pictorial representation of these models is provided in Fig. 6.

Given realistic parameter values, the two models numerically behave very similarly over most of the human lifetime: they predict that cancer incidence should be approximated by a power function of age, where the power is equal to the number of necessary mutations minus one. When both age and predicted cancer incidence are plotted on a logarithmic scale, an approximately straight line is produced. These models fit the spontaneous age-dependent cancer incidence data for many adult-onset solid tumors reasonably well, particularly in the age range of 20–70. This observation led to the term "log–log cancers" (Moolgavkar

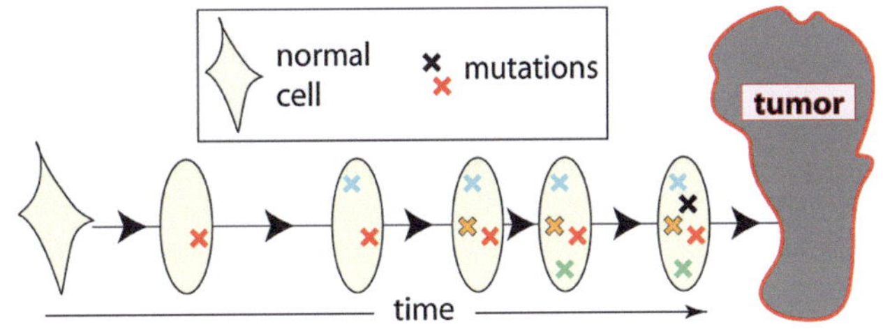

Fig. 6 A schematic representation of the assumptions for the Armitage-Doll model. The various mutations in the stem cell lineage produce pre-malignant changes. The last (*black*) mutation produces a fully malignant cell, which can grow into a tumor (*grey mass*)

1986), referring to the fact that the age-specific incidence of these cancers can be described by a power function of age.

The number of mutations needed for full malignancy is usually considered an adjustable parameter in the Nordling and Armitage-Doll models. Fitting the models to spontaneous cancer incidence data suggests that this number is on the order of 5–6 for many solid tumors. This estimate agrees with experimental evidence in some cases (Tahara 2004; Tamura 2006; Midorikawa et al. 2007; Feitelson et al. 2004; Bockmuhl and Petersen 2002; Trosko 2006; Michor et al. 2004, 2005).

Variants of the Armitage-Doll model intended for prediction of radiation-induced cancer risk have been applied to data sets such as the Japanese atomic bomb survivors (Pierce and Mendelsohn 1999; Pierce and Vaeth 2003). The main finding is that the effect of relatively low acute radiation doses, such as those experienced by survivors of the Hiroshima and Nagasaki bombings, can be approximated based on the assumption that radiation effectively "accelerates" normal aging. In other words, a given dose of radiation is roughly equivalent to a certain amount of time with spontaneous mutation rates (Fig. 7). The excess cancer risk is described solely as a function of age and radiation dose, and variables such as age at exposure and time since exposure are not individually important. After irradiation, the ERR decreases approximately as the reciprocal of age. These conclusions are reasonably well supported by atomic bomb survivor data.

3.2 Two-Stage Models with Clonal Expansion

The models in this class are based on the broad paradigm of initiation, promotion, transformation, and progression in carcinogenesis, which has been applied to numerous studies of chemically induced and radiation-induced tumors in experimental animals. They are also sometimes motivated by the concept of "two-hit" recessive oncogenesis, developed by Knudson to describe the data on sporadic and inherited forms of human retinoblastoma (Knudson 1971).

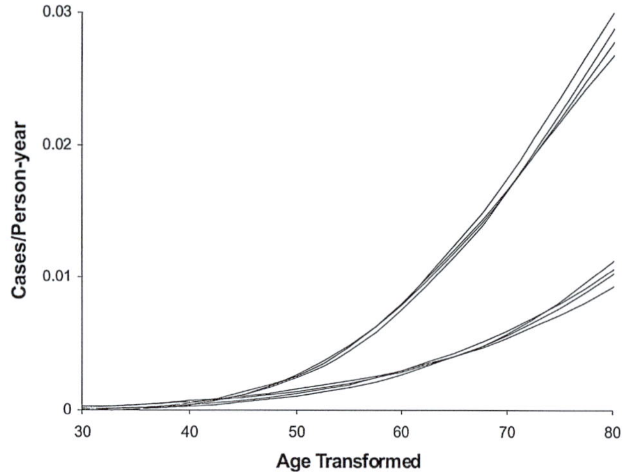

Fig. 7 Male and female age-specific cancer rates on transformed age scales, using the Pierce-Mendelsohn model (a derivative of the Armitage-Doll model), for the four dose categories of 0, 0.005, 0.5, and 1 Sv. The data are for non-sex-specific solid tumors in atomic bomb survivors. The four *upper curves* are for males, with age scale age + 4.1 dose, and *lower curves* are for females with age scale age + 6.4 dose. The figure and caption are reproduced from Pierce and Vaeth (2003)

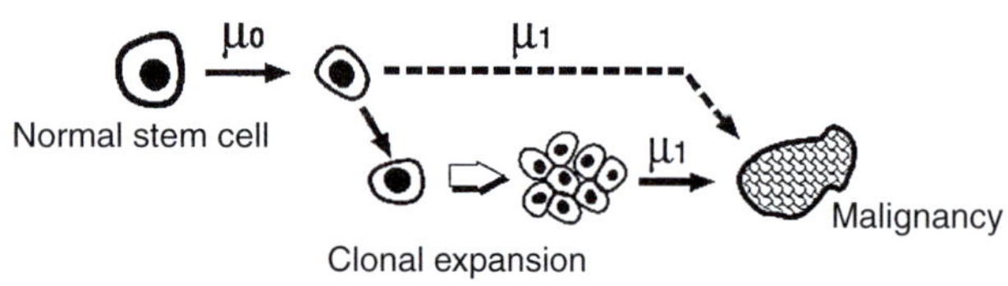

Fig. 8 A representation of the TSCE model, adapted from Luebeck and Hazelton (2002), Curtis et al. (2006). μ_0 and μ_1 are rate constants for initiation or transformation, respectively

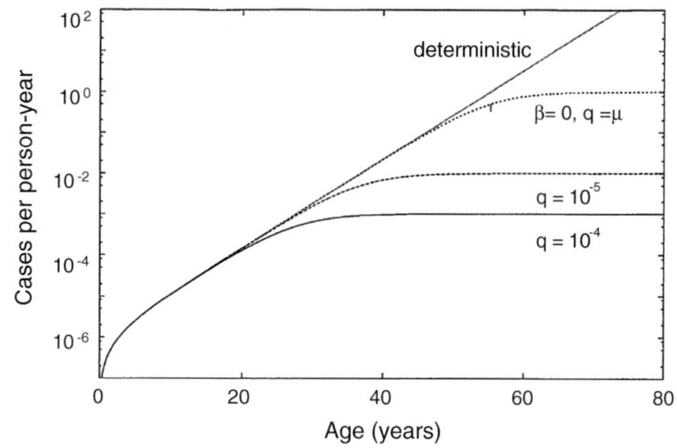

Fig. 9 The spontaneous cancer hazard function as function of age predicted by the TSCE model with various parameter values, from Heidenreich and Hoogenveen (2001). The deterministic version refers to the simplified case where clonal expansion is modeled deterministically, rather than stochastically, i.e., using only a net expansion rate instead of individual birth and death rates

The most widely used representative of this class is the TSCE model (Moolgavkar 1978, 1980). It assumes that a stem cell which has acquired a single relevant mutation has a slight growth or survival advantage relative to normal cells (e.g., can proliferate at a faster rate and/or is more resistant to apoptotic signals). Over time, the growth advantage leads to clonal expansion of the mutated pre-malignant cell. When any cell within the clone acquires a second oncogenic mutation, it becomes a fully malignant cell, which can grow into a clinical cancer. Acquisition of the first mutation, leading from a normal to a pre-malignant cell, is called initiation. Clonal expansion of the pre-malignant cells is called promotion. Acquisition of the second mutation, leading from a pre-malignant to a malignant cell, is called transformation. Exogenous agents such as chemicals or ionizing radiation can affect these three processes, e.g., by initiating more normal cells and/or accelerating clonal expansion of the mutant ones. The general TSCE model assumptions are shown in Fig. 8.

As its name implies, the TSCE model therefore considers only two stages (i.e. initiation that makes pre-malignant cells and transformation that makes malignant cells) on the pathway to cancer. It focuses on tracking over time the number of once-mutated, initiated, pre-malignant cells. Usually this is done stochastically, i.e. an initiated cell can proliferate or die/differentiate or transform with certain probabilities per unit time. Thc clonal cxpansion rate is approximately the difference between the birth and death probabilities. Incidence of malignant cells is proportional to the number of initiated cells. A malignant cell gives rise to clinical cancer after a lag period, which is sometimes assumed to be constant (e.g., 10 years).

The TSCE model has been fitted to numerous data sets on spontaneous and carcinogen-induced tumors in animals and humans (Heidenreich et al. 1999, 2002, 2007; Heidenreich and Paretzke 2001). Spontaneous cancer incidence in humans over the age range of 20–70 is typically described very well, marginally better than by the previously discussed multistage models without clonal expansion, although the small differences in quality of fit are typically not statistically significant. The mechanistic implications are, however, different: In the models without clonal expansion, the "slope" of the spontaneous age-dependent cancer incidence curve is determined by the number of stages (mutations) on the pathway toward cancer. In the TSCE model, it is determined mainly by the net clonal expansion rate of initiated cells (i.e., by the difference between proliferation and death/differentiation rates for these cells). The typical cancer hazard function predicted by the TSCE model is shown in Fig. 9.

The TSCE model has also been applied to radiogenic cancer risks in atomic bomb survivors, and many other radiation-related data sets. The fits have generally been good. The mechanistic interpretations of the observed patterns are, as for the spontaneous tumors, different from those using

Armitage-Doll-type models: The radiogenic risk depends on age at exposure and time since exposure, and also on the degree to which radiation affects initiation versus promotion. If radiation affects predominantly (or exclusively) the initiation step, as is sometimes assumed, ERR decreases with age at exposure. If it affects predominantly promotion (i.e. accelerates the clonal expansion of already initiated cells), ERR is much less dependent on age at exposure. Predominance of initiation modulation is often inferred from analysis of atomic bomb survivors, although the possible role of promotion by low-LET photon radiation has recently drawn more attention (Heidenreich et al. 2007). Predominance of promotion modulation is usually inferred from analysis of long-term exposure to high-LET radiation, e.g., radon-exposed underground miners (Curtis et al. 2001).

The TSCE model explicitly addresses clonal expansion of pre-malignant cells, which has been observed or presumed in many organs, e.g., colon (Leedham and Wright 2008; Leedham et al. 2005; McDonald et al. 2006), liver (Kohle 2008; Rusyn et al. 2006), skin (Brash 2006; Brash et al. 2005), esophagus (Maley 2007; Maley and Reid 2005), bladder (Spiess and Czerniak 2006), and others (Perez-Ordonez et al. 2006), supporting the general conclusion that hyperplasia is a common property of pre-malignant cells. The ability of certain nongenotoxic substances (promoters) to produce cancers by inducing proliferation of already initiated cells also supports an important role for clonal expansion during carcinogenesis (Kohle 2008; Shaw and Jones 1994; Yamasaki 1992).

The TSCE model does not consider the possibly important effects of limitations of clonal expansion, e.g., due to tissue architecture (Michor et al. 2004; Leedham and Wright 2008; Leedham et al. 2005; Michor et al. 2003a; Calabrese et al. 2004; Komarova and Cheng 2006; Bennett et al. 2003; Potten and Booth 2002; Slack 2000) and diffusion-based size restrictions for pre-angiogenic tumors (Almog et al. 2006; Brem et al. 1977; Thomlinson and Gray 1955; Naumov et al. 2006; Hlatky et al. 1996). A recent TSL model (Sachs et al. 2005) attempts to include these factors.

3.3 Multistage Models with Genomic Instability

It is well known that cells in many tumors are genomically unstable. There are different types of genomic instability, such as chromosomal instability (CIN), which leads to loss or duplication of large pieces of chromosomes, and microsatellite instability (MIN), which leads to accumulation of more subtle DNA sequence changes. In either case, mutation rates throughout the genome can be elevated by several orders of magnitude above the normal values (Nowak et al. 2002, 2006). Presumably, this phenotype greatly accelerates the acquisition of mutations relevant for carcinogenesis, such as activation of oncogenes and loss of tumor suppressor genes. However, it remains unclear at what point, i.e., early or late, genomic instability usually appears during cancer development (Michor et al. 2003a, b; Nishimura et al. 2000; Finley et al. 2006). If it appears early, in the form of the so-called "mutator phenotype", it may be a very important driving force for carcinogenesis because it accelerates subsequent mutation rates. If it appears late, by the time most of the mutational steps toward cancer have already occurred, it is probably less important, although destabilization of the genome even at a late stage may affect properties of the tumor such as resistance to therapy and acquisition of metastatic potential.

Many recent models of spontaneous carcinogenesis (Michor et al. 2004, 2005) focus on genomic instability. It has also been included in models of radiation-induced cancers (Little and Li 2007; Little and Wright 2003; Ohtaki and Niwa 2001). Typically, in such models genomic instability is added to a multistage framework that essentially represents an extension of the concepts used in both the stochastic TSCE model and the Armitage-Doll model. The number of stages is an adjustable parameter, as for the Armitage-Doll model. The cells in each stage, however, can clonally expand by a stochastic process of births and deaths, as in the TSCE model. At some point, genomic instability can be acquired, presumably by a random mutation in some genome-guardian gene(s) (e.g., genes responsible for DNA repair, cell cycle checkpoints, etc.). Once this occurs, the unstable cell clone can proceed more quickly to subsequent stages leading to malignancy.

Because they include several phenomena, i.e., multiple mutational stages, clonal expansion, and genomic instability, such models are very flexible and can involve a very large number of potentially adjustable parameters (e.g., number of stages, mutation, and clonal expansion rates for each stage with or without genomic instability). Consequently, it is not surprising that they can adequately fit the data on age-dependent spontaneous cancer incidence. However, the quality of fit is usually no better than (or sometimes marginally worse than) that for simpler models such as the TSCE model (Little and Li 2007). This occurs in part because the simpler models already fit the data very well, so further improvement will always be marginal and may not reach statistical significance. This phenomenon is illustrated in Fig. 10. A more detailed discussion of some conclusions that can be drawn from comparing the fits of different models to spontaneous cancer incidence curves is presented below, in Sect. 4.

Some inference about the potential role of genomic instability in radiation-induced cancers can be made using available data. One consequence of genomic instability is the prediction that cancer ERR should increase with time

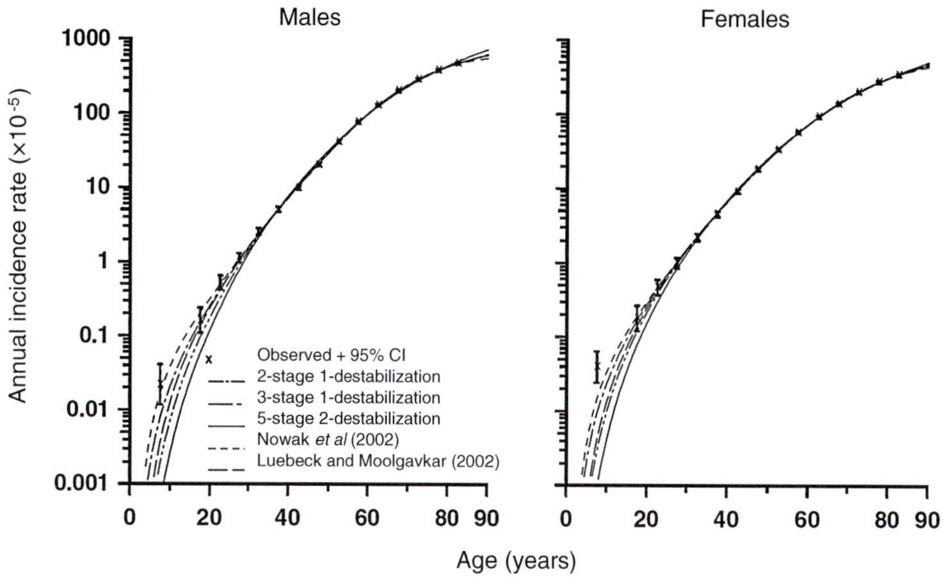

Fig. 10 Spontaneous colon cancer hazards predicted by models of Nowak et al. (2002) (with two cancer-stage mutations and one destabilizing mutation), of Luebeck and Moolgavkar (2002) (with four cancer-stage mutations and no destabilizing mutations), and of Little and Wright (2003) (with two cancer-stage mutations and one destabilizing mutation, three cancer-stage mutations and one destabilizing mutation, five cancer-stage mutations and two destabilizing mutations), with stem cell population fixed to 10^8 cells, fitted to SEER colon cancer data. The figure and caption are reproduced from Little and Li (2007)

since exposure because the mutation rate(s) would remain elevated. This intuitive conclusion is supported by mathematical results (Little and Wright 2003). The data from atomic bomb survivors generally do not support this: in the long run ERR for most cancers remains constant or decreases with time since exposure. A plausible interpretation is that low-LET radiation may not induce genomic instability that persists long enough to substantially affect cancer incidence. This does not mean that genomic instability is unimportant in spontaneous incidence of the cancer in question—for example, instability could be already present before irradiation, and the exposure would have no substantial impact on this phenomenon. Also, an increase of ERR with time since exposure is suggested by some second cancer data sets, e.g., for colon cancer in radiotherapy-treated cervical cancer patients (Chaturvedi et al. 2007). Such findings may support the alternative interpretation that radiation-induced genomic instability may be important for carcinogenesis, at least for some tumor types.

3.4 Old Age Effects

As mentioned above, the incidence of typical adult-onset solid tumors rises quite steeply with age in the age range of 20–70. At older ages, however, the increase in incidence slows down and, for some cancers (e.g., breast, lung), is apparently reversed—incidence decreases for ages >80 (e.g. SEER database, http://seer.cancer.gov). Similar trends are seen in some animal cancer data sets (Pompei et al. 2001).

The reasons for these old age phenomena are not fully understood. For cancers of hormonally sensitive organs, such as the female breast, a decrease in incidence at old age may be due to large changes in hormonal status: e.g., clonal expansion of pre-malignant cells may slow down and many clones may become extinct when estrogenic stimulation is reduced. For cancers where population incidence is dominated by some exogenous risk factor, such as smoking in male lung cancer, cohort effects of different exposure to this factor may complicate true age effects: For example, individuals who are now in the oldest age groups may have, on average, smoked less during their lifetime than individuals in somewhat younger cohorts, producing an apparently lower cancer incidence at older ages. Variations in spontaneous carcinogenesis rates between individuals can also be important: If some individuals are more susceptible to getting cancer, e.g. because of some subtle defects in anti-neoplastic cell signaling or DNA repair capacity, they will get cancer at an earlier age. The oldest age groups will be depleted of these individuals, and enriched for those with lower cancer susceptibility (Fig. 11).

There may also be true physiological reasons for a turnover in cancer incidence at old age. A likely mechanism is senescence of stem cells and/or deterioration of stem cell function, or niche function, with age (Brunet and Rando 2007; Carlson and Conboy 2007; Sharpless and DePinho 2007). The number of viable normal stem cells may not necessarily decrease at old age, but their ability to proliferate may become impaired due to senescence of the stem

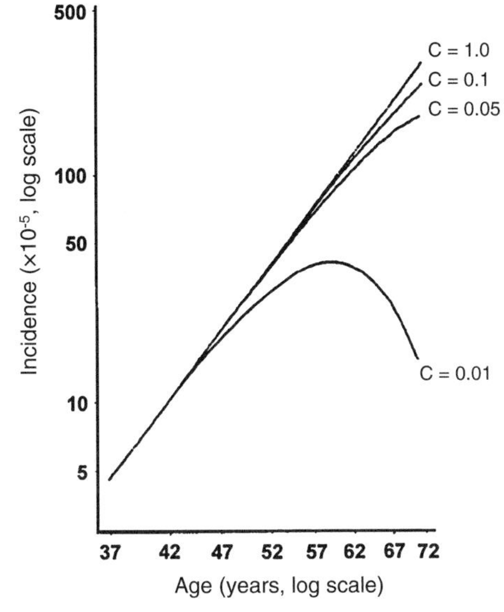

Fig. 11 Predicted cancer incidence trends with age using a model of heterogeneous cancer susceptibility by Cook et al. (1969), reproduced from Ritter et al. (2003). The variable *C* represents the fraction of cancer-susceptible individuals

cells themselves and/or loss of function of surrounding stem cell niche-forming cells (Fig. 12). Similar mechanisms may apply to some extent to mutated pre-malignant stem cells as well, leading to reduced carcinogenesis rates at old age.

The old age effects on cancer incidence are handled and explained differently in the context of the commonly used carcinogenesis models described above. For example, the Armitage-Doll model with realistic parameters predicts that cancer incidence should continue to increase roughly as a power of age for ages beyond 80 years. The TSCE and TSL models predict an asymptotic flattening of the incidence hazard function at old age. This prediction is somewhat at odds with the data mentioned before, which suggest a decrease in cancer incidence at very old ages. Such data are becoming progressively more difficult to ignore, because as more people survive to older ages, the incidence statistics for ages beyond 80 are becoming more accurate and more difficult to explain by poor diagnosis and incomplete adjustment for competing risks.

The mathematical structure of 2-stage and multistage cancer models discussed so far precludes them from predicting a decrease in cancer incidence at old ages (reviewed by Ritter et al. 2003). A new model which explicitly addresses this issue was developed by Pompei and Wilson (Pompei et al. 2001; Pompei and Wilson 2002; Harding et al. 2008). The model assumes that carcinogenesis proceeds according to Armitage-Doll multistage principles throughout most of the life span of an individual. At old ages, it is modified by a "cancer extinction" term, where the probability of nonextinction is described by the term $1 - \beta t$, where t is age and β is an adjustable parameter. Some fits of this model to spontaneous cancer data sets are shown in Fig. 13.

An important qualitative implication of the Pompei-Wilson model is that lifetime cancer incidence is predicted to be less than unity, i.e., cancer is not a certainty even in the absence of competing risks.

3.5 Some Generalizations

To summarize, the main biological concepts represented in current long-term models, often with different emphases, are:

(1) Solid tumor carcinogenesis involves accumulation of several—two or more—mutational/epigenetic events in target, e.g., stem, cells. To become fully malignant, a cell must contain all the critical mutations, not necessarily in one order.
(2) Some mutations may cause the cell to become genomically unstable, thereby making future mutations more likely.
(3) Cells that have undergone at least one mutational event, which are often called "initiated" or "pre-malignant" cells, may have some net proliferative/survival advantage over their normal counterparts, e.g., they are more resistant to apoptotic signals and/or less dependent on growth factors. Consequently, these pre-malignant cells can undergo clonal expansion over time. All cells in a clone contain the same mutations as the clone's founder, so as the number of cells in the clone grows, the clone becomes an ever larger target for accumulation of additional mutations on the pathway to full malignancy.

Available data on spontaneous carcinogenesis, though very extensive, are generally not sufficient to statistically reject any of the competing long-term models, because different mechanisms can predict similar realistic cancer incidence functions, i.e., a rapid increase in incidence with increasing age over a wide range of ages (Little and Li 2007; Heidenreich et al. 2002; Kopp-Schneider and Portier 1991). For example, fits of comparable quality are generated by:

(1) Models with multiple mutational stages (>2), but without genomic instability or clonal expansion (Nordling 1953; Armitage and Doll 1954; Armitage 1985).
(2) Models with fewer stages (e.g., 2), with genomic instability, with or without clonal expansion (Little and Li 2007; Little and Wright 2003; Ohtaki and Niwa 2001; Meza et al. 2008).
(3) Models with only 2 stages, with or without genomic instability, but with clonal expansion (Moolgavkar 1978, 1980, 1983; Moolgavkar and Knudson 1981; Sachs et al. 2005).

These different approaches produce numerically similar fits to spontaneous cancer incidence data because different

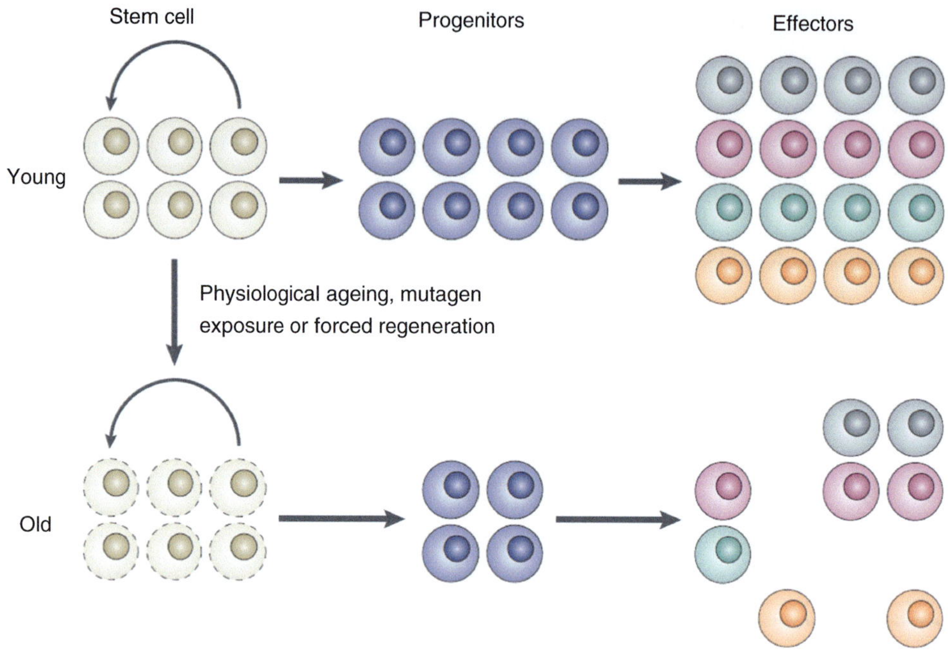

Fig. 12 A schematic representation of stem cell/stem cell niche aging, from Sharpless and DePinho (2007)

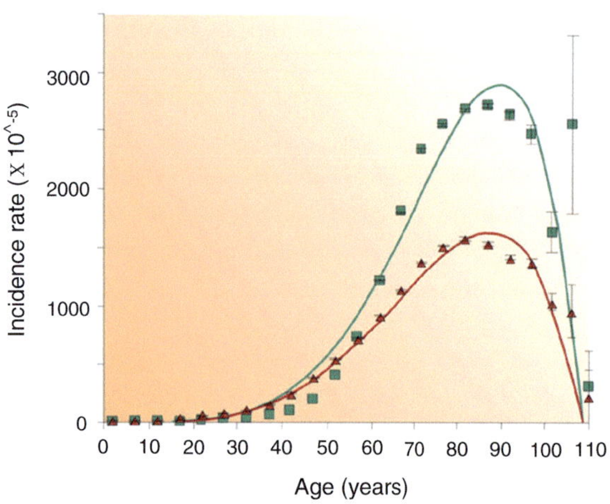

Fig. 13 Fits of the Pompei-Wilson model to the sum of all cancers for males (*green*) and females (*red*) using data from the SEER database. The *curves* in the figure are reproduced from Harding et al. (2008)

mechanisms can have approximately compensatory effects for one another. For example, increasing the number of necessary mutational stages and increasing the clonal expansion rate of mutant cells during some or all of these stages both have a roughly similar consequence—the predicted age-dependent cancer incidence curve becomes steeper. Increasing the mutation rate leading from a given stage to the next, e.g. by invoking genomic instability, has a roughly similar numerical effect to increasing the clonal expansion rate during this stage—i.e. the transition rate to the next stage is elevated either because the next mutation is more likely per cell per unit time, or because there are more cells in the target clone. Therefore, the number of mutational stages, clonal expansion, and genomic instability approximately compensate for one another—if one or two of these mechanisms are absent from a model, a reasonable fit to the data can still be produced by increasing the role of the remaining mechanism(s).

Modeling approaches also differ in the interpretation of old age effects on carcinogenesis rates. For example, in the Armitage-Doll model and its derivatives, the flattening or decrease of cancer incidence at old ages is explained solely by population heterogeneity and other exogenous factors (e.g. poor cancer diagnosis at old age). In other words, the old age effects are assumed not to occur in individuals, but result from population-level phenomena. In the TSCE and TSL models, these effects are explained by the stochastics of clonal expansion or by physiological constraints on the number of pre-malignant cells in an organ, respectively. Finally, some models (e.g., the Pompei-Wilson model) assume that cancer risks are explicitly affected by the age of the individual.

This situation shows that current understanding of the complex processes involved in carcinogenesis is quite limited. Experimental or epidemiological data which could help to elucidate the relative contributions of various processes such as clonal expansion and genomic instability are often limited as well. Therefore, the various models are usually applied to spontaneous or carcinogen-induced cancer incidence data, which represent only the ultimate net result of these processes. Although such data may not have adequate power to reject any of the models, they can allow some useful inferences.

One potentially important conclusion can be drawn from the fact that very simple models such as the TSCE model fit most data sets reasonably even though they ignore numerous biologically plausible aspects of carcinogenesis. Introducing some of these aspects, e.g., extending the models to more stages with or without genomic instability, usually does not improve the fit substantially (Little and Li 2007). This implies that some processes in carcinogenesis (e.g., clonal expansion) may dominate over others, so that capturing these key processes may be more important than increasing model complexity by incorporating numerous lesser contributors. Such an approach may be useful at the current stage of knowledge of carcinogenesis, where introducing too many mechanisms into the model has the principal effect of increasing the number of adjustable parameters, because there is often insufficient information to estimate the values of the extra parameters from sources independent of the data set being fitted.

4 Integration of Short-Term and Long-Term Models

The lack of detailed treatment of radiation-specific effects typically limits risk predictions from long-term models to exposure conditions where a known shape for the early dose–response relationship, e.g., a linear shape, holds. Situations where this dose–response relationship itself requires mechanistic analyses, such as at high fractionated radiotherapeutic doses, are difficult to describe solely with long-term models. Conversely, the more detailed dose responses produced by short-term models can be converted into cancer risk at much later times only by considering the effects of factors such as age at exposure and time since exposure, which are not explicitly taken into account by the short-term formalisms. Probably a unified approach of integrating short- and long-term formalisms is needed, where a detailed initial dose response for pre-malignant cell numbers is produced over a wide range of doses, and changes to the shape of this dose response over the latency period before the development of cancer are also analyzed. A schematic representation of model unification is provided in Fig. 14.

4.1 An Example of Short-Term and Long-Term Model Unification

Here we provide one specific example of unifying the two different model classes (Shuryak 2009a, b). The goal was to produce a simple formalism with the smallest possible number of adjustable parameters, which would illustrate the idea of a unified short-long-term approach and allow integrated analysis of background cancers, atomic bomb survivors, and second cancers. Alternative examples of unifying long- and short-term models are certainly possible.

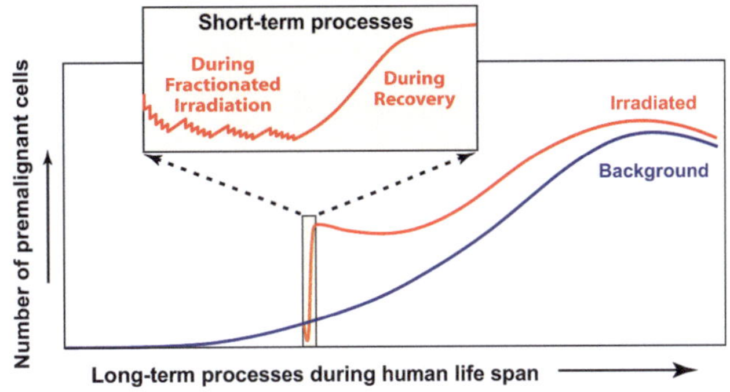

Fig. 14 A general scheme of short- and long-term processes governing the total number of pre-malignant cells, adapted from Shuryak et al. (2009). As an unirradiated individual ages, the number of viable pre-malignant cells grows, but may turn over and decrease at very old age (*blue line* in the main graph). Radiation exposure (e.g., radiotherapy for an existing cancer nearby) initially causes the number of pre-malignant cells to decrease due to cell killing (*red line*). After exposure stops, the irradiated tissues recover, allowing pre-malignant cells to repopulate and reach a number somewhat higher, than was present before irradiation, i.e., a net excess radiogenic cancer risk is produced. Fluctuations in the number of pre-malignant cells throughout the irradiation and recovery periods (i.e., during the short-term processes) are shown in the inset graph. The number of pre-malignant cells determines the incidence of malignant cells and thereby cancer incidence later

The long-term part of the model approximates carcinogenesis by a two-stage process, where normal stem cells can be initiated to become pre-malignant cells, which can clonally expand and mutate into fully malignant cells, which then give rise to cancer after some lag period. The basic assumptions are similar to those of several models discussed above, including the TSCE model. However, the long-term formalism differs from the TSCE model in three main ways:

(1) Normal and pre-malignant stem cells are considered as localized in distinct stem cell niches or compartments (Bennett et al. 2003; Potten and Booth 2002; Slack 2000; Borthwick et al. 2001; Fuchs et al. 2004; Ghazizadeh and Taichman 2005; Li and Xie 2005). The number of such niches per organ, and the number of stem cells per niche, are homeostatically regulated (Fuchs et al. 2004; Li and Xie 2005). Niche boundaries can affect the rate of clonal expansion of pre-malignant cells (Brash et al. 2005; Zhang et al. 2001). By comparison, the TSCE model and previously discussed multi-stage models do not directly consider the effects of tissue compartmentalization or homeostatic regulation of pre-malignant cells.

(2) Pre-malignant cells in all niches are assumed to lose their carcinogenic potential with age, so that at old age they have a progressively smaller probability of being transformed to malignant cells. This assumption is suggested by a decrease in incidence of most cancers at very old age, e.g., >80 years in humans (SEER database, http://seer.cancer.gov; see Fig. 13) and >800 days

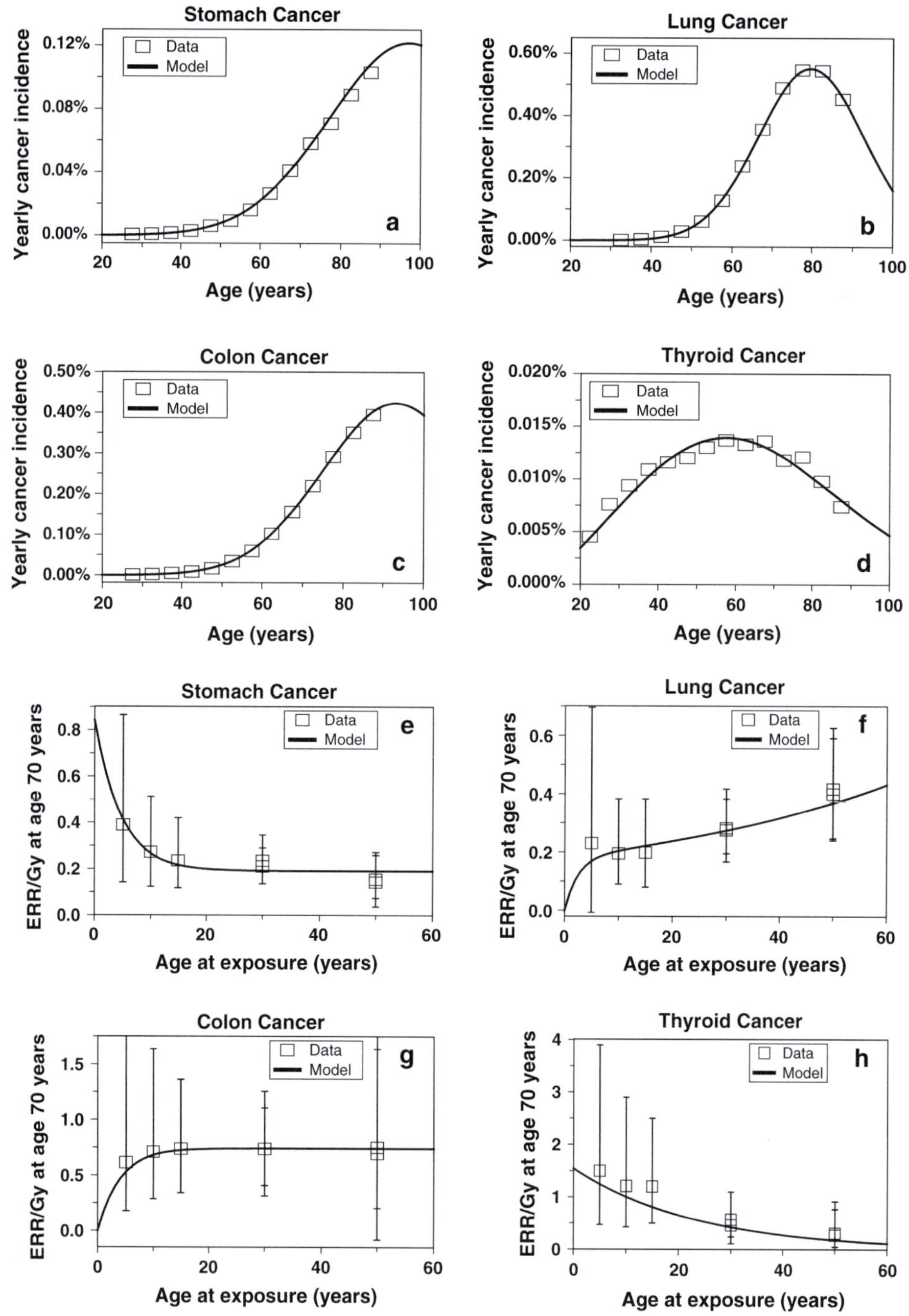

Fig. 15 Fits of the unified model of Sect. 4.1 to spontaneous and radiation-induced incidence of selected cancers: stomach, lung, colon, and thyroid. **a–d** Spontaneous cancer incidence from SEER. **e–h** The radiation-induced cancer ERRs for atomic bomb survivors. **i–l** The ERRs for high-dose radiotherapy-induced second cancers

in mice (Pompei et al. 2001). The likely mechanism is senescence of stem cells and/or deterioration of stem cell function, or niche function, with age (Brunet and Rando 2007; Carlson and Conboy 2007; Sharpless and DePinho 2007). As discussed above, standard two-stage and multistage models cited above do not reproduce this trend very well. The unified formalism addresses this issue by introducing an age-dependent senescence probability for pre-malignant cells, which mathematically differs from one used by Pompei and Wilson (Pompei et al. 2001; Pompei and Wilson 2002), so that a prediction of negative cancer incidence at very old age is removed.

(3) To reduce the number of adjustable model parameters, clonal expansion of pre-malignant stem cells is treated deterministically, using a net proliferation rate. In other words, clonal expansion is estimated by a deterministic "exponential model", instead of the stochastic TSCE model. Until the onset of old age, both approaches produce numerically similar results with realistic parameter values (Heidenreich and Hoogenveen 2001). At old age, the stochastic TSCE model predicts a

Fig. 15 continued

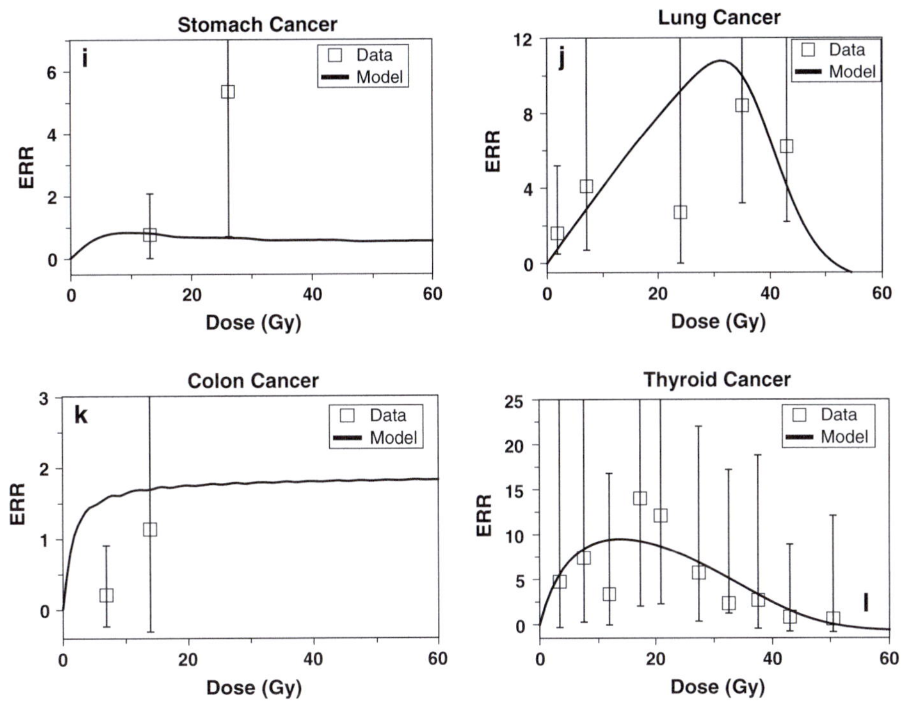

plateau in the cancer hazard, whereas the deterministic approximation predicts further growth. However, in the unified formalism, the hazard at old age decreases due to the senescence assumption mentioned above. So, the stochastically generated plateau is not necessary to explain old age effects and was neglected because its analysis would require an extra adjustable parameter.

The short-term part of the model is based on the stochastic initiation-inactivation-proliferation (*iip*) model cited earlier (Sachs et al. 2007). Some improvements relative to previous *iip* models are introduced: in mathematical approach, by using analytic solutions for stochastic birth–death processes in place of Monte-Carlo simulations; and in biological assumptions, by emphasizing pre-malignant niches and clones, rather than individual pre-malignant cells.

The model was applied to data for several common solid cancer types. For each tumor type, the data included spontaneous US cancer incidence from SEER and radiogenic excess risks in atomic bomb survivors at doses of a few Gy or less, and in radiotherapy-treated patients at much higher fractionated doses. Model fits to clinical data for some selected cancer types are shown in Fig. 15. The goal of the figure is to display the various age, time and dose patterns of spontaneous and radiogenic cancer risks, and the ability of the model to describe these patterns using one set of parameters for each cancer.

Because the unified model integrates some features of short- and long-term modeling approaches, it should, in principle, share the advantages of both: i.e., it can predict spontaneous and radiogenic cancer risks over a wide range of radiation doses at any point during the lifetime of the individual. Its main disadvantages are those common to all two-stage carcinogenesis models, namely very simplistic treatment of many aspects of carcinogenesis such as multiple mutational stages.

4.2 Model Comparisons

A comparison of the unified model of Sect. 4.1 with some commonly used carcinogenesis models described above, by fitting models to spontaneous cancer incidence data for selected sites, is shown in Fig. 16. Colon cancer in males was chosen as an example where the rate of increase of cancer incidence slows down at old age, but absolute incidence does not decline. Lung cancer in males was chosen as an example of the opposite case, where incidence does peak and declines at very old age.

In the first case, exemplified by colon cancer, all the carcinogenesis models tested here fit the data quite well (Fig. 16a). They differ only in their predictions at very old age, beyond the range of the data set: some predict continued increase in cancer incidence (e.g., the Armitage-Doll model), other predict a plateau (e.g., the TSCE model), and yet others predict a decline (e.g., the unified and Pompei-Wilson models). In the second case exemplified by lung cancer, where incidence declines at old ages, the best fits are understandably generated by those models that can accommodate such a decline (Fig. 16c).

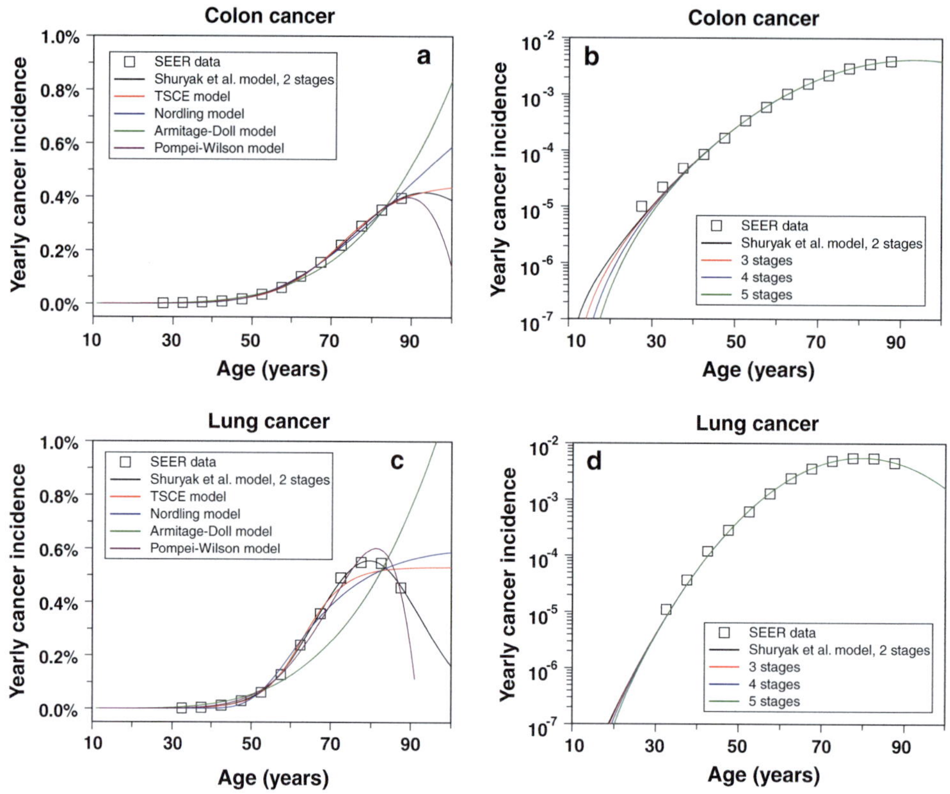

Fig. 16 Best fits of several carcinogenesis models to spontaneous cancer incidence data from SEER for selected cancer types. **a**, **b** Data and model fits for colon cancer in males, and **c**, **d** the analogous information for male lung cancer

Panels b and d in Fig. 16 refer to extensions of the unified model to more than two stages, designed to explore the effects of multiple mutations. Clearly, the differences between the versions with different numbers of stages are marginal. The simplest two-stage version fits the data essentially no worse than, or even marginally better than, those with more stages. This result is in qualitative agreement with those of (Little and Li 2007; Little and Wright 2003), cited earlier, where several two-stage and multistage models were also compared on the same data. Mechanistically, this finding may imply that one of the mutational stages is dominant in determining the rate of carcinogenesis. For example, this key stage may be the first to result in a growth advantage, leading to clonal expansion, which increases the probability of subsequent mutations by increasing the target cell number. In general, it may be that one or a few events produce sufficient deregulation of cell signaling/proliferation, so that further deregulation proceeds as a cascade leading towards cancer.

5 Radiation-Induced Leukemia

The previous sections dealt exclusively with cancers of solid organs. Radiation-induced leukemia (Curtis et al. 1994, 2006; Travis et al. 2000; Weiss et al. 1995; Inskip et al. 1993; Boice et al. 1987; Little et al. 1999) needs to be considered separately. For example, the period between radiation exposure and the development of leukemia is typically only a few years (Curtis et al. 1994), much less than for the development of most solid tumors (Boice et al. 1988), which may imply certain mechanistic differences between these two cancer classes, e.g., the number of mutations needed for malignancy and/or the proliferation kinetics of pre-malignant cells.

Many epidemiological studies of leukemia risks after radiation therapy have been reported. However, treatment techniques for radiation therapy are changing rapidly, particularly with increasing use of escalated treatment doses, altered dose fractionation or protraction, and altered dose distributions in normal tissues (Zelefsky et al. 2002; Nguyen and Ang 2002; Hall and Wuu 2003). Thus, as with the solid tumors, results from these epidemiological studies, which typically analyze data from treatments that took place several decades ago, cannot be applied directly to modern-day protocols. Thus evaluating leukemia risks associated with modern-day and future treatments also requires the development of mechanistic models that use organ doses or dose distributions as the basis for predicting cancer risks.

The *iip* approach described above for solid tumors was shown to be superior in fitting recent second cancer data on solid tumors at high doses, compared with the older linear quadratic exponential (LQE) approach, which neglected cell proliferation and underestimated the risks at these doses

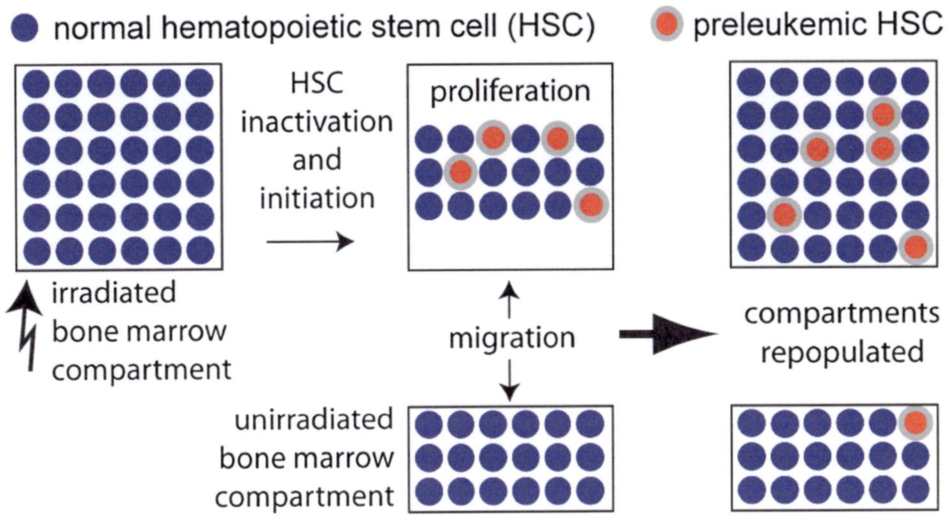

Fig. 17 A schematic representation of the concepts of initiation, inactivation, proliferation and migration of normal and pre-leukemic mutated stem cells in bone marrow compartments and blood. Adapted from Shuryak et al. (2006)

(Sachs and Brenner 2005). However, measured ERRs for radiation therapy-induced leukemia are lower than those predicted by the *iip* model, although still higher than those predicted by the LQE model (Travis et al. 2000; Little 2001). A potential reason for this difference between the risk patterns for high-dose radiation-induced solid tumors and leukemias is the difference in repopulation mechanisms for the relevant target cells. For solid tumors, the target cells are assumed to be the stem cells for that organ; for leukemias, the cells at risk for radiation-induced initiation to a preleukemic state are probably hematopoietic stem cells (HSCs) and/or pluripotent progenitor cells. Like other stem cells, HSCs in a given location can repopulate by symmetric proliferation; unlike other stem cells, they can also repopulate by migrating through the blood stream from distant locations (Hanks 1964; Croizat et al. 1980; Fliedner et al. 2002). Migration of HSCs, occurring primarily through the blood stream, is more rapid and longer ranged than migration of solid organ stem cells (Fliedner et al. 2002; Fliedner 1998). A substantial fraction of the repopulating HSCs will, therefore, originate far from the radiation treatment volume, in regions in which they were much less likely to have been initiated by radiation to become preleukemic HSCs (Fig. 17). In contrast, repopulating stem cells in solid organs will generally have originated in heavily irradiated regions and would, therefore, include an appreciable fraction of premalignant cells. Thus, long-range HSC migration would partially offset the carcinogenic effects of proliferation and would be expected to result in an ERR for leukemia associated with high-dose radiation that is intermediate between the ERR predicted by the *iip* model, which neglects migration, and the ERR predicted by the standard LQE model, which neglects both proliferation and migration. In fact, such an intermediate ERR has been observed in epidemiologic studies (Travis et al. 2000; Little 2001). Consequently, the *iip* approach was extended to apply to leukemias, by adding an analysis of long-range HSC migration to improve the accuracy of risk estimation for leukemias associated with radiation therapy, and to increase mechanistic understanding of radiation leukemogenesis (Shuryak 2009a, b). In this model, the bone marrow is divided into several compartments, corresponding to skeletal regions. Each compartment contains some number of target stem cells, estimated from the literature. The blood is considered as an additional compartment. With some probability per unit time, some stem cells can exit from a given bone marrow compartment, remain transiently in the blood, and return to some bone marrow compartment. The compartments of origin and return do not have to be the same. For example, it is possible for a stem cell to migrate through the bloodstream from the femur to the ribs.

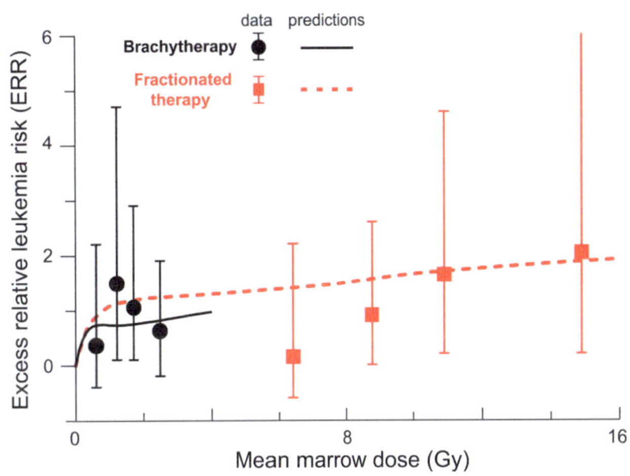

Fig. 18 Model predictions from Shuryak et al. (2006), using parameter values estimated from the literature, compared with epidemiological data on radiation-induced leukemia after radiotherapy for uterine cancer from Curtis et al. (1994)

Table 1 A comparison of the properties of some biologically based models potentially useful for radiotherapy-induced second-cancer risk estimation

Model	References	Short-term processes			Long-term processes				
		Init	Inact	Prolif	NS	CE	GI	TA	OA
LQE	Bennett et al. (2004), Dasu et al. (2005)	+	+						
Schneider et al.	Schneider and Kaser-Hotz (2005), Schneider and Walsh (2008)	+	+	+					
iip	Lindsay et al. (2001), Sachs and Brenner (2005), Sachs et al. (2007), Wheldon et al. (2000)	+	+	+					
Nordling, Armitage-Doll	Nordling (1953), Armitage (1954, 1985)	+			>2				
TSCE	Moolgavkar (1978, 1980, 1983)	+	+	+	2	+			
Little-Wright	Little and Li (2007), Little and Wright (2003)	+		+	≥2	+	+	+	
Pompei-Wilson	Pompei et al. (2001), Pompei and Wilson (2002)	+			>2				+
Shuryak et al.	Shuryak (2009a, b)	+	+	+	≥2	+		+	+

Details of the model assumptions are discussed in the main text. The + symbols indicate that the model focuses on this particular aspect of carcinogenesis. In most cases, models including more effects or more stages have more adjustable parameters

Init initiation, *Inact* cell inactivation, *Prolif* cell repopulation through proliferation

NS number of stages, *CE* clonal expansion, *GI* genomic instability, *TA* tissue architecture effects, *OA* old age effects

Without excess radiation exposure, the rate of such migration is relatively small. However, when radiation kills a substantial proportion of stem cells in some compartment(s), the cells in other compartments, even in distant ones, are assumed to exit into the bloodstream and home into the damaged compartments with the goal of repopulating them. In other words, the entire hematopoietic system is considered as a single integrated unit that attempts to maintain a homeostatically determined total number of HSCs in the body. When a certain bone marrow region is depopulated by radiation, the system responds in two ways: (1) by local proliferation of surviving cells in the damaged region and (2) by accelerated migration of cells from undamaged regions to the damaged one. These concepts are schematically illustrated in Fig. 17.

This initiation, inactivation, proliferation, and migration model of radiogenic leukemia can explain the ERR dose responses observed for inhomogeneous high-dose fractionated irradiation, which occurs during cancer radiotherapy (Fig. 18). In this situation, some bone marrow regions, which are in close proximity to the radiotherapy field, receive very high radiation doses. In contrast, other more distant regions receive essentially zero doses. The mean dose to the bone marrow, which is frequently estimated in epidemiological studies, is, therefore, of limited utility in predicting the excess cancer risk, if the dose distribution is not known. When the distribution is known, the model predicts the observed risks adequately even without fitting to the data, using only biologically plausible parameter values on stem cell radiosensitivity, proliferation, migration etc., obtained from independent sources (Fig. 18).

The main disadvantages of the model are the same as for the general short-term model class, to which it belongs. Specifically, to account for the effects of age at exposure and time since exposure on leukemia risk, the model relies on proportionality factors derived from additional data, i.e., from atomic bomb survivors.

6 Conclusions

A comparison of the properties of some models discussed in this chapter is provided in Table 1. Although the field of mathematical modeling of spontaneous and radiation-induced carcinogenesis has existed for a half-century, the current models are still far from being able to explain many complexities of this process. Because multiple phenomena in carcinogenesis are still poorly understood and their quantitative contributions under various conditions are difficult to estimate experimentally or epidemiologically, incorporating them into mathematical models is difficult. When several such phenomena are included in a single model, the consequence is often "overfitting", i.e., the model contains numerous adjustable parameters, many combinations of which can adequately fit the available data sets. This situation leads to models that focus only on a few specific aspects of carcinogenesis and explain the observed patterns only in light of these aspects. Unfortunately, models that focus on quite different mechanisms, e.g., genomic instability versus clonal expansion of pre-malignant cells, can describe usual data sets approximately equally well, making it difficult to discriminate between the more and less important mechanisms.

Despite their shortcomings, mechanistic mathematical models of carcinogenesis are important conceptual and quantitative tools, for which, in some situations, there are no good alternatives. They are particularly useful whenever cancer risks must be estimated under exposure situations for which no data yet exist, e.g., for novel and prospective radiotherapy protocols. Direct extrapolation from existing data is often not possible due to complex differences between the data sets, but mathematical models can accommodate such extrapolation. Of course, the level of confidence in model-based extrapolations depends on how well the model describes existing data, and on how biologically plausible are its mechanistic assumptions.

For second cancers, such modeling has already suggested two preliminary but important insights:

(1) Additional minimization of regions outside the primary tumor experiencing high doses, comparable to the treatment dose, may be as important as minimizing the much larger volumes experiencing small doses, contrary to the idea that, due to cell killing, very high doses do not contribute much to the second cancer risk.

(2) Radiotherapy-induced second cancer risks are generally particularly relevant for patients treated in childhood because their expected survival time can be sufficiently long for second cancers to develop. However, the radiotherapy-induced risks in adults can also be substantial, particularly if radiation acts by promotion of the growth of background pre-malignant cells.

References

Almog N, Henke V, Flores L et al (2006) Prolonged dormancy of human liposarcoma is associated with impaired tumor angiogenesis. Faseb J 20:947–949

Anonymous (2004) Cancer survivors: living longer, and now, better. Lancet 364:2153–2154

Armitage P (1985) Multistage models of carcinogenesis. Environ Health Perspect 63:195–201

Armitage P, Doll R (1954) The age distribution of cancer and a multistage theory of carcinogenesis. Br J Cancer VIII:1–12

BEIR VII Report, Phase 2 (2005) Health risks from exposure to low levels of ionizing radiation. The National Academic Press, Washington

Bennett WR, Crew TE, Slack JM et al (2003) Structural-proliferative units and organ growth: effects of insulin-like growth factor 2 on the growth of colon and skin. Development 130:1079–1088

Bennett J, Little MP, Richardson S (2004) Flexible dose-response models for Japanese atomic bomb survivor data: Bayesian estimation and prediction of cancer risk. Radiat Environ Biophys 43:233–245

Bockmuhl U, Petersen I (2002) DNA ploidy and chromosomal alterations in head and neck squamous cell carcinoma. Virchows Arch 441:541–550

Boice JD Jr, Blettner M, Kleinerman RA et al (1987) Radiation dose and leukemia risk in patients treated for cancer of the cervix. J Natl Cancer Inst 79:1295–1311

Boice JD Jr, Engholm G, Kleinerman RA et al (1988) Radiation dose and second cancer risk in patients treated for cancer of the cervix. Radiat Res 116:3–55

Borthwick DW, Shahbazian M, Krantz QT et al (2001) Evidence for stem-cell niches in the tracheal epithelium. Am J Respir Cell Mol Biol 24:662–670

Brash DE (2006) Roles of the transcription factor p53 in keratinocyte carcinomas. Br J Dermatol 154(Suppl 1):8–10

Brash DE, Zhang W, Grossman D et al (2005) Colonization of adjacent stem cell compartments by mutant keratinocytes. Semin Cancer Biol 15:97–102

Brem SS, Gullino PM, Medina D (1977) Angiogenesis: a marker for neoplastic transformation of mammary papillary hyperplasia. Science 195:880–882

Brenner DJ, Hahnfeldt P, Amundson SA et al (1996) Interpretation of inverse dose-rate effects for mutagenesis by sparsely ionizing radiation. Int J Radiat Biol 70:447–458

Brenner DJ, Curtis RE, Hall EJ et al (2000) Second malignancies in prostate carcinoma patients after radiotherapy compared with surgery. Cancer 88:398–406

Brenner DJ, Shuryak I, Russo S et al (2007) Reducing second breast cancers: a potential role for prophylactic mammary irradiation. J Clin Oncol 25:4868–4872

Brunet A, Rando TA (2007) Ageing: from stem to stern. Nature 449:288–291

Calabrese P, Tavare S, Shibata D (2004) Pretumor progression: clonal evolution of human stem cell populations. Am J Pathol 164:1337–1346

Carlson ME, Conboy IM (2007) Loss of stem cell regenerative capacity within aged niches. Aging Cell 6:371–382

Chaturvedi AK, Engels EA, Gilbert ES et al (2007) Second cancers among 104,760 survivors of cervical cancer: evaluation of long-term risk. J Natl Cancer Inst 99:1634–1643

Cook PJ, Doll R, Fellingham SA (1969) A mathematical model for the age distribution of cancer in man. Int J Cancer 4:93–112

Croizat H, Frindel E, Tubiana M (1980) The effect of partial body irradiation on haemopoietic stem cell migration. Cell Tissue Kinet 13:319–325

Curtis SB (1986) Lethal and potentially lethal lesions induced by radiation—a unified repair model. Radiat Res 106:252–270

Curtis RE, Boice JD Jr, Stovall M et al (1994) Relationship of leukemia risk to radiation dose following cancer of the uterine corpus. J Natl Cancer Inst 86:1315–1324

Curtis SB, Luebeck EG, Hazelton WD et al (2001) The role of promotion in carcinogenesis from protracted high-LET exposure. Phys Med 17(Suppl 1):157–160

Curtis R, Freedman D, Ron E et al (2006) New malignancies among cancer survivors: SEER Cancer Registries, 1973–2000. National Cancer Institute, Bethesda

Dale RG (1986) The application of the linear-quadratic model to fractionated radiotherapy when there is incomplete normal tissue recovery between fractions, and possible implications for treatments involving multiple fractions per day. Br J Radiol 59:919–927

Dasu A, Toma-Dasu I, Olofsson J et al (2005) The use of risk estimation models for the induction of secondary cancers following radiotherapy. Acta Oncol 44:339–347

Feitelson MA, Pan J, Lian Z (2004) Early molecular and genetic determinants of primary liver malignancy. Surg Clin North Am 84:339–354

Finley JC, Reid BJ, Odze RD et al (2006) Chromosomal instability in Barrett's esophagus is related to telomere shortening. Cancer Epidemiol Biomarkers Prev 15:1451–1457

Fliedner TM (1998) The role of blood stem cells in hematopoietic cell renewal. Stem Cells 16(Suppl 1):13–29

Fliedner TM, Graessle D, Paulsen C et al (2002) Structure and function of bone marrow hemopoiesis: mechanisms of response to ionizing radiation exposure. Cancer Biother Radiopharm 17:405–426

Fuchs E, Tumbar T, Guasch G (2004) Socializing with the neighbors: stem cells and their niche. Cell 116:769–778

Ghazizadeh S, Taichman LB (2005) Organization of stem cells and their progeny in human epidermis. J Invest Dermatol 124:367–372

Gray LH (1957) Radiobiology and cancer. Nature 179:991–994

Hahnfeldt P, Hlatky L (1996) Resensitization due to redistribution of cells in the phases of the cell cycle during arbitrary radiation protocols. Radiat Res 145:134–143

Hahnfeldt P, Hlatky L (1998) Cell resensitization during protracted dosing of heterogeneous cell populations. Radiat Res 150:681–687

Hall EJ, Wuu CS (2003) Radiation-induced second cancers: the impact of 3D-CRT and IMRT. Int J Radiat Oncol Biol Phys 56:83–88

Hanks GE (1964) In vivo migration of colony-forming units from shielded bone marrow in the irradiated mouse. Nature 203:1393–1395

Harding C, Pompei F, Lee EE et al (2008) Cancer suppression at old age. Cancer Res 68:4465–4478

Heidenreich WF, Hoogenveen R (2001) Limits of applicability for the deterministic approximation of the two-step clonal expansion model. Risk Anal 21:103–105

Heidenreich WF, Paretzke HG (2001) The two-stage clonal expansion model as an example of a biologically based model of radiation-induced cancer. Radiat Res 156:678–681

Heidenreich WF, Jacob P, Paretzke HG et al (1999) Two-step model for the risk of fatal and incidental lung tumors in rats exposed to radon. Radiat Res 151:209–217

Heidenreich WF, Luebeck EG, Hazelton WD et al (2002) Multistage models and the incidence of cancer in the cohort of atomic bomb survivors. Radiat Res 158:607–614

Heidenreich WF, Cullings HM, Funamoto S et al (2007) Promoting action of radiation in the atomic bomb survivor carcinogenesis data? Radiat Res 168:750–756

Hlatky L, Hahnfeldt P, Tsionou C et al (1996) Vascular endothelial growth factor: environmental controls and effects in angiogenesis. Br J Cancer Suppl 27:S151–S156

Hodgson DC, Koh ES, Tran TH et al (2007) Individualized estimates of second cancer risks after contemporary radiation therapy for Hodgkin lymphoma. Cancer 110:2576–2586

Hofmann W, Crawford-Brown DJ, Fakir H et al (2006) Modeling lung cancer incidence in rats following exposure to radon progeny. Radiat Prot Dosimetry 122:345–348

Inskip PD, Kleinerman RA, Stovall M et al (1993) Leukemia, lymphoma, and multiple myeloma after pelvic radiotherapy for benign disease. Radiat Res 135:108–124

Ivanov VK, Gorski AI, Tsyb AF et al (2004) Solid cancer incidence among the Chernobyl emergency workers residing in Russia: estimation of radiation risks. Radiat Environ Biophys 43:35–42

Knudson AG Jr (1971) Mutation and cancer: statistical study of retinoblastoma. Proc Natl Acad Sci U S A 68:820–823

Koh ES, Tran TH, Heydarian M et al (2007) A comparison of mantle versus involved-field radiotherapy for Hodgkin's lymphoma: reduction in normal tissue dose and second cancer risk. Radiat Oncol 2:13

Kohle C, Schwarz M, Bock KW (2008) Promotion of hepatocarcinogenesis in humans and animal models. Arch Toxicol 82:623–631

Komarova NL, Cheng P (2006) Epithelial tissue architecture protects against cancer. Math Biosci 200:90–117

Kopp-Schneider A, Portier CJ (1991) Distinguishing between models of carcinogenesis: the role of clonal expansion. Fundam Appl Toxicol 17:601–613

Lange CS, Mayer PJ, Reddy NM (1997) Tests of the double-strand break, lethal-potentially lethal and repair-misrepair models for mammalian cell survival using data for survival as a function of delayed-plating interval for log-phase Chinese hamster V79 cells. Radiat Res 148:285–292

Leedham SJ, Wright NA (2008) Expansion of a mutated clone—from stem cell to tumour. J Clin Pathol 61(2):164–171

Leedham SJ, Schier S, Thliveris AT et al (2005) From gene mutations to tumours–stem cells in gastrointestinal carcinogenesis. Cell Prolif 38:387–405

Li L, Xie T (2005) Stem cell niche: structure and function. Annu Rev Cell Dev Biol 21:605–631

Lindsay KA, Wheldon EG, Deehan C et al (2001) Radiation carcinogenesis modelling for risk of treatment-related second tumours following radiotherapy. Br J Radiol 74:529–536

Little MP (2001) Comparison of the risks of cancer incidence and mortality following radiation therapy for benign and malignant disease with the cancer risks observed in the Japanese A-bomb survivors. Int J Radiat Biol 77:431–464

Little MP (2007) A multi-compartment cell repopulation model allowing for inter-compartmental migration following radiation exposure, applied to leukaemia. J Theor Biol 245:83–97

Little MP, Li G (2007) Stochastic modelling of colon cancer: is there a role for genomic instability? Carcinogenesis 28:479–487

Little MP, Wright EG (2003) A stochastic carcinogenesis model incorporating genomic instability fitted to colon cancer data. Math Biosci 183:111–134

Little MP, Weiss HA, Boice JD Jr et al (1999) Risks of leukemia in Japanese atomic bomb survivors, in women treated for cervical cancer, and in patients treated for ankylosing spondylitis. Radiat Res 152:280–292

Luebeck EG, Hazelton WD (2002) Multistage carcinogenesis and radiation. J Radiol Prot 22:A43–A49

Luebeck EG, Moolgavkar SH (2002) Multistage carcinogenesis and the incidence of colorectal cancer. Proc Natl Acad Sci U S A 99:15095–15100

Maley CC (2007) Multistage carcinogenesis in Barrett's esophagus. Cancer Lett 245:22–32

Maley CC, Reid BJ (2005) Natural selection in neoplastic progression of Barrett's esophagus. Semin Cancer Biol 15:474–483

McDonald SA, Preston SL, Greaves LC et al (2006) Clonal expansion in the human gut: mitochondrial DNA mutations show us the way. Cell Cycle 5:808–811

Mebust M, Crawford-Brown D, Hofmann W et al (2002) Testing extrapolation of a biologically based exposure-response model from in vitro to in vivo conditions. Regul Toxicol Pharmacol 35:72–79

Meza R, Jeon J, Moolgavkar SH et al (2008) Age-specific incidence of cancer: phases, transitions, and biological implications. Proc Natl Acad Sci U S A 105:16284–16289

Michor F, Iwasa Y, Komarova NL et al (2003a) Local regulation of homeostasis favors chromosomal instability. Curr Biol 13:581–584

Michor F, Frank SA, May RM et al (2003b) Somatic selection for and against cancer. J Theor Biol 225:377–382

Michor F, Iwasa Y, Rajagopalan H et al (2004) Linear model of colon cancer initiation. Cell Cycle 3:358–362

Michor F, Iwasa Y, Lengauer C et al (2005) Dynamics of colorectal cancer. Semin Cancer Biol 15:484–493

Midorikawa Y, Makuuchi M, Tang W et al (2007) Microarray-based analysis for hepatocellular carcinoma: from gene expression profiling to new challenges. World J Gastroenterol 13:1487–1492

Moolgavkar SH (1978) The multistage theory of carcinogenesis and the age distribution of cancer in man. J Natl Cancer Inst 61:49–52

Moolgavkar S (1980) Multistage models for carcinogenesis. J Natl Cancer Inst 65:215–216

Moolgavkar SH (1983) Model for human carcinogenesis: action of environmental agents. Environ Health Perspect 50:285–291

Moolgavkar SH (1986) Carcinogenesis modeling: from molecular biology to epidemiology. Annu Rev Public Health 7:151–169

Moolgavkar SH, Knudson AG Jr (1981) Mutation and cancer: a model for human carcinogenesis. J Natl Cancer Inst 66:1037–1052

Naumov GN, Bender E, Zurakowski D et al (2006) A model of human tumor dormancy: an angiogenic switch from the nonangiogenic phenotype. J Natl Cancer Inst 98:316–325

NCRP Report 136 (2001) Evaluation of the linear-nonthreshold dose-response model for ionizing radiation. The National Academic Press, Washington

Neglia JP, Robison LL, Stovall M et al (2006) New primary neoplasms of the central nervous system in survivors of childhood cancer: a report from the Childhood Cancer Survivor Study. J Natl Cancer Inst 98:1528–1537

Nguyen LN, Ang KK (2002) Radiotherapy for cancer of the head and neck: altered fractionation regimens. Lancet Oncol 3:693–701

Nilsson P, Thames HD, Joiner MC (1990) A generalized formulation of the 'incomplete-repair' model for cell survival and tissue response to fractionated low dose-rate irradiation. Int J Radiat Biol 57:127–142

Nishimura M, Furumoto H, Kato T et al (2000) Microsatellite instability is a late event in the carcinogenesis of uterine cervical cancer. Gynecol Oncol 79:201–206

Nordling CO (1953) A new theory on the cancer inducing mechanism. Br J Cancer 7:68–72

Nowak MA, Komarova NL, Sengupta A et al (2002) The role of chromosomal instability in tumor initiation. Proc Natl Acad Sci U S A 99:16226–16231

Nowak MA, Michor F, Iwasa Y (2006) Genetic instability and clonal expansion. J Theor Biol 241:26–32

Ohtaki M, Niwa O (2001) A mathematical model of radiation carcinogenesis with induction of genomic instability and cell death. Radiat Res 156:672–677

Ottolenghi A, Ballarini F, Merzagora M (1999) Modelling radiation-induced biological lesions: from initial energy depositions to chromosome aberrations. Radiat Environ Biophys 38:1–13

Perez-Ordonez B, Beauchemin M, Jordan RC (2006) Molecular biology of squamous cell carcinoma of the head and neck. J Clin Pathol 59:445–453

Pierce DA, Mendelsohn ML (1999) A model for radiation-related cancer suggested by atomic bomb survivor data. Radiat Res 152:642–654

Pierce DA, Vaeth M (2003) Age-time patterns of cancer to be anticipated from exposure to general mutagens. Biostatistics 4:231–248

Pompei F, Wilson R (2002) A quantitative model of cellular senescence influence on cancer and longevity. Toxicol Ind Health 18:365–376

Pompei F, Polkanov M, Wilson R (2001) Age distribution of cancer in mice: the incidence turnover at old age. Toxicol Ind Health 17:7–16

Potten CS, Booth C (2002) Keratinocyte stem cells: a commentary. J Invest Dermatol 119:888–899

Radivoyevitch T, Kozubek S, Sachs RK (2001) Biologically based risk estimation for radiation-induced CML. Inferences from BCR and ABL geometric distributions. Radiat Environ Biophys 40:1–9

Ritter G, Wilson R, Pompei F et al (2003) The multistage model of cancer development: some implications. Toxicol Ind Health 19:125–145

Ron E (2006) Childhood cancer—treatment at a cost. J Natl Cancer Inst 98:1510–1511

Ronckers CM, Sigurdson AJ, Stovall M et al (2006) Thyroid cancer in childhood cancer survivors: a detailed evaluation of radiation dose response and its modifiers. Radiat Res 166:618–628

Rossi HH, Kellerer AM (1986) The dose rate dependence of oncogenic transformation by neutrons may be due to variation of response during the cell cycle. Int J Radiat Biol Relat Stud Phys Chem Med 50:353–361

Rusyn I, Peters JM, Cunningham ML (2006) Modes of action and species-specific effects of di-(2-ethylhexyl)phthalate in the liver. Crit Rev Toxicol 36:459–479

Sachs RK, Brenner DJ (2005) Solid tumor risks after high doses of ionizing radiation. Proc Natl Acad Sci U S A 102:13040–13045

Sachs RK, Chan M, Hlatky L et al (2005) Modeling intercellular interactions during carcinogenesis. Radiat Res 164:324–331

Sachs RK, Shuryak I, Brenner D et al (2007) Second cancers after fractionated radiotherapy: stochastic population dynamics effects. J Theor Biol 249:518–531

Schneider U, Kaser-Hotz B (2005) Radiation risk estimates after radiotherapy: application of the organ equivalent dose concept to plateau dose-response relationships. Radiat Environ Biophys 44:235–239

Schneider U, Walsh L (2008) Cancer risk estimates from the combined Japanese A-bomb and Hodgkin cohorts for doses relevant to radiotherapy. Radiat Environ Biophys 47:253–263

Schollnberger H, Mitchel RE, Crawford-Brown DJ et al (2002) Nonlinear dose-response relationships and inducible cellular defence mechanisms. J Radiol Prot 22:A21–A25

Sharpless NE, DePinho RA (2007) How stem cells age and why this makes us grow old. Nat Rev Mol Cell Biol 8:703–713

Shaw IC, Jones HB (1994) Mechanisms of non-genotoxic carcinogenesis. Trends Pharmacol Sci 15:89–93

Shuryak I, Sachs RK, Hlatky L et al (2006) Radiation-induced leukemia at doses relevant to radiation therapy: modeling mechanisms and estimating risks. J Natl Cancer Inst 98:1794–1806

Shuryak I, Hahnfeldt P, Hlatky L, Sachs RK, Brenner DJ (2009a) A new view of radiation-induced cancer: integrating short- and long-term processes. Part I: approach. Radiat Environ Biophys 48(3):263–274 (Erratum in: Radiat Environ Biophys 50(4): 607–608)

Shuryak I, Hahnfeldt P, Hlatky L, Sachs RK, Brenner DJ (2009b) A new view of radiation-induced cancer: integrating short- and long-term processes. Part II: second cancer risk estimation. Radiat Environ Biophys 48(3):275–286 (Erratum in: Radiat Environ Biophys 50(4):607–608)

Slack JM (2000) Stem cells in epithelial tissues. Science 287:1431–1433

Sontag W (1997) A discrete cell survival model including repair after high dose-rate of ionizing radiation. Int J Radiat Biol 71:129–144

Spiess PE, Czerniak B (2006) Dual-track pathway of bladder carcinogenesis: practical implications. Arch Pathol Lab Med 130:844–852

Stewart RD (2001) Two-lesion kinetic model of double-strand break rejoining and cell killing. Radiat Res 156:365–378

Tahara E (2004) Genetic pathways of two types of gastric cancer. IARC Sci Publ 157:327–349

Tamura G (2006) Alterations of tumor suppressor and tumor-related genes in the development and progression of gastric cancer. World J Gastroenterol 12:192–198

Thames HD (1985) An 'incomplete-repair' model for survival after fractionated and continuous irradiations. Int J Radiat Biol Relat Stud Phys Chem Med 47:319–339

Thomlinson RH, Gray LH (1955) The histological structure of some human lung cancers and the possible implications for radiotherapy. Br J Cancer 9:539–549

Tobias CA (1985) The repair-misrepair model in radiobiology: comparison to other models. Radiat Res Suppl 8:S77–S95

Travis LB, Andersson M, Gospodarowicz M et al (2000) Treatment-associated leukemia following testicular cancer. J Natl Cancer Inst 92:1165–1171

Travis LB, Gospodarowicz M, Curtis RE et al (2002) Lung cancer following chemotherapy and radiotherapy for Hodgkin's disease. J Natl Cancer Inst 94:182–192

Travis LB, Hill DA, Dores GM et al (2003) Breast cancer following radiotherapy and chemotherapy among young women with Hodgkin disease. JAMA 290:465–475

Trosko JE (2006) From adult stem cells to cancer stem cells: Oct-4 Gene, cell–cell communication, and hormones during tumor promotion. Ann N Y Acad Sci 1089:36–58

Upton AC (2003) The state of the art in the 1990's: NCRP Report No. 136 on the scientific bases for linearity in the dose-response relationship for ionizing radiation. Health Phys 85:15–22

Weiss HA, Darby SC, Fearn T et al (1995) Leukemia mortality after X-ray treatment for ankylosing spondylitis. Radiat Res 142:1–11

Wheldon EG, Lindsay KA, Wheldon TE (2000) The dose-response relationship for cancer incidence in a two-stage radiation carcinogenesis model incorporating cellular repopulation. Int J Radiat Biol 76:699–710

Yakovlev A, Polig E (1996) A diversity of responses displayed by a stochastic model of radiation carcinogenesis allowing for cell death. Math Biosci 132:1–33

Yamasaki H, Mesnil M, Nakazawa H (1992) Interaction and distinction of genotoxic and non-genotoxic events in carcinogenesis. Toxicol Lett 64–65 Spec No:597–604

Zaider M, Wuu CS (1995) The effects of sublethal damage recovery and cell cycle progression on the survival probability of cells exposed to radioactive sources. Br J Radiol 68:58–63

Zelefsky MJ, Fuks Z, Hunt M et al (2002) High-dose intensity modulated radiation therapy for prostate cancer: early toxicity and biochemical outcome in 772 patients. Int J Radiat Oncol Biol Phys 53:1111–1116

Zhang W, Remenyik E, Zelterman D et al (2001) Escaping the stem cell compartment: sustained UVB exposure allows p53-mutant keratinocytes to colonize adjacent epidermal proliferating units without incurring additional mutations. Proc Natl Acad Sci U S A 98:13948–13953

The Bioepidemiology of Multiple Primary Cancers

Lois B. Travis and Andrea K. Ng

Contents

L. B. Travis (✉)
Department of Radiation Oncology, University of Rochester Medical Center, 265 Crittenden Boulevard, Rochester, NY CU 420318, USA
e-mail: lois_travis@urmc.rochester.edu

A. K. Ng
Department of Radiation Oncology, Harvard Medical School, Brigham and Women's Hospital, Dana-Farber Cancer Institute, 75 Francis Street ASB1-L2, Boston, MA 02115, USA

Abstract

- The number of cancer survivors with second or higher order cancers is increasing, with these malignancies now comprising about 16 % (or 1 in 6) incident cancers reported to the population-based registries of the National Cancer Institute's (NCI's) Surveillance, Epidemiology, and End Results (SEER) Program.
- In a recent review of over two million cancer survivors who were reported to the NCI's SEER Program (1973–2000), the relative risk of subsequent neoplasms was significantly elevated (Observed to expected ratio = 1.14; 95 % C.I. = 1.14–1.15.). Twenty-five years after first cancer diagnosis, the cumulative incidence of all second cancers was 13.7 %.
- Second cancers can reflect the late effects of therapy, the impact of lifestyle choices (e.g., tobacco use), host factors, environmental determinants, and the operation of joint effects, including gene–environment and gene–gene interactions. A sizable proportion of all subsequent cancers in the review of the SEER program data developed among cancer survivors with initial cancers that are strongly related to tobacco and/or alcohol use.
- In the SEER program review, cancer treatment among all older adults taken together did not appear to be linked with a sizable excess of subsequent cancers, but children and young adults appeared to be particularly susceptible to the carcinogenic effects of therapy. In the present chapter, we highlight recent analytic studies of subsequent malignancies following HL and testicular cancer as well as cancers of breast and prostate.

1 Introduction

Significant improvements in cancer detection, supportive care, and treatment in the past few decades have resulted in increasing numbers of cancer survivors. In the U.S. alone in

P. Rubin et al. (eds.), *ALERT – Adverse Late Effects of Cancer Treatment*, Medical Radiology. Radiation Oncology,
DOI: 10.1007/978-3-540-72314-1_15, © Springer-Verlag Berlin Heidelberg 2014

2005, there were an estimated 10.8 million cancer survivors, who have a 5-year relative survival rate overall of almost 66 % (Ries et al. 2007). In view of the improved survival for increasing numbers of patients (Anonymous [No authors listed] 2004), the identification and quantification of the late sequelae of cancer and its treatment have become imperative. The development of a new primary malignancy is one of the most serious events experienced by cancer survivors, with an increasing number of survivors diagnosed with second or higher order cancers, which now comprise about 16 % (or 1 in 6) incident cancers reported to the National Cancer Institute's (NCI's) Surveillance, Epidemiology, and End Results (SEER) program (Ries et al. 2007). Further, second solid cancers are a leading cause of death among several populations of long-term survivors, especially those with Hodgkin lymphoma (HL) (Dores et al. 2005). Second cancers can reflect the late effects of therapy, the influence of lifestyle choices (e.g., tobacco or excessive alcohol use), host factors, environmental determinants, and the operation of joint effects, including gene–environment and gene–gene interactions (Travis et al. 2006). Travis et al. (2006) recently categorized second primary cancers into three major groups according to predominant etiologic factor i.e., therapy-related; syndromic; and those due to shared etiologic influences. These authors underscored the non-exclusivity of these groups.

In the present chapter, we summarize the overall results of a systematic review of subsequent cancers conducted among over 2 million cancer survivors reported to the population-based cancer registries which comprise the NCI SEER Program, 1973–2000 (Curtis et al. 2006). Methodologic issues involved in this form of cohort study (as well as case–control investigations) will also be summarized. In addition, we highlight recent findings of subsequent malignancies following Hodgkin lymphoma, testicular cancer, breast cancer, and prostate cancer, malignancies for which a relatively large amount of data has been generated. Second tumors among childhood cancers were recently described by Bhatia et al. (2003). For additional information, the reader is referred to comprehensive reviews of multiple primary cancers (Travis 2002; Bhatia and Landier 2005; Behrens et al. 2000), including discussions of possible underlying genetic mechanisms (Travis et al. 2006; Allan and Travis 2005).

2 Methods to Evaluate Second Cancer Risk

2.1 Cohort Studies

Two epidemiologic study designs (cohort and case–control) have been applied in most studies of therapy-related cancers. In a cohort study, a group of cancer patients is identified by means of specified inclusion criteria, e.g., all one-year survivors of testicular cancer reported to selected population-based cancer registries (Travis et al. 2005). These patients can then be either prospectively or retrospectively followed for a diagnosis of second cancer. Sources of cohort investigations include population-based cancer registries such as the NCI SEER Program and nation-wide cancer registries in Scandinavia. Strengths of these registries include the large numbers of subjects, which allows detection of even small second cancer risks, the evaluation of site-specific risks, and the opportunity to describe the effect(s) of latency, sex, and age at first and at second cancer diagnosis (Travis et al. 2005). Moreover, the observed and expected numbers of second cancers are derived from the same population. The population-based nature of the registries precludes the selection or referral bias that may confound clinical series. A major weakness of these registries, however, is that cancer treatment data are limited, usually comprising only the initial course of therapy, and then in terms of broad categories, such as radiotherapy or chemotherapy. Data for radiotherapy fields or the names and doses of cytotoxic drugs are not collected. Further, information on additional courses of therapy is not gathered. Although underascertainment of second cancers can result from migration of patients from SEER Program catchment regions, this is an almost negligible concern in nation-wide registries, such as those in Scandinavia. Information derived from population-based registries facilitate an evaluation of site-specific second cancer risk according to a number of relevant parameters and enable observation of trends in risk as cancer therapies evolve (Schonfeld et al. 2006). Registries also serve as a foundation for nested case–control investigations in which thorough evaluations of treatment effects, including a description of dose–response relations with radiation and chemotherapy, can be undertaken.

Other sources of patient cohorts in which second cancer risks can be evaluated include hospital-based cancer registries and clinical trials. Hospital-based cancer registries provide the advantage of detailed patient data, although inconsistent follow-up, administration of differing therapies, and underascertainment of second cancers can restrict the usefulness of these sources. If follow-up is more complete for patients with second cancers than for patients who remain well, elevated risks result. Strengths of clinical trial data include the availability of detailed data for protocol treatments, and the potential for direct comparisons between treatment effectiveness and second cancer risk in randomized groups. Weaknesses include the lack of information on off-protocol therapy, limited follow-up, and frequently incomplete ascertainment of long-term adverse events, including second cancers. The relatively small number of patients in many clinical trials also does not permit adequate statistical power to accurately evaluate long-term treatment sequelae.

Several risk measures can be estimated from cohort studies. A commonly used comparison in relation to the general population is the observed to expected ratio (O/E) [or standardized incidence ratio (SIR)] of second cancers. Person-years of observation in the cohort, stratified by age, sex, calendar year, etc., are used to estimate the expected numbers of second cancers, based on cancer incidence rates in the general population. The observed number of second cancers is then compared with the number expected. A second type of calculation is the excess absolute risk (EAR), which is calculated by subtracting the expected number of second cancers from the observed number, dividing by the person-years at risk, and then multiplying by 10,000. In order to allow for a refined adjustment of the effects of age at first and second cancer diagnosis, latency, and calendar year, multivariable statistical methods have been effectively applied (Travis et al. 2005).

Even a large O/E ratio can translate into a small absolute risk, if the second cancer is rare in the general population. For example, in an international registry-based study of HL (Dores et al. 2002), the EAR of acute myeloid leukemia (AML) was about 6 excess cases per 10,000 patients per year, although the SIR was over 20. Thus, the EAR is especially useful in demonstrating which second cancers account for the largest disease burden in a population, and facilitates comparison with other late sequelae.

Other methods to measure risk in cohort studies involve actuarial techniques in which censored data methods are used to evaluate in-cohort risk, e.g., the proportion of patients in whom a second cancer is diagnosed in a specified time period. A standard measure is the cumulative risk, in which methods that allow for competing risks (Gooley et al. 1999) are usually used, since a patient may die of another cause before a second cancer is diagnosed. Even with actuarial estimation procedures, second cancer risk may be overestimated if follow-up is more complete for patients with complications who re-enter the health care system than for those who remain well.

2.2 Case–Control Studies

Nested case–control studies of cancer survivors provide an efficient approach to investigate in detail the role of treatment in second cancer risk, including quantification of the dose–response relation with radiation or cumulative drug dose (Travis et al. 2003; van Leeuwen et al. 2003). In this type of study design, the diagnoses of second cancers (cases) are ascertained in a well-defined cohort of cancer survivors. Controls are a stratified, random matched sample of subjects without a second cancer derived from the same cohort. Therapies between cases and matched controls are then compared. One drawback of case–control studies is that statistical methods require specification of a reference group. An optimal group would be non-exposed patients, however, this choice is usually unavailable. An alternative approach is to choose patients managed with surgery only or a low-dose exposure group, bearing in mind that with the latter choice, the estimates may be diminished. An alternative approach is to use continuous variables (e.g., radiation dose) to model second cancer risk (Gilbert et al. 2003). A potential weakness of nested case–control studies is overmatching. The intent of matching is to ensure comparability of cases and controls on confounding variables. Overmatching occurs when a matching factor is not a confounder, such as cancer stage, since stage commonly influences therapy. The drawbacks of overmatching include diminished statistical power to detect associations and larger standard errors. A bias in the relative risk estimates typically does not occur.

3 Selected Results in the NCI SEER Program, 1973–2000

3.1 Overview

In late 2006, the NCI published a systematic review of all subsequent neoplasms among cancer survivors reported from 1973 through 2000 to the nine original cancer registries of the SEER Program (the states of Connecticut, Hawaii, Iowa, New Mexico, and Utah; and the metropolitan areas of Detroit, Atlanta, Seattle-Puget Sound, and San Francisco) (Curtis et al. 2006). These areas cover more than 10 % of the U.S. population. This comprehensive review provided information on more than 2 million cancer patients who survived at least 2 months, with nearly 390,000 patients surviving at least 10 years, and 76,000 patients surviving 20 or more years. Almost 11 million person-years at risk were accrued over the follow-up period.

The NCI monograph (Curtis et al. 2006) reported on the risk of subsequent cancers following first primary cancers, with one chapter each devoted to first cancers of the following sites: buccal cavity and pharynx; digestive tract (excluding colorectal cancer); colon, rectum, and anus; respiratory tract, breast cancer; uterine cervix, vagina, and vulva; uterine corpus and ovary; male genital tract; urinary tract; bone, soft tissue, and Kaposi sarcoma; melanoma; brain and central nervous system; thyroid and other endocrine glands; Hodgkin lymphoma, non-Hodgkin lymphoma, and myeloma; leukemia; and childhood cancer. The risks of subsequent cancers were evaluated by gender, age at diagnosis of the initial cancer, and time since diagnosis, as well as the initial treatment and histologic type for selected cancers.

Table 1 Risk of subsequent primary cancer after any initial cancer, by age at initial diagnosis, SEER 1973–2000

	Total			Males			Females		
Age at initial diagnosis	O	O/E	EAR	O	O/E	EAR	O	O/E	EAR
All ages	185,407	1.14[a]	21	100,428	1.11[a]	22	84,979	1.17[a]	21
00–17	351	6.13[a]	15	176	6.44[a]	15	175	5.84[a]	15
18–29	1,401	2.92[a]	22	562	3.39[a]	22	839	2.67[a]	23
30–39	4,909	2.37[a]	39	1,530	2.88[a]	40	3,379	2.20[a]	38
40–49	13,537	1.61[a]	39	4,466	1.83[a]	52	9,071	1.52[a]	34
50–59	34,159	1.27[a]	32	15,957	1.33[a]	46	18,202	1.21[a]	24
60–69	62,286	1.13[a]	23	35,986	1.11[a]	25	26,300	1.14[a]	22
70–79	52,321	1.02[a]	4	32,419	1.00	0	19,902	1.05[a]	9
80–115	16,443	0.92[a]	−19	9,332	0.92[a]	−26	7,111	0.93[a]	−14

Notes All first primary cancers, except for non-melanoma skin, are included in the analysis. Subsequent cancers include second, third, and later primaries and encompass all cancer sites, except for non-melanoma skin and subsequent prostate cancers following first primary prostate cancer. Due to their large impact on subsequent cancer risks for males, O, O/E, and EAR were adjusted by excluding observed and expected numbers of subsequent prostate cancers following an initial prostate cancer (O = 44, E = 15,185). The population at risk includes 2,036,597 patients who survived 2 or more months after initial diagnosis during 1973–2000 (1,038,089 males and 998,508 females, 9 SEER registries). Numbers of patients surviving at least 5, 10, and 20 years were 789, 221, 387, 436, and 75,859 patients, respectively. The age distribution at initial diagnosis was 3.4, 14.2, 44.2, 25.6, and 12.6 % for age groups <30, 30–49, 50–69, 70–79, and $\geq$80 years, respectively. The average age at initial cancer diagnosis was 64.6 years for men and 62.5 years for women

O observed number of subsequent (second, third, etc.) primary cancers, *E* expected numbers of subsequent cancers, *O/E* ratio of observed to expected cancers, *PYR* person-years at risk, *EAR* excess absolute risk (excess cancers per 10,000 person-years, calculated as [(O-E)/PYR]×10,000)

[a] $P < 0.05$

Reproduced from (Curtis et al. 2006), which is a U.S. government work that may be reproduced or copied without permission

3.2 Summary of Overall Risks of Subsequent Cancers

Overall, 185,404 new primary cancers were observed compared with 162,602 expected (O/E = 1.14; 95 % C.I. = 1.14–1.15; excess absolute risk (EAR) 21 excess subsequent cancer cases per 10,000 person-years) (Table 1). A sizable percentage (93 %) of patients with multiple cancers had microscopic confirmation of each malignancy, ensuring a low probability that metastasis from the first malignancy would be misclassified as a new primary cancer.

Notable differences were apparent by age at first cancer diagnosis with 6-fold relative risks for survivors of childhood cancer (O/E = 6.13) (Table 1), 2- to 3-fold increased risks for patients diagnosed as young adults (ages 18–39 years), and 1.2- to 1.6-fold elevated risks for ages 40–59 years. However, the largest burden of new malignancies in general was experienced by patients initially diagnosed with cancer at ages 30–49 years, with an EAR of 39 per 10,000 person-years.

For all cancers considered together, almost 14 % of SEER patients were diagnosed with a second cancer by 25 years of follow-up (cumulative incidence of 5.0, 8.4, 10.8, and 13.7 % at 5, 10, 15, and 25 years, respectively). Cumulative incidence of second cancer also varied by age at first cancer diagnosis, and was highest among those diagnosed between 50 and 69 years of age (16.4 % at 25 years of follow-up). Although children (ages <18 years) demonstrated a 3.5 % cumulative incidence of second cancer at 25 years, it is expected that risk will continue to rise as these patients enter the age period of increasing cancer incidence.

3.3 Overall Patterns of Multiple Primary Cancers

Tobacco and Alcohol. The risk of subsequent cancers following initial primary cancers that have been typically associated with tobacco and/or alcohol (e.g., cancers of oral cavity/pharynx, esophagus, larynx, and lung) is shown in Table 2. It should be noted that over 11,000 of the 24,688 subsequent cancers among these patients similarly developed at these sites (O/E = 3.62). Curtis et al. (2006) pointed out that tobacco/alcohol-related cancer sites accounted for more than 35 % of the total excess cancers occurring in the SEER Program. The rate of excess cancers (EAR) was estimated at 114 cases per 10,000 person-years. Curtis and colleagues also reported a differential influence of tobacco or alcohol when the initial cancers were evaluated by histologic type (e.g., squamous cell carcinoma versus adenocarcinoma of the esophagus), by cancer subsite (e.g., renal pelvis versus renal parenchyma), or by earlier age at initial diagnosis (e.g., age <70 versus older ages). Further, the known impact of tobacco and alcohol on second

Table 2 Risk of subsequent primary cancers following first primary cancers that are strongly related to tobacco and/or alcohol exposure (oral cavity and pharynx, esophagus, larynx, lung, and bronchus), by sex, SEER 1973–2000

	Total			Males			Females		
Subsequent primary cancer	O	O/E	EAR	O	O/E	EAR	O	O/E	EAR
All subsequent cancers	24,688	1.64[a]	114	17,491	1.58[a]	120	7,197	1.82[a]	105
Oral/pharynx, esophagus, larynx, and lung/bronchus	11,593	3.62[a]	99	8,184	3.20[a]	105	3,409	5.33[a]	90
Oral/pharynx	2,510	9.04[a]	26	1,742	7.78[a]	28	768	14.29[a]	23
Larynx, lung/broncus	8,084	2.95[a]	63	5,704	2.62[a]	66	2,380	4.26[a]	59
Esophagus	999	5.49[a]	10	738	4.74[a]	11	261	9.94[a]	8
Bladder, renal pelvis, ureter, and kidney parenchyma	1,772	1.44[a]	6	1,449	1.39[a]	8	323	1.71[a]	4
Bladder, renal pelvis, ureter	1,325	1.42[a]	5	1,116	1.38[a]	6	209	1.68[a]	3
Kidney parenchyma	447	1.48[a]	2	333	1.40[a]	2	114	1.78[a]	2
Pancreas	531	1.36[a]	2	346	1.28[a]	1	185	1.55[a]	2
Cervix uteri	60	1.16	<1	–	–	–	60	1.16	<1
Stomach	474	1.39[a]	2	395	1.44[a]	2	79	1.17	<1
All other cancers	10,258	1.05[a]	5	7,117	1.03[a]	4	3,141	1.08[a]	8

Notes The population at risk includes 336,929 patients who survived 2 or more months after an initial diagnosis of cancer of the oral cavity/pharynx, esophagus, larynx, or lung/bronchus during 1973–2000 (221,000 males and 115,929 females, 9 SEER registries). Cancers of the oral cavity/pharynx are defined to include cancers of the tongue, tonsil, mouth/floor of mouth, oropharynx, and hypopharynx. All subsequent cancers include second, third, and later primaries and encompass all cancer sites, except for non-melanoma skin

O observed number of subsequent (second, third, etc.) primary cancers, *E* expected numbers of subsequent cancers, *O/E* ratio of expected cancers; *PYR* person-years at risk, *EAR* excess absolute risk (excess cancers per 10,000 person-years, calculated as [(O-E)-PYR]×10,000)

[a] $P < 0.05$

Reproduced from Curtis et al. (2006), which is a U.S. government work that may be reproduced or copied without permission

cancer risk is also shown by the risk reductions that have been observed with cessation of exposures following the initial cancer diagnosis (Do et al. 2004).

Therapeutic Effects. Based on the systematic review of all SEER program data, Curtis et al. (2006) concluded that cancer treatment among older adults did not appear to be linked with a sizable excess of subsequent cancers. In contrast, children and young adults appeared to be especially susceptible to the carcinogenic effects of intensive treatment, as reviewed earlier (Travis et al. 2008). In the SEER program, 5-year survivors of childhood cancer given radiotherapy initially had the largest risks of solid tumors, consistent with the long latency period associated with radiogenic solid cancers. Radiotherapy appeared to contribute to the heightened risk for solid tumors arising in areas in which high-dose, large-field radiotherapy had been used in the past, in particular, for second cancers of breast, lung, and other sites among patients with Hodgkin lymphoma, as reported previously (Travis et al. 2002, 2003, 2005, 2008; Gilbert et al. 2003). Elevated risks of acute leukemia were observed after radiotherapy for cancers of cervix and uterine corpus. Among patients treated with radiotherapy for breast cancer, excesses cancers of the lung and esophagus, as well as sarcomas, occurred.

Dietary Factors and Hormones. Information reported to the SEER program does not include lifestyle factors (such as obesity, physical inactivity, and diet) or reproductive information that may influence on cancer risk. However, these variables likely played a role in the increased risk of new malignancies among patients with cancers of the female breast, reproductive organs, and the upper and lower digestive tract. In particular, Curtis et al. (2006) pointed out that, in addition to tobacco and alcohol, a low intake of vegetables and fruits may have had an impact on the excesses of multicentric tumors along the upper aerodigestive tract. Moreover, it was suggested that physical inactivity, excess caloric intake, obesity, and reproductive variables likely influenced the patterns of hormone-dependent tumors (e.g., breast, uterine corpus, ovary, and prostate), as well as colon cancer (Curtis et al. 2006).

Genetic Predisposition. Several patterns of multiple primary cancers in the SEER Program appeared consistent with previously reported familial cancer syndromes. In children and young adults, the association of breast cancer, sarcoma, and other cancers was likely reflective of Li-Fraumeni syndrome, which has been mainly linked with germline mutations of p53 (reviewed in Travis et al. (2006)). Excess subsequent cancers of uterine corpus, ovary, bile ducts, small intestine, and renal pelvis observed among patients with early-onset colon cancer were consistent with hereditary nonpolyposis colon cancer (Lynch syndrome), due to inherited mutations in mismatch repair genes [reviewed in Travis et al. (2006)]. The sizable risks of contralateral breast and ovarian cancer among younger women with breast cancer are consistent with heritable syndromes associated with germline mutations of BRCA1/2.

Infection and Immunosuppression. Several constellations of cancers may have reflected the influence of viruses [e.g., human papillomavirus (HPV), human immunodeficiency virus, human herpesvirus 8, Epstein-Barr virus, hepatitis B and C, and Helicobacter pylori, together with immune dysregulation and inflammation (Hisada and Rabkin 2005; Morgan et al. 2006)]. For example, cancers of cervix and anogenital tract likely reflected a role of HPV infections. The immune dysfunction inherent to chronic lymphocytic leukemia probably contributed to the excess risks of cutaneous melanoma, as reported earlier (Travis et al. 1992).

4 Second Malignancies Among Survivors of Selected Adult Cancers

4.1 Hodgkin Lymphoma

Given the high curability of HL and the generally young age at diagnosis, a considerable body of work has documented the large risk of subsequent malignancies among these patients. The largest excesses of therapy-related leukemias in HL patients occur in the first decade after treatment (van Leeuwen and Travis 2005), with the initial reports dating back to the early 1970s (Arseneau et al. 1972). The elevated risk is largely accounted for by the antecedent alkylating agent chemotherapy, for which strong dose–response relationships have been documented (Kaldor et al. 1990; van Leeuwen et al. 1994). Data with regard to splenectomy for HL as well as the addition of radiation therapy to chemotherapy as additional risk factors for therapy-related leukemia are conflicting (Henry-Amar 1992; Andrieu et al. 1990). The prognosis after a diagnosis of secondary leukemia among HL patients is poor, with a median survival of less than 1 year (Ng et al. 2002). The replacement of mechlorethamine, vincristine, procarbazine, and prednisone (MOPP) combination chemotherapy by adriamycin, bleomycin, vinblastine, and dacarbazine (ABVD) has substantially reduced the risk of leukemia (Schonfeld et al. 2006). Possibly leukemogenic agents, however, are still given during salvage therapy, and are often included in newer regimens, such as bleomycin, etoposide, adriamycin, cyclophosphamide, procarbazine, and prednisone (BEACOPP) (Diehl et al. 2003). Thus, excess secondary leukemias may eventually occur in subgroups of HL patients given selected new chemotherapy regimens.

Although an elevated risk of non-Hodgkin's lymphoma (NHL) after HL has been reported (van Leeuwen and Travis 2005), the relationship with prior therapy is unclear. Patients with lymphocyte predominant HL have been shown to be at higher risk for developing NHL than those with other histologic types. The prognosis of NHL after HL appears to be comparable to patients with de novo advanced-stage NHL (Rueffer et al. 2001).

Solid tumors have emerged as the major type of second malignancy after HL, comprising up to 75–80 % of all cases (Hodgson et al. 2007). Radiotherapy-associated solid tumors usually develop after a considerably longer latency period (at least 5–9 years) from the time of primary treatment of HL than do secondary leukemias, with increased risks persisting for at least three decades (Hodgson et al. 2007). The majority of second primary solid cancer arise within or at the edges of prior HL radiotherapy fields, supporting an important role for antecedent irradiation. Recent studies have also reported significant relationships with radiation dose for HL to the site of second tumor occurrence for selected solid cancers. In a large international case–control investigation of women treated for HL before age 30 years who developed breast cancer (105 cases; 266 matched controls), radiation dose to the area of the breast where the tumor developed in the case (and a comparable area in matched controls) was estimated for each case–control set (Travis et al. 2003). Breast cancer risk increased significantly with increasing radiation dose to reach 8-fold for the highest category (median dose 42 Gy) compared to the lowest dose group (<4 Gy) (p trend for dose <0.001). In a separate Dutch study of women treated for HL before the age of 40 years (van Leeuwen et al. 2003), similar results were found, with most of the latter patients also included in the international investigation (Travis et al. 2003). In both studies (Travis et al. 2003; van Leeuwen et al. 2003), women who received both chemotherapy and radiation therapy had a significantly reduced risk (about 50 %) compared to women given with radiation therapy alone; moreover, the radiation-associated risks were decreased among women given alkylating agents and/or who received a radiation dose of 5 Gy or more to the ovaries. The Dutch study, in particular, clearly showed that the marked risk reduction associated with chemotherapy was secondary to the high number of women who developed premature menopause. Findings in both investigations indicated that ovarian hormones are an important influence in promoting tumorigenesis, with radiation producing an initiating event (Travis et al. 2003; van Leeuwen et al. 2003).

A highly significant dose–response relationship with radiation has similarly been shown for the development of lung cancer after HL. In an international study by Travis et al. (2002), lung cancer risk increased with increasing radiation dose to the area of the lung in which cancer developed, even among HL patients who received 40 or more Gy (p trend with dose <0.001); risk reached 7- to 9-

fold at doses of 30 or more Gy. All risks were calculated in relation to patients who received <5 Gy to the area of the lung in which cancer developed.

It should be pointed out that the data on solid tumors after radiotherapy for HL are based on patients treated in an era during which large treatment fields and very high radiation doses were used. In contrast, radiation treatment fields are now significantly smaller with the current standard consisting of involved-field radiation therapy given as part of combined modality therapy. Further, ongoing investigations are examining the effect of further reductions in radiation treatment dose for HL. Both these dose reductions and the trend toward the use of involved-node radiation therapy will result in additional reductions in the exposure of normal tissue to radiation (Girinsky et al. 2006). Thus, it is likely that HL patients who receive radiotherapy in the modern treatment era will incur a lower risk of solid tumors.

Given the historically important role of radiation therapy in the treatment of HL, there is a deficit of long-term data on late effects in those patients treated with chemotherapy alone. In a British survey of 1,693 HL patients given chemotherapy only, the relative risk of lung cancer was elevated 3-fold (RR = 3.3; 95 % C.I., 2.2–4.7) (Swerdlow et al. 2000). The increased risk of lung cancer was comparable in magnitude to HL patients who received either radiation therapy alone (RR, 2.9, 95 % C.I., 1.9–4.1) or combined modality therapy (RR, 4.3, 95 % C.I., 2.9–6.2). Most HL patients in this study were treated with alkylating-agent based chemotherapy. The important role of alkylating agents given for HL in the subsequent occurrence of lung cancer was confirmed in a case–control study by the same British group (Swerdlow et al. 2001), and in the NCI-international case–control study described above (Travis et al. 2002); both investigations demonstrated significant dose–response relationships between cumulative amount of alkylating agent chemotherapy and lung cancer risk.

Age is an important modifying factor in the risk of selected treatment-related second cancers after HL. Young age at mantle irradiation has consistently been shown to be associated with a significantly increased risk of breast cancer in patients with HL (Travis et al. 2003; Ng et al. 2002; Hodgson et al. 2007; van Leeuwen et al. 2000), which is not consistent with the known radiosensitivity of the breast in young women. In a recent population-based cohort study by Hodgson et al., the absolute risks of breast cancer in women diagnosed with HL at ages 15–25 were 34–47 per 10,000 person-years at 10 years, which was higher than the absolute risks of women in the general population between 50 and 54 years, the typical age at which screening mammography is recommended (Hodgson et al. 2007).

The increasing awareness of the substantial excesses of breast cancer after therapy for HL at a young age has prompted a need for informed counseling. Estimates of the cumulative absolute risk of breast cancer among young women treated for HL at age 30 years or younger, however, have varied widely ranging from 4.2 to 34 % at 20–25 years after treatment (Bhatia et al. 2003; Swerdlow et al. 2000; Aisenberg et al. 1997; Sankila et al. 1996). Most estimates have not taken into account the influence of alkylating agent therapy, which can reduce breast cancer risk (Travis et al. 2003; van Leeuwen et al. 2003), or the effect of competing causes of mortality (Gooley et al. 1999). Accurate projections of breast cancer risk, as available for women in the general population (Gail et al. 1989), are important to predict the disease burden among the growing population of HL survivors treated with past regimens and to facilitate the development of risk-adapted long-term follow-up recommendations. Estimates of the cumulative absolute risk of breast cancer for women treated for HL at age 30 years or younger were recently provided in terms of measures of radiation dose and chemotherapy recorded in medical charts (Travis et al. 2005). The estimates also took into account age and calendar year of HL diagnosis, age at counseling, baseline breast cancer incidence rates, and competing causes of mortality. For example, a HL survivor treated at age 25 years with a chest radiation dose of at least 40 Gy without alkylating agents had an estimated cumulative absolute risks of breast cancer by age 35, 45, and 55 years of 1.4, 11.1, and 29.0 %, respectively. Cumulative absolute risks were predictably lower in women also treated with alkylating agents used in the past, which frequently caused in ovarian failure. In comparison, in the general population the absolute risks of breast cancer in white women from age 20 years to ages 30, 40, 50, and 60 years are, respectively, 0.04, 0.5, 2.0, and 4.3 %. Travis et al. (2005) emphasized that the risk estimates are most relevant for HL survivors treated with past regimens, and should be used circumspectly in women treated with more recent approaches, including limited-field radiotherapy and/or ovary-sparing chemotherapy.

Tobacco use is another important factor that modifies the risk of treatment-related lung cancer among HL survivors. In the NCI-International case–control study of lung cancer described above (Travis et al. 2002), in which the reference (comparison) group was comprised of HL patients with minimal radiation exposure and who were non-smokers or light smokers, those patients given either alkylating agent chemotherapy alone or 5 or more Gy of radiation therapy alone to the region of the lung in which cancer developed later experienced 4.3- and 7.2-fold increased risks of lung cancer, respectively. These relative risks increased to 16.8- and 20.2-fold, respectively, among those HL patients who also smoked at least one pack of cigarettes per day. For those cigarette smokers (at least one pack per day) also given alkylating agent chemotherapy and 5 or more Gy of radiation therapy to the area of the lung in which cancer developed, a significantly increased 50-fold relative risk of lung cancer was evident, consistent with a multiplicative effect of smoking on the risk of treatment-related lung cancer.

As data on second malignancy risk after HL therapy have been generated, increasing research and clinical efforts have been directed toward the development of programs for early detection and prevention of a new cancer and for risk factor modification (e.g., smoking cessation) as well as treatment refinements (described above) (Mauch et al. 2005). These iterative efforts may provide a useful model for managing survivors of other primary cancers for whom long-term data on excess second malignancies are only now emerging.

4.2 Testicular Cancer

Testicular cancer is highly curable and largely affects young patients, who currently have a 95 % 5-year relative survival rate. Past treatments for testicular cancer included the use of relatively large radiotherapy fields, and second malignancies are an important cause of death among these patients (Schairer et al. 2007; van den Belt-Dusebout et al. 2007).

Increased risks for secondary leukemias have been reported in survivors of testicular cancer, as well as excess solid tumors, including malignant mesothelioma, and cancers of the lung, thyroid, esophagus, stomach, pancreas, colon, rectum, kidney, bladder, and connective tissue (Travis et al. 2005). Excess contralateral testicular cancers have also been observed, which are likely due to underlying predisposition rather than treatment. In a large population-based study of 29,515 U.S. testicular cancer survivors, the 15-year cumulative risk of contralateral testicular cancer was 1.9 %, and represented a 12.4-fold higher risk than that expected in the general population (Fossa et al. 2005).

Many solid tumors which follow testicular cancer, depending on site, are likely due in part to the historical use of para-aortic and pelvic radiation therapy for testicular cancer; mediastinal irradiation was also given through the 1970s. In the largest international population-based study of testicular cancer survivors to date, Travis et al. described site-specific solid tumor risk among 40,576 testicular cancer patients (Travis et al. 2005) who were followed for an average of 11.8 years. The relative risks of developing a solid tumor were significantly increased after both radiation therapy alone and chemotherapy alone (RR, 2.0 and 1.8, respectively). Although the relative risk was somewhat higher among patients who received both chemotherapy and radiation therapy (RR, 2.9), the risk did not differ significantly from those patients treated with single-modality therapy. For the group of infradiaphragmatic solid tumors that were likely related to prior radiation treatment (based on anatomic site of development), the relative risks increased significantly with increasing follow-up time.

Excess leukemias after testicular cancer have been linked to both antecedent chemotherapy and radiation therapy (van den Belt-Dusebout et al. 2007; Travis et al. 2000; Pedersen-Bjergaard et al. 1991; Kollmannsberger et al. 1999). Chemotherapeutic agents that have been associated with the development of leukemia in testicular cancer patients include cisplatin and etoposide (Travis et al. 2000; Pedersen-Bjergaard et al. 1991; Kollmannsberger et al. 1999). An international population-based study by Travis et al. examined treatment-associated leukemia in 18,567 men with testicular cancer who had survived at least one year. The risk of leukemia increased significantly with increasing radiation field size, which was reflected in total dose to active bone marrow. Further, after taking into account the dose of radiation to active bone marrow, the risk of leukemia was also significantly associated with cumulative amount of cisplatin (Travis et al. 2000), with too few patients exposed to etoposide to reliably evaluate risk.

4.3 Breast Cancer

Women with breast cancer comprise about 20 % of all cancer survivors. An extensive amount of data exist for contralateral breast cancer, which is related in large part to pre-existing breast cancer risk factors (Kirova et al. 2007; Boice et al. 1992; Storm et al. 1992). Prior radiation therapy may also contribute to excess risks, especially among women treated at a young age. Endometrial cancer is another second malignancy that is related to both shared risk factors and breast cancer therapy, in particular, tamoxifen. Lung cancer and sarcoma are other solid tumors that have been reported in breast cancer survivors, with risks largely related to radiotherapy exposure. An increased risk of leukemia after breast cancer has been associated with antecedent chemotherapy and radiation therapy.

The risk of contralateral breast cancer is increased 2- to 5-fold among breast cancer survivors (Boice et al. 1992). Conflicting information exists on the contribution of radiation therapy to the excess risks (Kirova et al. 2007; Boice et al. 1992; Gao et al. 2003; Hill-Kayser et al. 2006). In a case–control study by Boice et al., the overall relative risk of contralateral breast cancer was not significantly elevated after radiation therapy (RR, 1.19, 95 % C.I., 0.94, 1.15) (Boice et al. 1992). Among those patients who were under 45 years of age at the time of irradiation, however, the relative risk was significantly elevated (RR, 1.59; 95 % C.I. 1.07–2.36). In contrast, in a separate large case–control study undertaken in Denmark, there was no significant difference in the risk of contralateral breast cancer in women who did and did not receive radiation therapy, regardless of age at treatment (Storm et al. 1992). In the latter investigation, contralateral tumors were uniformly distributed in the medial, lateral, and central portions of the breast, a pattern which was also not consistent with a causal role of radiotherapy. In a report from the Early Breast Cancer Trialists' Collaborative Group, a significantly increased risk of contralateral breast cancer was reported after radiotherapy, primarily during the period 5–14 years after randomization (RR, 1.43, p = 0.00001), a latency pattern which is not consistent with the late effects of radiotherapy; significant excesses following radiotherapy were reported even among women aged 50 years or older (RR, 1.25, p = 0.002) (Clarke et al. 2005). A recent large survey of 13,472 breast cancer patients treated at the Institut Curie did not demonstrate an increased overall risk of contralateral tumors among women who received radiation therapy compared to those who did not receive irradiation (RR, 1.1, 95 % C.I., 0.96–1.27); however, analyses by patient age were not performed (Kirova et al. 2007).

Tamoxifen, which is prescribed as adjuvant therapy for many breast cancer patients with estrogen-receptor positive tumors, has been shown to reduce the risk of contralateral tumors by 30–40 % (Fisher et al. 2005). Nonetheless, a number of large studies have clearly shown a 2- to 4-fold increased risk of endometrial cancer after tamoxifen therapy (Fisher et al. 1994, 1998). Whereas early studies suggested that endometrial cancer after tamoxifen therapy might have a more favorable prognosis compared with de novo tumors, more recent data have suggested that tamoxifen-related endometrial cancers may demonstrate more aggressive behavior (Magriples et al. 1993; Bergman et al. 2000; Saadat et al. 2007). However, because most endometrial cancers that develop after tamoxifen therapy are detected at an early stage and are thus able to be surgically resected (Saadat et al. 2007), these cancers do not appear to be associated with poorer endometrial cancer-specific survival.

Radiation therapy is an important modality in the treatment of breast cancer, either as part of breast-conserving therapy or as post-mastectomy radiation therapy. Other solid tumors have also been linked to radiotherapy for breast cancer, including lung cancer, soft tissue sarcoma, and esophageal cancer. In a number of studies (Kirova et al. 2007; Roychoudhuri et al. 2004; Neugut et al. 1993), women who received radiation therapy have been shown to be at a 1.5- to 3-fold increased risk of developing lung cancer compared to women who did not receive radiation therapy. The increased risk appeared to be more clearly related to post-mastectomy radiation therapy, in which the target volume often also includes the supraclavicular, axillary and/or internal mammary nodal region, thus exposing a larger volume of underlying lung tissue to radiation, while the existence of any increased risk after post-lumpectomy radiation therapy is less certain (Zablotska and Neugut 2003; Deutsch et al. 2003). The observation that lung cancer after breast cancer therapy is more frequently found in the ipsilateral lung also supports a contributing role of radiation therapy to the elevated risk (Zablotska and Neugut 2003). Several studies showed an even greater increase in lung cancer risk among smokers given breast irradiation (Neugut et al. 1994; Ford et al. 2003), although any interaction between tobacco exposure and prior radiation therapy on subsequent lung cancer risk is not as well-delineated as in HL survivors.

The 15-year cumulative incidence of sarcoma after breast cancer is low (<0.5 %), although the relative risk has been estimated to be as high as 7-fold, given the low background incidence in the general population (Kirova et al. 2005, 2007; Huang and Mackillop 2001; Karlsson et al. 1998). In an Italian study of breast cancer survivors conducted by Rubino et al. (2003), all subsequent sarcomas were either localized to the previously irradiated fields or to the upper extremity of the arm ipsilateral to the treated breast among women given radiotherapy. By estimating the initial radiation dose to the site of sarcoma development, using a dose of ≤14 Gy as reference, women who received 14–44 Gy had a 1.6-fold increased risk of sarcoma, while those who received ≥45 Gy to the site had a 30.6-fold increased risk (p trend for dose <0.001). Angiosarcoma after breast cancer was initially shown to be associated with chronic lymphedema following radical mastectomy (Jessner et al. 1952). Given the increasing use of radiotherapy with breast-conserving surgery, a growing number of reports now document the occurrence of cutaneous angiosarcoma of the breast arising in the radiation field (Kirova et al. 2005; Esler-Brauer et al. 2007; Virtanen et al. 2007; Simonart and Heenen 2004). Dissimilar to other radiation-related soft tissue sarcomas, breast angiosarcoma appears to have a short latency period, with diagnoses documented in the first 5 years after therapy.

Excess leukemias following breast cancer are related to prior chemotherapy and radiation therapy (Boice et al. 1992; Curtis et al. 1992; Praga et al. 2005; Campone et al. 2005). In a population-based, nested case–control study of women treated for breast cancer between 1973 and 1985, Curtis et al. (1992) showed that compared to women who did not receive alkylating agent chemotherapy or radiation therapy, the relative risks of acute myelogenous leukemia after radiation therapy alone, alkylating chemotherapy alone, and both chemotherapy and radiation therapy were 2.4, 10.0, and 17.4, respectively. A significant dose–response relation was observed for either cumulative dose of melphalan, cyclophosphamide, or radiation to the active bone marrow, and subsequent leukemia risk. This study, however, was conducted in a period when higher cumulative doses of chemotherapy and larger field radiation therapy were used than are presently given. Further, melphalan-containing regimens are no longer used in the treatment of breast cancer. Recent data demonstrate that the risk of secondary acute leukemia is more significantly related to the dose-intensity of cyclophosphamide than with cumulative dose (Smith et al. 2003), an observation which is noteworthy in view of the increasing trend toward the use of dose-intensified regimens for breast cancer. Even as evolutions in systemic chemotherapy for breast cancer may eventually affect the risk of second malignancies, recent advances in radiation therapy, including the use of intensity modulated therapy radiation, and the growing interest in partial breast irradiation (Chen and Vicini 2007) may also influence the risk profile. The degree to which second cancer risk will be affected by these newer radiation therapy approaches and techniques will have to be documented through long-term follow-up of sufficiently large cohorts of breast cancer survivors, which will enable sufficient statistical power for the detection of increased risks.

4.4 Prostate Cancer

Given the large number of prostate cancer survivors, the issue of the late effects of cancer and its treatment have become critically important. In recent years, an increasing number of reports have documented an increased risk of second cancers after radiation therapy for prostate cancer [reviewed in van Leeuwen and Travis (2005)]. In an early report (Neugut et al. 1997), the risk of second cancers following radiotherapy for prostate carcinoma was evaluated among patients reported to the population-based registries which comprise the NCI's Surveillance, Epidemiology, and End Results (SEER) program (1973–1990). Patients treated with radiation therapy had significant excesses of bladder cancer after a latent period of 8 years (RR, 1.5, 95 % C.I., 1.1–2.0), while excesses were not apparent among men who did not receive radiation therapy. In a more recent survey, utilizing the Mayo Clinic Cancer Registry (Chrouser et al. 2005), the overall relative risk of bladder cancer after radiation therapy was not significantly increased. However, among those men given adjuvant radiation therapy after a radical prostatectomy, the relative risk of bladder cancer was 5-fold higher than expected ($p = 0.05$), which may reflect the larger volume of bladder tissue exposed to radiation in the post-operative setting.

In an updated study of prostate cancer patients reported to the SEER Program (1973–1993), second cancer risks among men who were initially given radiation therapy were compared with those observed after surgery alone (Brenner et al. 2000). Men given radiotherapy demonstrated significant excesses of sarcoma and cancers of lung, bladder, and rectum. The elevated risks of lung cancer were hypothesized to reflect low scatter doses of radiation to the lungs. This finding may be more relevant to men given Cobalt irradiation to the whole pelvis, although the SEER program does not collect data on type of radiotherapy. A more recent investigation using the linked SEER-Medicare database studied a larger group of prostate cancer patients, including those treated in the more recent era (Moon et al. 2006). Men given external beam radiotherapy demonstrated significantly increased risks of malignant melanoma, and cancers of bladder, rectum, colon, brain, stomach, and lung, with odds ratios ranging from 1.25 to 1.85, when compared with men who did not receive external beam radiation therapy. Patients who received radioactive implants with or without external beam radiation therapy, however, did not show significant excesses of second cancers, when compared with those who did not receive radiation.

Another updated survey of prostate cancer patients reported to the SEER program (1973–2001) focused on the risk of rectal cancer following irradiation (Kendal et al. 2006). Unlike previous studies, a significant association between radiation therapy and subsequent excesses of rectal cancer were not found. Results of Cox proportional hazards analysis (with prostate irradiation, prostate surgery and age at diagnosis entered as covariates) showed that only increasing age was associated with an increased risk of subsequent rectal cancer.

Among prostate cancer patients given radiotherapy and reported to the British Columbia Tumor Registry (Pickles and Phillips 2002), significantly increased risks of sarcoma ($RR = 1.7$, $p < 0.05$), colorectal cancer ($RR = 1.21$, $p < 0.01$), and pleural cancer ($RR = 2.28$, $p < 0.01$) were observed. Although significant bladder cancer excesses were not apparent in the radiotherapy cohort, risks for both bladder cancer ($RR = 1.32$, $p < 0.01$) and testicular cancer ($RR = 2.82$, $p < 0.05$) were significantly increased in the non-irradiated cohort, which were attributed to heightened surveillance.

Most of the investigations to date that evaluate the risk of malignancies among prostate cancer survivors are based on data reported to population-based tumor registries. The conflicting observations with regard to the contribution of radiotherapy to various second malignancies after prostate cancer may reflect a number of factors, including the standard procedure of most registries to gather data only on initial course of therapy, the incomplete registration of this initial treatment, and misclassification. Moreover, selection bias may be operant in decisions to manage patients with either surgery alone or radiation therapy, and the limited data available in most population-based registries do not permit the identification of confounding factors. Patients with significant co-morbid illnesses and/or a history of heavy tobacco use may not be treated with surgery and may be more likely to be given radiation therapy. Further, among prostate cancer patients given radiation therapy, treatment-related sequelae such as cystitis, hematuria, proctitis, and rectal bleeding may lead to additional cystoscopies or colonoscopies, which can then result in an apparent increase in the incidence of urologic and colorectal cancers.

In those studies that show significant excesses of cancers after radiotherapy for prostate cancer, the overall risk appears to be low. In the investigation by Brenner and colleagues, which included prostate cancer patients given larger field Cobalt irradiation, the risk of developing a second malignancy was estimated at 1 in 290 (Brenner et al. 2000). In the last few years, intensity modulated radiation therapy (IMRT) has been increasingly utilized to treat prostate cancer in order to permit more conformal dose distribution and dose escalation (Guckenberger and Flentje 2007). Depending on treatment energy, IMRT is associated with a 3- to 5-fold higher number of monitor units as compared with conventional treatment. Applying risk coefficients from the National Council of Radiation Protection and Measurements for specific anatomic sites to this configuration, the risks of second malignancy using IMRT techniques have been estimated to be 2–3 times higher than that after conventional radiation therapy (Kry et al. 2005). These preliminary estimates remain to be confirmed in epidemiologic studies which include large numbers of patients given IMRT who have been followed for sufficient periods of time to permit detection of any increased radiotherapy-associated risk.

5 Comment

In view of the increasing numbers of cancer survivors, the development of second malignant neoplasms has emerged as a significant complication that can affect quality of life and long-term survival. It is critical to continue to describe and quantify the site-specific risks of second malignancies. Moreover, the evolving patterns have important implications for patient counseling and the recommendation of behavioral changes (e.g., smoking cessation), cancer screening and prevention strategies. Where efficacious screening methods (e.g., mammographic examination) are available, these modalities should be included in patient follow-up, as indicated, e.g., for women treated for HL at a young age with the wide-field, high-dose chest radiotherapy treatments of the past [reviewed in Travis et al. (2008)]. Preventive approaches will also decrease the risk of selected second cancers, and cancer survivors should be strongly advised to implement practices consistent with a healthy lifestyle. An improved recognition and understanding of second malignancies can inform changes in regimens to minimize exposure to cytotoxic agents. Modification or reduction of current treatments that have established efficacy, however, should not be undertaken outside the context of clinical trials. Further, it is important to remember that second malignancies are a consequence of success, and not observed unless a patient survives an initial cancer diagnosis. Thus, it must be kept in mind that the survival benefits provided by many cancer treatments greatly outweigh the risk of developing a second primary cancer. Moreover, as so clearly shown in the recent systematic review of the SEER program data (Curtis et al. 2006), lifestyle choices such as alcohol or tobacco use have a sizable impact on the risk of second cancers, as well as on the occurrence of first primary cancers. Results in the SEER program also confirm that multiple primary cancers can reflect the late effects of therapy, the influence of other factors including nutrition and hormones, infections and immunosuppression, genetic predisposition, other host factors, environmental determinants, and the operation of joint effects, including gene–environment and gene–gene interactions (Travis et al. 2006; Travis 2002).

References

Aisenberg AC, Finkelstein DM, Doppke KP et al (1997) High risk of breast carcinoma after irradiation of young women with Hodgkin's disease. Cancer 79:1203–1210

Allan JM, Travis LB (2005) Mechanisms of therapy-related carcinogenesis. Nat Rev Cancer 5:943–955

Andrieu JM, Ifrah N, Payen C et al (1990) Increased risk of secondary acute nonlymphocytic leukemia after extended-field radiation therapy combined with MOPP chemotherapy for Hodgkin's disease. J Clin Oncol 8:1148–1154

Anonymous [No authors listed] (2004) Cancer survivors: living longer, and now, better [editorial]. Lancet 364:2153–2154

Arseneau JC, Sponzo RW, Levin DL et al (1972) Nonlymphomatous malignant tumors complicating Hodgkin's disease. Possible association with intensive therapy. N Engl J Med 287:1119–1122

Behrens C, Travis LB, Wistuba II et al (2000) Molecular changes in second primary lung and breast cancers after therapy for Hodgkin's disease. Cancer Epidemiol Biomark Prev 9:1027–1035

Bergman L, Beelen ML, Gallee MP et al (2000) Risk and prognosis of endometrial cancer after tamoxifen for breast cancer. Comprehensive cancer centres' ALERT group. Assessment of liver and endometrial cancer risk following tamoxifen. Lancet 356:881–887

Bhatia S, Landier W (2005) Evaluating survivors of pediatric cancer. Cancer J 11:340–354

Bhatia S, Yasui Y, Robison LL et al (2003) High risk of subsequent neoplasms continues with extended follow-up of childhood Hodgkin's disease: report from the late effects study group. J Clin Oncol 21:4386–4394

Boice JD Jr, Harvey EB, Blettner M et al (1992) Cancer in the contralateral breast after radiotherapy for breast cancer. N Engl J Med 326:781–785

Brenner DJ, Curtis RE, Hall EJ et al (2000) Second malignancies in prostate carcinoma patients after radiotherapy compared with surgery. Cancer 88:398–406

Campone M, Roche H, Kerbrat P et al (2005) Secondary leukemia after epirubicin-based adjuvant chemotherapy in operable breast cancer patients: 16 years experience of the French adjuvant study group. Ann Oncol 16:1343–1351

Chen PY, Vicini FA (2007) Partial breast irradiation. Patient selection, guidelines for treatment, and current results. Front Radiat Ther Oncol 40:253–271

Chrouser K, Leibovich B, Bergstralh E et al (2005) Bladder cancer risk following primary and adjuvant external beam radiation for prostate cancer. J Urol 174:107–110, discussion 110–101

Clarke M, Collins R, Darby S et al (2005) Effects of radiotherapy and of differences in the extent of surgery for early breast cancer on local recurrence and 15-year survival: an overview of the randomised trials. Lancet 366:2087–2106

Curtis RE, Boice JD Jr, Stovall M et al (1992) Risk of leukemia after chemotherapy and radiation treatment for breast cancer. N Engl J Med 326:1745–1751

Curtis RE, Ron E, Hankey BA et al (2006) New malignancies following breast cancer. In: Curtis RE, Freedman DM, Ron E et al (eds) New malignancies among cancer survivors: SEER cancer registries, 1973–2000. NIH publication no. 05-5302. National Cancer Institute, Bethesda, pp 181–205

Deutsch M, Land SR, Begovic M et al (2003) The incidence of lung carcinoma after surgery for breast carcinoma with and without postoperative radiotherapy. Results of national surgical adjuvant breast and bowel project (NSABP) clinical trials B-04 and B-06. Cancer 98:1362–1368

Diehl V, Franklin J, Pfreundschuh M et al (2003) Standard and increased-dose BEACOPP chemotherapy compared with COPP-ABVD for advanced Hodgkin's disease. N Engl J Med 348:2386–2395

Do KA, Johnson MM, Lee JJ et al (2004) Longitudinal study of smoking patterns in relation to the development of smoking-related secondary primary tumors in patients with upper aerodigestive tract malignancies. Cancer 101:2837–2842

Dores GM, Metayer C, Curtis RE et al (2002) Second malignant neoplasms among long-term survivors of Hodgkin's disease: a population-based evaluation over 25 years. J Clin Oncol 20:3484–3494

Dores G, Schonfeld S, Chen J et al (2005) Long-term cause-specific mortality among 41–146 one-year survivors of Hodgkin lymphoma (HL). Proc Am Soc Clin Oncol 23:562S

Esler-Brauer L, Jaggernauth W, Zeitouni NC (2007) Angiosarcoma developing after conservative treatment for breast carcinoma: case report with review of the current literature. Dermatol Surg 33:749–755

Fisher B, Costantino JP, Redmond CK et al (1994) Endometrial cancer in tamoxifen-treated breast cancer patients: findings from the national surgical adjuvant breast and bowel project (NSABP) B-14 [see comments]. J Natl Cancer Inst 86:527–537

Fisher B, Costantino JP, Wickerham DL et al (1998) Tamoxifen for prevention of breast cancer: report of the national surgical adjuvant breast and bowel project P-1 Study [see comments]. J Natl Cancer Inst 90:1371–1388

Fisher B, Costantino JP, Wickerham DL (2005) Effects of chemotherapy and hormonal therapy for early breast cancer on recurrence and 15-year survival: an overview of the randomised trials. Lancet 365:1687–1717

Ford MB, Sigurdson AJ, Petrulis ES et al (2003) Effects of smoking and radiotherapy on lung carcinoma in breast carcinoma survivors. Cancer 98:1457–1464

Fossa SD, Chen J, Schonfeld SJ et al (2005) Risk of contralateral testicular cancer: a population-based study of 29,515 U.S. men. J Natl Cancer Inst 97:1056–1066

Gail MH, Brinton LA, Byar DP et al (1989) Projecting individualized probabilities of developing breast cancer for white females who are being examined annually. J Natl Cancer Inst 81:1879–1886

Gao X, Fisher SG, Emami B (2003) Risk of second primary cancer in the contralateral breast in women treated for early-stage breast cancer: a population-based study. Int J Radiat Oncol Biol Phys 56:1038–1045

Gilbert ES, Stovall M, Gospodarowicz M et al (2003) Lung cancer after treatment for Hodgkin's disease: focus on radiation effects. Radiat Res 159:161–173

Girinsky T, van der Maazen R, Specht L et al (2006) Involved-node radiotherapy (INRT) in patients with early Hodgkin lymphoma: concepts and guidelines. Radiother Oncol 79:270–277

Gooley TA, Leisenring W, Crowley J et al (1999) Estimation of failure probabilities in the presence of competing risks: new representations of old estimators. Stat Med 18:695–706

Guckenberger M, Flentje M (2007) Intensity-modulated radiotherapy (IMRT) of localized prostate cancer: a review and future perspectives. Strahlenther Onkol 183:57–62

Henry-Amar M (1992) Second cancer after the treatment for Hodgkin's disease: a report from the International Database on Hodgkin's Disease. Ann Oncol 3(Suppl 4):117–128

Hill-Kayser CE, Harris EE, Hwang WT et al (2006) Twenty-year incidence and patterns of contralateral breast cancer after breast conservation treatment with radiation. Int J Radiat Oncol Biol Phys 66:1313–1319

Hisada M, Rabkin CS (2005) Viral causes of cancer. In: Shields PG (ed) Cancer risk assessment. Taylor and Francis, Boca Raton, pp 287–311

Hodgson DC, Gilbert ES, Dores GM et al (2007) Long-term solid cancer risk among 5-year survivors of Hodgkin's lymphoma. J Clin Oncol 25:1489–1497

Huang J, Mackillop WJ (2001) Increased risk of soft tissue sarcoma after radiotherapy in women with breast carcinoma. Cancer 92:172–180

Jessner M, Zak FG, Rein CR (1952) Angiosarcoma in postmastectomy lymphedema (Stewart-Treves syndrome). AMA Arch Dermatol Syphilol 65:123–129

Kaldor JM, Day NE, Clarke EA et al (1990) Leukemia following Hodgkin's disease. N Engl J Med 322:7–13

Karlsson P, Holmberg E, Samuelsson A et al (1998) Soft tissue sarcoma after treatment for breast cancer—a Swedish population-based study. Eur J Cancer 34:2068–2075

Kendal WS, Eapen L, Macrae R et al (2006) Prostatic irradiation is not associated with any measurable increase in the risk of subsequent rectal cancer. Int J Radiat Oncol Biol Phys 65:661–668

Kirova YM, Vilcoq JR, Asselain B et al (2005) Radiation-induced sarcomas after radiotherapy for breast carcinoma: a large-scale single-institution review. Cancer 104:856–863

Kirova YM, Gambotti L, De Rycke Y et al (2007) Risk of second malignancies after adjuvant radiotherapy for breast cancer: a large-scale, single-institution review. Int J Radiat Oncol Biol Phys 68:359–363

Kollmannsberger C, Hartmann JT, Kanz L et al (1999) Therapy-related malignancies following treatment of germ cell cancer. Int J Cancer 83:860–863

Kry SF, Salehpour M, Followill DS et al (2005) The calculated risk of fatal secondary malignancies from intensity-modulated radiation therapy. Int J Radiat Oncol Biol Phys 62:1195–1203

Magriples U, Naftolin F, Schwartz PE et al (1993) High-grade endometrial carcinoma in tamoxifen-treated breast cancer patients. J Clin Oncol 11:485–490

Mauch P, Ng A, Aleman B et al (2005) Report from the Rockefellar Foundation Sponsored International Workshop on reducing mortality and improving quality of life in long-term survivors of Hodgkin's disease. Bellagio, Italy, 9–16 July 2003. Eur J Haematol (supp):68–76

Moon K, Stukenborg GJ, Keim J et al (2006) Cancer incidence after localized therapy for prostate cancer. Cancer 107:991–998

Morgan GJ, Linet MS, Rabkin CS (2006) Immunologic factors. In: Schottenfeld D, Fraumeni JFJ (eds) Cancer epidemiology and prevention. Oxford University Press, New York, pp 549–561

Neugut AI, Robinson E, Lee WC et al (1993) Lung cancer after radiation therapy for breast cancer [see comments]. Cancer 71:3054–3057

Neugut AI, Murray T, Santos J et al (1994) Increased risk of lung cancer after breast cancer radiation therapy in cigarette smokers [see comments]. Cancer 73:1615–1620

Neugut AI, Ahsan H, Robinson E et al (1997) Bladder carcinoma and other second malignancies after radiotherapy for prostate carcinoma. Cancer 79:1600–1604

Ng AK, Bernardo MV, Weller E et al (2002) Second malignancy after Hodgkin disease treated with radiation therapy with or without chemotherapy: long-term risks and risk factors. Blood 100:1989–1996

Pedersen-Bjergaard J, Daugaard G, Hansen SW et al (1991) Increased risk of myelodysplasia and leukemia after etoposide, cisplatin, and bleomycin for germ-cell tumours. Lancet 338:359–363

Pickles T, Phillips N (2002) The risk of second malignancy in men with prostate cancer treated with or without radiation in British Columbia, 1984–2000. Radiother Oncol 65:145–151

Praga C, Bergh J, Bliss J et al (2005) Risk of acute myeloid leukemia and myelodysplastic syndrome in trials of adjuvant epirubicin for early breast cancer: correlation with doses of epirubicin and cyclophosphamide. J Clin Oncol 23:4179–4191

Ries L, Melbert D, Krapcho M et al (2007) SEER cancer statistics review, 1975–2004. National Cancer Institute, Bethesda

Roychoudhuri R, Evans H, Robinson D et al (2004) Radiation-induced malignancies following radiotherapy for breast cancer. Br J Cancer 91:868–872

Rubino C, de Vathaire F, Shamsaldin A et al (2003) Radiation dose, chemotherapy, hormonal treatment and risk of second cancer after breast cancer treatment. Br J Cancer 89:840–846

Rueffer U, Josting A, Franklin J et al (2001) Non-Hodgkin's lymphoma after primary Hodgkin's disease in the German Hodgkin's lymphoma study group: incidence, treatment, and prognosis. J Clin Oncol 19:2026–2032

Saadat M, Truong PT, Kader HA et al (2007) Outcomes in patients with primary breast cancer and a subsequent diagnosis of endometrial cancer : comparison of cohorts treated with and without tamoxifen. Cancer 110:31–37

Sankila R, Garwicz S, Olsen JH et al (1996) Risk of subsequent malignant neoplasms among 1,641 Hodgkin's disease patients diagnosed in childhood and adolescence: a population-based cohort study in the five Nordic countries. Association of the Nordic Cancer Registries and the Nordic Society of Pediatric Hematology and Oncology. J Clin Oncol 14:1442–1446

Schairer C, Hisada M, Chen BE et al (2007) Comparative mortality for 621 second cancers in 29,356 testicular cancer survivors and 12,420 matched first cancers. J Natl Cancer Inst 99:1248–1256

Schonfeld SJ, Gilbert ES, Dores GM et al (2006) Acute myeloid leukemia following Hodgkin lymphoma: a population-based study of 35,511 patients. J Natl Cancer Inst 98:215–218

Simonart T, Heenen M (2004) Radiation-induced angiosarcomas. Dermatology 209:175–176

Smith RE, Bryant J, DeCillis A et al (2003) Acute myeloid leukemia and myelodysplastic syndrome after doxorubicin-cyclophosphamide adjuvant therapy for operable breast cancer: the national surgical adjuvant breast and bowel project experience. J Clin Oncol 21:1195–1204

Storm HH, Andersson M, Boice JD Jr et al (1992) Adjuvant radiotherapy and risk of contralateral breast cancer. J Natl Cancer Inst 84:1245–1250

Swerdlow AJ, Barber JA, Hudson GV et al (2000) Risk of second malignancy after Hodgkin's disease in a collaborative British cohort: the relation to age at treatment. J Clin Oncol 18:498–509

Swerdlow AJ, Schoemaker MJ, Allerton R et al (2001) Lung cancer after Hodgkin's disease: a nested case-control study of the relation to treatment. J Clin Oncol 19:1610–1618

Travis LB (2002) Therapy-associated solid tumors. Acta Oncol 41:323–333

Travis LB, Curtis RE, Hankey BF et al (1992) Second cancers in patients with chronic lymphocytic leukemia. J Natl Cancer Inst 84:1422–1427

Travis LB, Andersson M, Gospodarowicz M et al (2000) Treatment-associated leukemia following testicular cancer. J Natl Cancer Inst 92:1165–1171

Travis LB, Gospodarowicz M, Curtis RE et al (2002) Lung cancer following chemotherapy and radiotherapy for Hodgkin's disease. J Natl Cancer Inst 94:182–192

Travis LB, Hill DA, Dores GM et al (2003) Breast cancer following radiotherapy and chemotherapy among young women with Hodgkin disease. JAMA 290:465–475

Travis LB, Fossa SD, Schonfeld SJ et al (2005a) Second cancers among 40,576 testicular cancer patients: focus on long-term survivors. J Natl Cancer Inst 97:1354–1365

Travis LB, Hill D, Dores GM et al (2005b) Cumulative absolute breast cancer risk for young women treated for Hodgkin lymphoma. J Natl Cancer Inst 97:1428–1437

Travis LB, Rabkin CS, Brown LM et al (2006) Cancer survivorship—genetic susceptibility and second primary cancers: research strategies and recommendations. J Natl Cancer Inst 98:15–25

Travis LB, Hodgson D, Allan J et al (2008) Second cancers. In: Cancer: Principles and practice of oncology. Lippincott Williams and Wilkins, Philadelphia (in press)

van den Belt-Dusebout AW, de Wit R, Gietema JA et al (2007) Treatment-specific risks of second malignancies and cardiovascular disease in 5-year survivors of testicular cancer. J Clin Oncol 25:4370–4378

van Leeuwen FE, Travis LB (2005) Second cancers. In: DeVita VT Jr et al (eds) Cancer: principles and practice of oncology, 7th edn. Lippincott Williams & Wilkins, Philadelphia, pp 2575–2602

van Leeuwen FE, Chorus AM, van den Belt-Dusebout AW et al (1994) Leukemia risk following Hodgkin's disease: relation to cumulative dose of alkylating agents, treatment with teniposide combinations, number of episodes of chemotherapy, and bone marrow damage. J Clin Oncol 12:1063–1073

van Leeuwen FE, Klokman WJ, Veer MB et al (2000) Long-term risk of second malignancy in survivors of Hodgkin's disease treated during adolescence or young adulthood. J Clin Oncol 18:487–497

van Leeuwen FE, Klokman WJ, Stovall M et al (2003) Roles of radiation dose, chemotherapy, and hormonal factors in breast cancer following Hodgkin's disease. J Natl Cancer Inst 95:971–980

Virtanen A, Pukkala E, Auvinen A (2007) Angiosarcoma after radiotherapy: a cohort study of 332,163 Finnish cancer patients. Br J Cancer 97:115–117

Zablotska LB, Neugut AI (2003) Lung carcinoma after radiation therapy in women treated with lumpectomy or mastectomy for primary breast carcinoma. Cancer 97:1404–1411

Radiation-Related Second Primary Cancers: Clinical Perspectives

David C. Hodgson, Andrea Ng, and Lois B. Travis

Contents

D. C. Hodgson (✉)
Department of Radiation Oncology, University of Toronto, Princess Margaret Hospital, 610 University Ave, Toronto, ON M5G 2M9, Canada
e-mail: David.Hodgson@rmp.uhn.on.ca

A. Ng
Department of Radiation Oncology, Harvard Medical School, Brigham and Women's Hospital and Dana-Farber Cancer Institute, 75 Francis street L2, Boston, MA 02115, USA

L. B. Travis
Department of Radiation Oncology, University of Rochester, James P. Wilmot Cancer Center, 265 Crittenden Boulevard; CU 420318, Rochester, NY 14642-0318, USA

Abstract

Radiation therapy (RT) is a major treatment used in the curative management of many cancer types. As survival rates for many forms of cancer continue to improve, there is increasing clinical attention being directed toward the risk of delayed radiation-induced second cancer (SC). Survivors of Hodgkin lymphoma, leukemia, cervix cancer, and breast cancer treated with RT have been shown, to varying degrees, to experience increased risks of SC. Important improvements in the analysis of risk can aid clinical interpretation: in particular, emphasis on the cumulative incidence of SC, and appropriate adjustment for competing causes of death can provide more clinically meaningful insight into the burden of SC than descriptions of the relative risk. The nature of the dose-risk relationship for normal tissues exposed to intermediate and high dose is uncertain, although there are emerging data that the risk may increase with increasing dose above 10 Gy. A better understanding of the risk associated with doses in this range will be an important component of developing RT treatments that limit the risk of SC and also for understanding the potential risk associated with newer treatments, such as intensity modulated radiation therapy (IMRT). Further research is required to better understand how the interaction of RT and chemotherapy or biologic agents may affect SC risk, and to identify the genetic contributors to the development of SC.

1 Introduction

There are an estimated 10.7 million cancer survivors in the United States, and this population is growing by roughly 2 % annually (Ries et al. 2006). As more patients experience prolonged survival after an initial cancer diagnosis, the late effects of treatment have emerged as an increasingly important clinical concern.

P. Rubin et al. (eds.), *ALERT – Adverse Late Effects of Cancer Treatment*, Medical Radiology. Radiation Oncology,
DOI: 10.1007/978-3-540-72314-1_16, © Springer-Verlag Berlin Heidelberg 2014

One of the most serious late effects of cancer and its treatment is the development of second cancers (SC), which accounted for approximately 16 % of incident malignancies reported to the National Cancer Institute's (NCI's) Surveillance, Epidemiology, and End Results (SEER) Program in 2003 (Ries et al. 2006). SC are also a leading cause of mortality among several populations of long-term survivors (Bhatia et al. 2003; Capra et al. 2007; Guerin et al. 2007; Hodgson et al. 2007a, b; Travis et al. 2005; Travis and Gilbert 2005; Tward et al. 2007). Development of a SC can reflect the cellular and tissue damage caused by cancer treatment, as well as the influence of environmental exposures, biological determinants, and combinations of effects, including gene-environment and gene–gene interactions (Travis et al. 2006).

The focus of this chapter will be the influence of radiation therapy (RT) on the risk of SC. RT is associated with elevated risks of second cancer among survivors of Hodgkin lymphoma (Aleman et al. 2003; Bhatia et al. 2003; Capra et al. 2007; Hodgson et al. 2007), non-Hodgkin lymphoma (Bluhm et al. 2008; Sacchi et al. 2008; Travis et al. 1991, 1993), testicular cancer (Kaldor et al. 1987; Schairer et al. 2007; Travis et al. 2005; van Leeuwen et al. 1993), cervix cancer (Boice et al. 1985; Chaturvedi et al. 2007) and breast cancer (Brown et al. 2007; Deutsch et al. 2007; Gao et al. 2003; Schaapveld et al. 2008) as well as several forms of childhood cancer. (Bassal et al. 2006; Dinu et al. 2008; Neglia et al. 2001). Increased risks of second cancer have also been reported among patients receiving RT for prostate cancer, (Brenner et al. 2000; Moon et al. 2006; Pickles and Phillips 2002; Rapiti et al. 2008) and cancer of the nasopharynx, (Kong et al. 2006) reflecting in part the increasing awareness and concern regarding late effects of treatment as the control of the primary disease improves.

2 Analytic Issues Influencing the Clinical Interpretation of Second Cancer Studies

2.1 Relative versus Absolute Risks

Elevated risks of SC are often expressed as the ratio of observed number of cases/expected number cases (O/E ratio), where the expected number of cases is typically based on the cancer incidence reported in the general population, standardized to the sex, age, race, and calendar year distribution of the study cohort. This ratio is also referred to as the standardized incidence ratio (SIR).

One limitation of the SIR as a measure of risk is its sensitivity to the baseline incidence of the cancer type being evaluated: for uncommon cancers (such as leukemia) a small number of excess cases can produce a large increase in SIR. In contrast, the SIR may be lower for more common cancers (e.g., breast cancer) that affect a greater number of patients in the general population. In this regard, the SIR may obscure the true excess morbidity caused by a particular second cancer. A more clinically meaningful expression of risk is the absolute excess risk (AER), typically defined as the number of excess cases occurring per 10,000 person-years of follow-up: (observed number of cases per year − expected number of cases per year)/total person-years at risk × 10,000). Since the AER better reflects the actual number of patients affected, it is generally considered to be a more clinically relevant indicator of the burden of morbidity caused by SC.

2.2 Cumulative Incidence and Competing Risks

Both SIR and AER present risks in terms different from those used to describe most other cancer-related clinical outcomes, such as 5-year disease-free survival or overall survival. This can make it a challenge to weigh the risks and benefits of treatment. For example, clinical trials have demonstrated that following chemotherapy for early stage HL, radiation therapy improves disease-free survival by about 5–10 % (Meyer et al. 2003; Nachman et al. 2002), while epidemiologic studies have reported that this treatment is associated with a 2- to 6-fold increased risk of second cancer (Dores et al. 2002; Ng et al. 2002). It is easier to make a clinically meaningful evaluation of risk–benefit concerns if the second cancer risk is also expressed as a cumulative incidence (e.g., the 20-year risk of second cancers after wide field mantle ± para-aortic RT is approximately 20 % (Ng et al. 2002).

The Kaplan–Meier method has been used to estimate the cumulative incidence of second cancers over time (Bhatia et al. 1996; Dores et al. 2002; Ng et al. 2002). Studies using this approach have typically censored patients who die prior to developing SC. However, one of the assumptions of the Kaplan–Meier estimate is that censored patients do not differ systematically from non-censored patients with regard to their risk of developing the outcome of interest (i.e., the assumption of "non-informative" censoring). This assumption is not met when deceased patients are censored, since they have no further risk of developing a SC. Clinical readers should be aware that the Kaplan–Meier estimate of cumulative incidence can significantly inflate the apparent risk of SC, particularly among patient groups with worse overall survival rates, and the magnitude of this overestimate increases with follow-up time. (Pintilie 2006) (Fig. 1). Notably, most estimates of the AER also censor patients at the time of death, and so multiplying the annual AER x the number of years of follow-up as an approximation of the

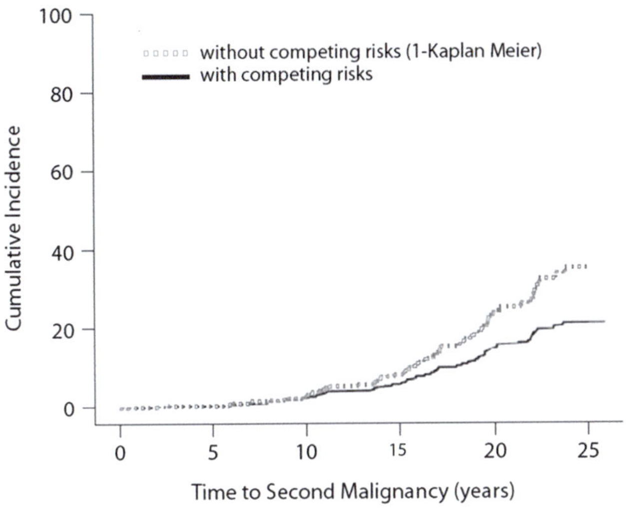

Fig. 1 Cumulative incidence of second cancers among patients treated at the Princess Margaret Hospital for Hodgkin lymphoma, aged ≥30 -years at HL diagnosis. The Kaplan–Meier method does not adequately account for competing causes of death that can occur prior to developing a second cancer. As a result, the cumulative incidence of second cancers is overestimtated compared to models that account for competing risks, particularly with prolonged follow-up. Reproduced with permission from Neglia et al. 2006

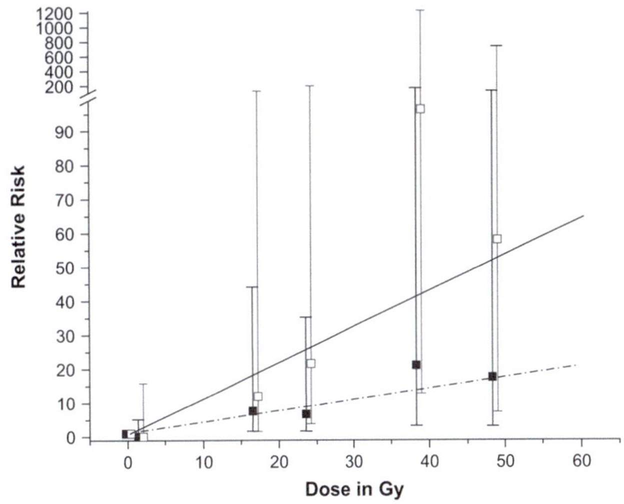

Fig. 2 Relative risk of subsequent glioma and meningioma within the Childhood Cancer Survivor Study cohort by radiation dose (*open boxes*, mean observed relative risk for meningioma; *closed boxes*, mean observed relative risk for glioma; *solid line*, fitted line for meningioma risk; *hatched line*, fitted line for glioma risk). $P < 0.001$ (likelihood ratio test, two-sided). Reproduced with permission from Neglia et al. 2006

cumulative incidence also does not adequately account for competing causes of death.

Several methods to account for competing causes of death that may influence the cumulative incidence of late effects have been described (Pintilie 2006). While a detailed review of these methods are beyond the scope of this review, appropriate clinical interpretation of SC studies requires an understanding that competing risks should be accounted for in study analyses.

3 Radiation Dose-Risk Relationships and Implications for Radiation Therapy

The relationship between low-dose radiation exposures and cancer risk has been studied extensively in studies of Japanese atomic bomb survivors (Ron et al. 1994; Thompson et al. 1994), and those experiencing occupational radiation exposures (Cardis et al. 2007; Lie et al. 2008). Consequently, the relationship between radiation dose and cancer risk is better understood for low-dose exposures than for doses typically prescribed for RT. For most solid tumors and leukemia, there is an approximately linear increase in risk with increasing radiation dose up to about 5 Gy (Boice et al. 1988; Curtis et al. 1994; Preston et al. 2002). At higher doses, cell killing offsets the induction of malignancy in hematopoietic tissue, and the risk of developing leukemia declines (Boice et al. 1987). In part due to this observation, it has been a common clinical precept that second cancers occur at the edge of RT fields because increased cell killing results in lower SC risk for tissues in the "high dose" (i.e., >35 Gy) volume. However, analytic studies of selected second solid cancers among patients receiving RT have demonstrated that this is often not the case (Travis and Gilbert 2005; Travis et al. 2003; van Leeuwen et al. 2003). For example, following mediastinal RT for HL, the risks of breast- and lung cancer have been shown to increase with increasing doses above 30 Gy (Gilbert et al. 2003; Travis et al. 2002), although the slope of the dose-risk curve appears to be less steep in this dose range. Similarly, the risks of soft-tissue sarcoma (Rubino et al. 2005), osteosarcoma (Hawkins et al. 1996), glioma and meningioma (Neglia et al. 2006) have also been found to rise with increasing radiation doses above 20 Gy. In a CCSS study, increasing radiation dose-risk relationships were apparent for both glioma and meningioma, with no downturn of the risk at high doses. At radiation doses of 30–45 Gy to the site of CNS tumor development, the RRs of glioma and meningioma were 21.0 and 96.3, respectively, compared with exposure to less than 1 Gy (Fig. 2). The radiation dose response for glioma was significantly stronger for patients irradiated before age five (Neglia et al. 2006).

In contrast, radiation-induced thyroid cancer risk appears to increase with increasing doses up to 10–20 Gy (Ron et al. 1995; Sigurdson et al. 2005), and then plateaus or declines with increasing dose. The dose-risk relationship for radiation-induced leukemia is quite different from that seen for solid tumor induction: the risk of leukemia is much higher at low doses, and there is little or no increased risk at higher dose (i.e. >20 Gy), likely due to bone marrow ablation (Curtis et al. 1992; Little et al. 1999).

These findings suggest two clinically important conclusions relating to RT-related SC risk. First, no single dose-risk relationship will apply to all exposed tissues: there is variation in the sensitivity of different tissues with regard to cancer induction by radiation. Second, for many tissues, the risk of radiation-induced SC increases with increasing doses up to and exceeding doses typically occurring at the edge of treatment fields.

4 Intensity Modulated Radiation Therapy and Second Cancer Risk

An understanding of the radiation dose-risk relationship has important implications when considering the potential therapeutic gains that may be achieved with intensity modulated radiation therapy (IMRT). Compared to conventional RT, IMRT typically achieves more conformal (i.e., smaller) high-dose volumes at the expense of exposing a larger volume of normal tissues to low/intermediate doses. This occurs in part because IMRT often employs more treatment fields than conventional RT, thereby exposing additional tissue to intermediate-dose radiation from these added fields. Further, IMRT may be associated with long "beam on" times (i.e. more monitor units) than conventional RT, and can thereby increase the low-dose total body exposure caused by radiation leakage during treatment (Hall 2006). Finally, use of high energy beams (e.g., 18 MV) may increase total body neutron dose due to the interaction of high energy X-rays with the components of the linear accelerator. A small number of studies have predicted that, in spite of the improved conformality of the high-dose volume, the additional low-dose exposure may increase the risk of second cancers compared to conventional RT (Hall 2006; Schneider 2006).

Radiation oncologists prescribing IMRT should be aware of these issues when weighing the merits of different RT plans. In many cases, a well-designed IMRT plan can deliver an integral dose to the irradiated volume comparable to a non-IMRT plan, with a larger low/intermediate dose volume, but a smaller high-dose volume. In view of the dose-risk data presented above, it remains to be determined how increasing low-dose tissue volume while decreasing the high-dose volume will affect the overall increase in SC risk with IMRT. Also, since externally mounted beam modifying devices (e.g., wedges) attenuate the RT beam, segmented IMRT beams may in some cases require comparatively less "beam on" time to treat the same volume than older techniques. Furthermore, these wedges are often placed in close proximity to the patient and are a source of scatter dose to the patient. (Woo et al. 2006) Consequently, it is not a necessary feature of IMRT that it increases total body exposure compared to conventional RT given historically. (See Fig. 3 comparing IMRT vs. conventional tangent RT for breast cancer treatment).

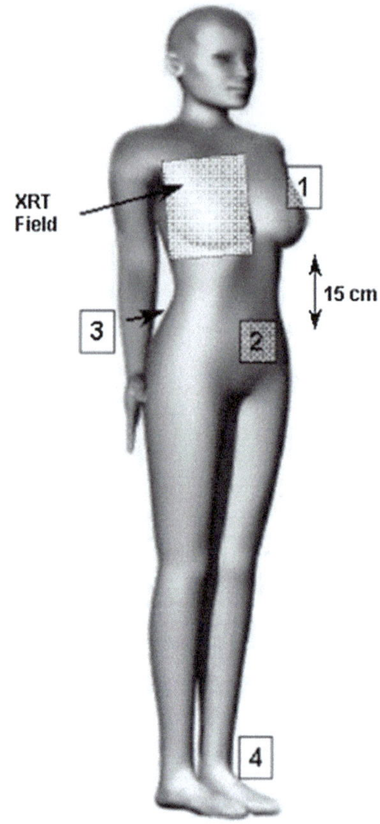

	Contralateral breast	Abdomen	Back	Contralateral ankle
	Mean Dose, Gy (SD)	Mean Dose, Gy (SD)	Mean Dose, Gy (SD)	Mean Dose, Gy (SD)
Treatment type				
Physical wedge	2.37 (0.55)	1.20 (0.31)	1.10 (0.34)	0.038 (0.011)
Dynamic wedge or breast IMRT	0.96 (0.36)	0.36 (0.13)	0.40 (0.20)	0.010 (0.007)

Fig. 3 Scatter dose to normal tissues associated with breast RT, comparing physical wedges and dynamic wedges/IMRT. Because physical wedges are placed close to the patient, they can produce greater scatter dose to normal tissues than techniques that employ segmented multileaf collimation to modify beam intensity. Reproduced with permission from Woo et al. (2006)

Appropriate utilization of IMRT requires both the consideration of primary tumor control as well as the risk of other radiation-related toxicities. The potential increase in absolute risk of SC associated with IMRT over conventional RT (estimated to be <3 % for patients with prostate IMRT (Kry et al. 2007)), should be considered within the context of a patient's competing risk of death from the primary cancer, and the potential benefit that IMRT may provide in properly treating the primary tumor and reducing the risk of serious chronic organ damage (e.g., xerostomia, rectal toxicity, osteopenia/bone fractures). In particular, clinicians should be aware of the potential for IMRT to increase SC risk, and the features of an IMRT plan that may influence this risk, such as dose to the entire irradiated volume, and the number of monitor units required to deliver treatment. Further research is required to quantify the potential for IMRT to increase the risk of SC compared to conventional RT in order to facilitate more thoughtful balancing of the potential risks and benefits.

5 Second Malignancy Risk in Survivors of Adult-Onset Cancers

Radiation therapy plays a central role as part of curative treatment in a considerable number of adult-onset malignancies. Most of the data on radiation-related second malignancy risks derive from patients with primary cancers in whom RT is routinely (or was historically) used as definitive or adjuvant treatment, and on primary cancers that tend to affect young patients, have a high cure rate, and/or a long natural history. Among survivors of various adult-onset malignancies, the largest amount of data with regard to SC risk exist for survivors of Hodgkin lymphoma. Data on radiation-related second malignancy risks are also available in survivors of testicular cancer, cervical cancer, and more recently breast cancer and prostate cancer.

5.1 Radiation-Related Malignancies After Hodgkin Lymphoma

The cure of Hodgkin lymphoma (HL) using large-field radiation therapy was first demonstrated over 50 years ago (Peters and Middlemiss 1958), with ensuing decades witnessing a considerable evolution of treatment. Excess second malignancies after successful treatment of Hodgkin lymphoma were first reported in the early 1970s (Arseneau et al. 1972). These early reports focused mostly on increased leukemia risks that were largely related to the use of alkylating chemotherapy in a dose-dependent manner. The use of large-field radiation therapy was also initially suggested as a contributing factor to excess leukemias. However, in a case–control study by van Leeuwen et al. (van Leeuwen et al. 1994), the addition of RT to chemotherapy did not significantly increase the risk of leukemia (relative risks of chemotherapy alone versus combined modality therapy: 44.6 vs. 20.9. $p = 0.16$). Although total-nodal irradiation in combination with chemotherapy was associated with a 2.5-fold elevated risk of leukemia compared with patients treated with chemotherapy alone, the increase was not statistically significant ($p = 0.39$).

Unlike leukemias after Hodgkin lymphoma, which typically arise within the first 10 years after treatment, solid tumors are associated with a longer latency, ranging from 5 to over 15 years, depending on the subtype of solid tumors. In addition, the risks appear to persist for prolonged periods of time. In more recent studies with longer follow-up time, solid tumors account for over three-quarters of all cases of second malignancies after Hodgkin lymphoma.

The contribution of RT to the development of SC after Hodgkin lymphoma is supported by several studies demonstrating increased risks among patients receiving RT as part of their initial treatment (Aleman et al. 2003; Bhatia et al. 2003; Capra et al. 2007; Hodgson et al. 2007). As noted previously, studies have reported a significant radiation dose–response relationship in the development of specific types of solid tumors after HL. Two case–control studies examined in detail the relationship between radiation dose and the risk of breast cancer after Hodgkin lymphoma therapy (Travis et al. 2003; van Leeuwen et al. 2003). In both studies, the radiation dose at the site of the breast cancer was estimated in the case patients and compared to the dose in a comparable location in the control subjects. In the study by van Leeuwen et al., which consisted of 48 cases of breast cancer and 175 matched controls, the breast cancer risk was significantly increased only after a radiation dose of 38.5 Gy or higher, but not at lower doses (van Leeuwen et al. 2003). In the large, international case–control study by Travis et al. (Travis et al. 2003), which consisted of 105 breast cancer cases and 266 matched controls, a radiation dose of >4 Gy to the breast was associated with a 3.2-fold breast cancer risk compared with women who received lower doses of radiation and no alkylating chemotherapy. The risk increased to 8-fold for women who received >40 Gy to the breast (p trend < 0.001). The comparable results of these studies is due in part to overlap of breast cancer cases evaluated in the Dutch study (40 of 48 cases) (van Leeuwen et al. 2003) that were also included in the international series by Travis et al. (2003).

A significant radiation dose–response relationship has similarly been shown for the development of lung cancer after Hodgkin lymphoma. Travis et al. conducted a case–control study of 222 cases of lung cancer and 444 matched controls in patients who had been treated for Hodgkin lymphoma (Travis et al. 2002). Using patients who received <5 Gy to the area of the lung in which the cancer developed as the reference group, the lung cancer risk increased with increasing dose to the lung (p trend $< .001$), although the increased risk was statistically significant only after exposure to doses of 30 Gy or higher.

A number of factors have modifying effects on radiation-related second malignancy after Hodgkin lymphoma. For breast cancer after Hodgkin lymphoma, young age at mantle irradiation has consistently been shown to be associated with significantly increased risk for breast cancer in women (Ng et al. 2002; Travis et al. 2003). In addition to age at treatment, ovarian hormonal exposures also have a significant modifying effect on breast cancer risk after Hodgkin lymphoma therapy. In the studies by both Travis et al. 2003 and van Leeuwen et al. 2003 patients who received chemotherapy and radiation therapy had significantly a reduced risk of breast cancer compared with those treated with radiation therapy alone, and the radiation-related risks were also attenuated by a radiation dose of 5 Gy or more delivered to the ovaries. The Dutch study also clearly showed that the substantial risk reduction associated with chemotherapy was attributable to the high frequency of premature menopause in chemotherapy-treated patients (van Leeuwen et al. 2003). Taken together, results in both studies showed that ovarian hormones play a critical role in promoting breast tumorigenesis once radiation has produced an initiating event.

The striking effect of smoking on the treatment-related risk for lung cancer among HL survivors merits emphasis. In a case–control study by Travis and colleagues (2002), in which the reference group consisted of patients who had HL who had minimal radiation exposure and who were nonsmokers or light smokers, those patients who received either alkylating agent chemotherapy alone or 5 Gy or more of radiation therapy alone to the area of the lung in which cancer developed later experienced 4.3-fold and 7.2-fold increased risks for lung cancer, respectively. These relative risks increased to 16.8-fold and 20.2-fold, respectively, in those patients who also smoked at least one pack of cigarettes per day. For cigarette smokers (at least one pack per day) who had also received alkylating chemotherapy and 5 Gy or more of radiation therapy to the area of the lung in which cancer developed, the relative risk for subsequent lung cancer was 49.1, consistent with a multiplicative effect of tobacco use on the risk for treatment-related lung cancer. In view of these findings, clinicians should be diligent in facilitating smoking cessation among both new HL patients and survivors.

In considering SC risk after Hodgkin lymphoma, it should be noted that while RT is a major contributor to excess risks, a number of other factors also influence risk, including chemotherapy (Swerdlow et al. 2000; Travis et al. 2002), underlying immune dysfunction and genetic predisposition. Further, much of the data on solid tumors after radiation therapy for Hodgkin lymphoma was based on patients treated in an era when large treatment fields and higher radiation doses were routinely employed. A significantly reduced volume of normal tissue is exposed with the current standard of care, which includes involved-field radiation therapy as part of combined modality therapy (Fig. 4). A comparative study of mantle RT fields versus contemporary IFRT for patients with mediastinal disease found that the latter was associated with a reduction in radiation dose to female breast tissue of approximately 65, and a 35 % reduction in lung dose (Koh et al. 2007). Radiobiologic modeling predicted comparable reductions in the breast- and lung cancer risks associated with the transition from mantle RT to IFRT (Hodgson et al. 2007). A meta-analysis showed that the risk of breast cancer is significantly higher after extended-field than involved-field radiation therapy (OR, 3.25, $p = 0.04$), which is likely related to the reduced amount of breast tissue in a more limited treatment field (e.g., exclusion of the axillae) (Franklin et al. 2006). Ongoing clinical efforts are exploring the possibility of further reductions in radiation treatment doses for HL. More recently, there is a trend toward involved-node radiation therapy that further reduces the exposure of normal tissue to radiation (Girinsky et al. 2006). It is thus expected that patients who receive RT in the modern era will likely experience lower risks for second malignancies than those reported in long-term follow-up studies of now outdated treatment.

5.2 Radiation-Related Malignancies After Testicular Cancer

Historically, treatment for testicular cancer included the use of large-field radiation therapy including treatment to the mediastinum and paraaortic and pelvic lymph nodes. Similar to Hodgkin lymphoma, testicular cancer typically affect young adults and has a high cure rate. In addition, as in survivors of Hodgkin lymphoma, second malignancy has been associated with excess mortality among selected long-term survivors of testicular cancer (Schairer et al. 2007). The types of second malignancy documented in survivors of testicular cancer include leukemia and several solid tumors, including mesothelioma, cancers of the lung, thyroid, esophagus, stomach, pancreas, colon, rectum, kidney, bladder, and connective tissue (Pedersen-Bjergaard et al. 1991; Travis et al. 2005; van den Belt-Dusebout et al. 2007). Much of the existing data on treatment-related second malignancy after testicular cancer may reflect the historical routine use of large field RT, although chemotherapy has also been shown to contribute to the risk. An excess risk for contralateral testicular cancer has also been observed, which is likely related to underlying predisposition rather than prior treatment (Fossa et al. 2005).

A population-based case–control study by Travis et al. explored treatment-associated leukemia in men with testicular cancer who had survived at least one year (Travis et al. 2000). The risk for leukemia increased significantly with increasing radiation field size, which was reflected in dose to active bone marrow. In addition, after taking into

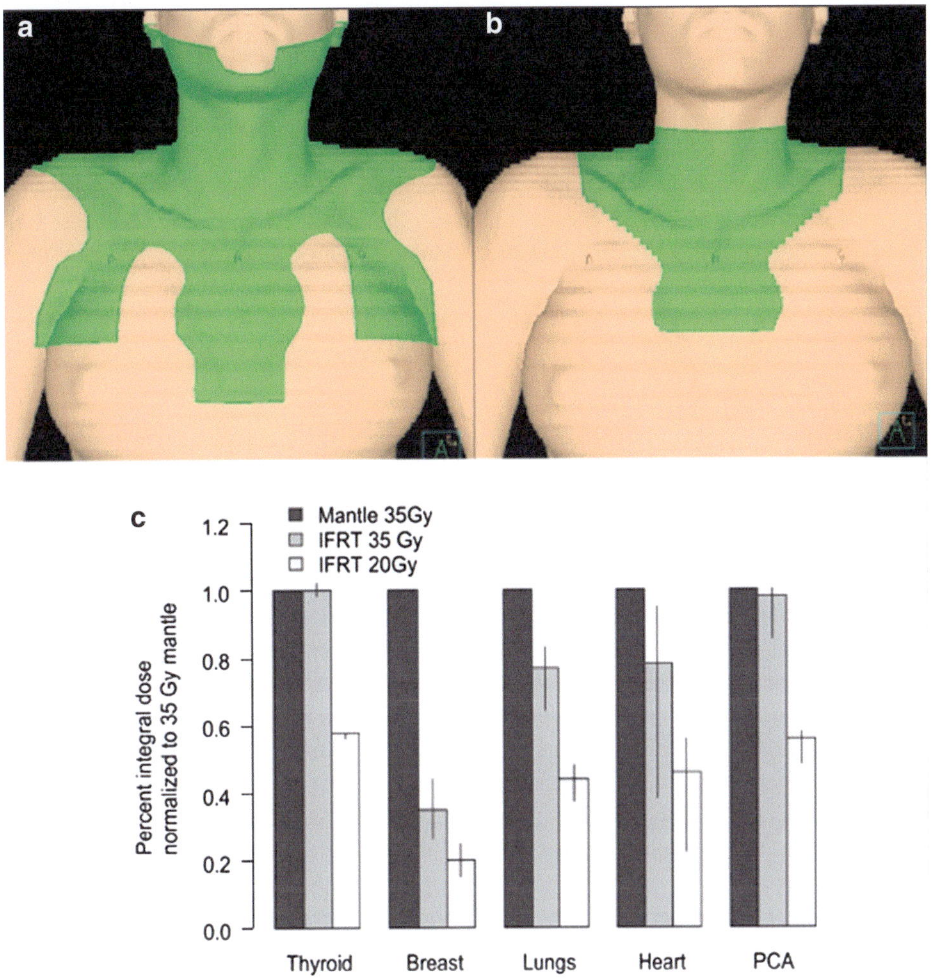

Fig. 4 Dose to normal tissues associated with mantle field (**a**) and involved-field RT (**b**) for a female patient with mediastinal HL. Historically used mantle fields contributed significant dose to normal tissue by electively treating the axillae. Restriction of RT to lymph node regions initially involved with disease can significantly reduce normal tissue exposure (**c**). Many north american pediatric protocols also reduce dose to ≈20 Gy, further reducing normal tissue dose compared to 35 Gy mantle RT. Reproduced with permission from Koh et al. (2007), and Hodgson et al. (2007b)

account the amount of radiation exposure to active bone marrow, the risk for leukemia was also significantly associated with cumulative dose of cisplatin received.

In the largest cohort study on testicular cancer survivors to date, Travis et al. reported on the solid tumor risk among 40,576 patients (Travis et al. 2005). At a mean follow-up of 11.8 years, the relative risks of developing a solid tumor were significantly increased after both radiation therapy and chemotherapy alone (RR, 2.0 and 1.8, respectively). Among 10-year survivors of testicular cancer initially treated with radiation therapy, the relative risks of solid tumors at sites included in typical infradiaphragmatic fields (e.g., bladder, stomach, pancreas, and kidneys) were considerably higher than those at sites not in field. Significantly increased risks of cancers of the esophagus, pleura, or lung were also found, likely reflecting the historical use of prophylactic mediastinal irradiation. In a cohort study from the Netherlands based on 1,909 patients with testicular cancer, the relative risk of second malignancy was 1.6 (95 % CI, 1.3–2.1) (Travis et al. 1993). Patients who had received radiation therapy to the paraaortic lymph nodes and who survived testicular cancer for more than 5 years were at particularly high risk of developing stomach cancer (RR, 6.9; 95 % CI, 3.3–12.7). In a update from the same group based on 2,707 5-year testicular cancer survivors (van den Belt-Dusebout et al. 2007), followed for a median of 17.6 years, the relative risk of second malignancy was 1.7 (95 % C.I., 1.5–1.9), with subdiaphragmatic radiotherapy being strongly associated with increased risk of SC.

5.3 Radiation-Related Malignancy After Cervical Cancer

Both definitive RT and radical surgery are accepted options in the treatment of nonbulky early-stage cervical cancer, while primary RT is typically the treatment of choice for women with bulky stage IB and IIA cervical cancer. Survivors of cervical cancer are at increased risk for developing several second malignancies, some of which can be explained by shared infectious causes or environmental risk factors, whereas others are attributable to previous treatment exposures. Kleinerman and colleagues were among the first to report on the risk of second malignancies following cervical cancer (Kleinerman et al. 1982). Compared with the general population, survivors of cervical cancer had a 1.4-fold increased risk for a second malignancy. A history of radiation therapy was associated with significant excesses of several cancers arising in the pelvic radiation field, including tumors of bladder, kidney, rectum, corpus uteri, and ovary. Since then, several studies have confirmed these findings (Boice et al. 1985; Chaturvedi et al. 2007). Chaturvedi and colleagues updated and expanded these data based on 104,760 1-year survivors of cervical cancer reported to 13 population-based cancer registries in Denmark, Finland, Norway, Sweden, and the United States (Chaturvedi et al. 2007). In this larger study with longer follow-up time, a significantly elevated relative risk (RR = 1.3; 95 % CI, 1.28–1.33) for second malignancy was again found. Moreover, the authors showed that following radiation therapy for cervical cancer, the risks for second cancers of the rectum/anus, colon, urinary bladder, ovary, and other female genital sites remained significantly elevated for more than 40 years. Several second cancers were likely related to shared etiologic factors rather than radiation therapy, because an increased risk was also observed among the non-radiation therapy cohort. These included cancers of the pharynx, genital sites, and rectum/anus, which are related to human papillomavirus infections; and cancers of the lungs, pancreas, and urinary bladder, which are related to tobacco use. In this study, younger age at cervical cancer treatment was associated with a significantly higher cumulative risk for second cancer. After adjustment for competing mortality, the 40-year cumulative risk of any second cancer was higher among women diagnosed with cervical cancer before age 50 than among women diagnosed after age 50 (22.2 vs. 16.4 %).

5.4 Radiation-Related Malignancy After Breast Cancer

Radiation therapy is an important modality in the treatment of breast cancer, either as part of breast-conserving therapy or postmastectomy treatment. Among the various types of second cancers observed in survivors of breast cancer, the largest amount of data exists for contralateral breast cancer, which is partly related to preexisting breast cancer risk factors (Boice et al. 1992; Gao et al. 2003; Hemminki et al. 2007; Kirova et al. 2007; Storm et al. 1992). The increased risk has been estimated to range from two- to five-fold among breast cancer survivors, with conflicting data on the contribution of RT to these excesses. In a case–control study by Boice and colleagues (1992), the overall relative risk for contralateral breast cancer was not significantly increased after radiation therapy (RR = 1.19; 95 % CI, 0.94–1.15). Among women who were younger than 45 years of age at the time of irradiation, however, the relative risk was significantly elevated (RR 1.59; (95 % CI, 1.07–2.36). In the Early Breast Cancer Trialists' Collaborative Group report, which evaluated the effects of RT, a significantly increased risk for contralateral breast cancer was found, mainly during the period 5 –14 years after randomization (RR = 1.43; P = .00001), and the increased risk associated with RT was significant elevated among women aged 50 years or older when randomized (RR = 1.25; P = .002) (Clarke et al. 2005). In contrast, in another large case–control study from Denmark, there was no significant difference in the risk for contralateral breast cancer in women who did and did not receive RT, regardless of age at treatment (Storm et al. 1992). In the Danish study, it was found that the second breast cancers were evenly distributed in the medial, lateral, and central portions of the breast, which also argued against a causal role of radiotherapy in tumorigenesis. A large-scale, single-institution study from Institut Curie which included 13,472 women, similarly failed to show an increased risk for contralateral breast cancer when comparing women who did or did not receive radiation therapy (RR = 1.1; 95 % CI, 0.96–1.27). Analysis by age, however, was not performed in that study (Kirova et al. 2007).

In addition to contralateral breast cancer, several other solid tumors have also been linked to a history of radiation therapy for breast cancer. These include cancers of the lung, thyroid and esophagus, and soft tissue sarcoma (Huang and Mackillop 2001; Huang et al. 2001; Levi et al. 2005; Neugut et al. 1993; Roychoudhuri et al. 2004; Zablotska and Neugut 2003). An increased risk for leukemia after breast cancer has also been observed, which is associated with exposure to both chemotherapy and radiation therapy.

Women who receive RT for breast cancer have been shown to be at a 1.5- to 3-fold increased risk for developing lung cancer compared with women who did not receive radiation therapy (Neugut et al. 1993; Zablotska and Neugut 2003). The increased risk seemed to be more clearly related to postmastectomy radiation therapy, in which the radiation target volume often also include the supraclavicular, axillary, or internal mammary nodal region, thus exposing a larger volume of underlying lung tissue to the radiation, whereas the risk after post-lumpectomy RT is less certain (Deutsch et al. 2003; Zablotska and Neugut 2003). The observation that lung cancer after breast cancer therapy is more frequently found in the ipsilateral lung also supports the contributing role of radiation to the risk (Zablotska and Neugut 2003). Several studies showed further increases in the risk for lung cancer among smokers who received breast irradiation (Ford et al. 2003; Neugut et al. 1994), although the interaction between tobacco exposure and prior radiation therapy on subsequent lung cancer risk is not as well elucidated as in survivors of HL.

Adjuvant radiation therapy for breast cancer has also been related to excess esophageal cancers (Levi et al. 2005; Roychoudhuri et al. 2004). In a cohort study from the Thames Cancer Registry on 64,782 cases of breast cancer diagnosed between 1961 and 2000, the incidence of esophageal cancer among the 33,763 patients who received radiation therapy and the 31,019 patients who did not receive radiation therapy was compared (Roychoudhuri et al. 2004). The relative risk for esophageal cancer was found to be significantly increased at 2.19 (95 % C.I. 1.10–4.62) at 15 or more years after initial breast cancer treatment. A significantly increased excess risk of esophageal cancer after breast cancer therapy with increasing follow-up time from initial diagnosis was also demonstrated in other population-based studies (Ahsan and Neugut 1998; Levi et al. 2005).

Sarcoma after breast cancer is a rare event, with a 15 year incidence rate of less than 0.5 %, although the relative risk has been estimated to be as high as seven, because of the low background incidence in the general population (Huang and Mackillop 2001; Kirova et al. 2005). In a study by Rubino and colleagues (2005), all observed sarcomas occurred among women who had initially received radiation therapy, and in all cases the sarcomas were located in the irradiated fields or in the upper extremity of the arm ipsilateral to the treated breast. Further, a significant dose–response relationship was demonstrated. By estimating the initial radiation dose to the site of sarcoma development, using a dose of 14 Gy or less to the site as reference, women who received 14–44 Gy had a 1.6-fold increased risk for sarcoma, whereas those who received 45 Gy or more to the site had a 30.6-fold increased risk ($P < .001$). Angiosarcoma was initially shown to be associated with chronic lymphedema following radical mastectomy (Jessner et al. 1952). With the increasing use of radiation therapy, there have been a growing number of reports of cutaneous angiosarcoma of the breast arising in the radiation field (Brenn and Fletcher 2005; Esler-Brauer et al. 2007; Fodor et al. 2006; Virtanen et al. 2007). Unlike other radiation-related soft tissue sarcoma, angiosarcoma has a short latency and can occur in the first 5 years after therapy.

The increased risk for leukemia following breast cancer is related to both chemotherapy and RT (Campone et al. 2005; Curtis et al. 1992; Praga et al. 2005; Smith et al. 2003). In a case–control study by Curtis and colleagues of women treated for breast cancer between 1973 and 1985 (Curtis et al. 1992), 90 women who developed leukemia and 264 matched controls were studied. Compared with women who did not receive alkylating chemotherapy or radiation therapy, the relative risk for acute myelogenous leukemia after radiation therapy alone, alkylating chemotherapy alone, and both chemotherapy and radiation therapy were 2.4, 10.0, and 17.4, respectively. With regard to the contribution of radiation therapy, a significant dose–response effect was observed for the cumulative dose of radiation to the active bone marrow and the subsequent risk for leukemia.

There has been significant progress in the radiation treatment techniques for breast cancer. Much of the data on second malignancy risks were based on outdated treatment including use of large-field treatments, such as the hockey-stick technique (Harris and Hellman 1988), which has since been abandoned, and cobalt therapy. In addition, advances in radiation therapy (Chen and Vicini 2007), including use of intensity modulated therapy radiation (IMRT), and the growing interest in partial breast irradiation may also alter the second malignancy risk of breast cancer survivors. The risks associated with these newer radiation therapy approaches and techniques remain to be clarified.

5.5 Radiation-Related Malignancy After Prostate Cancer

Radiation therapy has a curative role in selected patients with localized disease. Patients are also routinely offered adjuvant radiation therapy for rising prostate specific antigen after radical prostatectomy in the absence of evidence of distant metastasis. There has been increasing attention to the risk for SC after radiation therapy for prostate cancer (Brenner et al. 2000; Chrouser et al. 2005; Liauw et al. 2006; Moon et al. 2006; Neugut et al. 1997; Pickles and Phillips 2002). Neugut and colleagues were the first to report on the effect of RT for prostate carcinoma on the risk for second cancers in a population-based study using data from the SEER program (Neugut et al. 1997). Men who received radiation therapy had a significantly increased risk for developing bladder cancer after a latent period of 8 years (RR = 1.5; 95 % CI, 1.1–2.0), whereas the risk was not increased among men who did not receive RT. An increased risk for rectal cancer or leukemia after RT was not seen (Neugut et al. 1997). In a more recent study based on the Mayo Clinic Cancer Registry (Chrouser et al. 2005), whereas the overall relative risk for bladder cancer after radiation therapy was not significantly increased, among the subset of patients who received adjuvant radiation therapy after a radical prostatectomy the relative risk for bladder cancer was fivefold higher than expected ($P = 0.05$), which may be because of the larger volume of bladder exposed to the radiation in the postoperative setting.

In a subsequent study by Brenner and colleagues (Brenner et al. 2000), which also used data from the SEER program, men who were treated initially with radiation therapy were compared with men treated with surgery alone. Patients who received radiation therapy had a significantly increased risk for bladder cancer, rectal cancer, sarcoma, and lung cancer. The finding of a significant association between irradiation for prostate cancer and lung cancer risk was attributed to low scatter doses of radiation to the lungs. This observation may be more pertinent in patients who received cobalt irradiation to the whole pelvis. A study using the linked SEER-Medicare database included a larger number of patients, including those treated in the more recent era (Moon et al. 2006). Men who received external beam radiation therapy had a statistically significantly increased risk for developing cancers of the bladder, rectum, colon, brain, stomach, and lung, and melanoma, with odds ratios ranging from 1.25 to 1.85, when compared with men who did not receive external beam radiation therapy. Patients who received radioactive implants with or without external beam radiation therapy, however, did not have a significantly increased risk for second cancer when compared with those not receiving RT.

In a study from the British Columbia Tumor Registry, among patients who received RT, significantly elevated risks for colorectal cancer (RR = 1.21; $P < .01$), pleural cancer (RR = 2.28; $P < .01$) and sarcoma (RR = 1.7; $P < .05$) were observed. Although the bladder cancer risk was not significantly increased in the radiation therapy cohort, the risks for bladder cancer (RR = 1.32; $P < .01$) and testicular cancer (RR = 2.82; $P < .05$) were significantly increased in the non-irradiation cohort, which was believed to be related to heightened surveillance (Pickles and Phillips 2002).

Another report also based on data from the SEER program focused on the risk for rectal cancer after prostatic irradiation (Kendal et al. 2006). Unlike previous studies, a significant association between radiation therapy and a subsequently increased risk for rectal cancer was not found. Results of Cox proportional hazards analysis (with prostate irradiation, prostate surgery, and age at diagnosis entered as covariates) showed that only age was associated with an increased risk for subsequent rectal cancer.

Most studies on malignancies after prostate cancer therapy used data from population-based registries. The conflicting findings on the contribution of radiation therapy to various second malignancies after prostate cancer may reflect the fact that most registries collect data only on initial course of therapy, registration of initial treatment is incomplete in some registries, and selection criteria differ for patients given surgery versus radiation therapy. Moreover, given the limited data available in most population-based registries, it is not possible to identify or to control for confounding factors. Incomplete adjustment for attained age is the most obvious of these: patients who receive RT for prostate cancer are consistently older than those who undergo surgery alone. Since advancing age is associated with increasing risk of malignancy, incomplete adjustment for the age differences between patients undergoing RT versus surgery will erroneously elevate the apparent SC risk associated with RT. Similarly, patients who have significant comorbid illnesses or heavy smoking histories may not be selected for surgery and may be more likely to undergo radiation therapy. Consequently, increased risks of lung cancer may in part relate to unmeasured confounders such as smoking status. Further, among patients who received radiation therapy, treatment-related effects, including proctitis, rectal bleeding, cystitis, and hematuria may lead to additional colonoscopies or cystoscopies, which in turn can produce a detection bias and an apparent increased incidence of colorectal or other urologic cancers. Even so, radiation is a known carcinogen, and the risk of SC among long-term survivors of prostate RT should be considered in the clinical context in which prostate cancer treatment decisions are being made.

In studies that demonstrate a significant risk for cancers after radiation therapy for prostate cancer, the absolute incidence seems to be low. In the study by Brenner and colleagues that included patients who received larger-field cobalt irradiation, the risk for developing a radiation-associated second malignancy was estimated at 1 in 290 (Brenner et al. 2000). In the last several years, IMRT has been increasingly adopted in the treatment of prostate cancer to allow more conformal dose distribution and dose escalation (Guckenberger and Flentje 2007). Depending on treatment energy, IMRT is associated with a 3- to 5 -fold larger number of monitor units as compared with conventional treatment. Using the National Council of Radiation Protection and Measurements risk coefficients for specific anatomic sites, the risk for second malignancy using IMRT techniques has been estimated to be two to three times higher than that after conventional radiation therapy (Kry et al. 2007). These estimates are yet to be confirmed in epidemiologic studies with sufficient follow-up time for those patients who have received IMRT.

6 Pediatric Malignancies

Second cancer risk in survivors of childhood malignancy have been the subject of large cohort studies in North America and Europe (de Vathaire et al. 1999; Neglia et al. 2001; Olsen et al. 1993). The Childhood Cancer Survivor Study (CCSS) (Neglia et al. 2001), reported SC risks in a cohort of 13,581 five-year survivors of childhood and adolescent cancer, diagnosed between 1970 and 1986. The risk of developing a second malignancy was increased 6.4-fold compared with the general population, and the cumulative risk was 3.2 % at 20 years (median follow-up time of 15 years). In a population-based British cohort of 16,541 three-year survivors of childhood cancer, the absolute excess risk of SC was 12 per 10,000 patients per year, and the 28-year cumulative risk was 4.2 % (Jenkinson et al. 2004). Similarly, a population-based European study of 30,880 children diagnosed 1943–1987 reported a 3.6-fold increased risk of SC (95 % CI: 3.1–4.1) and a 35-year cumulative incidence of 3.7 % (Olsen et al. 1993). The largest RRs have been reported for second primary bone tumors, soft tissue sarcoma, leukemia, and cancers of the brain, thyroid, and breast.

Notably, some young adult survivors of pediatric malignancy appear to be at increased risk of cancers typically diagnosed in late adulthood, and the excess relative risk of radiation-related cancers of the breast, lung, thyroid, and gastrointestinal tract are greater for children and adolescents than for adults.

For example, the CCSS found significant excess risks of cancers of the breast (RR = 12.5) (Kenney et al. 2004), nonmelanoma skin (RR = 6.3 after RT) (Perkins et al. 2005), head and neck (RR = 13.6), kidney (RR = 10.6), colon and rectum (RR = 2.7), lung (RR = 3.1), and bladder (RR = 5.1). Remarkably, the median age at diagnosis of these adult-type carcinomas was 27 years (Bassal et al. 2006).

A complete review of the risks of SC following each primary malignancy of childhood is beyond the scope of this chapter. However, examination of SC risk following acute lymphoblastic leukemia and retinoblastoma reveals issues specific to the pediatric population.

6.1 Risk of Second Cancer in Survivors of Acute Lymphoblastic Leukemia

Since ALL is the most common childhood cancer, and has a high cure rate, risks of SC among ALL survivors have been studied extensively. Several investigations have demonstrated an increased risk of SC, and central nervous system tumors in particular (Bhatia et al. 2002; Loning et al. 2000; Maule et al. 2007; Pui et al. 2003; Walter et al. 1998). A German study of 5,006 ALL patients treated between 1979 and 1995 reported a 15-year cumulative incidence of SC of 3.3 % following completion of initial treatment (Loning et al. 2000). Cranial radiation increases the risk of high-grade astrocytomas, particularly during the first decade after treatment, but can also increase the risk of low-grade brain tumors or meningiomas among 10-year survivors of ALL (Walter et al. 1998). As noted above, the risk of a second brain tumor increases with increasing cranial radiation dose (Walter et al. 1998). The CCSS study reported 20-year cumulative risks of 1.0 %, 1.7 %, and 3.2 % for patients who received radiation doses of 10–21 Gy, 21–30 Gy, and greater than 30 Gy, respectively. Risk of CNS tumors is higher in children 5 years of age or younger at first treatment (Loning et al. 2000; Walter et al. 1998).

In part due to these concerns, prophylactic cranial RT has been largely replaced by intrathecal chemotherapy and high-dose intravenous methotrexate in contemporary ALL treatment protocols. A study of SC among 8,831 ALL survivors treated on risk-based Children's Cancer Group protocols between 1983 and 1995 (i.e. using intensive chemotherapy and limited use of radiation) reported a RR of second cancer of 7.2-fold, with a cumulative risk of 1.2 % at 10 years (Bhatia et al. 2002). Notably, this result is not dramatically different from prior studies, and in other clinical situations, chemotherapy alone or in combined modality regimens may also increase this risk of solid cancers (Menu-Branthomme et al. 2004). Longer follow-up will be needed to fully elucidate the extent to which risk-adapted treatments using high dose methotrexate will reduce the risk of SC among ALL survivors.

In ALL survivors, treatment with epipodophyllotoxin agents (e.g., etoposide) has been associated with the development of acute myeloid leukemia (AML). A study of 734 children with ALL who received epipodophyllotoxin maintenance reported a 6-year cumulative incidence of AML of 3.8 % (Pui et al. 1991). Continual treatment is major risk factor: patients who received weekly or twice-weekly doses of epipodophyllotoxins had a significantly greater risk of AML than those treated less frequently (e.g., courses lasting 3–5 consecutive days given every 3–4 weeks) (Le Deley et al. 2003; Pui et al. 1991).

6.2 Retinoblastoma

Only a portion of the excess second cancer risk in survivors of childhood cancer is related to treatment. Largely uncharacterized biologic variability in the population is thought to substantially modify the risk of treatment-related SC. Retinoblastoma (RB) is a classic example: familial retinoblastoma is caused by inherited mutations of the RB-1 tumor suppressor gene, which is located on the long arm of chromosome 13q14 (Friend et al. 1986). In a study of 1,604 one-year survivors of RB, the risk of SC was increased 19-fold in hereditary retinoblastoma survivors (88 % of whom had received RT) while the risk was not elevated in non-hereditary patients (RR = 1.2), compared to the general population. Fifty years after retinoblastoma diagnosis, the cumulative incidence of second malignancy, adjusting for competing risks of death, was 36 % in hereditary patients, and 5.7 % in nonhereditary patients (Wong et al. 1997). In patients with hereditary retinoblastoma, RT significantly increases the cumulative incidence of second cancers to approximately 40 % at 50 years, versus 20 % in nonirradiated patients. RT does not appear to significantly affect risk in nonhereditary retinoblastoma patients (Kleinerman et al. 2005; Wong et al. 1997).

While RB is a classic example genetic defect associated with an increased risk of SC, very few SC can be attributed to the presence of such high-penetrance genetic changes. There is some evidence that patients with neurofibromatosis Type 1 treated for optic pathway gliomas have and increased incidence of second central nervous system tumors, and particularly after receiving RT (Sharif et al. 2006). Mutations in the ataxia-telangiectasia (ATM) gene are associated with increased radiation sensitivity, however existing studies indicate ATM mutation carriers do not account for a significant proportion of patients with radiation-induced second cancers following HL treatment (Broeks et al. 2000; Nichols et al. 1999). A better understanding of the influence of common low-penetrance genetic factors on the risk of treatment-related SC could potentially be an important advance in tailoring cancer treatments to not only maximize initial cure rates, but to also reduce the resulting late toxicity for the majority of patients (Travis et al. 2006).

7 Summary

As increasing numbers of patients who have cancer are cured, the occurrence of SC has emerged as a problem limiting long-term survival and quality of life, particularly among young patients. A significant proportion of cancer survivors do not receive routine screening examinations (e.g., mammography), in spite of routine contact with the health care system. At a minimum, these should be performed as part of follow-up, in accordance with accepted guidelines. Survivor-specific guidelines for follow-up care are emerging (Children's Oncology Group, 2008). although the evidence base supporting many of these guidelines is weak, especially in survivors of adult-onset cancers. Future refinement of observational studies, with greater focus on absolute risks among identifiable patient groups, will assist patient counseling and rational screening strategies among cancer survivors. Further, improved understanding of therapy-related second malignancies can guide the development of new treatment regimens that have the potential to minimize late effects while maintaining or improving initial cure rates.

References

Ahsan H, Neugut AI (1998) Radiation therapy for breast cancer and increased risk for esophageal carcinoma. Ann Intern Med 128:114–117

Aleman BM et al (2003) Long-term cause-specific mortality of patients treated for Hodgkin's disease. J Clin Oncol 21:3431–3439

Arseneau JC et al (1972) Nonlymphomatous malignant tumors complicating Hodgkin's disease. Possible association with intensive therapy. N Engl J Med 287:1119–1122

Bassal M et al (2006) Risk of selected subsequent carcinomas in survivors of childhood cancer: a report from the childhood cancer survivor study. J Clin Oncol 24:476–483

Bhatia S et al (1996) Breast cancer and other second neoplasms after childhood Hodgkin's disease. N Engl J Med 334:745–751

Bhatia S et al (2002) Low incidence of second neoplasms among children diagnosed with acute lymphoblastic leukemia after 1983. Blood 99:4257–4264

Bhatia S et al (2003) High risk of subsequent neoplasms continues with extended follow-up of childhood hodgkin's disease: report from the late effects study group. J Clin Oncol 21:4386–4394

Bluhm EC et al (2008) Cause-specific mortality and second cancer incidence after non-Hodgkin lymphoma: a report from the childhood cancer survivor study. Blood 111:4014–4021

Boice JD Jr et al (1985) Second cancers following radiation treatment for cervical cancer. An international collaboration among cancer registries. J Natl Cancer Inst 74:955–975

Boice JD Jr et al (1987) Radiation dose and leukemia risk in patients treated for cancer of the cervix. J Natl Cancer Inst 79:1295–1311

Boice JD Jr et al (1988) Radiation dose and second cancer risk in patients treated for cancer of the cervix. Radiat Res 116:3–55

Boice JD Jr et al (1992) Cancer in the contralateral breast after radiotherapy for breast cancer. N Engl J Med 326:781–785

Brenn T, Fletcher CD (2005) Radiation-associated cutaneous atypical vascular lesions and angiosarcoma: clinicopathologic analysis of 42 cases. Am J Surg Pathol 29:983–996

Brenner DJ et al (2000) Second malignancies in prostate carcinoma patients after radiotherapy compared with surgery. Cancer 88:398–406

Broeks A et al (2000) Increased risk of breast cancer following irradiation for Hodgkin's disease is not a result of ATM germline mutations. Int J Radiat Biol 76:693–698

Brown LM et al (2007) Risk of second non-hematological malignancies among 376,825 breast cancer survivors. Breast Cancer Res Treat 106:439–451

Campone M et al (2005) Secondary leukemia after epirubicin-based adjuvant chemotherapy in operable breast cancer patients: 16 years experience of the french adjuvant study group. Ann Oncol 16:1343–1351

Capra M et al (2007) Long-term outcome in children with Hodgkin's lymphoma: the united kingdom children's cancer study group HD82 trial. Eur J Cancer 43:1171–1179

Cardis E et al (2007) The 15-country collaborative study of cancer risk among radiation workers in the nuclear industry: estimates of radiation-related cancer risks. Radiat Res 167:396–416

Chaturvedi AK et al (2007) Second cancers among 104,760 survivors of cervical cancer: evaluation of long-term risk. J Natl Cancer Inst 99:1634–1643

Chen PY, Vicini FA (2007) Partial breast irradiation. Patient selection, guidelines for treatment, and current results. Front Radiat Ther Oncol 40:253–271

Children's Oncology Group (2008) http://www.survivorshipguidelines.1062_org/. Accessed April, 2013

Chrouser K, et al. (2005) Bladder cancer risk following primary and adjuvant external beam radiation for prostate cancer. J Urol 174: 107–110, (discussion 110–111)

Clarke M et al (2005) Effects of radiotherapy and of differences in the extent of surgery for early breast cancer on local recurrence and 15-year survival: an overview of the randomised trials. Lancet 366:2087–2106

Curtis RE et al (1992) Risk of leukemia after chemotherapy and radiation treatment for breast cancer. N Engl J Med 326:1745–1751

Curtis RE et al (1994) Relationship of leukemia risk to radiation dose following cancer of the uterine corpus. J Natl Cancer Inst 86:1315–1324

de Vathaire F et al (1999) Second malignant neoplasms after a first cancer in childhood: temporal pattern of risk according to type of treatment. Br J Cancer 79:1884–1893

Deutsch M et al (2007) An association between postoperative radiotherapy for primary breast cancer in 11 National Surgical Adjuvant Breast and Bowel Project (NSABP) studies and the subsequent appearance of pleural mesothelioma. Am J Clin Oncol 30:294–296

Deutsch M et al (2003) The incidence of lung carcinoma after surgery for breast carcinoma with and without postoperative radiotherapy. Results of National Surgical Adjuvant Breast and Bowel Project (NSABP) clinical trials B-04 and B-06. Cancer 98:1362–1368

Dinu I et al (2008) Prediction of second malignant neoplasm incidence in a large cohort of long-term survivors of childhood cancers. Pediatr Blood Cancer 50:1026–1031

Dores GM et al (2002) Second malignant neoplasms among long-term survivors of Hodgkin's disease: a population-based evaluation over 25 years. J Clin Oncol 20:3484–3494

Esler-Brauer L et al (2007) Angiosarcoma developing after conservative treatment for breast carcinoma: case report with review of the current literature. Dermatol Surg 33:749–755

Fodor J et al (2006) Angiosarcoma after conservation treatment for breast carcinoma: our experience and a review of the literature. J Am Acad Dermatol 54:499–504

Ford MB et al (2003) Effects of smoking and radiotherapy on lung carcinoma in breast carcinoma survivors. Cancer 98:1457–1464

Fossa SD et al (2005) Risk of contralateral testicular cancer: a population-based study of 29,515 U.S. men. J Natl Cancer Inst 97:1056–1066

Franklin J et al (2006) Second malignancy risk associated with treatment of Hodgkin's lymphoma: meta-analysis of the randomised trials. Ann Oncol 17:1749–1760

Friend SH et al (1986) A human DNA segment with properties of the gene that predisposes to retinoblastoma and osteosarcoma. Nature 323:643–646

Gao X et al (2003) Risk of second primary cancer in the contralateral breast in women treated for early-stage breast cancer: a population-based study. Int J Radiat Oncol Biol Phys 56:1038–1045

Gilbert E et al (2003) Lung cancer after treatment for Hodgkin's disease: focus on radiation effects. Radiat Res 159(2):161–173

Girinsky T et al (2006) Involved-node radiotherapy (INRT) in patients with early Hodgkin lymphoma: concepts and guidelines. Radiother Oncol 79:270–277

Group CsO (2006) www.survivorshipguidelines. Accessed Nov 2007

Guckenberger M, Flentje M (2007) Intensity-modulated radiotherapy (IMRT) of localized prostate cancer: a review and future perspectives. Strahlenther Onkol 183:57–62

Guerin S et al (2007) Treatment-adjusted predisposition to second malignant neoplasms after a solid cancer in childhood: a case-control study. J Clin Oncol 25:2833–2839

Hall EJ (2006) Intensity-modulated radiation therapy, protons, and the risk of second cancers. Int J Radiat Oncol Biol Phys 65:1–7

Harris JR, Hellman S (1988) Put the "hockey stick" on ice. Int J Radiat Oncol Biol Phys 15:497–499

Hawkins MM et al (1996) Radiotherapy, alkylating agents, and risk of bone cancer after childhood cancer. J Natl Cancer Inst 88:270–278

Hemminki K et al (2007) Risks for familial and contralateral breast cancer interact multiplicatively and cause a high risk. Cancer Res 67:868–870

Hodgson DC et al (2007a) Long-term solid cancer risk among 5-year survivors of Hodgkin's lymphoma. J Clin Oncol 25:1489–1497

Hodgson DC et al (2007b) Individualized estimates of second cancer risks after contemporary radiation therapy for Hodgkin lymphoma. Cancer 110:2576–2586

Huang J, Mackillop WJ (2001) Increased risk of soft tissue sarcoma after radiotherapy in women with breast carcinoma. Cancer 92:172–180

Huang J et al (2001) Risk of thyroid carcinoma in a female population after radiotherapy for breast carcinoma. Cancer 92:1411–1418

Jenkinson HC et al (2004) Long-term population-based risks of second malignant neoplasms after childhood cancer in Britain. Br J Cancer 91:1905–1910

Jessner M et al (1952) Angiosarcoma in postmastectomy lymphedema (Stewart-Treves syndrome). AMA Arch Derm Syphilol 65:123–129

Kaldor JM et al (1987) Second malignancies following testicular cancer, ovarian cancer and Hodgkin's disease: an international collaborative study among cancer registries. Int J Cancer 39:571–585

Kendal WS et al (2006) Prostatic irradiation is not associated with any measurable increase in the risk of subsequent rectal cancer. Int J Radiat Oncol Biol Phys 65(3):661–668

Kenney L et al (2004) Breast cancer after childhood cancer: a report from the Childhood Cancer Survivor Study. Ann Intern Med 141(8):590–597

Kirova YM et al (2007) Risk of second malignancies after adjuvant radiotherapy for breast cancer: a large-scale, single-institution review. Int J Radiat Oncol Biol Phys 68:359–363

Kirova YM et al (2005) Radiation-induced sarcomas after radiotherapy for breast carcinoma: a large-scale single-institution review. Cancer 104:856–863

Kleinerman RA et al (1982) Second cancers following radiotherapy for cervical cancer. J Natl Cancer Inst 69:1027–1033

Kleinerman RA et al (2005) Risk of new cancers after radiotherapy in long-term survivors of retinoblastoma: an extended follow-up. J Clin Oncol 23:2272–2279

Koh ES et al (2007) A comparison of mantle versus involved-field radiotherapy for Hodgkin's lymphoma: reduction in normal tissue dose and second cancer risk. Radiat Oncol 2:13

Kong L et al (2006) The risk of second primary tumors in patients with nasopharyngeal carcinoma after definitive radiotherapy. Cancer 107:1287–1293

Kry SF et al (2007) Uncertainty of calculated risk estimates for secondary malignancies after radiotherapy. Int J Radiat Oncol Biol Phys 68:1265–1271

Le Deley MC et al (2003) Risk of secondary leukemia after a solid tumor in childhood according to the dose of epipodophyllotoxins and anthracyclines: a case-control study by the Societe Francaise d'Oncologie Pediatrique. J Clin Oncol 21:1074–1081

Levi F et al (2005) Increased risk of esophageal cancer after breast cancer. Ann Oncol 16:1829–1831

Liauw SL et al (2006) Second malignancies after prostate brachytherapy: incidence of bladder and colorectal cancers in patients with 15 years of potential follow-up. Int J Radiat Oncol Biol Phys 66:669–673

Lie JA et al (2008) Ionizing radiation exposure and cancer risk among Norwegian nurses. Eur J Cancer Prev 17:369–375

Little MP et al (1999) Risks of leukemia in Japanese atomic bomb survivors, in women treated for cervical cancer, and in patients treated for ankylosing spondylitis. Radiat Res 152:280–292

Loning L et al (2000) Secondary neoplasms subsequent to Berlin-Frankfurt-Munster therapy of acute lymphoblastic leukemia in childhood: significantly lower risk without cranial radiotherapy. Blood 95:2770–2775

Maule M et al (2007) Risk of second malignant neoplasms after childhood leukemia and lymphoma: an international study. J Natl Cancer Inst 99:790–800

Menu-Branthomme A et al (2004) Radiation dose, chemotherapy and risk of soft tissue sarcoma after solid tumours during childhood. Int J Cancer 110:87–93

Meyer R et al (2003) A Randomized phase III comparison of single - modality ABVD with a strategy that includes radiation therapy in patients with early-stage Hodgkins disease: The HD-6 trial of the national cancer institute of canada clinical trials group. abstr 81. J Clin Oncol (accepted for publication)

Moon K et al (2006) Cancer incidence after localized therapy for prostate cancer. Cancer 107:991–998

Nachman JB et al (2002) Randomized comparison of low-dose involved-field radiotherapy and no radiotherapy for children with Hodgkin's disease who achieve a complete response to chemotherapy. J Clin Oncol 20:3765–3771

Neglia JP et al (2001) Second malignant neoplasms in five-year survivors of childhood cancer: childhood cancer survivor study. J Natl Cancer Inst 93:618–629

Neglia JP et al (2006) New primary neoplasms of the central nervous system in survivors of childhood cancer: a report from the childhood cancer survivor study. J Natl Cancer Inst 98:1528–1537

Neugut AI et al (1997) Bladder carcinoma and other second malignancies after radiotherapy for prostate carcinoma. Cancer 79:1600–1604

Neugut AI et al (1994) Increased risk of lung cancer after breast cancer radiation therapy in cigarette smokers. Cancer 73:1615–1620

Neugut AI et al (1993) Lung cancer after radiation therapy for breast cancer. Cancer 71:3054–3057

Ng AK et al (2002) Second malignancy after Hodgkin disease treated with radiation therapy with or without chemotherapy: long-term risks and risk factors. Blood 100:1989–1996

Nichols KE et al (1999) Heterozygous germline ATM mutations do not contribute to radiation-associated malignancies after Hodgkin's disease. J Clin Oncol 17:1259

Olsen JH et al (1993) Second malignant neoplasms after cancer in childhood or adolescence. Nordic society of paediatric haematology and oncology association of the nordic cancer registries. BMJ 307:1030–1036

Pedersen-Bjergaard J et al (1991) Increased risk of myelodysplasia and leukaemia after etoposide, cisplatin, and bleomycin for germ-cell tumours. Lancet 338:359–363

Perkins JL et al (2005) Nonmelanoma skin cancer in survivors of childhood and adolescent cancer: a report from the childhood cancer survivor study. J Clin Oncol 23:3733–3741

Peters MV, Middlemiss KC (1958) A study of Hodgkin's disease treated by irradiation. Am J Roentgenol Radium Ther Nucl Med 79:114–121

Pickles T, Phillips N (2002) The risk of second malignancy in men with prostate cancer treated with or without radiation in British Columbia, 1984–2000. Radiother Oncol 65:145–151

Pintilie M (2006) Competing risks: a practical perspective. Wiley, West Sussex

Praga C et al (2005) Risk of acute myeloid leukemia and myelodysplastic syndrome in trials of adjuvant epirubicin for early breast cancer: correlation with doses of epirubicin and cyclophosphamide. J Clin Oncol 23:4179–4191

Preston DL et al (2002) Radiation effects on breast cancer risk: a pooled analysis of eight cohorts. Radiat Res 158:220–235

Pui CH et al (2003) Extended follow-up of long-term survivors of childhood acute lymphoblastic leukemia. N Engl J Med 349:640–649

Pui CH et al (1991) Acute myeloid leukemia in children treated with epipodophyllotoxins for acute lymphoblastic leukemia. N Engl J Med 325:1682–1687

Rapiti E et al (2008) Increased risk of colon cancer after external radiation therapy for prostate cancer. Int J Cancer 123:1141–1145

Ries L et al (2006) SEER cancer statistics review 1975–2003. National Cancer Institute, Bethesda

Ron E et al (1995) Thyroid cancer after exposure to external radiation: a pooled analysis of seven studies. Radiat Res 141:259–277

Ron E et al (1994) Cancer incidence in atomic bomb survivors. Part IV: Comparison of cancer incidence and mortality. Radiat Res 137:S98–S112

Roychoudhuri R et al (2004) Radiation-induced malignancies following radiotherapy for breast cancer. Br J Cancer 91:868–872

Rubino C et al (2005) Radiation dose and risk of soft tissue and bone sarcoma after breast cancer treatment. Breast Cancer Res Treat 89:277–288

Sacchi S et al (2008) Secondary malignancies after treatment for indolent non-Hodgkin's lymphoma: a 16-year follow-up study. Haematologica 93:398–404

Schaapveld M et al (2008) Risk of new primary nonbreast cancers after breast cancer treatment: a Dutch population-based study. J Clin Oncol 26:1239–1246

Schairer C et al (2007) Comparative mortality for 621 second cancers in 29356 testicular cancer survivors and 12420 matched first cancers. J Natl Cancer Inst 99(16):1248–1256

Schneider U (2006) Calculated risk of fatal secondary malignancies from intensity-modulated radiotherapy: In regard to Kry et al. (Int J Radiat Oncol Biol Phys 2005;62:1195–1203). Int J Radiat Oncol Biol Phys 64: 1290; (author reply 1290–1291)

Sharif S et al (2006) Second primary tumors in neurofibromatosis 1 patients treated for optic glioma: substantial risks after radiotherapy. J Clin Oncol 24:2570–2575

Sigurdson AJ et al (2005) Primary thyroid cancer after a first tumour in childhood (the childhood cancer survivor study): a nested case-control study. Lancet 365:2014–2023

Smith RE et al (2003) Acute myeloid leukemia and myelodysplastic syndrome after doxorubicin-cyclophosphamide adjuvant therapy for operable breast cancer: the national surgical adjuvant breast and bowel project experience. J Clin Oncol 21:1195–1204

Storm HH et al (1992) Adjuvant radiotherapy and risk of contralateral breast cancer. J Natl Cancer Inst 84:1245–1250

Swerdlow AJ et al (2000) Risk of second malignancy after Hodgkin's disease in a collaborative British cohort: the relation to age at treatment. J Clin Oncol 18:498–509

Thompson DE et al (1994) Cancer incidence in atomic bomb survivors. Part II: solid tumors, 1958–1987. Radiat Res 137:S17–S67

Travis LB et al (1991) Second cancers following non-Hodgkin's lymphoma. Cancer 67:2002–2009

Travis LB et al (1993) Second cancers among long-term survivors of non-Hodgkin's lymphoma. J Natl Cancer Inst 85:1932–1937

Travis LB et al (2000) Treatment-associated leukemia following testicular cancer. J Natl Cancer Inst 92:1165–1171

Travis LB et al (2002) Lung cancer following chemotherapy and radiotherapy for Hodgkin's disease. J Natl Cancer Inst 94:182–192

Travis LB et al (2003) Breast cancer following radiotherapy and chemotherapy among young women with Hodgkin disease. JAMA 290:465–475

Travis LB, Gilbert E (2005) Lung cancer after Hodgkin lymphoma: the roles of chemotherapy, radiotherapy and tobacco use. Radiat Res 163:695–696

Travis LB et al (2005a) Second cancers among 40,576 testicular cancer patients: focus on long-term survivors. J Natl Cancer Inst 97:1354–1365

Travis LB et al (2005b) Cumulative absolute breast cancer risk for young women treated for Hodgkin lymphoma. J Natl Cancer Inst 97:1428–1437

Travis LB et al (2006) Cancer survivorship—genetic susceptibility and second primary cancers: research strategies and recommendations. J Natl Cancer Inst 98:15–25

Tward J et al (2007) Incidence, risk factors, and pathogenesis of second malignancies in patients with non-Hodgkin lymphoma. Leuk Lymphoma 48:1482–1495

van den Belt-Dusebout AW et al (2007) Treatment-specific risks of second malignancies and cardiovascular disease in 5-year survivors of testicular cancer. J Clin Oncol 25:4370–4378

van Leeuwen FE et al (1994) Second cancer risk following Hodgkin's disease: a 20-year follow-up study. J Clin Oncol 12:312–325

van Leeuwen FE et al (2003) Roles of radiation dose, chemotherapy, and hormonal factors in breast cancer following Hodgkin's disease. J Natl Cancer Inst 95:971–980

van Leeuwen FE et al (1993) Second cancer risk following testicular cancer: a follow-up study of 1,909 patients. J Clin Oncol 11:415–424

Virtanen A et al (2007) Angiosarcoma after radiotherapy: a cohort study of 332,163 Finnish cancer patients. Br J Cancer 97:115–117

Walter AW et al (1998) Secondary brain tumors in children treated for acute lymphoblastic leukemia at st jude children's research hospital. J Clin Oncol 16:3761–3767

Wong FL et al (1997) Cancer incidence after retinoblastoma. Radiation dose and sarcoma risk. JAMA 278:1262–1267

Woo TC et al (2006) Body radiation exposure in breast cancer radiotherapy: impact of breast IMRT and virtual wedge compensation techniques. Int J Radiat Oncol Biol Phys 65:52–58

Zablotska LB, Neugut AI (2003) Lung carcinoma after radiation therapy in women treated with lumpectomy or mastectomy for primary breast carcinoma. Cancer 97:1404–1411

The Psychosocial and Functional Impact of Radiation Therapy

Jason Q. Purnell, Karen Mustian, Pascal Jean-Pierre, Oxana Palesh, Luke J. Peppone, Supriya G. Mohile, Tom V. Darling, and Gary R. Morrow

Contents

J. Q. Purnell (✉)
The Brown School/Institute for Public Health, Washington University in St. Louis, Campus Box 1196, Brown Hall, Room 215,One Brookings Drive, St. Louis, MO 63130, USA
e-mail: jpurnell@wustl.edu

K. Mustian
Departments of Radiation Oncology & Community and Preventive Medicine, University of Rochester Medical Center, 601 Elmwood Avenue, Box 704 Rochester, NY 14642, USA

P. Jean-Pierre
Department of Psychology, University of Notre Dame, 109 Haggar Hall, Notre Dame, IN 46556, USA

O. Palesh
Department of Psychiatry & Behavioral Sciences, Stanford School of Medicine, 401 Quarry Road, Stanford, CA 94305, USA

L. J. Peppone · T. V. Darling
Department of Kinesiology and Physical Education, Valdosta State University, 1500 N. Patterson St., Valdosta, GA 31698, USA

S. G. Mohile
Department of Medical Hematology/Oncology, USA, 601 Elmwood Avenue, Rochester, NY 14642, USA

G. R. Morrow
Departments of Radiation Oncology & Psychiatry, DirectorUniversity of Rochester Cancer Center Community Clinical Oncology Program Research Base, 601 Elmwood Avenue, Rochester, NY 14642, USA

Abstract

- Cancer treatment, including radiation therapy, can cause immediate side effects as well as persistent disruptions across several domains of functioning.
- Symptoms, and side effects related to radiation therapy should be conceptualized, assessed, and addressed as co-occurring rather than in isolation.
- Cancer-related fatigue and sleep problems associated with radiation therapy are increasingly amenable to behavioral and pharmacological treatments, however, more research is needed to establish standards of care.
- Psychological problems, while significant for some cancer patients, appear to abate during and after treatment. Radiation oncologists are encouraged to assess for psychological problems and refer patients for appropriate treatment.
- Patient anxiety regarding radiation therapy can be alleviated to a significant extent by providing appropriate information throughout the treatment process.
- Cancer-related cognitive dysfunction has also been associated with radiotherapy, but systematic interventions for cancer patients are still lacking.
- Racial and ethnic minorities and other underserved populations face unique challenges that can be addressed by radiation oncology.

1 Introduction

This year alone, more than 1.4 million Americans will be diagnosed with cancer Jemal et al. (2008). Cancer and its treatments can produce multiple distressing symptoms and

P. Rubin et al. (eds.), *ALERT – Adverse Late Effects of Cancer Treatment*, Medical Radiology. Radiation Oncology, DOI: 10.1007/978-3-540-72314-1_17, © Springer-Verlag Berlin Heidelberg 2014

impairments in function: patients often experience physical and psychological symptoms both during and after aggressive cancer treatments. Those undergoing radiation and chemotherapy suffer from a myriad of physical side effects, including nausea, alopecia, pain, and fatigue, as well as a variety of psychiatric problems such as depression and anxiety. Improvements in medical technologies, development and availability of more effective drugs, and technological innovations in radiotherapy equipment and delivery have facilitated more timely identification and management of malignancies. Progress in oncology research and clinical practice has contributed to increased survival rates for patients with many types of cancer. Unfortunately, the effective management of cancer creates side effects (e.g., cognitive dysfunction, fatigue, nausea, and vomiting) that affect important dimensions of patients' psychosocial functioning and quality of life (Ahles et al. 2002; Bender et al. 2001; Saykin et al. 2003).

2 Symptom Burden During Radiation Therapy

Symptom burden is a quantitative measure of the overall effect of symptoms on a patient's function and health-related quality of life (HRQOL). Early recognition of, and effective intervention directed against, treatment-related symptoms is essential, as these symptoms can lead to treatment delays or early discontinuation. Symptom control is an integral component of cancer care during and after treatment.

HRQOL, as utilized in cancer care, is a multidimensional construct that includes four dimensions: physical function, psychological function, social role function, and disease- or treatment-related symptoms. Patient ratings of symptom severity and their impact on function are important subsets of HRQOL. Unlike objective "signs" of disease noted on physical examination or imaging scans, symptoms are dependent on the observations of the patient and can only be elicited through patient report. It is often difficult to define or characterize symptoms because the underlying etiology could derive from the disease, the treatment, comorbid medical conditions, or a combination thereof. Whereas many symptoms are caused by the underlying cancer, treatment may lead to commonly recognized side effects including fatigue, neuropathy, insomnia, cognitive dysfunction, psychological distress, and depression. While these symptoms may occur during treatment, residual treatment-related symptoms can persist even after effective treatment has been completed. All causes of discomfort play a part in the total symptom burden, which consists of the patient's global impressions of disease or treatment burden and the impact of these symptoms on daily activities (Cleeland et al. 2007).

Although symptoms of cancer and cancer treatment have been studied as single entities, certain symptoms occur together and can influence one another. Multiple symptoms additively and synergistically affect overall quality of life (Cleeland et al. 2000, 2007; Dodd et al. 2001). Dodd et al. (2001) defined a "symptom cluster" as three or more concurrent symptoms that are related to each other. Typical symptoms that co-occur include fatigue, pain, insomnia, anorexia, and psychological distress. Given et al. reported that clusters of symptoms, such as insomnia, fatigue, and pain in 826 elderly patients had a consistent and significant effect on QOL unrelated to the type of cancer, treatment, stage of disease, or comorbid conditions (Given et al. 2001). It has been hypothesized that symptoms may occur together due to common underlying inflammatory or neuroimmunologic mechanisms (Cleeland et al. 2003; Lee et al. 2004). Symptoms may not always occur in the same patterns and may not develop or disappear with the same temporal course, making necessary thoughtful longitudinal studies to identify coexisting symptoms.

Several multiple-symptom assessment scales have been developed and validated to assess not only the most frequent symptoms but also symptoms that co-occur, and the interference of symptoms with quality of life and daily activities. The ideal scale is brief, easy to understand, and able to be administered for both clinical and research purposes (Cleeland et al. 2000, 2007). Kirkova et al. (2006) systematically reviewed cancer symptom assessments and identified 21 tools most appropriate for clinical use in cancer patients. Although this review did not identify any that met all the criteria of an ideal instrument, thirteen of the available symptom assessment tools evaluated more than five symptoms and also assessed interference of symptoms with overall quality of life and daily activities. The M.D. Anderson Symptom Inventory (MDASI) is one such tool frequently utilized to rate the severity of 13 symptoms common in cancer patients and the impact of these symptoms on various aspects of a patient's life. Research investigating the properties of the inventory revealed that the most severe symptoms (i.e., fatigue, insomnia, lack of appetite, pain, psychological distress) were similar regardless of cancer type (Cleeland et al. 2000).

Several studies have assessed the prevalence of symptoms and the impact of overall symptom burden on the QOL of cancer patients undergoing radiotherapy (RT). In a study evaluating the longitudinal relationship between chemoradiation for non-small-cell lung cancer and patient symptoms, 63 % of patients suffered from moderate to severe levels of multiple symptoms by the end of treatment (Wang et al. 2006). While all symptoms interfered with daily activities, fatigue, distress, and sadness caused the most

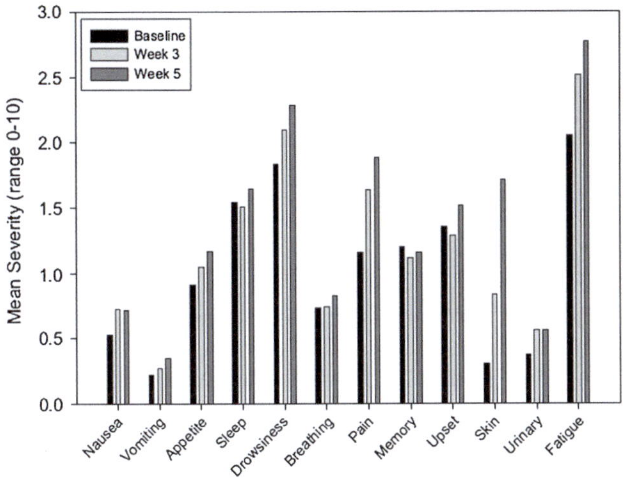

Fig. 1 Mean severity of symptoms at baseline and at weeks 3 and 5 during the course of RT (n = 419) (with permission from Hickok et al. 2005a)

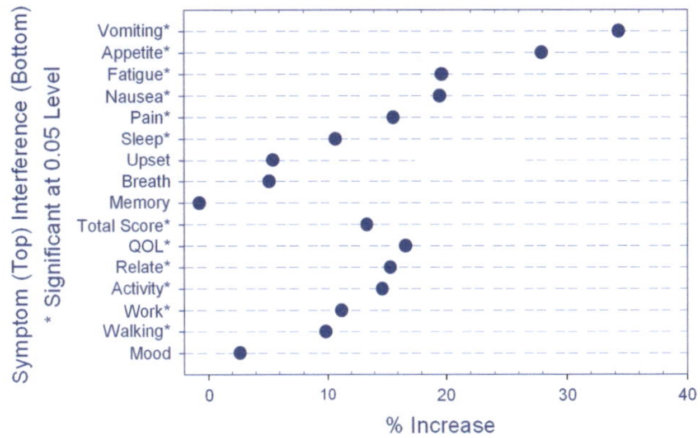

Fig. 2 Percentage increase in symptom interference following radiation therapy

significant disruption to daily life. Investigators at the University of Rochester characterized the longitudinal course of 12 common symptoms in 1,129 consecutive patients during radiotherapy (Hickok et al. 2005a). Eighty-four percent of patients experienced symptoms before treatment. During the five-week course of treatment, the 419 patients who completed both pre- and post-RT assessments reported that the frequency of all symptoms increased significantly (Fig. 1). In another study by the same investigators, fatigue was highly prevalent in patients undergoing RT; only 13 % reported no fatigue (Hickok et al. 2005b).

The same University of Rochester research team recently utilized a modified version of the MDASI to assess the prevalence of multiple symptoms and their interference with daily life activities in patients undergoing radiotherapy. The primary goals were to determine the prevalence and the pattern of change in specific symptoms during and after radiation therapy and to evaluate the impact of symptoms on QOL and daily activities. All age groups and tumor types were included in the analysis. The investigators found a significant increase in the severity of almost all symptoms and their impact on QOL and daily activities. The overall symptom burden score (a sum of the individual symptom scores) significantly increased post-radiotherapy (Fig. 2). In addition, higher symptom burdens correlated with deficits in patients' impressions of their own QOL.

The majority of previous symptom research has focused on individual symptoms, yet in reality patients often experience many different symptoms simultaneously. Research in patients undergoing radiotherapy has illustrated a high prevalence of symptoms that significantly impact QOL and daily activities. Moreover, high symptom burden and specific symptom clusters can have a deleterious effect on patient outcomes due to delays or discontinuation of treatment (Miaskowski et al. 2004). Given the negative effects of high symptom burden on daily activities and HRQOL, more research is necessary to evaluate the effect of interventions that target common symptom clusters rather than individual symptoms. Ideally, the development of such interventions will lead to a reduction of overall symptom burden in cancer patients.

3 Cancer-Related Fatigue

Cancer-related fatigue (CRF) is a global term used to refer to fatigue resulting from cancer and/or its treatments including surgically-induced, chemotherapy-induced, and radiation-induced fatigue. CRF is a multifaceted, psychosocial and physiological state characterized by an overwhelming sensation of exhaustion that is accompanied by a decreased capacity for mental and physical energy expenditure (Ahlberg et al. 2003; Barton-Burke and Barton-Burke 2006; Berger 1998; Broeckel et al. 1998; Carroll et al. 2007; Cella 1998; Cella et al. 1998, 2001, 2002; Curt et al. 2000; Escalante 2003; Hickok et al. 2003, Hickok et al. 2005b; Hofman et al. 2004, 2007; Irvine et al. 1991; Jacobsen et al. 2007; Jean-Pierre et al. 2007; Jereczek-Fossa et al. 2001; Kroenke et al. 1988; Mock 2004; Mock and Olsen 2003; Morrow 2007; Morrow et al. 2002, 2005; Mustian et al. 2007; National Comprehensive Cancer Network 2008; Piper et al. 1987; Portenoy and Itri 1999; Ryan et al. 2007). CRF is differentiated from the fatigue experienced by healthy individuals because of its severity, persistence, and impact on quality of life among cancer patients and survivors (Carroll et al. 2007; Hofman et al. 2007; Morrow 2007; Mustian et al. 2007; Ryan et al. 2007). Unlike the fatigue stemming from physical or mental exertion that can be relieved with rest or sleep, CRF is not alleviated by resting or sleeping (Carroll et al. 2007; Hofman et al. 2007; Morrow 2007; Mustian et al. 2007; National comprehensive

Cancer Network 2008; Ryan et al. 2007). Cancer patients and survivors report that CRF begins with diagnosis, worsens during the course of treatment, and can persist for months and years after treatments are completed (Carroll et al. 2007; Hofman et al. 2007; Morrow 2007; Mustian et al. 2007; Ryan et al. 2007). CRF can also immerge for the first time months or years after treatments are completed (Carroll et al. 2007; Hofman et al. 2007; Morrow 2007; Mustian et al. 2007; National Comprehensive Cancer Network 2008; Ryan et al. 2007). As such CRF can be characterized as an acute or chronic side effect as well as an early or late side effect resulting from cancer and its treatments (Mustian et al. 2007).

From 60 to 100 % of cancer patients and survivors with a variety of diagnoses who are receiving different types of treatments report some degree of CRF, with 41 % or more indicating a severe level of CRF (0 = no CRF to 10 = CRF as bad as you can imagine; a score $\geq$7 = severe on this 11-point Likert Scale) during treatment (Ahlberg et al. 2003; Barton-Burke and Barton-Burke 2006; Berger 1998; Broeckel et al. 1998; Cella 1998; Cella et al. 1998, 2001, 2002; Curt et al. 2000; Escalante 2003; Hickok et al. 2001, 2003; Hofman et al. 2004; Irvine et al. 1991; Jereczek-Fossa et al. 2001; Kroenke et al. 1988; Mock 2004; Mock and Olsen 2003; Piper et al. 1987; Portenoy and Itri 1999). More than 80 % of cancer survivors report that the CRF they experience persists for months and even years after treatments are completed, with 17–38 % indicating that their CRF persists well beyond 6 months post-treatment (Barton-Burke and Barton-Burke 2006; Carroll et al. 2007; Frank-Stromberg and Wright 1984; Hofman et al. 2007; Jacobsen et al. 2007; Meyerowitz et al. 1983; Morrow 2007; Mustian et al. 2006; Mustian et al. 2007; Padilla and Grant 1985; Prue et al. 2006; Ryan et al. 2007). CRF is associated with a poorer prognosis among patients and often continues even when a survivor's cancer is undetectable or in remission (Carroll et al. 2007; Hofman et al. 2007; Jacobsen et al. 2007; Jean-Pierre et al. 2007; Morrow 2007; Mustian et al. 2007; Ryan et al. 2007).

CRF has a considerable negative impact on an individual's ability to perform important normal daily activities and overall QOL (Carroll et al. 2007; Hofman et al. 2007; Jacobsen et al. 2007; Jean-Pierre et al. 2007; Morrow 2007; Mustian et al. 2007, 2008; Ryan et al. 2007). This impact stems from the physiological and psychosocial signs and symptoms of CRF which typically include: anemia, hypothyroidism, shortness of breath, muscle atrophy, physical weakness, decreased aerobic capacity, decreased ability to walk, reduced capacity to bathe, dress or cook, sleep disruption, pain, self-reported tiredness, mood disturbance, depression, anxiety, hopelessness, negative outcome expectancies, impaired memory, the inability to concentrate, a reduction in patients' ability to participate in leisure activities, a reduced capacity to sustain meaningful relationships and activities with families, a reduced ability to continue working and a reduction in engagement in social and other activities (Carroll et al. 2007; Hofman et al. 2007; Jacobsen et al. 2007; Jean-Pierre et al. 2007; Meyerowitz et al. 1979; Mock 2004; Morrow 2007; Morrow et al. 2002, 2005; Mustian et al. 2007, 2008; National Comprehensive Cancer Network 2008; Rhodes et al. 1988; Ryan et al. 2007). These signs and symptoms occur both during and after treatment for cancer (Carroll et al. 2007; Hofman et al. 2007; Jacobsen et al. 2007; Jean-Pierre et al. 2007; Morrow 2007; Mustian et al. 2007, 2008; Ryan et al. 2007). CRF is often reported as more distressing and having a greater negative impact on patients' and survivors' daily activities and QOL than other cancer-related symptoms such as vomiting, nausea, pain, and depression (Carroll et al. 2007; Curt et al. 2001; Hofman et al. 2007; Jacobsen et al. 2007; Jean-Pierre et al. 2007; Mock 2004; Morrow 2007; Morrow et al. 2002, 2005; Mustian et al. 2007, 2008; National Comprehensive Cancer Network 2008; Ryan et al. 2007). While great advances have been made in cancer treatments over the past decade, the negative impact of CRF is magnified because life expectancy has increased among cancer survivors. The experience of CRF is prolonged and there is no effective cure (Carroll et al. 2007; Hofman et al. 2007; Jacobsen et al. 2007; Jean-Pierre et al. 2007; Morrow 2007; Mustian et al. 2007, 2008; Ryan et al. 2007).

Cancer-related fatigue was first acknowledged as an official diagnosis in the International Classification of Disease (ICD-10) in 1998. The National Comprehensive Cancer Network (NCCN) published the first set of guidelines for the management of CRF in 2000. These guidelines were based on a synthesis of the best and most currently available research and clinical experience in oncology. These NCCN Practice Guidelines were recently updated in 2008 and provide concise, up-to-date, evidence-based and clinically-based recommendations for the management of CRF based on current knowledge of the symptom and development of new therapies (National Comprehensive Cancer Network 2008).

The current NCCN guidelines for the management of CRF (National Comprehensive Cancer Network 2008) suggest that clinicians frequently screen for CRF in patients with cancer and, when present, first treat possible contributing factors (e.g., pain, emotional distress, sleep disruption, anemia, nutrition, physical activity levels), including comorbid conditions (e.g., infection, cardiac dysfunction, pulmonary dysfunction, renal dysfunction, hepatic dysfunction, neurologic dysfunction, endocrine dysfunction, hypothyroidism), which is typically done via pharmacologic therapies (National Comprehensive Cancer Network 2008). Many patients with cancer continue to experience CRF even after successful clinical management of these contributing factors (Carroll et al. 2007; Hofman et al. 2007; Jacobsen et al. 2007; Jean-Pierre et al. 2007; Morrow 2007; Mustian et al. 2007, 2008; Ryan et al. 2007). Patients may also experience CRF in the absence of any clinically discernable contributing factors (Carroll et al. 2007; Hofman et al. 2007; Jacobsen et al. 2007; Jean-Pierre et al. 2007; Morrow 2007; Mustian et al. 2007, 2008; Ryan et al. 2007). In instances where no specific causal factors can be identified, or when the patient continues to have moderate-to-severe fatigue and/or persistent chronic fatigue after treatments for the cancer are complete and the other possible contributing factors have been clinically treated, the NCCN guidelines (National Comprehensive Cancer Network 2008) recommend that physicians consider both pharmacologic interventions and nonpharmacologic behavioral interventions including maintaining physical activity, psychosocial therapies, and other integrative therapies. Some of the most promising therapies that are still under investigation include exercise (Jacobsen et al. 2007; Mustian et al. 2007), psychosocial therapies (Jacobsen et al. 2007; Mustian et al. 2007), and Modafinil (Morrow et al. 2008).

Despite the existence of the NCCN guidelines and a growing body of literature that has identified some promising treatments, there is currently no evidence-based, effective cure for CRF, and there is no specific standard of care for CRF in the medical community. Moreover, very little attention has been given to the unique pathophysiological and treatment nuances of CRF as an acute versus chronic side effect or an early versus late effect. More scientific research is needed to discern the pathophysiology of all types of CRF and to develop effective cures for all types of CRF. This knowledge will provide the evidence upon which the standards of care for CRF in oncology will eventually be based.

4 Sleep Problems During Radiation Therapy

Relatively little attention has been devoted to sleep disturbance, one of the most distressing symptoms patients experience (Savard and Morin 2001). The spectrum of sleep disorders ranges from insomnia to sleep apnea, parasomnias, restless leg syndrome, and circadian rhythm disorders. Insomnia is defined as difficulty falling asleep, staying asleep or waking up earlier than intended, resulting in daytime complaints of fatigue or sleepiness for at least 1 month and not due to another mental disorder. Insomnia is prevalent; several epidemiological studies report that 15–20 % of the population has insomnia (Ohayon 2007). In general, population sleep loss and/or insomnia are associated with several negative physical and psychiatric consequences including fatigue, psychiatric illness (e.g., major depression and anxiety), physical complaints, substance abuse, reduced quality of life, and cognitive impairment (Breslau et al. 1996; Katz and Mchorney 2002; Lee et al. 2005; Leger et al. 2001, 2002; Ohayon and Zulley 2001; Walsh and Engelhardt 1999; Zee and Walsleben 2004). Some data also suggest that sleep difficulty may negatively influence cardiovascular conditions, reduce immune function, and affect the respiratory and musculoskeletal systems (Burgos et al. 2006; Katz and Mchorney 2002; Schwartz et al. 1999; Suka et al. 2003). Katz and Mchorney (2002) report that insomnia is independently associated with reduced health-related quality of life to the same extent as other serious chronic conditions such as diabetes and heart disease.

Although the full impact of insomnia on cancer patients and on disease progression is largely unknown, it is reasonable to assume that it would create similar adverse psychiatric and physiological consequences in cancer patients as in the general population. Insomnia may exacerbate other cancer-related symptoms (i.e., fatigue, nausea, depressive mood, pain, and/or reduced pain tolerance), and disrupted circadian rhythms may influence disease incidence, progression, and survival (Anderson et al. 2003; Fortner et al. 2002; Koopman et al. 2002; Mormont et al. 2000; Spiegel and Sephton 2002).

While the literature on the prevalence of insomnia in cancer patients is scant, two early studies found that the proportion of people who had difficulty staying asleep was significantly higher among cancer patients (40–45 %) than among healthy controls (14–25 %) (Kaye et al. 1983; Malone et al. 1994). Although both of these studies underscored the importance of studying sleep in cancer patients, the sample size in Kaye et al. (1983) was insufficient to draw any definitive conclusions about insomnia in cancer patients, and Malone et al. (1994) failed to undertake a detailed examination of sleep concerns.

A more recent study conducted by Savard and colleagues in 2001 focused specifically on the prevalence, clinical characteristics, and risk factors for insomnia in the context of breast cancer. They surveyed 300 breast cancer survivors with a median time since diagnosis of 49 months (Savard et al. 2001). Nearly 51 % reported insomnia symptoms, 19 % met diagnostic criteria for insomnia disorder, 33 % reported that insomnia occurred after they were diagnosed with cancer, and for 58 % of patients, insomnia became worse during the course of their cancer. This study was one of the first to note that insomnia prevalence is significantly higher in women with breast cancer than in the general population. Savard and colleagues also identified risk factors for the development of insomnia in breast cancer patients. The study found that unemployment, being on sick leave, and being widowed were significant contributors to the development of insomnia in this population. In addition, they reported that chemotherapy either caused or aggravated sleep difficulties. The authors hypothesized that the spike in symptoms during chemotherapy might be explained either by the antiemetic drugs used in treatment or the onset of menopause brought on by chemotherapy.

The most comprehensive insomnia prevalence study (Davidson et al. 2002) included 982 cancer patients (with a mean age of 65 years) with six different types of cancer (gastrointestinal, gynecologic, genitourinary, breast, lung, and nonmelanoma skin). Patients completed a "Sleep Survey" questionnaire that was used to evaluate the presence or absence of various sleep problems (e.g., insomnia, restless leg syndrome, fatigue) and to define their type of sleep problem (i.e., difficulty falling asleep, difficulty staying asleep, or waking up too early) (Davidson et al. 2002). Three hundred patients reported insomnia (30.5 %), and the majority (76 %) reported the greatest difficulty with frequent awakening. The authors found that the prevalence of insomnia was highest in the surgery group (45 %), followed by chemotherapy (34.5 %) and radiation (29.5 %); these differences, however, were not statistically significant. The authors also noted that cancer patients who reported marked fatigue were 2.5 times more likely to have insomnia than others.

The most recent study, conducted by Mao and colleagues, describes the symptom burden in cancer survivors (Mao et al. 2007). The author's evaluated data collected from 1904 cancer survivors from the 2002 National Health Interview Survey. Nearly 52 % of the survivors were six or more years past their initial diagnosis of cancer, and nearly 30 % reported insomnia symptoms, compared to 17 % of healthy controls. Younger patients (age < 50 years) had an increased symptom burden compared to older patients (age > 64 years), and the adjusted odds ratios for insomnia were 2.7 and 1.44, respectively.

A recent study conducted by the URCC CCOP group (Palesh et al. 2007) surveyed 648 cancer patients (mean age = 61) who completed questionnaires evaluating fatigue, pain, depression, and difficulty sleeping. Sixty percent received chemotherapy and 40 % received radiation therapy. Participants rated the severity of their symptoms at their worst on an 11-point Likert Scale (0 = *Not present* to 10 = *As bad as you can imagine*) prior to treatment, during treatment, and 6 months following treatment. Patients reported significantly more sleep problems during treatment (median = 4) than either prior to or following treatment (both, median = 2). Women reported more sleep problems than men before, during, and after treatment (all $p < 0.01$). Younger patients (age ≤ 60) reported more problems with sleep at all time points (all $p < 0.001$). Patients receiving chemotherapy had more difficulties with sleep at all time points than patients undergoing radiation alone (all $p < 0.001$) (Fig. 3). These results show that women, younger patients, and patients undergoing chemotherapy

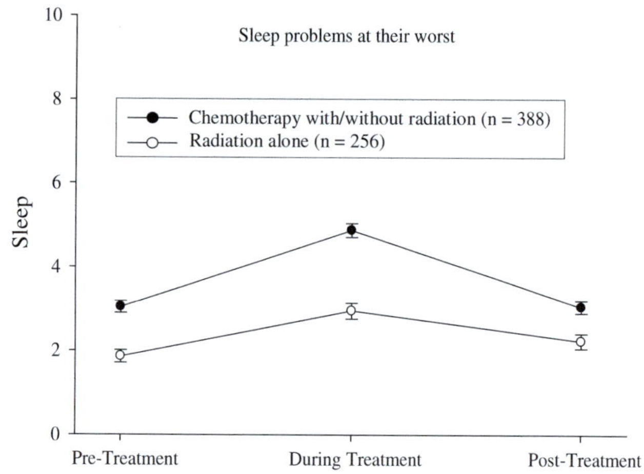

Fig. 3 Sleep problems by treatment type

versus radiation are at higher risk for developing sleep problems and, furthermore, that difficulties with sleep increase during cancer treatment.

All of these studies taken together indicate that insomnia is a prevalent and distressing symptom for cancer patients. Multiple studies indicate that insomnia rates among cancer patients are two to three times higher than rates in the general population. Increasing evidence suggests that cancer treatment might cause or exacerbate existing insomnia complaints and that the use of radiation and/or chemotherapy may cause these complaints to increase. To date, no definitive studies have evaluated insomnia in cancer patients undergoing radiation. It is still unclear whether insomnia precedes cancer or whether insomnia develops as a result of cancer diagnosis and/or treatment. Diagnosis and treatment of cancer and concerns about survival are severe stressors that in themselves might precipitate the development of insomnia; multiple additional biological and psychological "insults" (e.g., tumor biology, anti-cancer medications, early menopause, and fatigue) might also precipitate the development of insomnia symptoms. Given the high rate of insomnia in cancer patients, more investigation into its precipitating and perpetuating factors is needed in order to design effective interventions.

Within the general population, insomnia is highly treatable with pharmacological and psychological therapies (i.e., zolpidem and cognitive-behavioral therapy for insomnia). Several studies conducted in cancer survivors indicate that pharmacological and behavioral interventions are also effective in this group (Espie et al. 2008; Jacobsen et al. 1994; Savard et al. 2005). Additional research is needed to uncover physiological, psychological, and behavioral factors that contribute to the development of insomnia during radiation. Such studies will increase understanding of the natural course of insomnia disorder and allow the development of effective interventions.

5 Radiation Oncology and Psychological Functioning

A cancer diagnosis and its subsequent treatment represent major sources of stress that can lead to a variety of psychological difficulties (Dunn et al. 2004; Steginga et al. 1998). Two major themes characterize the psychological distress of cancer patients: first, the fear of the unknown, and second, the patient's belief that the treatment will cause pain, discomfort, and/or adverse effects (Poroch 1995). While no consensus exists on the prevalence of psychological morbidity among cancer patients, seminal research in this area places the estimate as high as 47 % (Derogatis et al. 1983). Major depression, the most investigated psychiatric disorder in cancer, has been reported in 0–38 % of patients, and "depression spectrum disorders" in 0–58 % (Massie 2004). This wide range of prevalence estimates is largely due to the highly variable methods of assessment (e.g., self-report paper-and-pencil instruments, structured interviews, clinical interviews, and DSM diagnoses) and the differences in study design used by research teams since the 1960s. Investigation has also focused on anxiety disorders, with prevalence estimates ranging from 1.7–23 % and similar patterns of variability in study approach (Stark and House 2000).

Though other psychiatric illnesses (e.g., Posttraumatic Stress Disorder and Adjustment Disorder) have also received research attention, depression and anxiety are widely considered the most important comorbidities for cancer patients because of their potential for interference with treatment and association with poor health outcomes (Frick et al. 2007). Anxiety and stress have been associated with reduced survival and poorer prognosis, although the association is inconsistent (De Boer et al. 1999). There is also evidence that depression predicts progression and mortality and can affect immune function (Spiegel and Giese-Davis 2003). Psychological comorbidities may impair adherence to medical treatment, which could account for poorer outcomes (Spiegel and Giese-Davis 2003). Psychological distress among cancer patients has also been linked to impaired social functioning, nausea, and vomiting (Smith et al. 2003), all of which have a negative effect on quality of life (Frick et al. 2007; Smith et al. 2003).

In terms of psychological distress in response to radiation treatment (RT), an instructive review of the literature has been conducted by Stiegelis et al. (2004). They divided 45 studies, obtained through Medline and Psychlit databases between 1980 and 2002, into four categories representing studies that assessed psychological functioning: (a) prior to RT, (b) during RT, (c) after RT, and (d) using longitudinal designs. The studies included patients receiving both curative and palliative external radiation therapy with a range of cancer sites (e.g., breast, head and neck, prostate, bladder, cervix) and other adjuvant treatments (e.g., chemotherapy and hormone therapy).

Prior to RT, the studies reported that 10–20 % of patients had anxiety symptoms and only 1.5–8 % had depressive symptoms. The authors attribute the difference to anticipatory anxiety about treatment and its side effects prior to treatment and suggest that the absence of treatment side effects may account for relatively low levels of depression (Stiegelis et al. 2004).

During RT, anxiety symptoms were reported in 21–54 % of patients; these symptoms, however, showed relatively consistent declines as treatment progressed. For example, Rahn et al. (1998) showed that 40 % of patients were anxious on the first day of treatment, while only 19 % were still anxious by the last day. It is likely that patients' anxiety decreased as they gained more familiarity with treatment. In contrast to the pre-treatment phase, depressive symptoms were relatively high during RT, with 12-31 % of patients reporting such symptoms.

Data were less consistent in studies examining anxiety and depression following radiation treatment. Reports of anxiety symptoms ranged from 0 to 52 % of patients, with assessments of anxiety covering time points from immediately after RT to as many as 13 years post-treatment. There was also significant variability in depression, ranging from 8 to 48 % of patients. However, most studies found that between 8 and 21.5 % of patients reported depressive symptoms. The authors suggest that, in some instances, differences in cut-off scores and response format may have elevated reporting (Stiegelis et al. 2004).

Longitudinal studies also showed inconsistencies, with some (Monga et al. 1999) finding an improvement in depressive symptoms over the course of RT and others (Chawla et al. 1999) finding a worsening of symptoms. Stiegelis and colleagues suggest that this difference may be attributable to varying baseline levels of psychological functioning and point to Andersen and Tewfik's (1985) observation that: (a) patients with high levels of anxiety at baseline are more likely to see a substantial decrease in symptoms; (b) patients with low anxiety are likely to worsen; and (c) patients with moderate anxiety are unlikely to see much change in symptoms. However, the majority of both cross-sectional and longitudinal studies found declines in anxiety, depressive symptoms, and psychological distress after RT compared to the periods prior to and during treatment.

The literature has also addressed the particular distress that may accompany the end of RT (Deshields et al. 2005). This treatment termination distress may be occasioned both by the loss of support from medical staff, family, and friends once treatment is completed and by anxiety about returning to a regular routine (Culver et al. 2002; Lampic et al. 1994; Leedham and Ganz 1999). In a study of breast cancer patients at the end of RT, Deshields and colleagues found elevated levels of depression and somewhat diminished quality of life, but lower levels of anxiety compared to healthy population norms. Consistent with the studies reviewed by Steigelis et al., the authors speculate that anxiety associated with diagnosis and treatment had subsided by the end of RT. In addition, both depression and quality of life improved substantially within 2 weeks of the end of treatment.

Despite the evidence that depression, anxiety, and quality of life concerns are significant problems for cancer patients, especially in the early phases of diagnosis and treatment, barriers remain in terms of recognition and treatment of these symptoms in radiation oncology practice. These barriers include lack of communication about emotional issues between oncologists and their patients (Pollak et al. 2007), stigmatization and devaluation of mental health concerns and treatment (Holland 2003), belief that psychological problems are a "natural" part of the cancer experience (Spiegel 1996), and a tendency to dismiss somatic complaints thought to be associated with the cancer itself that may be indicative of psychological distress (Hahn et al. 2004; Jackson and Jackson 2007). Addressing these barriers to treatment of psychological problems in radiation oncology requires the concerted efforts of oncologists to properly assess these symptoms and to intervene when necessary.

Hahn et al. (2004) have demonstrated the effectiveness of the Beck Depression Inventory-II for identifying clinically depressed patients and strongly urge its routine use. Jackson and Jackson (2007) offer a helpful review of comorbid depression in adult oncology and note that both psychotherapeutic and pharmacologic treatments have been shown to be effective in this patient population. Similar brief measures and interventions are available for treatment of anxiety. In an historical retrospective on the field of psycho-oncology, Holland (2003) notes that the number of empirically supported psychosocial interventions has never been as great as it is now, making it relatively easy for radiation oncologists to refer patients for the appropriate treatment for psychological distress. These treatments not only increase patient quality of life but enhance compliance with treatment, which may affect survival.

6 Patient Information Needs During Radiation Therapy

One way to ameliorate psychological distress and improve quality of life for cancer patients is by providing appropriate information regarding the disease and its treatment. Educational and informational materials have been used to ease psychological distress for a variety of medical procedures including dental surgery, postoperative recovery, and MRI usage (Davis et al. 1994; Hartfield et al. 1982; Mogan et al. 1985; Selim 2001; Sime and Libera 1985). Early informational and educational programs were implemented in trials among cancer patients, with some success (Lilja et al. 1998; Mcquellon et al. 1998; Wells et al. 1995; Williams and Schreier 2004; Wilson et al. 2006). More recent research has shown that providing information and education to patients on both the disease and the course of treatment can improve psychological well-being (Helgeson et al. 1999; Helgeson et al. 2001).

The desire of cancer patients to be informed and educated about their treatment is well-documented. Information and education are particularly significant in the case of RT, because the treatment is frequently misunderstood by the general public (Chapman et al. 2003; Dunn et al. 2004). Research has shown that patients undergoing RT have fears directly related to the treatment itself and its perceived negative side-effects (Andersen et al. 1984; Frith 1991; O'rourke 1999). One study found that of 50 patients who were prescribed curative RT, the majority did not expect it to be effective (Haggmark et al. 2001). Of patients who considered themselves "well informed," over two-thirds wanted more information, while only 2 % did not want any information on their treatment or its potential side effects (Cassileth et al. 1980). When providing informational materials to patients, clinicians must consider a number of factors (e.g., gender, age, ability to comprehend, family support) that influence patients' preferences (Meredith et al. 1996). The lack of information and educational materials can intensify existing fears resulting from the initial diagnosis and can cause patients to misinterpret symptoms and the side effects of treatments (Cimprich and Ronis 2001; Peck and Boland 1977).

Harrison et al. assessed the information needs of breast cancer patients over their first course of radiation therapy (Harrison et al. 1999). Thirty-three women were interviewed about their informational needs and preferences during the first, third, and final week of treatment and again 1 month post-treatment. In general, patients had high information needs throughout the entire course of RT. This study also demonstrated that most women undergoing RT had a strong desire for information on both the disease and the treatment. Based on these findings, the authors recommend continually assessing the informational needs of patients throughout the course of their treatment.

There is also evidence that the provision of appropriate information has an impact on treatment-related side effects. A randomized trial conducted in 2002 examined the effects of information on the severity of treatment side effects in 152 RT patients (Kim et al. 2002). The intervention took place during the first and fifth radiation treatments and provided patients with specific, objective information about what to expect during treatment, while the control group was given only general information. The results demonstrated that the brief, targeted information was successful in reducing both fatigue and sleep problems among those who received it. This trial demonstrated that targeted information can have a positive impact on certain side effects, which may represent a method of improving quality of life among those receiving RT.

The timing of information dissemination can affect how patients use that information. A trial conducted in 2000 sought to determine the optimal timing of information provision to radiotherapy patients (D'haese et al. 2000). Sixty-eight patients were randomized to receive either a description of RT procedures and sensations or teaching sheets with treatment-site information. Patients received the information either all at once or in a stepwise manner. The analyses revealed that patients who received all the information at once were more anxious and less satisfied with their radiation therapy. The authors believed this negative outcome resulted from the timing of the intervention. Receiving the information only a short time before the commencement of RT did not give the patients the opportunity to discuss the information with a clinician. The authors also noted that it was important to maintain contact with the patients post-treatment, since some evidence suggests that anxiety increases during this period.

A recent trial of 525 patients undergoing RT assessed the impact of different forms of information on anxiety (Jones et al. 1999). This randomized trial utilized two groups who each received information via computer. One group received personalized information while the other group received only general information. The patients assigned the personalized information found they learned something new and were more likely to share the information with others. In addition, those who received the personalized information showed a greater reduction in anxiety than those receiving the general information. The authors suggest that clinicians should offer personalized information via computer as a cost-effective way to educate patients and possibly reduce patient anxiety.

The next two studies used informational audio- and videotapes to educate patients undergoing radiation therapy. The first study was a quasi-experimental design of 92 patients beginning RT, which assessed the effects of a patient education video on psychological distress (Dunn et al. 2004). The study found those in the intervention group reported high levels of utilization and satisfaction. Nevertheless, the video had no effect on coping or psychological distress throughout the course of treatment. A 1996 study used informational audiotapes to increase knowledge and self-care behaviors in those undergoing RT (Hagopian 1996). Seventy-five patients were assigned to receive standard care or standard care plus an information audiotape. The results demonstrated that patients who received the audiotapes were more knowledgeable, used more self-care measures, and practiced more helpful self-care behaviors than the control group. The audiotapes had a positive effect because of their convenience; patients could receive the information at the time and place of their choosing.

Clinicians can use a variety of information media, rather than just the standard printed materials. A recent clinical trial randomized 310 patients beginning radiotherapy to receive standard care or standard care plus a 15-minute educational videotape, a 12-page informational booklet, and an audiotape of relaxation techniques (Krischer et al. 2007). The results did not show an overall reduction in psychological distress for the informational intervention versus standard care, but they did show a reduction in psychological distress among those who had higher levels of psychological distress at baseline. These findings demonstrate that informational and educational materials can benefit patients with heightened distress.

A diagnosis of cancer and its subsequent treatment are stressful, life-changing events. The anxiety and depression that result can have detrimental effects. The evidence is clear that patients have a strong desire for informational and educational materials concerning their diagnosis and course of treatment. Unfortunately, these informational needs are often unmet. Research has shown the importance of providing patients with information both before they begin treatment and throughout treatment. All media (booklets, audiotapes, videotapes) can be effective, as long as the patient can comprehend the message. Personalized information is more effective than general information. In certain studies, education reduced side effects and increased self-care measures. Nevertheless, although information eased psychological distress in some studies, none has linked the provision of information to improved prognosis or survival. However, it is clear that providing information to patients has positive effects during treatment and may help to alleviate anxiety.

7 Radiotherapy and Cognitive Functioning

Cancer-related cognitive dysfunction (CRCD) is an incapacitating and enduring side effect of cancer treatment (e.g., radiation therapy) with critical social/relational and economic implications. Many cancer patients have reported mild to moderate CRCD in important neuropsychological and cognitive domains of attention, concentration, processing speed, and memory (Paraska and Bender 2003). Incidence rates of CRCD range from 17 to 75 %. Previous studies have reported a higher incidence of cognitive dysfunction among cancer patients than in matched healthy controls (Brezden et al. 2000). A recent prospective, longitudinal study reported that 61 % of patients undergoing cancer treatment demonstrated diminished neuropsychological function in multiple domains of cognition 6 months following initiation of treatment (Wefel et al. 2004).

Many hypotheses have been put forth to explain the etiologies of CRCD. Some of the hypotheses include a genetic predisposition, such as an absence of epoetin alfa (O'shaughnessy 2002, 2003; Weiss 2003), direct and/or indirect toxic effects of cancer treatment on the central nervous system (Ahles et al. 2002; Meyers et al. 2005; Wefel et al. 2004), differences in estrogen secretion (Bender et al. 2007), the effects of cytokine activities in the brain, microvasculature obstruction, and infarction of brain tissue (Meyers 2000). Other psychologically-based explanations include the relationship between CRCD and cancer-related fatigue and mood states such as anxiety and depression (Bender et al. 2001; Saykin et al. 2003; Staat and Segatore 2005; Tannock et al. 2004).

CRCD has been associated with radiotherapy for malignant tumors with primary sites within (e.g., brain) and outside the central nervous system (e.g., lung, breast). Researchers have classified the negative effects of radiotherapy on the central nervous system (CNS) in three broad categories: acute reactions, short-term delayed reactions, and long-term delayed reactions (Lilja et al. 2001). Acute reactions occur within hours or days immediately following radiotherapy and are associated with increased intracranial pressure. Short-term delayed reactions occur within a few weeks or months after completion of radiotherapy. Last, long-term delayed reactions occur from months to years after completion of radiotherapy.

Both prophylactic and therapeutic whole brain radiotherapy (WBRT) are associated with cognitive problems in cancer patients. Welzel et al. (2008) conducted a prospective study comparing the effects of prophylactic and therapeutic RT (WBRT) on memory function among adults with and without brain metastases. The authors performed serial cognitive evaluations of patients before (T0), after starting (T1), at the end of treatment (T2), and at 6–8 weeks after completion of radiotherapy (RT) (T3). The sample included small-cell lung cancer patients treated with prophylactic cranial irradiation, patients with brain metastases treated with therapeutic cranial irradiation (TCI), and breast cancer patients treated with RT to the breast (control group). Interestingly, the authors reported that before therapy, patients treated with prophylactic cranial irradiation performed worse on most tests than patients treated with TCI and patients from the control group. The findings also showed a significant relationship between pretreatment cognitive status and verbal memory function during and after WBRT. Specifically, during and after WBRT verbal memory function was primarily influenced by pretreatment cognitive status and to a lesser extent by WBRT. Acute (T1) radiation effects on verbal memory function were only observed in TCI patients, whereas subacute (T3) radiation effects on verbal memory function were observed in both TCI and prophylactic cranial irradiation patients. Visual memory and attention, however, were not influenced by WBRT. Welzel et al. (in press) reported that observed effects of irradiation were more pronounced in patients with the above-average performance at baseline. WBRT causes cognitive dysfunction immediately after the beginning of radiation therapy only in patients with brain metastases.

Lilja et al. (2001) examined the short-term effects of radiotherapy (RT) on attention and memory performance in patients with primary brain tumors. Participants were subjected to neuropsychological assessment at baseline (before RT, which lasted for 6 weeks), within 2 weeks after the completion of radiotherapy, and at 3 months after the completion of radiotherapy. Healthy control individuals were assessed at baseline and follow-up. The findings showed that at baseline, cancer patients scored significantly lower than the controls in tests of semantic memory, visuoconstructive skill, and visual and verbal memory. Cancer patients performed significantly more poorly than individuals in the control group on a two-choice reaction time test, a subtraction test, and a vigilance test. The authors concluded, however, that RT was not associated with negative short-term effects in attention and memory function in patients with brain tumors who received a radiation dose of 54.5 grays. They noted that the cognitive deficits experienced by cancer patients were evident at baseline, before RT. Therefore, they concluded that the observed problems in cognitive performance were associated with the malignancy itself and/or prior surgical procedures.

CRCD is a significant problem for many cancer patients. As with other cancer and treatment-related side effects such as cancer-related fatigue, CRCD can have an enduring negative effect on psychosocial performance (Ahles et al. 2002). Despite increasing recognition of the negative impact of CRCD on patients' well-being and psychosocial functioning, systematic interventions to control CRCD are still lacking. Patients with CRCD could benefit from behavioral interventions, and longitudinal studies to inform the development of neuropsychological therapies to control CRCD are needed. In the meantime, neuropsychological and cognitive techniques that have been applied to help improve cognitive performance in other populations with a similar profile of cognitive dysfunction (e.g., mild cognitive impairment) could be adapted for cancer patients struggling with CRCD.

8 Psychosocial Effects of Cancer Among Ethnic Minorities and Underserved Populations

The impact of cultural beliefs on cancer treatment and survival is evident in a number of cultures. Culture can affect psychosomatic processes, which can have a negative impact on cancer survival. In a study of 28,169 Chinese Americans, researchers discovered that those who had a specific combination of disease and birth year considered ill-fated by Chinese astrology died younger than the control population, and that individuals with stronger Chinese traditions died even earlier (Phillips et al. 1993). While these study results cannot be fully explained, investigators concluded that the findings were partly due to psychosomatic processes. The findings seemed consistent with other studies (Dean and Surtees 1989; Derogatis et al. 1979; Greer 1991; Greer et al. 1979; Hislop et al. 1987) that found that cancer patients who displayed stoic acceptance or helplessness/hopelessness about their disease died earlier than patients without these psychological characteristics.

A cultural study of cancer beliefs among American Samoans (Hubbell et al. 2005) produced several unexpected answers to the basic questions: (1) *What is cancer?*, (2) *What causes cancer?*, and (3) *What can you do to prevent cancer?* Answers included the following: (1) Cancer is not a Samoan disease, but a new illness brought by the Westerners (there is no word for cancer in the Samoan language); (2) Departure from the Samoan lifestyle *fa'aSamoa* is a major factor in causing cancer (including eating nontraditional foods such as canned goods or refrigerated items); (3) Lifestyle modifications can prevent cancer but prevention is not part of the Samoan culture (the majority depend on traditional remedies and traditional healers; few see medical doctors, and only if symptoms are severe).

The impact of cultural beliefs, mores, and norms on the cancer experience is understudied (Aziz and Rowland 2002). Studies suggest that cultural beliefs and attitudes toward cancer, seem to affect the individual sufficiently to produce measurable change in physiological outcomes (advanced cancer stage and diminished survival). Research is needed to confirm these findings, and new investigations examining cultural influences may aid in the overall understanding of cancer disparities.

Of course, culture is just one aspect of the cancer experience for many minorities and underserved individuals. There is a growing consensus that socioeconomic status is a greater determinant of cancer disparities than either ethnicity or race (American Cancer Society 2000). Poor individuals, regardless of race or ethnic background, have a 10–15 % lower five-year cancer survival rate than individuals of higher socioeconomic status (American Cancer Society 2000). Poverty is commonly associated with lower levels of education, low-paying jobs and unemployment, lack of health insurance and limited access to healthcare, inadequate transportation and resources, lack of adequate health information, risky health behaviors, and various other factor that can result in advanced cancer stage and a diminished health status (Haynes and Smedley 1999; Smedley et al. 2003). Factors associated with poverty make quality cancer care difficult for both the healthcare professional and the patient.

A panel discussion (Dana-Farber Cancer Institute and Beth Israel Deaconess Medical Center) presented several examples of cancer experiences in minority and underrepresented communities (Gilligan et al. 2003). Cancer survivors from different racial and ethnic backgrounds used their personal experiences to address many of the issues and concerns regarding cancer care disparities. The general mistrust of healthcare providers, was repeatedly mentioned during discussions. One individual reported that she was so worried about staff attitudes toward minority patients that she avoided calling for assistance at night while in the hospital. Another individual stated that "people are frightened when they come for care." She explained that many people, specifically women from other countries, will not see male physicians and will not return if they are assigned a male provider. Conversely, men from some countries may not respect female doctors, and many may refuse service.

The panel moderators addressed specific cancer disparity issues (access to medical care, poverty, outreach and educational programs, screening, research, and personal support). Specific comments from cancer survivors included:

Access: "Some patients cannot afford the cost of treatments; a few cannot even afford a cab. Also, medical services occur at night…but taxicabs are reluctant to come into our communities."

Poverty: "People on hourly wages live from paycheck to paycheck, so they cannot afford to take time off. If there are children, child care is needed in order for parents to come."

Language: "For the Hispanic population, the language barrier is an obvious obstacle to communicating effectively with healthcare professionals. Having providers learn to speak other languages is not a viable solution. I think that we should expand resources for teaching immigrants to learn English."

Screening: "After my surgery for prostate cancer, I met with my three brothers in Spain to discuss PSA examinations. My youngest brother left the room, because he didn't want to listen, and my older brothers had little to say. The cultural norm in Spain is that you go for medical tests only when you are sick."

Research: "Minority communities are often skeptical of these trials…Many members of my support group are skeptical, because treatments might not be effective. Also, they do worry about being harmed by the new medicines."

While these statements do not describe the entire cancer experience for ethnic minorities and underserved groups, they certainly send a strong message that cancer care disparities do exist. Additionally, cancer experiences may differ within ethnic and racial subgroups, and these differences magnify the complexity of providing high quality and equitable cancer care.

The combination of certain cultural and socioeconomic factors leads to a variety of negative cancer experiences, which contribute to inadequate and unequal cancer care. The challenges for healthcare professionals and cancer patients include identifying current and potential causes of cancer care disparities, increasing awareness among healthcare providers of various cultural and socioeconomic influences, targeting and developing strategies for improvement, implementing effective programs, and monitoring success.

Radiation oncology is a "fertile ground for conducting disparities research" (Greenwood 2005). The following are study findings regarding disparities in radiation oncology:

- Case study: 41-year-old African American female with schizophrenia received several interruptions in radiation treatment and less than half of the recommended chemotherapy regimen due to missed appointments (Garner 2003).
- Women with disabilities do not receive standard post-surgical therapy including radiation therapy, resulting in a higher risk for recurrence and cancer-related morbidity (Beth Israel Deaconess Medical Center 2006).
- Among older patients with rectal cancer, blacks are 23 % less likely to receive radiation therapy than whites (Morris et al. 2008).
- In a study of 93 Native American radiation therapy patients the median one-way travel distance for treatment was 109 miles, 37 % traveled at least 150 miles; 28 % had treatment delays of six or more days; 15 % had delays of 11 or more days; 50 % experienced grade 2 radiation treatment toxicities; and 10 patients had grade 3 radiation treatment toxicities (Rogers and Petereit 2005).
- Significant disparities occur in the management of early-stage breast cancer among Asian Americans and Pacific Islanders, with Japanese, Hawaiians, and Filipinos being particularly less likely to receive standard-of-care treatment (i.e., breast conserving surgery, radiation therapy, and chemotherapy) (Gelber et al. 2006).
- Black women who had a lumpectomy were 7 % less likely than whites to receive radiation therapy. Black men diagnosed with prostate cancer were 11 % less likely to get surgical or radiation treatment (Dunham 2008).
- Although black and white rectal cancer patients were equally likely to consult an oncologist, the use of adjuvant therapy was significantly different. Radiation therapy was administered for 73.7 % of black patients versus 83.4 % of white patients (Morris et al. 2008).

Results from these studies point to opportunities to improve treatment for underserved and minority patients in radiation oncology, an imperative that has been recognized as a national priority. Interventions designed to aid clinicians in provision of optimal treatment and to encourage patient acceptance of such treatment is sorely needed.

References

Ahlberg K et al (2003) Assessment and management of cancer-related fatigue in adults [Review] [140 refs]. Lancet 362:640–650

Ahles TA et al (2002) Neuropsychologic impact of standard-dose systemic chemotherapy in long-term survivors of breast cancer and lymphoma. J Clin Oncol 20:485–493

American Cancer Society (2000) Fighting cancer in the poor and underserved. American Cancer Society, New York

Andersen BL, Tewfik HH (1985) Psychological reactions to radiation therapy: reconsideration of the adaptive aspects of anxiety. J Pers Soc Psychol 48:1024–1032

Andersen BL et al (1984) Anxiety and cancer treatment: response to stressful radiotherapy. Health Psychol 3:535–551

Anderson KO et al (2003) Fatigue and sleep disturbance in patients with cancer, patients with clinical depression, and community-dwelling adults. J Pain Symptom Manag 25:307–318

Aziz NM, Rowland JH (2002) Cancer survivorship research among ethnic minority and medically underserved groups. Oncol Nurs Forum 29:789–801

Barton-Burke M, Barton-Burke M (2006) Cancer-related fatigue and sleep disturbances. Further research on the prevalence of these two symptoms in long-term cancer survivors can inform education, policy, and clinical practice. [Review] [31 refs]. Am J Nurs 106:72–77

Bender CM et al (2001) Cognitive function and reproductive hormones in adjuvant therapy for breast cancer: a critical review. J Pain Symptom Manag 21:407–424

Bender CM et al (2007) Memory impairments with adjuvant anastrozole versus tamoxifen in women with early-stage breast cancer. Menopause J North Am Menopause Soc 14:995–998

Berger AM (1998) Patterns of fatigue and activity and rest during adjuvant breast cancer chemotherapy. Oncol Nurs Forum 25:51–62

Beth Israel Deaconess Medical Center (2006) Press release: disparities in breast cancer treatment for women with disabilities. Beth Israel Deaconess Medical Center, Boston

Breslau N et al (1996) Sleep disturbance and psychiatric disorders: a longitudinal epidemiological study of young adults. Biol Psychiatry 39:411–418

Brezden CB et al (2000) Cognitive function in breast cancer patients receiving adjuvant chemotherapy. J Clin Oncol 18:1–7

Broeckel JA et al (1998) Characteristics and correlates of fatigue after adjuvant chemotherapy for breast cancer. J Clin Oncol 16:1689–1696

Burgos I et al (2006) Increased nocturnal interleukin-6 excretion in patients with primary insomnia: a pilot study. Brain Behav Immun 20:246–253
Carroll JK et al (2007) Pharmacologic treatment of cancer-related fatigue. Oncologist 12(Suppl 1):43–51
Cassileth BR et al (1980) The effect of experience on radiation therapy patients' desire for information. Int J Radiat Oncol Biol Phys 6:493–496
Cella D (1998) Factors influencing quality of life in cancer patients: anemia and fatigue. Semin Oncol 25:43–46
Cella D et al (1998) Progress toward guidelines for the management of fatigue. Oncology 12:369–377
Cella D et al (2001) Cancer-related fatigue: prevalence of proposed diagnostic criteria in a United States sample of cancer survivors. J Clin Oncol 19:3385–3391
Cella D et al (2002) Fatigue in cancer patients compared with fatigue in the general United States population. Cancer 94:528–538
Chapman K et al (2003) Lay understanding of terms used in cancer consultations. Psychonosology 12:557–566
Chawla S et al (1999) Temporal assessment of quality of life of head and neck cancer patients receiving radical radiotherapy. Qual Life Res 8:73–78
Cimprich B, Ronis DL (2001) Attention and symptom distress in women with and without breast cancer. Nurs Res 50:86–94
Cleeland CS et al (2000) Assessing symptom distress in cancer patients: the M.D Anderson symptom inventory. Cancer 89:1634–1646
Cleeland CS et al (2003) Are the symptoms of cancer and cancer treatment due to a shared biologic mechanism? A cytokine-immunologic model of cancer symptoms. Cancer 97:2919–2925
Cleeland CS et al (2007) Symptom burden: multiple symptoms and their impact as patient-reported outcomes. J Natl Cancer Inst Monogr 37:16–21
Culver JL et al (2002) Coping and distress among women under treatment for early stage breast cancer: comparing African Americans, Hispanics and non-Hispanic whites. Psycho-Oncology 11:495–504
Curt GA et al (2000) Impact of cancer-related fatigue on the lives of patients: new findings from the fatigue coalition. Oncologist 5:353–360
Curt GA et al (2001) Impact of cancer-related fatigue on the lives of patients: new findings from the fatigue coalition. In: Marty M, Pecorelli S (eds) Fatigue and cancer. Elsevier, Amsterdam, pp 3–16
Davidson JR et al (2002) Sleep disturbance in cancer patients. Social Sci Med 54:1309–1321
Davis TM et al (1994) Undergoing cardiac catheterization: the effects of informational preparation and coping style on patient anxiety during the procedure. Heart Lung 23:140–150
De Boer MF et al (1999) Psychosocial correlates of cancer relapse and survival: a literature review. Patient Educ Couns 37:215–230
Dean C, Surtees PG (1989) Do psychological factors predict survival in breast cancer? J Psychosom Res 33:561–569
Derogatis LR et al (1979) Psychological coping mechanisms and survival time in metastatic breast cancer. JAMA 242:1504–1508
Derogatis LR et al (1983) The prevalence of psychiatric disorders among cancer patients. JAMA 249:751–757
Deshields T et al (2005) Ending treatment: the course of emotional adjustment and quality of life among breast cancer survivors immediately following radiation therapy. Support Care Cancer 13:1018–1026
D'haese S et al (2000) The effect of timing of the provision of information on anxiety and satisfaction of cancer patients receiving radiotherapy. J Cancer Educ 15:223–227
Dodd MJ et al (2001) Symptom clusters and their effect on the functional status of patients with cancer. Oncol Nurs Forum 28:465–470
Dunham W (2008) Racial disparities persist in U.S. cancer treatment. National Prostate Cancer Coalition, Reuters
Dunn J et al (2004) Evaluating patient education materials about radiation therapy. Patient Educ Couns 52:325–332
Escalante CP (2003) Treatment of cancer-related fatigue: an update. Support Care Cancer 11:79–83
Espie CA et al (2008) Randomized controlled clinical effectiveness trial of cognitive behavior therapy compared with treatment as usual for persistent Insomnia in patients with cancer. J Clin Oncol 26:1–9
Fortner BV et al (2002) Sleep and quality of life in breast cancer patients. J Pain Symptom Manag 24:471–480
Frank-Stromberg M, Wright P (1984) Ambulatory cancer patients' perception of the physical and psychosocial changes in their lives since the diagnosis of cancer. Cancer Nurs 7:117–130
Frick E et al (2007) Anxiety, depression and quality of life of cancer patients undergoing radiation therapy: a cross-sectional study in a community hospital outpatient centre. Eur J Cancer Care 16:130–136
Frith B (1991) Giving information to radiotherapy patients. Nurs Stand 5:33–35
Garner EI (2003) Cervical cancer: disparities in screening, treatment, and survival. Cancer Epidemiol Biomarkers Prev 12:242s–247s
Gelber RP et al (2006) Ethnic disparities in breast cancer management among Asian Americans and Pacific Islanders. Ann Surg Oncol 13:977–984
Gilligan TD et al (2003) Cancer survivorship issues for minority and underserved populations. Cancer Epidemiol Biomarkers Prev 12:284s–286s
Given CW et al (2001) Predictors of pain and fatigue in the year following diagnosis among elderly cancer patients. J Pain Symptom Manag 21:456–466
Greenwood A (2005) NCI radiation oncology program tackles cancer disparaties www.cancer.gov 2(6):16–26
Greer S (1991) Psychological response to cancer and survival. Psychol Med 21:43–49
Greer S et al (1979) Psychological response to breast cancer: effect on outcome. Lancet 2:785–787
Haggmark C et al (2001) Effects of information supply on satisfaction with information and quality of life in cancer patients receiving curative radiation therapy. Patient Educ Couns 45:173–179
Hagopian GA (1996) The effects of informational audiotapes on knowledge and self-care behaviors of patients undergoing radiation therapy. Oncol Nurs Forum 23:697–700
Hahn CA et al (2004) Routine screening for depression in radiation oncology patients. Am J Clin Oncol Cancer Clin Trials 27:497–499
Harrison DE et al (1999) Information needs and preference for information of women with breast cancer over a first course of radiation therapy. Patient Educ Couns 38:217–225
Hartfield MT et al (1982) Effects of information about a threatening procedure on patients' expectations and emotional distress. Nurs Res 31:202–206
Haynes A, Smedley B (1999) The unequal burden of cancer: an assessment of NIH research and programs for ethnic minorities and the medically underserved. National Academy Press, Washington
Helgeson VS et al (1999) Education and peer discussion group interventions and adjustment to breast cancer. Arch Gen Psychiatry 56:340–347
Helgeson VS et al (2001) Long-term effects of educational and peer discussion group interventions on adjustment to breast cancer. Health Psychol 20:387–392

Hickok JT, Morrow GR, Roscoe JA, Pierce HI, Rosenbluth RJ (2001) Prevalence and severity of acute and delayed NV associated with 3 highly emetogenic chemotherapies. In: Supportive care in cancer, 13th international symposium 9, 289

Hickok JT, Roscoe JA, Morrow GR Bushunow P, Shelke AR, Matteson S, Dakhil SR, Flynn PJ (2003) Occurrence of severe nausea in 194 women treated with doxorubicin for breast cancer. Support Care Cancer 11:393

Hickok JT et al (2005a) Occurrence, severity, and longitudinal course of twelve common symptoms in 1129 consecutive patients during radiotherapy for cancer. J Pain Symptom Manag 30:433–442

Hickok JT et al (2005b) Frequency, severity, clinical course, and correlates of fatigue in 372 patients during 5 weeks of radiotherapy for cancer. Cancer 104:1772–1778

Hislop TG et al (1987) The prognostic significance of psychosocial factors in women with breast cancer. J Chronic Dis 40:729–735

Hofman M et al (2004) Cancer patients' expectations of experiencing treatment-related side effects: a university of Rochester cancer center–community clinical oncology program study of 938 patients from community practices. Cancer 101:851–857

Hofman M et al (2007) Cancer-related fatigue: the scale of the problem. Oncologist 12:4–10

Holland JC (2003) Psychological care of patients: psycho-oncology's contribution. J Clin Oncol 21:253S–265S

Hubbell FA et al (2005) Exploring beliefs about cancer among American Samoans: focus group findings. Cancer Detect Prev 29:109–115

Irvine DM et al (1991) A critical appraisal of the research literature investigating fatigue in the individual with cancer. Cancer Nurs 14:188–199

Jackson CW, Jackson KH (2007) Comorbid depression in adult oncology. J Pharm Pract 20:360–367

Jacobsen PB et al (1994) Hypnotic efficacy and safety of Triazolam administered during the postoperative period. Gen Hosp Psychiatry 16:419–425

Jacobsen PB et al (2007) Systematic review and meta-analysis of psychological and activity-based interventions for cancer-related fatigue [Review] [70 refs]. Health Psychol 26:660–667

Jean-Pierre P et al (2007) Assessment of cancer-related fatigue: implications for clinical diagnosis and treatment. Oncologist 12:11–21

Jemal A et al (2008) Cancer statistics, 2008. CA Cancer J Clin 58:71–96

Jereczek-Fossa BA et al (2001) Radiotherapy-related fatigue: how to assess and how to treat the symptom: a commentary. Tumori 87:147–152

Jones R et al (1999) Randomised trial of personalised computer based information for cancer patients. BMJ 319:1241–1247

Katz DA, McHorney CA (2002) The relationship between insomnia and health-related quality of life in patients with chronic illness. J Fam Pract 51:229–235

Kaye J et al (1983) Sleep patterns in patients with cancer and patients with cardiac disease. J Psychol 114:107–113

Kim Y et al (2002) The effects of information and negative affect on severity of side effects from radiation therapy for prostate cancer. Support Care Cancer 10:416–421

Kirkova J et al (2006) Cancer symptom assessment instruments: a systematic review. J Clin Oncol 24:1459–1473

Koopman C et al (2002) Sleep disturbances in women with metastatic breast cancer. Breast J 8:362–370

Krischer MM et al (2007) Self-administered stress management training in patients undergoing radiotherapy. J Clin Oncol 25:4657–4662

Kroenke K et al (1988) Chronic fatigue in primary care. Prevalence, patient characteristics, and outcome. JAMA 260:929–934

Lampic C et al (1994) Anxiety and cancer-related worry of cancer-patients at routine follow-up visits. Acta Oncol 33:119–125

Lee B-N et al (2004) A cytokine-based neuroimmunologic mechanism of cancer-related symptoms. Neuroimmunomodulation 11:279–292

Lee KA et al (2005) Critical components of a sleep assessment for clinical practice settings [Review] [27 refs]. Issues Ment Health Nurs 26:739–750

Leedham B, Ganz PA (1999) Psychosocial concerns and quality of life in breast cancer survivors. Cancer Invest 17:342–348

Leger D et al (2001) SF-36: Evaluation of quality of life in severe and mild insomniacs compared with good sleepers. Psychosom Med 63:49–55

Leger D et al (2002) Medical and socio-professional impact of insomnia. Sleep 25:625–629

Lilja Y et al (1998) Effects of extended preoperative information on perioperative stress: an anaesthetic nurse intervention for patients with breast cancer and total hip replacement. Intensive Crit Care Nurs 14:276–282

Lilja AM et al (2001) Short-term effects of radiotherapy on attention and memory performances in patients with brain tumors. Cancer 91:2361–2368

Malone M et al (1994) Assessment of the impact of cancer on work, recreation, home management and sleep using a general health status measure. J R Soc Med 87:386–389

Mao JJ et al (2007) Symptom burden among cancer survivors: impact of age and comorbidity. J Am Board Fam Med 20:434–443

Massie MJ (2004) Prevalence of depression in patients with cancer. J Natil Cancer Inst Monogr 32:57–71

McQuellon RP et al (1998) Reducing distress in cancer patients with an orientation program. Psychooncology 7:207–217

Meredith C et al (1996) Information needs of cancer patients in west Scotland: cross sectional survey of patients' views. BMJ 313:724–726

Meyerowitz BE et al (1979) Adjuvant chemotherapy for breast carcinoma. Cancer 43:1613–1618

Meyerowitz BE et al (1983) Quality of life for breast cancer patients receiving adjuvant chemotherapy. Am J Nurs 83:232–235

Meyers CA (2000) Neurocognitive dysfunction in cancer patients. Oncology 14:75–79

Meyers CA et al (2005) Cognitive impairment, fatigue, and cytokine levels in patients with acute myelogenous leukemia or myelodysplastic syndrome. Cancer 104:788–793

Miaskowski C et al (2004) Symptom clusters: the new frontier in symptom management research. J Natl Cancer Inst Monogr 32:17–21

Mock V (2004) Evidence-based treatment for cancer-related fatigue [Review] [70 refs]. J Natl Cancer Inst Monogr 32:112–118

Mock V, Olsen M (2003) Current management of fatigue and anemia in patients with cancer [Review] [33 refs]. Semin Oncol Nurs 19:36–41

Mogan J et al (1985) Effects of preoperative teaching on postoperative pain: a replication and expansion. Int J Nurs Stud 22:267–280

Monga U et al (1999) Prospective study of fatigue in localized prostate cancer patients undergoing radiotherapy. Radiat Oncol Investig 7:178–185

Mormont MC et al (2000) Marked 24-h rest/activity rhythms are associated with better quality of life, better response, and longer survival in patients with metastatic colorectal cancer and good performance status. Clin Cancer Res 6:3038–3045

Morris AM, Billingsley KG, Hayanga AJ, Matthews B, Baldwin LM, Birkmeyer JD (2008) Residual treatment disparities after oncology referral for rectal cancer. J Natl Cancer Inst 100:738–744

Morrow GR (2007) Cancer-related fatigue: causes, consequences, and management. Oncologist 12:1–3

Morrow GR et al (2002) Fatigue associated with cancer and its treatment. Support Care Cancer 10:389–398

Morrow GR et al (2005) Management of cancer-related fatigue. Cancer Invest 23:229–239

Morrow GR, Jean-Pierre P, Roscoe JA, Heckler CE, Schwartzenberger PO, Giguere JK, Dakhil SRA (2008) Phase III randomized, placebo-controlled, double-blind trial of a eugeroic agent in 642 cancer patients reporting fatigue during chemotherapy: a URCC CCOP study. J Clin Oncol 26:504s

Mustian KM, Hofman M Morrow GR, Griggs JJ, Jean-Pierre P, Kohli S, Roscoe JA, Simondet J, Bushunow P (2006) Cancer-related fatigue and shortness of breath among cancer survivors: a prospective URCC CCOP study. In: NCI cancer survivorship conference

Mustian KM et al (2007) Integrative nonpharmacologic behavioral interventions for the management of cancer-related fatigue. Oncologist 12:52–67

Mustian KM et al (2008) Cancer-related fatigue interferes with activities of daily living among 753 patients receiving chemotherapy: a URCC CCOP study. J Clin Oncol 26:(May 20 suppl; abstr 9500)

National Comprehensive Cancer Network (2008) National comprehensive cancer network practice guidelines. Cancer related fatigue panel 2008 guidelines. National comprehensive cancer network version 1 (March 2004; Rockledge, PA)

Ohayon MM (2007) Prevalence and comorbidity of sleep disorders in general population. Rev Prat 57:1521–1528

Ohayon MM, Zulley J (2001) Correlates of global sleep dissatisfaction in the German population. Sleep 24:780–787

O'Rourke ME (1999) Narrowing the options: the process of deciding on prostate cancer treatment. Cancer Invest 17:349–359

O'Shaughnessy JA (2002) Effects of epoetin alfa on cognitive function, mood, asthenia, and quality of life in women with breast cancer undergoing adjuvant chemotherapy. Clin Breast Cancer Suppl 3:S116–S120

O'Shaughnessy JA (2003) Chemotherapy-induced cognitive dysfunction: a clearer picture. Clin Breast Cancer Suppl 2:S89–S94

Padilla G, Grant M (1985) Quality of life as a cancer nursing outcome variable. Adv Nurs Sci 8:45–49

Palesh O, Mustian K, Roscoe JA, Morrow G, Perlis M, Issel B, Banerjee T, Delmore JE (2007) Prevalence and severity of sleep disturbance in 596 cancer patients: a URCC CCOP study. J Clin Oncol 25:18S

Paraska K, Bender CM (2003) Cognitive dysfunction following adjuvant chemotherapy for breast cancer: Two case studies. Oncol Nurs Forum 30:473–478

Peck A, Boland J (1977) Emotional reactions to radiation treatment. Cancer 40:180–184

Phillips DP et al (1993) Psychology and survival. Lancet 342:1142–1145

Piper BF et al (1987) Fatigue mechanisms in cancer patients: developing nursing theory. Oncol Nurs Forum 14:17–23

Pollak KI et al (2007) Oncology communication about emotion during visits with patients with advanced cancer. J Clin Oncol 25:5748–5752

Poroch D (1995) The effect of preparatory patient education on the anxiety and satisfaction of cancer patients receiving radiation therapy. Cancer Nurs 18:206–214

Portenoy RK, Itri LM (1999) Cancer-related fatigue: guidelines for evaluation and management. Oncologist 4:1–10

Prue G et al (2006) Cancer-related fatigue: a critical appraisal [Review] [84 refs]. Eur J Cancer 42:846–863

Rahn AN et al (1998) Influence of radiotherapy on psychological health in breast cancer patients after breast conserving surgery. Anticancer Res 18:2271–2273

Rhodes VA et al (1988) Patients' descriptions of the influence of tiredness and weakness on self-care abilities. Cancer Nurs 11:186–194

Rogers D, Petereit DG (2005) Cancer disparities research partnership in Lakota country: clinical trials, patient services, and community education for the Oglala, Rosebud, and Cheyenne River Sioux tribes. Am J Public Health 95:2129–2132

Ryan JL et al (2007) Mechanisms of cancer-related fatigue. Oncologist 12:22–34

Savard J, Morin CM (2001) Insomnia in the context of cancer: a review of a neglected problem. J Clin Oncol 19:895–908

Savard J et al (2001) Prevalence, clinical characteristics, and risk factors for insomnia in the context of breast cancer. Sleep 24:583–590

Savard J et al (2005) Randomized study on the efficacy of cognitive-behavioral therapy for insomnia secondary to breast cancer, part I: Sleep and psychological effects. J Clin Oncol 23(25):6083–6096

Saykin AJ et al (2003) Mechanisms of chemotherapy-induced cognitive disorders: neuropsychological, pathophysiological, and neuroimaging perspectives. Semin Clin Neuropsychiatry 8:201–216

Schwartz S et al (1999) Insomnia and heart disease: a review of epidemiologic studies. J Psychosom Res 47:313–333

Selim MA (2001) Effect of pre-instruction on anxiety levels of patients undergoing magnetic resonance imaging examination. East Mediterr Health J 7:519–525

Sime AM, Libera MB (1985) Sensation information, self-instruction and responses to dental surgery. Res Nurs Health 8:41–47

Smedley B, Stith A, Nelson A (2003) Unequal treatment: confronting racial and ethnic disparities in healthcare. National Academic Press, Washington

Smith EM et al (2003) Assessing the independent contribution to quality of life from anxiety and depression in patients with advanced cancer. Palliat Med 17:509–513

Spiegel D (1996) Cancer and depression. Br. J Psychiatry Suppl 109-116

Spiegel D, Giese-Davis J (2003) Depression and cancer: mechanisms and disease progression. Biol Psychiatry 54:269–282

Spiegel D, Sephton S (2002) Re: night shift work, light at night, and risk of breast cancer. J Natl Cancer Inst 94:530–533

Staat K, Segatore M (2005) The phenomenon of chemobrain. Clin J Oncol Nurs 9:713–721

Stark DPH, House A (2000) Anxiety in cancer patients. Br J Cancer 83:1261–1267

Steginga S et al (1998) Domains of distress: the experience of breast cancer in Australia. Oncol Nurs Forum 25:1063–1070

Stiegelis HE et al (2004) Psychological functioning in cancer patients treated with radiotherapy. Patient Educ Couns 52:131–141

Suka M et al (2003) Persistent insomnia is a predictor of hypertension in Japanese male workers. J Occup Health 45:344–350

Tannock IF et al (2004) Cognitive impairment associated with chemotherapy for cancer: report of a workshop. J Clin Oncol 22:2233–2239

Walsh JK, Engelhardt CL (1999) The direct economic costs of insomnia in the United States for 1995. Sleep 22:S386–S393

Wang XS et al (2006) Longitudinal study of the relationship between chemoradiation therapy for non-small-cell lung cancer and patient symptoms. J Clin Oncol 24:4485–4491

Wefel JS et al (2004) 'Chemobrain' in breast carcinoma? A prologue. Cancer 101:466–475

Weiss MJ (2003) New insights into erythropoietin and epoetin alfa: mechanisms of action, target tissues, and clinical applications. Oncologist 8:18–29

Wells ME et al (1995) Reducing anxiety in newly diagnosed cancer patients: a pilot program. Cancer Pract 3:100–104

Welzel G, Fleckenstein K, Schaefer J, Hermann B, Kraus-Tiefenbacher U, Mai SK, Wenz F (2008) Memory function before and after whole brain radiotherapy in patients with and without brain metastases. Int J Radiat Oncol Biol Phys 72:1311–1318

Williams SA, Schreier AM (2004) The effect of education in managing side effects in women receiving chemotherapy for treatment of breast cancer. Oncol Nurs Forum 31:E16–E23

Wilson RW et al (2006) Pilot study of a self-administered stress management and exercise intervention during chemotherapy for cancer. Support Care Cancer 14:928–935

Zee P, Walsleben J (2004) Toward optimal health: the experts discuss sleep sufficiency and health. J Women's Health 13:764–769

Nursing

Sheila Judge Santacroce and Madelyn Rubin

Contents

S. J. Santacroce · M. Rubin (✉)
Yale University School of Nursing,
100 Church Street South PO, New Haven,
CT, Box 974006536-0740, USA
e-mail: Madelyn.Rubin@yale.edu

Abstract

Nursing is a discipline that comprises a sizeable number of the qualified health professionals who interact with survivors throughout the cancer continuum. Nurses can also exert great influence in alleviating the personal and societal burdens attributable to cancer through the integration of clinical care, education, and research. With increasing survival rates and the growing numbers of long-term survivors, the mild to life-threatening consequences of cancer treatment regimens have become more evident. Through systematic collaborative research, more associations are now known about the relationship between treatment exposures and late effects, thus highlighting the need for life-long follow-up care. Pediatric oncology nursing has established guidelines for risk-based monitoring and standardized survivorship education, allowing for the nursing care of adult cancer survivors to be built upon what has already been implemented in pediatrics. Nurses and nurse practitioners (NPs) are well equipped to play a key role in survivorship care plan (SCP) management, including the promotion of health behaviors, treatment adherence, and regular screening for prompt recognition of potential late effects.

1 Introduction

With approximately 12 million people living with a history of cancer, understanding and attending to the needs of cancer survivors is a major public health concern. According to the National Cancer Institute (NCI), National Coalition of Cancer Survivors, and the Lance Armstrong Foundation (LAF), individuals are cancer survivors from the day of diagnosis through the rest of their lives. Nursing, a discipline that comprises a sizeable number of the qualified health professionals who come in contact with survivors throughout the cancer continuum, can wield great influence in alleviating the personal and societal burdens

P. Rubin et al. (eds.), *ALERT – Adverse Late Effects of Cancer Treatment*, Medical Radiology. Radiation Oncology,
DOI: 10.1007/978-3-540-72314-1_18, © Springer-Verlag Berlin Heidelberg 2014

that are attributable to cancer and its treatment. The usual roles of nurses and nurse practitioners (NP) in clinical care, education, and research can be put into practice with diverse populations of adult cancer survivors using, as Rowland has suggested (Rowland 2005), the pediatric oncology experience as a model.

2 The Pediatric Oncology Experience

2.1 Treatment Advancements and Recognition of Late Effects

Foremost among advancements in the treatment and control of cancer are those that have been made in childhood cancer. Currently, 5-year survival is expected for roughly 80 % and 10-year survival is likely for about 75 % of children newly diagnosed with cancer (Rowland et al. 2004). As survival rates and the number of long-term survivors increased, mild to life-threatening persistent or late onset consequences of effective regimens became evident, and later, through systematic collaborative research, associations were made between treatment exposures and late effects. Early on, the late effects of radiation therapy were understood to be subtler in nature and later in onset than those of surgery and possibly chemotherapy, thus life-long follow-up of patients who received this therapy is required for early detection of late effects and to guide therapy to the minimum necessary to attain cure (D'Angio 1975).

2.2 Establishment of Late Effects Clinics

The necessity of "late effects clinics" that could provide methodical evaluation and treatment as indicated for the continuously expanding population of childhood cancer survivors was recognized in the early 1980s (Meadows 2006), and the first one was established in 1983 at The Children's Hospital of Philadelphia. Since then, the number of such clinics and the scope of their services have greatly expanded aided by nursing (Institute of Medicine 2006; Hobbie and Hollen 1993). At least 50 long-term follow-up (LTFU) programs for childhood cancer survivors exist in the United States (Childhood Cancer Guides 2007). Key qualities of these programs are shown in Table 1. The usual referral pattern is that a survivor is referred by the treatment team to an LTFU program at the treating institution when he or she is 3–5 years post-diagnosis and/or 2 years post-treatment completion with no evidence of active disease. Some childhood cancer survivors may have been lost to follow-up for many years and self-refer when life circumstances, for example, thinking about marriage and childbearing, bring concerns about late effects to the forefront. The children's oncology group (COG) Nursing Discipline and Late Effects Committee (Children's Oncology Group Nursing Discipline and Late Effects Committee Children's Oncology Group Nursing Discipline and Late Effects Committee 2007) have created a guide to develop comprehensive LTFU clinical programs. This guide can also steer development of LTFU programs for adult cancer survivors.

2.3 Clinical Care of Childhood Cancer Survivors

Clinical care of childhood cancer survivors includes attention to parental caregivers and indirect care of the population of survivors and the community through education advocacy (Hobbie and Hollen 1993). As with pediatrics in general (Rowland 2005), pediatric oncology nurses take development and function into account. Their nursing care is informed by: (a) knowledge about typical development and important functions for the various age-stage groups they encounter, including adults, (b) sensitivity to how development and function can be altered by the cancer experience, and (c) the design and application of nursing actions that aim to support favorable developmental and functional outcomes. Characteristically, pediatric oncology nurses conduct anticipatory guidance and monitor for potential difficulties with regards to physical, psychological, developmental, and social outcomes of childhood cancer and its treatment.

2.3.1 Long-Term Follow-up Guidelines for the Care of Childhood Cancer Survivors

Recognizing the importance of anticipation in limiting adverse outcomes, that is, late effects, the COG Nursing Discipline and Late Effects Committee collaborated to develop LTFU Guidelines for Survivors of Child, Adolescent, and Young Adult Cancers (Children's Oncology Group Nursing Discipline and Late Effects Committee 2009; Landier et al. 2004). These guidelines, which are organized by the therapeutic exposure, are derived from evidence about associations between exposures and late effects. They are then integrated with opinions from clinical experts to establish risk-based, exposure-related recommendations about monitoring for potential late effects. Most (88%) guidelines recommend minimal assessments that can be obtained via thorough history and physical examination (Landier et al. 2004). Further evaluation is performed as indicated for survivors with concerning screening results or signs and symptoms. To extend the impact of the clinical visits and standardize the health education and anticipatory guidance, the COG Nursing Discipline and Late Effects Committee also created *Health Links*, Health Links is

Table 1 Key qualities of long-term follow-up programs

Draws on a philosophy of care that attends to
The whole person
The effects of the cancer experience on the family
Wellness versus illness
Staffed by multidisciplinary team consisting of but not limited to
Nurse practitioner and physician with expertize in late effects
Nurse coordinator/case manager
Medical social worker
Services include
Medical record abstraction and treatment summary preparation
Risk-based screening of individuals for physiological and psychosocial late effects
Referrals to other providers for evaluation and treatment as clinically indicated
Care coordinator
Patient and family education about
cancer diagnosis and treatment, potential late effects
current health status including actual late effects
recommendations regarding risk-reduction and regular monitoring
Help obtaining insurance, and educational and vocational services
Opportunities for participation in survivorship research
Assistance with transitioning to another care setting
Tracking of survivors post-transition in case there is need to notify
Education of providers-in-training and non-oncology providers about late effects

comprised of, standardized patient and family educational materials on 33 topics including risk-reduction behaviors to help control potential late affects (Landier et al. 2004). This tool can empower childhood cancer survivors and their caregivers to take steps in daily life to control late effects. One concern about the COG guidelines is that, although they are based on evidence regarding associations between treatments and late effects, the efficacy of the recommended screenings suggested risk-reduction behaviors have not been well evaluated (Institute of Medicine 2006; Landier et al. 2004). Pediatric oncology health professionals nonetheless agree that is reasonable to recommend that survivors adopt behaviors that have been shown to reduce health risks in the general population.

2.4 Models of Care for Childhood Cancer Survivors

As LTFU for childhood cancer survivors has matured, four basic models of care have been developed especially for adolescent and young adult survivors: (a) pediatric oncology directed care within the general program or through a distinct but allied LTFU program, (b) transitional care that aims to assist with the shift to adult oncology or community-based care, (c) adult oncology care, and (d) community-based care by an adult primary care provider in consultation with the pediatric oncology treatment team or LTFU program (Bhatia and Meadows 2006). Additional models of LTFU have been developed based on the individual survivor's level of complexity of need for care/care coordination or risk for late effects. For example, a model of care that offers same-day, same-clinic access to multiple subspecialists has been developed for survivors with actual late effects or at highest risk for late effects based on treatment intensity (Carlson et al. 2008). In contrast, mail and telephone follow-up have been used with childhood cancer survivors who do not attend LTFU (Parkes et al. 2007), and has been proposed for use with childhood cancer survivors who are at low risk for late effects (Skinner et al. 2007).

2.5 Summary

To summarize, increasing rates of survival and numbers of childhood cancer survivors made late effects and the need for long-term follow-up apparent. Nursing care of childhood cancer survivors includes family caregivers, uses a developmental perspective and is anticipatory. Pediatric oncology nursing has played critical roles in establishing and carrying out LTFU including development of guidelines for risk-based monitoring and standardized health education. Despite the lack of evidence about the efficacy of screening, nursing care of adult survivors of adult cancer can rapidly advance by building on what has been done in pediatrics.

3 Nursing Roles in the Care of Adult Cancer Survivors

The implications for nurses and nurse practitioners in the realm of cancer survivorship care are plentiful. Nurses already play a key role in the application and delivery of treatment summaries and care plans. Additionally, the incorporation of holistic wellness promotion and disease prevention counseling is a natural part of the nursing scope of practice (Ganz et al. 2008). With the growing number of cancer survivors and the accompanying shortage of oncologists, the burden of cancer symptom management and supportive survivorship care is starting to fall on primary care providers and nurse practitioners (Potosky et al. 2011; Rowland and Ganz 2011). The 2006 IOM survivorship report acknowledged that survivorship care planning is congruent with the education and skill set of nurse practitioners and that they are very willing to assume the role, but that they are concerned about the continuously changing nature of cancer surveillance guidelines (Hewitt et al. 2007, p. 38). Primary care NPs and oncology NPs are well versed in routine health maintenance, and can help by advising cancer survivors on issues such as nutrition, exercise, weight management, mental health, smoking cessation, alcohol consumption and cancer screening. Furthermore, nurse practitioners are well suited to provide cancer survivorship care through the integration of clinical care, education and research. With the Affordable Care Act, combined with the growing number of cancer survivors and the increased need for medical providers, nurse practitioners will be assuming more roles and responsibilities, so their involvement in survivorship care planning is critical.

3.1 Clinical Care

Compared to pediatrics, clinical programs that address the needs of adult cancer survivors are emergent. Model clinical programs for adult survivors exist in a few academic centers and the development of eight of these, starting with a pilot at University of Pennsylvania have been supported in part by funding from the LIVESTRONG™ Survivorship Center of Excellence (COE) Network initiative of the LAF. This Network was created to focus attention on adult cancer survivors, its primary goal being to develop and disseminate best clinical practices. Each Network member is located at a (NCI)-designated comprehensive cancer center where it is responsible for coordinating the design, development, evaluation, and integration of programs that aim to meet the needs of cancer survivors into the range of services offered (Lance Armstrong Foundation 2008). Names and locations of Network member institutions and where to access more information about them are shown in Table 2. To address needs that have been largely unmet by conventional oncology or primary care, the focus of the Network to date has been those survivors who have completed therapy (Shapiro et al. 2009).

Three models of clinical care for adult cancer survivors are being tested by the Network (Shapiro et al. 2009), and the NP carries out key clinical care roles in each of them. In the first model, the "consult model", the survivor is seen once by an NP or physician with survivorship expertize. The visit typically includes universal screening for psychosocial late effects, treatment-specific clinical assessments (medical and family history, review of systems, physical examination, clinical laboratory evaluation, imaging and other studies) with referrals and other follow-up as clinically indicated. Following the visit, a form of the individualized *SCP* and results of any assessments are sent to the patient, referring primary care provider, and oncology treatment team. The goal is to empower survivors with information about their cancer treatment, their future health risks, and what can be done to manage those risks including healthy behaviors and regular health care. Responsibility for the care of the survivor remains with the oncology treatment team and/or primary care provider, who through the consultation are also educated about the survivor's treatment history and health risks and can apply the consultant's recommendations about regular monitoring. In the second model, the "ongoing care model", the oncology treatment team hands responsibility for the care of the survivor over to a survivorship nurse practitioner or physician, at an established point in time post-treatment completion. The patient is seen on a regular basis, usually annually, by the survivorship health professional for ongoing monitoring and education about survivorship issues. Communication is maintained between treatment teams and primary care providers. In the third model, the "integrated care model", survivorship care is provided by the oncology treatment team. An *SCP* is prepared when the patient completes treatment, and then discussed with the patient at a subsequent "survivorship" visit and annually thereafter by a treatment team NP. Responsibility for the care of the survivor remains with the treatment team in the short term. Patients who are at low risk for late onset versus persistent treatment effects can be identified and eventually transitioned to primary care with recommendations for regular screenings and ongoing communication between providers (Shapiro et al. 2009).

Table 2 LIVESTRONG™ survivorship center of excellence network members

Institution/Location	Web address
University of Pennsylvania (UPenn) Abramson Cancer Center Philadelphia PA	http://www.penncancer.org/cancerprograms_detail2.cfm?id=56
Dana Farber Cancer Institute (DFCI) Boston MA	www.dana-farber.org/pat/surviving
Fred Hutchinson Cancer Research Center (FHCRC) Seattle WA	http://www.fhcrc.org/patient/support/survivorship/
University of California at Los Angeles (UCLA) Jonsson Comprehensive Cancer Center Los Angeles CA	http://www.cancer.ucla.edu/Index.aspx?page=221
Memorial Sloan Kettering Cancer Center (MSKCC) New York NY	www.mskcc.org/mskcc/html/58022.cfm
Ohio State University (OSU) Comprehensive Cancer Center Columbus OH	http://www.jamesline.com/patientsandvisitors/survivorship/Pages/index.aspx
University of North Carolina (UNC) Lineberger Comprehensive Cancer Center Chapel Hill NC	http://cancer.med.unc.edu/patient/support/carolinawel
University of Colorado (UC) Comprehensive Cancer Center Denver CO	www.uccc.info/for-healthcare-professional/cancercenter/prevention/survivorship/uccc-livestrong.aspx

Although yet to be systematically evaluated through research, the integrated model of care for adults with cancer may have disadvantages that resemble those previously observed, in the care of childhood cancer survivors. Some of disadvantages could be that: (a) the needs of patients in active treatment are prioritized over survivors' typically non-urgent needs, and more so as the number of patients in active treatment continues to grow (Shulman 2009), (b) the main area of concern at treatment completion is disease recurrence and so when information about late effects is presented at the end of treatment survivorship visit, patients and family caregivers may not absorb it, (c) survivors can feel social pressure to express only gratitude for successful treatment completion, and therefore lack willingness to discuss negative aspects of their treatment with those who delivered it. Furthermore, as the literature expands, oncology nurses and other health professionals may find it challenging to keep up with innovations in treatments and growing knowledge about survivorship. The benefits of the integrated approach include increased opportunities for direct communication and collaboration among health professionals.

Nurse Practitioners who provide clinical care for survivors can examine the survivor's treatment summary to determine his or her cancer-related health risks, and thus offer an approach to clinical care. Survivors who are at low risk for late effects might participate in annual postal assessments apropos to health-related quality of life and risk-based interim history. Postal assessments are reviewed by the nurse or NP who then initiates clinical evaluation for the patients reporting concerning signs and symptoms. At the other end of the risk spectrum, the NP may do ongoing symptom management and care coordination for survivors whose actual or potential late effects are numerous or complex, for example, survivors who have been treated with cranial or mantle radiation.

The role of the nurse to date has been fairly constant across COE clinical programs. Ideally, following the IOM recommendations (Institute of Medicine 2006), a treatment summary is completed and distributed to the patient at the completion of therapy. Therefore, a role for nursing in the clinical care of cancer survivors within the realm of medical record review and abstraction is to create a treatment summary. Network members have created institution-specific treatment summary templates that are intended to be completed by an oncology health professional such as a nurse, and if at all possible may become part of the survivor's electronic medical record. Alternatively, "A Prescription for Living" (Haylock et al. 2007), is a generic template that any nurse or survivor can use to create an individualized treatment summary based on the official medical record or the survivor's personal records. Along these same lines, the Network is collaborating with University of Pennsylvania's OncoLink to expand its Web-based treatment summary and *Survivorship Care Plan (SCP)* (see Table 3), which is called OncoLife™ (Shapiro et al. 2009).

In creating the treatment summary, the nurse should address all of the essential elements including: the cancer diagnosis and date, treating oncologist(s), elements of the treatment regimen (type and date of any surgeries to control the cancer; chemotherapy agents, routes of administration, and total dose when indicated; radiation type, field, fractionation, and total dose; transplant type and date), major acute treatment effects including psychosocial difficulties, date of treatment completion, current health status including

Table 3 Sources for clinical practice guidelines related to adult cancer

Resource	Organization	Web address
"Putting evidence into practice"	Oncology Nursing Society (ONS)	http://www.ons.org/outcomes/
Clinical practice guidelines	American Society of Clinical Oncology (ASCO)	http://www.asco.org
Clinical practice guidelines	National Comprehensive Cancer Network (NCCN)	http://www.nccn.org

non-cancer related comorbid conditions, and persistent treatment effects and known late effects. Essential elements of the *SCP* include all of the components of the treatment summary plus recommendations about cancer and treatment-specific screenings, advice about lifestyle changes to optimize the survivor's health, and information about the availability of psychosocial resources and referrals (Institute of Medicine 2007).

Unlike pediatrics, widely accepted exposure driven evidence-based or consensus-based guidelines are not yet available to guide creation of the *SCP* for adult cancer survivors. Based on the need for consensus-based guidelines, work is in progress through the American Society of Clinical Oncology (ASCO) and the National Comprehensive Cancer Network (see Table 3), to standardize care and study its effects has been recognized (Earle 2007).

3.1.1 "Upstreaming" Survivorship

Aside from the initial diagnosis, the transition from active treatment can be the most frightening and warrants special attention to survivorship care planning (Institute of Medicine 2006; Campbell 2008). It is a time when "upstreaming" of nursing attention to survivorship must occur, just as conversations about palliative care should commence at diagnosis and not end-of-life (Ferrell et al. 2008). Toward this goal, several Network members led by MSKCC are conducting educational programs for their office practice and hospital-based oncology nurses in anticipation of stimulating a shift in thinking about the timing of nursing attention to survivorship. With today's treatment regimens, about 65 % of newly diagnosed adult patients overall will survive their cancer for 5 years or more. Thus, it is reasonable to encourage, beginning at diagnosis, a forward-looking perspective that allows attention to maintenance or development of behaviors that can optimize health and well-being during active treatment and survivorship. Consistent messages from nurses that convey a sense of hope for the future can be a source of comfort and focus during treatment (Thorne et al. 2008), and may enhance a patient's outcomes by reducing risks for late effects. Furthermore, helping patients and their family caregivers to maintain or increase healthy behaviors and lessen risky behaviors at "teachable moments" (Demark-Wahnefried et al. 2005) earlier in the cancer continuum may be more achievable than later on in survivorship.

3.1.2 Health Behaviors

Nursing care of cancer patients, survivors, and their family caregivers should include regular assessments of tobacco use and second-hand smoke exposure, alcohol consumption, lifestyle, weight, and diet (American Cancer Society 2008; Mayer et al. 2008). During active treatment, nurses can help patients avoid unhealthy weight and physical deconditioning that can complicate therapy in the short term and ultimately compromise survival. Nurses and NPs are in an ideal position to provide guidance and support concerning diet and physical activity, direction to established guidelines and, for patients who need them, referrals to nutritionists, dietitians, and physical therapists. They can also counsel patients on the importance of immunizations a regular health screenings.

3.1.3 Treatment Adherence

Treatment adherence is fundamental to survivorship. Nurses can expect that patients will experience difficulties achieving at least 95 % adherence, and should therefore conduct regular assessments using an understanding and hopeful approach (Williams 2001). Acknowledging that patients and their family caregivers are doing their best given the complexities of life while employing a non-judgmental approach to problem-solving is important to establish patient-provider relationships aimed to optimize adherence (Thorne et al. 2004). At diagnosis and on a regular basis, nurses should encourage patients and their family caregivers to discuss their understanding of the cancer and its prognosis, treatment goals, and beliefs about treatment efficacy, and to define their various roles and responsibilities in adherence (Malbasa et al. 2007). Nurses can also help patients establish acceptable and supportive roles for their family caregivers and other concerned individuals with regards to supporting adherence. Nurses can also help patients to access medications and other aspects of their treatment regimen, as well as help them develop reminders systems (Malbasa et al. 2007). Nurses should supply precise written information about treatment and copies of treatment calendars and instructions, and may consider providing regular reminders via cell phone and other electronic means (Puccio et al. 2006).

3.1.4 Symptoms and Symptom Clusters

Related to adherence, nurses should conduct regular assessments of symptoms and/or symptom clusters that can emerge as side effects of cancer and its treatment and that may compromise adherence. Symptom clusters are groupings of two or more symptoms that commonly occur together and may share causation (Barsevick 2007), an example being the cluster of pain, depression, and fatigue. Such symptom/symptom clusters can produce distress and impact key functions such as the ability to work or do activities of daily living across the cancer continuum.

Nurses should use widely available standardized measures to conduct symptom assessments. Kirkova and colleagues have identified 21 instruments that are available and appropriate for clinical assessment of specific symptoms or groups of symptoms that have been related to cancer and its treatment (Kirkova et al. 2006). Moreover, the Patient-Reported Outcomes Measurement Information System (PROMIS) Network is developing what will be a publicly available resource of standardized accurate and efficient measures of physical symptoms, emotional distress, physical function, and social function. This measure can be used to assess responses to medical treatment and supportive care across the cancer continuum (Monti et al. 2008). Symptoms including depression, anxiety, posttraumatic stress, sleep disturbances, fatigue, and pain have been shown to occur in family caregivers and may affect the caregiver's ability to provide key aspects of care (Garcia et al. 2007). Nurses can identify the patient's primary family caregivers, conduct regular assessments of caregiver symptoms, and encourage referral to a primary care and/or mental health provider as indicated.

Assessments can be used to target and also evaluate outcomes of nursing interventions aimed at symptom management. Nurses should apply or recommend evidence-based symptom management interventions when possible. The Oncology Nursing Society (ONS) has developed a set of evidence-based resources, "Putting Evidence into Practice (PEP)", intended for use by nurses, NPs, and nurse researchers in the evidence-based care of people with cancer and their families (see Table 3). The PEP resources include reference cards, definitions, integrated reviews and meta-analyses, existing guidelines and standards, tables of instruments for measuring intervention outcomes and references, summaries of key evidence and gaps in evidence, recommendations, and links to current research and other relevant resources. Extant evidence-based guidelines are directed at anxiety, caregiver strain and burden, constipation, depression, dyspnea, fatigue, functional status, lymphedema, mucositis, nausea and vomiting, pain, peripheral neuropathy, nutritional status, and sleep-wake disturbances.

3.1.5 Complementary and Alternative Medicine

In addition to conventional medicine, cancer patients and survivors can make use of complementary and alternative medicine (CAM) as a means to manage symptoms including pain, symptoms of premature menopause, and psychosocial symptoms such as anxiety and depression. The use of CAM seems particularly prevalent among ethnic and racial minority group members and those whose beliefs and practices lack correspondence with prevailing approaches to care (Fletcher et al. 2008). Nurses should increase their knowledge about CAM therapies, explicitly ask cancer patients and survivors and family caregivers about their use of CAM, particularly considering the potential for detrimental supplement-drug herbal and dietary supplement interactions, and also consider recommending CAM therapies. For example, mindfulness-based stress reduction, art therapy, and music therapy that have reasonable mechanisms of action, are safe and have been shown to improve symptoms (Monti et al 2008).

3.1.6 A Special Clinical Population: Adolescent-Young Adult Cancer Patients and Survivors

Adolescent and young adult (AYA) cancer patients and survivors are an at risk population that deserves particular attention from nursing. The NCI AYA Oncology Group has defined the AYA population as including 15–39 year olds (Monti et al. 2008), based on SEER data showing that people in this age group have not shared in improvements in cancer survival to the same extent as others (Adolescent and Young Adult Oncology Progress Review Group 2006). This lack of progress has been attributed to AYA having low rates of enrollment in clinical trials, wherein much of the improvement in outcomes for children is attributed to clinical trials (O'Leary et al. 2006), and also to usual developmental characteristics of AYA.

Characteristically, AYA perceive their selves to be immortal and unique, and therefore not susceptible to cancer-related health threats or the consequences of risky health behaviors such as lack of adherence to medical recommendations. With normative increases in cognitive abilities, a central task for AYAs is to become independent. In pursuing independence, AYAs can be wary of parental assistance with health care communications, health care decision-making and adherence to medical recommendations. Moreover, AYAs can lack regular primary care providers who might provide crucial guidance in these matters. As an age group, AYA have the highest rates of being under- or uninsured (Bleyer et al. 2006).

Development tasks for AYA also include establishing a career, a sense of self as a sexual being, and commitment to another person (Albritton and Eden 2007). Achievements in these areas can be impeded by the effects of cancer and its treatment such as fatigue, changes in physical appearance, altered cognitive and psychological function, and problems with sexual functioning. Existential issues may be particularly intense for AYA who typically can grasp the potentially fatal nature of cancer but can lack the expectancy of personal vulnerability to cancer, substantial experience with health care, and the social support that can help them form a cognitive schema for making sense of their situation (Rowland 1990).

Nurses should endeavor to develop age-appropriate clinical environments that allow AYA patients and survivors to interact with their age-peers, convey a sense of hope for the future, and provide assistance with navigating health care, payment for care and educational systems. Nurses should also support AYA enrollment in clinical trials by introducing the option and helping them locate suitable treatment and supportive care clinical trials through resources such as that available online through the NCI at http://www.cancer.gov/clinicaltrials/search or LAF at: http://www.livestrong.org/site/c.khLXK1PxHmF/b.4012249/. Nurses should also advocate for the development of clinical trials that target issues of salience to AYA.

Given their age-based heightened risk for depression and posttraumatic stress disorder (PTSD), nurses should regularly assess AYA patients and survivors for these conditions and make referrals as clinically indicated (Santacroce 2010). Nurses should also ask methodically about current academic, work, social, and sexual functioning. Additionally, Nurses should repeatedly assess the concerns and information needs of AYA patients and survivors and their capacity for information processing; these can vary across the illness trajectory and with developmental advancement.

Nurses should assume that AYA patients and survivors are neither secure in their health care communications nor that they will ask even the most burning that they may have questions. Nurses can assist AYA patients and survivors by bringing up usual areas of concern for the age group, such as concerns about fertility preservation, and by helping AYA identify and write down their questions in anticipation of communications with physicians. When parents are involved, nurses should assume that AYA and parental perspectives and questions will differ, given differences in their developmental characteristics and tasks, understandings of cancer, and life experiences (Santacroce 2008).

Nurses must determine, as early as feasible, to what extent the AYA wishes to involve their parents in their care and decision making. Nurses can help AYA see that parental involvement is often necessary, principally during treatment. Nurses can help parents by guiding them on how to continue to support their AYA child's development in the context of cancer. Having permission from the AYA, the nurse could give information to the patient first and then, to the extent specified, to parents and patient together (Palmer et al. 2007). Nursing interventions for AYA could include those that promote functional coping and favorable development. Interventions that aim to enhance social support seem to have great potential to enhance outcomes for AYA (Rowland 1990).

3.2 Education

Education of cancer patients, survivors, and family caregivers about the potential effects of cancer and its treatment, and what can be done to manage them, is a central element of oncology clinical care and thus addressed throughout the previous section. As the population of cancer patients and survivors continues to grow with diagnostic and treatment advances, it is increasingly apparent that the oncology workforce is insufficient to supply all cancer-related care. (Shulman et al. 2009) Oncology nurses and NP can help expand this workforce by enhancing their communications with primary care providers as a means to educate them about issues for cancer patients and survivors including potential late effects and promote their involvement in survivorship care.

3.2.1 Education for Referring Primary Care Providers

After acute cancer treatment and initial follow-up visits, the care of cancer survivor patients is often transitioned from the oncologist to a primary care provider (PCP), however, the role of the PCP in survivorship care is currently not well defined (Haylock et al. 2007). Recent research highlights that when oncologists gradually become less involved in survivorship care, the patient's cancer-related surveilance, including late effects, declines significantly (Snyder et al. 2008). This finding implicates the need for a survivorship care plan (SCP) that explicitly outlines pertinent medical information and guidelines for how PCPs and oncologists are going to coordinate the follow-up care. Rather than requiring PCPs to extract brief summaries of care from multiple sources and synthesize the information themselves, it is preferable for the oncology team to provide a comprehensive summary and plan to facilitate a smooth transition (Horning 2008; Del Giudice et al. 2009). To illustrate this point, the 2006 Institute of Medicine (IOM) report on 'Implementing Cancer Survivorship Care Planning' found that out of all ambulatory cancer care visits, most are with primary care providers, but noted that many PCPs do not feel adequately prepared for the task. However, the perceived ability to care for cancer survivors increases when PCPs are given some form of treatment summary or SCP from oncologists. Unfortunately they rarely do receive these, and the transfer of care is continually rated very poorly (Hewitt and Ganz 2007, p.11; Nissen et al. 2007).

After the diagnostic evaluation is completed, the oncology nurse/NP should assure that the patient's primary care provider receive information about the diagnosis and treatment plan, potential acute effects of cancer and its treatment, implications of the diagnosis for other family members for example when there is a known genetic basis for the cancer, and available supportive care services. The oncology nurse/NP should encourage cancer patients and their family caregivers to maintain the patient's relationship with his or her primary care provider during cancer therapy for routine health maintenance and ongoing management of co-existing conditions not under specialty care. When treatment is completed, the oncology nurse/NP should assure that the patient's *SCP* is made available to the primary care provider. For survivors who in time are discharged from oncology care, the oncology nurse/NP should initiate explicit referrals back to primary care providers for regular monitoring for potential late effects according to an updated *SCP*, with a request for ongoing communication about the patient's health status and referral back to oncology if problems arise. The oncology nurse/NP can also conduct continuing education sessions about survivorship that target primary care providers and spotlight their roles. Equipped with education and up-to-date information, primary care providers will be well positioned to make important contributions to the care of cancer patients and survivors.

3.2.2 Education for Nurses

Survivorship has long been a subspecialty area within pediatric oncology nursing (Hobbie and Hollen 1993), and the same may happen in oncology nursing as a whole, potentially limiting interactions and knowledge exchange between oncology nurses who specialize in different aspects of the cancer continuum. However, nursing expertise in cancer survivorship and the care of survivors should inform cancer patients, for example, of the value of health education throughout the cancer continuum. Along with educating patients, families and primary care providers, nurses who specialize in survivorship should regularly conduct educational sessions for nurses who care for cancer patients during active treatment. Such sessions could be required as part of a required orientation program for oncology nursing staff and also a regular topic in Nursing Grand Rounds or unit-based educational programs. Nurses with expertise in survivorship should regularly participate in patient care rounds and treatment decision-making conferences where they can raise implications for survivorship. Finally, nurse faculty with expertise in survivorship should champion the addition of survivorship didactic content and clinical experiences in the curriculum at the baccalaureate level as well in Master's and clinical doctorate programs that prepare primary care and oncology NPs, and for inclusion of survivorship content on state licensure and national certification examinations.

3.3 Research

The scope of survivorship research has recently been redefined by Aziz 2007 as that which aims to: (a) identify, examine, prevent, and control the adverse effects of cancer and its treatment; (b) define and examine the effects of guidelines for follow-up and methods of surveillance for all cancer survivors; (c) prevent, control, and treat co-morbid conditions; (d) offer health promotion and lifestyle interventions as potential means to optimize health after cancer treatment; (e) explore the effects of the cancer experience on the family; and (f) reduce disparities in cancer outcomes that may be attributable to factors such as age, ethnicity, and income (Grinyer 2003). Opportunities for nursing to contribute to survivorship research are abundant.

Within their workplace or through nursing and multidisciplinary professional groups, nurses can collaborate in or lead research that looks at the nature and prevalence of late effects of established therapies, and work in partnership with colleagues from other disciplines to review and summarize the literature toward the development of evidence-based practice guidelines, or at least evidence-informed consensus-based recommendations, for the management of late effects. Nurses can also use the resultant guidelines to standardize nursing practices concerning the care of cancer survivors and then collaborate with nursing and other colleagues to evaluate the outcomes, costs, and implications of applying the guidelines to large numbers of survivors. Nurses should also conduct research on the creation and psychometric evaluation of measures that can be used in practice and in research to comprehensively assess cancer patients and survivors for symptoms that may indicate the development of acute and long-term effects of innovative therapies, especially symptoms which are nurse-sensitive, that is, can be influenced by nursing actions. Additionally, nurses can conduct intervention research that aims to establish best nursing practices for managing the range of symptoms that people can develop across the cancer continuum. Nurses should also do research that examines feasibility and effectiveness of translating evidence-based interventions into oncology nursing education and practice.

No standardized or evidence-based model of survivorship care exists (Aziz 2007), although the need for research that examines and compares outcomes for various models of care by oncologists and primary care physician is generally accepted. However, current third-party payment structures and other forces can pressure oncologists to focus on patients who are in active treatment versus survivors (Shulman et al. 2009), and nursing, predominantly the NP, has grown to be the core discipline providing survivorship clinical care across the various models. Yet there has been no call from nursing to examine and compare outcomes for various models of nurse-delivered survivorship care nor is much known about the economic feasibility of NP-provided survivorship care compared to care by an oncologist or primary care physician. Nursing must take the lead in conducting survivorship research that has to do with the nature, outcomes, and financial feasibility of nursing models of care.

Supporting adherence to medical recommendations concerning cancer treatment, participation in regular follow-up and primary care, adoption and maintenance of healthy lifestyle behaviors, and the management of co-morbid conditions is a means through which nursing can contribute to beneficial outcomes for survivors. Yet, research about the assessment of adherence, development, and evaluation of nursing interventions that aim to promote adherence and systematic incorporation of evidence-based interventions into usual oncology practice and educational programs has not been a major focus in oncology nursing. Adherence has a been a focus of nursing research about people with other chronic conditions notably diabetes. Thus an area through which nursing can be a factor in survivorship research is through research on the aforesaid aspects of adherence, and this research should build on what has been learned through nursing research on adherence in other chronic illness populations.

Nursing as a discipline characterized by concern with whole individuals including their social circumstances, in which the family and family caregivers can occupy a central position. As previously discussed, symptoms are prevalent in family caregivers in response to the caregiver burden, and these symptoms may compromise the caregiver's ability to provide care and thus outcomes for cancer patients and survivors. Nurses should conduct research that describes caregiver symptoms and associations with cancer outcomes, and also develop and test interventions that are intended to improve outcomes for cancer patients and survivors by preventing the development of or controlling caregiver symptoms.

In addition to developing symptoms in response to their cancer experience, family caregivers may be at risk for developing malignancy based on shared factors including genetic endowment. Another focus for nursing research is the development and testing of behavioral interventions that aim to: assist with decision making around cancer genetic testing, sharing of genetic information and potential responses to that information, participation in screenings that can facilitate early detection of cancers that have been linked to a genetic mutation and other behaviors that can minimize family members' risks for malignancy.

Social circumstances also include factors that can affect finances, for example, work and insurance. Work and insurance are especially salient issues for young adult cancer patients who may not yet be established in their careers or working fulltime at jobs with benefits that include health insurance and/or disability insurance, and potentially have many work years ahead of them. Yet symptoms such as fatigue, pain, and neuro-cognitive impairments have the potential to compromise their ability to complete essential educational programs and/or engage in work that in quantity and quality allows them to achieve financial security and other gratifications (Rowland 1990). Additionally, family caregivers may have to cut back on work for pay or decline opportunities for education and/or career advancement and higher pay in order to provide care. Similarly, their work performance may be adversely affected by the burdens or symptoms that can be associated with providing care for cancer patients and survivors. Nurses should conduct research that seeks to: (a) identify factors such as work and insurance that can affect financial security across the cancer continuum for individuals who have been diagnosed with cancer as well as their family caregivers, (b) describes potential barriers and facilitators of work, insurance, and other factors that can affect financial security, and (c) develop and test interdisciplinary inventions that aim to support financial security.

4 Conclusion

Cancer survivors and their family caregivers are at risk for adverse outcomes that can be related to cancer or its treatment. Nurses and NPs who care for people and their families who have been diagnosed with cancer must cultivate awareness and sensitivity to the potential for adverse outcomes throughout the cancer continuum. Nurses can educate patients and health professionals about these risks, and encourage the adoption of health behaviors that can prevent or minimize the severity of adverse outcomes. They can also conduct regular assessments including screening for potential late effects, apply evidence-based interventions, and conduct/collaborate in survivorship research that aims to maximize health and function after the diagnosis of cancer.

References

Adolescent and Young Adult Oncology Progress Review Group (2006). Closing the gap: research and care imperatives for adolescents and young adults with cancer. NCI , Bethesda, pp 06–6067

Albritton K, Eden T (2007) Access to care before and during therapy. In: Bleyer A, Barr R (eds) Cancer in Adolesc and Young Adults. Springer, New York, pp 61–69

American Cancer Society (2008) Cancer facts and figures. http://www.cancer.org/docroot/STT/content/STT_1x_Cancer_Facts_and_Figures_2008.asp?from=fast. Accessed 17 Jan 2009

Aziz N (2007) Cancer survivorship research: State of knowledge, challenges and opportunities. Acta Oncol 46:417–432
Barsevick A (2007) The concept of symptom cluster. Semin Oncol Nurs 23:89–98
Bhatia S, Meadows A (2006) Long-term follow-up of childhood cancer survivors: Future directions for clinical care and research. Pediatr Blood Cancer 46:143–148
Bleyer A, Budd T, Montello M (2006) Adolescents and young adults with cancer: the scope of the problem and criticality of clinical trials. Cancer 107:1645–1655
Campbell M, Mayer D, Abernethy A, Carroll S (2008) Cancer survivorship. NC Med J. 69:322–324
Carlson C, Hobbie W, Brogna M, Ginsburg J (2008) A multidisciplinary model of care for childhood cancer survivors with complex medical needs. J Pediatr Oncol Nurs 25:7–13
Childhood Cancer Guides. (2007) Survivorship resource center: follow-up clinics. http://www.acor.org/ped-onc/treatment/surclinics.html. Accessed 17 Jan 2009
Children's Oncology Group Nursing Discipline and Late Effects Committee (2007) Establishing and enhancing services for childhood cancer survivors: long–term follow up program resource guide. http://www.survivorshipguidelines.org/pdf/LTFUResourceGuide.pdf. Accessed 17 Jan 2009
Children's Oncology Group Nursing Discipline and Late Effects Committee (2007) Children's oncology group long-term follow-up guidelines for survivors of childhood, Adolescent, and Young Adult Cancers V.2. http://www.survivorshipguidelines.org/pdf/LTFUGuidelines.pdf. Accessed 17 Jan 2009
D'Angio G (1975) Pediatric cancer in perspective: cure is not enough. Cancer 35:866–870
Del Giudice ME, Grunfeld E, Harvey BJ, Piliotis E, Verma S (2009) Primary care physicians'views of routine follow-up care of cancer survivors. J Clin Oncol 27(20):3338–3345
Demark-Wahnefried W, Aziz N, Rowland J et al (2005) Riding the crest of teachable moments: promoting long-term health after the diagnosis of cancer. J Clin Oncol 23:5814–5830
Earle C (2007) Cancer survivorship research and guidelines: Maybe the cart should be beside the horse. J Clin Oncol 25:3800–3801
Ferrell B, Paice J, Koczywas M (2008) New standards and implications for improving the quality of supportive oncology practice. J Clin Oncol 23:3824–3831
Fletcher B, Dodd M, Schumacher K, Miakowski C (2008) Symptom experience of family caregivers of patients with cancer. Oncol Nurs Forum 35:23–44
Ganz PA, Casillas J, Hahn EE (2008) Ensuring quality care for cancer survivors: implementing the survivorship care plan. Sem Oncol Nurs 24(3):208–217
Garcia S, Cella D, Lauser S et al (2007) Standardizing patient-reported outcomes assessment in cancer clinical trials: a patient-reported outcomes measurement information system initiative. J Clin Oncol 32:5106–5112
Grinyer A (2003) Young adults with cancer: parent interactions with health care providers. Eur J Cancer Care. 33:622–630
Haylock PJ, Mitchell SA, Cox T, Temple SV, Curtiss CP (2007) The cancer survivor's prescription for living. Am J Nurs 107(4): 58–70
Hewitt ME, Greenfield S, Stovall E (eds), National Research Council, Institute of Medicine(2006) From cancer patient to cancer survivor: lost in transition. TheNational Academies Press, Washington
Hewitt ME, Ganz P (eds), Institute of Medicine (2007) Implementing cancer survivorship care planning: workshop summary. National Academies Press, Washington
Hobbie W, Hollen P (1993) Pediatric nurse practitioners specializing with survivors of childhood cancer. J Pediatr Health Care. 7:24–30
Horning SJ (2008) Follow-up of adult cancer survivors: new paradigms for survivorship care planning.Hematol Oncol Clin N Am 22:201–210
Institute of Medicine (2006) From cancer patient to cancer survivor: lost in transition. National Academies Press, Washington
Institute of Medicine (2007) Implementing cancer survivorship care planning. The National Academies Press, Washington
Kirkova J, Davis M, Walsh D et al (2006) Cancer symptom assessment instruments: A systematic review. J Clin Oncol 24:1459–1473
Lance Armstrong Foundation (2008) Survivorship centers http://www.livestrong.org/site/c.khLXK1PxHmF/b.2661103/k.7D72/Survivorship_Centers.htm. Accessed 17 Jan 2009
Landier W, Bhatia S, Eshelman D et al (2004) Development of risk-based guidelines for pediatric cancer survivors: The Children's Oncology Group Long-Term Follow-up Guidelines from the Children's Oncology Group Late Effects Committee and Nursing Discipline. J Clin Oncol 22:4979–4990
Malbasa T, Kodish E, Santacroce S (2007) Adolescent adherence to oral therapy for leukemia: a focus group study. J Pediatr Oncol Nurs 24:139–151
Mayer D, Terrin N, Menon U et al (2008) Health behaviors in cancer survivors. Oncol Nurs Forum 34:643–651
Meadows A (2006) Pediatric cancer survivorship: research and clinical care. J Clin Oncol 24:5160–5165
Monti D, Sulfian M, Peterson C (2008) Potential role of mind-body therapies in cancer survivorship. Cancer 2008(112):2607–2616
Nissen MJ, Beran MS, Lee MW, Mehta SR, Pine DA, Swenson KK (2007) Views of primary care providers on follow-up care of cancer patients. Fam Med 39(7):477–482
O'Leary M, Barr R, Ries LAG (eds) (2006) Cancer epidemiology in older adolescents and young adults 15 to 29 years of age, including SEER incidence and survival: 1975–2000. NCI, Bethesda
Palmer S, Mitchell S, Thompson K (2007) Unmet needs among adolescent cancer patients: a pilot study. Palliat Support Care. 5:127–134
Parkes S, Jenkinson H, Griffiths A, Kinch D (2007) Mann. Is postal follow-up of childhood cancer survivors worthwhile? Pediatr Blood Cancer 50:80–84
Potosky AL, Han PKJ, Rowland J, Klabunde CN, Smith T, Aziz N, Earle C et al (2011) Differences between primary care physician' and oncologists' knowledge, attitudes and practices regarding the care of cancer survivors. J Gen Intern Med 26(12):1403–1410
Puccio J, Belzer M, Olson J et al (2006) The use of cell phone reminder calls for assisting HIV infected adolescents and young adults to adhere to highly active antiretroviral therapy: a pilot study. AIDS Patient Care STD 20:438–444
Rowland J (1990) Developmental stage and adaptation: adult model. In: Holland JC, Rowland JH (eds) Psycho-oncology. Oxford University Press, New York
Rowland J (2005) Looking forward: beyond cure: pediatric cancer as a model. J Pediatr Psychol 30:1–3
Rowland J, Mariotto A, Aziz N et al (2004) Cancer survivorship-United States, 1971–2001. Morbid Mortal 53:526–530
Rowland JH, Ganz PA (eds) (2011) Cancer survivorship plans: a paradigm shift in the delivery of quality cancer care (Ch. 8). In: Feuerstein M, Ganz P (eds) Health services for cancer survivors. Springer Science & Business Media, LLC, New York
Rubin M (2012) Cancer survivorship in primary care (Unpublished N757 Research Paper Assignment). Yale University School of Nursing, New Haven
Santacroce S (2008) Late effects case report: the young adult childhood cancer survivor with symptoms of posttraumatic stress. Oncol Nurs Ed 22:22–30
Santacroce S, Zebrack B (2010) Adolescent and Young Adult Patients. In J. Holland, W.S. Breitbart, P.B. Jacobsen, M.S. Lederberg, M.J.

Loscalzo, R. McCorkle (eds.), Psycho-Oncology, New York, Oxford University Press

Shapiro C, McCabe M, Syrjala K et al (2009) The LIVESTRONG™ Survivorship center of excellence network. J Cancer Surviv (in press)

Shulman L, Jacobs L, Greenfield S, et al. (2009) Cancer care and cancer survivorship in the US: Will we be able to care for these patients in the future? JOP 5(3):119–123

Skinner R, Wallace W, Levitt G (2007) Long-term follow-up of children treated for cancer: why is it necessary, by whom, where and how? Arch Dis Child 92:257–260

Snyder CF, Earle CC, Herbert RJ, Neville BA, Blackford AL, Frick KD (2008) Preventive care for colorectal cancer survivors: a 5-year longitudinal study. J Clin Oncol 26(7):1073–1079

Thorne S, Harris S, Mahoney K, Con A, McGuinness L (2004) The context of health communication in chronic illness. Patient Educ Counsel. 54:299–306

Thorne S, Hislop T, Armstrong E, Oglov V (2008) Cancer care communication: the power to harm and the power to heal. Patient Educ Couns 71:34–40

Williams A (2001) Adherence to HIV regimens: 10 vital lessons. Am J Nurs 10:37–44

Economic Consequences of Late Effects

Andre Konski

Contents

Abstract

Late effects of cancer treatment can have economic consequences on patients and their families. The reduction in employment opportunities is directly related to the type of cancer and treatment received. Patients undergoing combinations of surgery, chemotherapy and radiotherapy experience far greater employment opportunities when compared to those patients surviving after having only single modality therapy. Employment status also can be influenced by social support provided by governments with patient's living in countries with more liberal social support not feeling as much pressure when compared to patients living in countries with very little support. In addition to reduced employment potential, survivors with late effects of cancer therapy will also require additional treatment to treat the late effects thereby increasing the cost of care. This too is also dependent upon type of cancer and treatment received.

1 Introduction

The adverse effect of radiation (RT) on normal tissues has been well documented. What have not been highlighted are the economic consequences these late effects have on patients and families. The direct economic cost of RT-induced late effects includes the cost of treatment to repair damaged tissue and organs as well as to ameliorate the symptoms of damage. For late effects occurring early in life, such as in the pediatric population, these costs would accumulate for longer periods of time with potentially staggering economic consequences to society. There are also the indirect medical costs to consider in addition to the direct cost of medical care.

The cost of transportation to/from hospitals/physician-offices and the cost of child or elder care to attend these visits are but two of many examples of indirect medical cost. The impact to society in general is even harder to

A. Konski (✉)
Department of Radiation Oncology,
Wayne State University School of Medicine
Barbara Ann Karmanos Cancer Center,
Detroit, Michigan, USA
e-mail: a_konski@fccc.edu

P. Rubin et al. (eds.), *ALERT – Adverse Late Effects of Cancer Treatment*, Medical Radiology. Radiation Oncology,
DOI: 10.1007/978-3-540-72314-1_19,

© Springer-Verlag Berlin Heidelberg 2014

quantify. Lost wages or reductions in potential earning capacity in patients unable to fully work can be difficult to measure but have been found to be less in long-term breast cancer survivors as a result of reduced work effort (Chirikos et al. 2002). A number of studies have investigated the relationship between symptoms and productivity reductions in survivors of breast cancer. A 3.1 % reduction in productivity was reported by breast cancer survivors compared to a healthy worker; with fatigue and hot flashers accounting for productivity reductions of 1.6–2.2 %, respectively (Lavigne et al. 2008). Another study found breast cancer survivors finding return to work difficult not because of discrimination by employers or colleagues but because of sequelae of their disease and it's treatment (Molina Villaverde et al. 2008).

This chapter will review the available literature pertaining to the cost of treating complications or late effects of cancer and its therapy. It is important to quantify the cost of treating complications or late effects as it is only then can the true total cost of cancer treatment be known for certain. In addition, knowing the exact cost of late effects is required for cost-effectiveness analyses of therapies to prevent or treat late effects.

2 Employment Reduction

2.1 Breast Cancer Survivors

The ability to work after a diagnosis of breast cancer was investigated in a cohort of Korean breast cancer survivors who had been working prior to the diagnosis of breast cancer. Compared to a group of 20–60-year-old Korean women without breast or any type of cancer, employment rates decreased from 47.6 % pretreatment to 33.2 % posttreatment (Ahn et al. 2009). Fatigue and exhaustion were the most frequent difficulties encountered during occupational work. There was no mention other than mastectomy on treatment-related factors affecting the survivor's ability to return to work. In another study, radiotherapy, shorter time since surgery and endocrine therapy predicted daily activity and work limitations due to sequelae in an age-stratified random sample of 2000 Danish female breast cancer survivors (Peuckmann et al. 2009). Bradley et al. on the other hand reported women surviving breast cancer had a 10 % less chance of working compared to women without breast cancer, but those women who did work were found to work on average approximately 3 more hours per week compared to women who did not have cancer (Bradley et al. 2002). Similarly, Berg et al. explored the work engagement of employed tumor free patients, including breast cancer survivors, compared to matched controls. They found no differences in work engagement rates between cancer survivors and normal matched controls although cancer survivors reported significantly poorer work ability, poorer health status, greater numbers of disease symptoms, more anxiety, and reduced physical quality of life (Berg Gudbergsson et al. 2008). An analysis of long-term costs associated with breast cancer in a population of Canadian women from 3 Quebec cities revealed that costs occurred over a long time period and were not borne by just the patient but by the whole family with wage losses being one of the principal cost sources (Lauzier et al. 2005). In another study from Quebec, women between 18 and 59 who were working at the time of the breast cancer diagnosis between 1996 and 1997 were studied and compared to a randomly selected group of patients without breast cancer. It was reported 85% of breast cancer survivors who remained free of disease during the 3-year study period were absent from work for 4 weeks or more when compared to 18% of the healthy women (Drolet et al. 2005). After 3 years, there was no difference between the two groups in work absence, although women with breast cancer who recurred had more eventual absences. This would cause a disruption in any workplace with higher cost to replace the sick worker and lower productivity for the company as part-time employees are never as productive as compared to full-time employees.

2.2 Lung Cancer Survivors

The impact of lung cancer on working lives was studied with the aid of a postal survey in Britain. Two hundred and sixty-seven eligible patients returned a consent form and questionnaire, for a response rate of 50 %. The majority of respondents were women with breast cancer but 6 % of the respondents had lung cancer. 82 % of the respondents did return to work and treatment modality (absence of surgery), i.e patients who did not receive surgery had the longest sick leave, and length of sick-leave were the only significant factors related to return to work (Amir et al. 2007). Males were more likely than females to return to work, and not take sick leave, but they were more likely to take longer periods of absence when they did.

A diagnosis of lung cancer, as well as blood, liver, and brain cancer, as well as older age, company employee, and lower income were significant predictors of early job loss or delayed re-employment in a study of Korean patients diagnosed with cancer (Park J.H. et al. 2008).

2.3 Head and Neck Cancer Survivors

The quality of life of 36 patients with primary squamous cell carcinoma of the base of the tongue treated with primary radiotherapy was evaluated with a variety of quality of life instruments. The annual incomes of these 36 patients at the time of follow-up were similar to the income at the time of presentation (Harrison et al. 1997). The majority of patients achieved excellent functional status and quality of life and could maintain their pre-diagnosis earning potential. What was not clear from the report was how these patients were selected from all of the patients treated between 1981 and 1990. Patients surviving head and neck cancer were among the highest to report an adjusted risk of disability or quitting work, however, among 1,433 patients surviving cancer and interviewed 1–5 years after completing treatment (Short et al. 2005).

Employment in head and neck survivors was studied in The Netherlands where they found 83% of patients initially employed at the time of diagnosis returned to work. At a median of 6 months after completing therapy, the majority of patients returned to the same type of work while 7/53 to adapted work and 9/53 to other work (Verdonck-de Leeuw IM et al 2012). It was reported that anxiety, oral dysfunction, trismus, problems with teeth and loss of appetite were some of the symptoms significantly associated with employment after treatment. This would be particularly problematic in patients who use oral communication skills in their line of work.

2.4 Gastric Cancer

Employment status and work-related difficulties comparing stomach cancer survivors and the general population was studied in 408 gastric cancer survivors in Korea. A greater percentage of nonworking was found among gastric cancer survivors, 46.6 %, compared to the general population, 36.5 % (Lee et al. 2008). In addition, survivors reported more fatigue, had reduced working hours, and had reduced work-related ability compared to the general population. This is most likely a result of the extent of surgery and subsequent treatment that occurs in patients with stomach cancer.

3 Pediatric Cancer Survivors

Functional outcomes and life satisfaction in long-term survivors of pediatric sarcomas was assessed in 32 participants in National Cancer Institute clinical trials. Eight patients reported cancer had negatively impacted work while 17 reported that it negatively impacted their vocational paths (Gerber L.H. et al 2006). Full-time employment was also found to be below the natural norms in a survey of 1,437 children who survived cancer treated at St. Jude's Research Hospital (Crom et al. 2007). This cohort was compared to normative data in the Medical Expenditure Panel Survey and the U.S. Census Bureau's Current Population Surveys. Full-time employment was normal, however, among survivors of hematologic malignancies who did not receive radiation. Hays et al, however, found with the exception of survivors treated for CNS tumors, patients treated between 1945 and 1975 had few economic sequelae of cancer or its therapy that extended beyond the first decades after treatment (Hays et al 1992). Fifty-six of 60 long-term survivors of pediatric brain tumors, exclusive of craniopharyngiomas and pituitary tumors, were evaluated a mean of 10 (range: 5–16) years after diagnosis. 66 % had no or mild disability compatible with active life and employment (Lannering et al 1990). Eighty-nine survivors of Ewing's sarcoma family tumors were compared to 97 sibling controls with the cancer survivors to be less likely to be employed full-time (Odds ratio 0.4, $p<0.01$) (Novakovic et al 1997). Education, employment, insurance, and marital status were studied among 694 survivors of pediatric lower extremity bone tumors in a long-term follow-up study of the Childhood Cancer Survivor Study. When compared with siblings, patients who had undergone amputation had significant deficits in education, employment, and health insurance (Nagarajan et al 2003).

3.1 General Economic Effects of Cancer Therapy

In a study of 964 cancer survivors in Denmark, a trend was noted that male cancer survivors were less likely than other men without cancer to be currently employed and more likely to be retired as compared to men without cancer (25.2% vs 29.7%, $p=0.06$ (Norredam et al. 2009). In addition to having less of an ability to return to work after being successfully treated for cancer, cancer survivors may not receive needed medical care because of financial concerns. In a study of data from the US National Health Interview Survey (NHIS) from 2003 to 2006, 6602 adult cancer survivors were identified and compared to 104,364 individuals without cancer. Approximately 8% of cancer survivors did not receive medical care because of cost, 9.9% did not fill prescriptions, 11.3% did not receive medical care and 2.7% did not receive mental care (Weaver et al. 2010). Challenges in obtaining employment after a cancer diagnosis and treatment were also noted in a cohort of patients with Hodgkin Lymphoma as compared to siblings. Patients with >4 physician visits within 2 years, <10 years from diagnosis, or with permanent hair loss from treatment were more likely to report inability to change jobs due to fear of losing insurance and compared to siblings, survivors of Hodgkin Lymphoma were more likely to face challenges in obtaining employment and insurance (Chen et al. 2012).

Another potential for additional economic cost is the cost associated with care provided by caregivers. This cost is not usually calculated or collected during the majority of economic studies of cancer care because it is time consuming and difficult to collect but the economic impact can be substantial. Patients with complications from cancer treatment can require increased care from not only healthcare providers but can require care from family members that is not captured. The opportunity cost of this care can be substantial as the caregivers may not be able to work while giving care to family members. Cost of caregiver care was tabulated from a national survey of caregivers of cancer patients between 2003 and 2006. On average, caregivers provided care for 8.3 hours per day for 13.7 months (Yabroff and Kim 2009). The number of months and daily hours spent caregiving were the highest for cancer survivors diagnosed with distant disease when compared to survivors with regional or localized disease, $p<0.05$. Cost of informal caregiver time over the 2-year period after diagnosis was highest for caregivers of patients with lung and ovarian cancer and lowest for caregivers of patients with breast cancer (Yabroff and Kim 2009).

4 Long-Term Economic Consequences of Cancer

A review of the literature found a significant number of articles dealing with the complications of therapy, but relatively few articles dealing with the cost of complications of cancer therapy, either radiation therapy, chemotherapy or surgery. One can extrapolate and use simple assumptions that patients with complications incur more healthcare costs compared to patients without complications but these data are not published as of yet. The available literature is highlighted below.

4.1 Genitourinary Cancer

Healthcare costs of men receiving androgen deprivation therapy were analyzed in a cohort of 8,577 men with prostate cancer; 3,055 who had initiated androgen deprivation therapy. The mean unadjusted total cost of health care during the 36-month period was $48,350 per person for men receiving androgen deprivation compared to men not receiving androgen deprivation (Krupski et al. 2007). After controlling for differences in health status, the majority of excess cost was attributable to the androgen deprivation, with a minority of cost attributable to fractures. Another study found radiation therapy to be the highest cost of treating a skeletal-related event (SRE) followed by pathologic fracture and then surgery in a retrospective claims analysis of 342 patients with a diagnosis of prostate cancer and at least 2 subsequent claims with a diagnosis of bone metastasis and 1 SRE (Lage et al. 2008). There was no mention as to how many patients were receiving androgen deprivation but one has to assume the great majority of patients must have been receiving androgen deprivation, since this is the standard treatment for bone metastasis in patient with prostate cancer.

Extreme variation in the cost of continuing care of patients with prostate cancer was thought to be responsible for potentially unnecessary excess cost to the health care system in an analysis of >100,000 patients diagnosed with prostate cancer between 1992-2005 in the SEER-Medicare database (Skolarus et al. 2010). Office visits and the use of androgen deprivation comprised the most physician-related payments for prostate cancer survivorship care (Skolarus et al 2010).

The lifetime costs of treating bladder cancer and associated complications were studied via a model in 208 patients with bladder cancer registered at MD Anderson Cancer Center between 1991 and 1999. Although the majority of cost was associated with surveillance and treatment of the primary malignancy, 30 % was attributable to treatment of complications (Avritscher et al. 2006). Unfortunately, the authors did not separate complication cost by procedure or treatment that was responsible for it.

4.2 Head and Neck Cancer

Head and neck cancer treatment can cause considerable morbidity, especially if combined with cytotoxic chemotherapy resulting in higher cost due to increased rates of hospitalization, opioid use and a greater need for fluid and nutritional support (Murphy et al. 2007). Higher costs were found in patients with head and neck cancer receiving radiochemotherapy experiencing severe mucositis/pharyngitis compared to patients without severe mucositis/pharyngitis, $39,313 versus $20,798, $p = 0.007$ (Nonzee et al. 2008). The total increased incremental cost for patients with mucositis was $17,244. This study technically, however, did not investigate the cost of *late* complications as data were collected from the initiation of radiochemotherapy to 2 months afterward. Similar results were noted in a study of 204 patients with head and neck cancer treated with RT with or without chemotherapy. Oral mucositis was found to be associated with an incremental increase of cost ranging between $1,700 and $6,000 depending upon on the mucositis grade (Elting et al. 2007). Once again, cost of treatment was measured from the start of RT to 6 weeks from completion of treatment. In a more recent observation, an increased risk of cerebrovascular disease was noted in older patients treated with head and neck cancer treated with definitive radiation (Smith et al. 2008). Although complication costs were not calculated, it is intuitive that patients

Table 1 Cost associated with treatment, recurrence, and complications for patients with medicare insurance treated on RTOG 91–11

	Treatment related costs	No recurrence and no complication n = 7	No recurrence but with complication n = 27	Recurrence but no complication n = 6	Recurrence and complication n = 26
RT only	$11,662	$21,770	$37,577	$61,804	$92,050
Induction chemotherapy and radiation	$17,439	$36,045	$43,958	$38,453	$65,208
Concurrent chemoradiation	$12,433	n/a	$58,224	$42,581	$50,576

experiencing cerebrovascular complications will exhibit higher healthcare costs compared to patients not exhibiting these complications.

It is also intuitive, but has never been fully substantiated, that patients with recurrences and complications cost more to treat as compared to patients who do not recur or experience a complication. This hypothesis was tested using Medicare Part A and Part B costs for patients with Medicare insurance treated on Radiation Therapy Oncology Group (RTOG) protocol 91-11 (Konski 2007). This clinical trial investigated three different treatments for larynx preservation in patients with locally advanced laryngeal cancer. Only 66 of the 547 patients randomized to the protocol had Medicare insurance. Patients were classified as having a complications if they had experienced a $\geq$ Grade 3 complication. Table 1 shows the costs by category and by treatment arm. Patients with no recurrence but with a complication had higher mean costs compared to treatment-related costs with no recurrence or complication. The costs were the highest for patients who received radiation only having experienced a recurrence and a complication and second highest for patients experiencing a recurrence but no complication. Likewise, the costs were also highest for patients receiving induction chemotherapy and radiation who experienced a recurrence and a complication. These results need to be further confirmed in other patient groups and treatment types..

4.3 Anemia/Neutropenic-Related Costs

Anemia secondary to anti-neoplastic treatment including radiotherapy can adversely affect treatment efficacy as well as decrease a patient's quality of life. Treatment of the anemia includes red blood cell (RBC) transfusions and use of growth factors such as epoetin. Epoetin beta with concomitant IV iron in anemic patients with lymphoproliferative malignancies not receiving chemotherapy resulted in better outcomes at lower cost compared to epoetin beta without iron (Hedenus et al. 2008). RBC transfusion in an oncology unit was studied in 118 patients in Norway. The annual cost of transfusions was calculated at Euro 1,069 (Norum and Moen 2008). Anemia treatment costs, erythropoietin versus blood transfusion, were analyzed in 12 patients with cervical cancer. Treatment was given either before or during the cancer therapy. Average transfusion-related costs were $990, compared to the projected erythropoietin-related costs of $3,869 (Kavanagh et al. 2001).

The impact of anemia and its treatment on employee disability and medical costs was evaluated in patients receiving chemotherapy within 6 months of cancer diagnosis. The data were also linked to their employer's short-term disability records. Twenty-five percent of patients had chemotherapy-induced anemia. The presence of anemia and longer length of transfusion therapy were associated with increased expenditures (Berndt et al. 2005). Longer length of erythropoietin alpha use, however, was associated with lower expenditures. The incremental cost of anemia was US $5,538 per month for the first 6 months following cancer diagnosis, 10.8 % of which were costs related to short-term disability leave (Berndt et al. 2005). Costs of neutropenic complications secondary to chemotherapy was evaluated using a US healthcare claims database. Costs of neutropenia-related care were $12,397 higher for neutropenia versus comparison patients (Weycker et al. 2008). Cost of all subsequent neutropenia-related care averaged $6,594 (Weycker et al. 2008). Cost of neutropenic complications in women with metastatic breast cancer treated with chemotherapy was studied in a retrospective cohort design and a US healthcare claims data. Chemotherapy-induced neutropenic complications were experienced in 11% of subjects with cost for inpatient care (88% of patients with complications) averaging $12,869 US Dollars, while the cost for outpatient care was significantly less at $2030 US Dollars (Weycker et al. 2012).

4.4 Targeted Agents

Newer agents targeting specific areas of the cell have gained increasing use in cancer care. They normally have few side effects but some have specific toxicities. Certain targeted agents result in dermatologic toxicity. A recent analysis of 132 patients treated between 2005 and 2008 having a cancer treated with 1 molecularly targeted agent showed patients with a dermatologic toxicity had a median of 3 visits for management of the dermatologic toxicity with a median cost of $1,920 US Dollars. Sorafenib had the highest overall median cost per patient ($2,509 per patient) while imatinib had the lowest overall median cost per patient ($1,263 per patient) (Borovicka et al. 2011). Although small in cost relative to other more costly complications, this is just the start of use of these type of agents and more informations will be forthcoming as their use increases.

Another recent analysis evaluated the economic burden of the use of monoclonal antibodies, bevacizumab, cetuximab, panitumumab, associated with treatment of metastatic colorectal cancer. The highest inpatient cost per event was for treatment of GI perforation ($32,443 US Dollars), followed by fistula ($29,062 US Dollars), and wound-healing complications ($13,240 US Dollars) (Burudpakdee et al. 2012). Inpatient costs to treat hypomagnesemia and skin rash were the lowest with outpatient treatment for skin rash was among the least costly at $185 US Dollars (Burudpakdee et al. 2012).

5 Conclusion

The economic cost of late effects of cancer therapy include not only the cost of treatment the actual complication, such as diarrhea, perforation or neutropenia, but also includes lost productivity of not being able to work and caregiver costs. Unfortunately, the economic consequences of radiotherapy late effects have not been studied extensively to date. With the advent of healthcare reform, studies documenting the economic effect of all cancer therapies, including late effects, need to be performed to decide which treatments provide the most economic use of scarce healthcare dollars.

References

Ahn E, Cho J, Shin DW, Park BW, Ahn SH, Noh DY, Nam SJ, Lee ES, Yun YH (2009) Impact of breast cancer diagnosis and treatment on work-related life and factors affecting them. Breast Cancer Res Treat 116(3):609–616

Amir Z, Moran T, Walsh L, Iddenden R, Luker K (2007) Return to paid work after cancer: a British experience. J Cancer Surviv 1(2):129–136

Avritscher EB, Cooksley CD, Grossman HB, Sabichi AL, Hamblin L, Dinney CP et al (2006) Clinical model of lifetime cost of treating bladder cancer and associated complications. Urology 68(3):549–553

Berg Gudbergsson S, Fossa SD, Dahl AA (2008) Is cancer survivorship associated with reduced work engagement? A NOCWO study. J Cancer Surviv 2(3):159–168

Berndt E, Crown W, Kallich J, Long S, Song X, Lyman GH (2005) The impact of anaemia and its treatment on employee disability and medical costs. Pharmacoeconomics 23(2):183–192

Borovicka JH, Calahan C, Gandhi M et al (2011) Economic burden of dermatologic adverse events induced by molecularly targeted cancer agents. Arch Dermatol 147(12):1403–1409

Bradley CJ, Bednarek HL, Neumark D (2002) Breast cancer and women's labor supply. Health Serv Res 37(5):1309–1328

Burudpakdee C, Zhao Z et al (2012) Economic burden of toxicities associated with metastatic colorectal cancer treatment regimens containing monoclonal antibodies. J MedEcon 15(2):371–377

Chen AB, Feng Y, Neuberg D, Recklitis C, Diller LR, Mauch PN, Ng AK et al (2012) Employment and insurance in survivors of Hodgkin lymphoma and their siblings: a questionnaire study. Leuk Lymphoma 53(8):1474–1480

Chirikos TN, Russell-Jacobs A, Cantor AB (2002) Indirect economic effects of long-term breast cancer survival. Cancer Pract 10(5): 248–255

Crom DB, Lensing SY, Rai SN, Snider MA, Cash DK, Hudson MM (2007) Marriage, employment, and health insurance in adult survivors of childhood cancer. J Cancer Surviv 1(3):237–245

Drolet M, Maunsell E, Mondor M, Brisson C, Brisson J, Masse B, et al (2005) Work absence after breast cancer diagnosis: a population-based study. CMAJ 173(7):765–71

Elting LS, Cooksley CD, Chambers MS, Garden AS (2007) Risk, outcomes, and costs of radiation-induced oral mucositis among patients with head-and-neck malignancies. Int J Radiat Oncol Biol Phys 68(4):1110–1120

Gerber LH, Hoffman K, Chaudhry U, Augustine E, Parks R, Bernad M et al (2006) Functional outcomes and life satisfaction in long-term survivors of pediatric sarcomas. Arch Phys Med Rehabil 87(12):1611–1617

Harrison LB, Zelefsky MJ, Pfister DG, Carper E, Raben A, Kraus DH et al (1997) Detailed quality of life assessment in patients treated with primary radiotherapy for squamous cell cancer of the base of the tongue. Head Neck 19(3):169–175

Hays DM, Landsverk J, Sallan SE, Hewett KD, Patenaude AF, Schoonover D et al (1992) Educational, occupational, and insurance status of childhood cancer survivors in their fourth and fifth decades of life. J Clin Oncol 10(9):1397–1406

Hedenus M, Nasman P, Liwing J (2008) Economic evaluation in Sweden of epoetin beta with intravenous iron supplementation in anaemic patients with lymphoproliferative malignancies not receiving chemotherapy. J Clin Pharm Ther 33(4):365–374

Kavanagh BD, Fischer BAT, Segreti EM, Wheelock JB, Boardman C, Roseff SD et al (2001) Cost analysis of erythropoietin versus blood transfusions for cervical cancer patients receiving chemoradiotherapy. Int J Radiat Oncol Biol Phys 51(2):435–441

Konski A, Bhargavan M, Owen J et al (2007) The price of failure: economic analysis of recurrence and complicaitons of patients treated on RTOG 91-11. Oncology (Williston Park) 21(5 Suppl. 2):3

Krupski TL, Foley KA, Baser O, Long S, Macarios D, Litwin MS (2007) Health care cost associated with prostate cancer, androgen deprivation therapy and bone complications. J Urol 178(4 Pt 1): 1423–1428

Lage MJ, Barber BL, Harrison DJ, Jun S (2008) The cost of treating skeletal-related events in patients with prostate cancer. Am J Manag Care 14(5):317–322

Lannering B, Marky I, Lundberg A, Olsson E (1990) Long-term sequelae after pediatric brain tumors: their effect on disability and quality of life. Med Pediatr Oncol 18(4):304–310

Lauzier S, Maunsell E, De Koninck M, Drolet M, Hebert-Croteau N, Robert J (2005) Conceptualization and sources of costs from breast

cancer: findings from patient and caregiver focus groups. Psychooncology 14(5):351–360
Lavigne JE, Griggs JJ, Tu XM, Lerner DJ (2008) Hot flashes, fatigue, treatment exposures and work productivity in breast cancer survivors. J Cancer Surviv 2(4):296–302
Lee MK, Lee KM, Bae JM, Kim S, Kim YW, Ryu KW et al (2008) Employment status and work-related difficulties in stomach cancer survivors compared with the general population. Br J Cancer 98(4):708–715
Molina Villaverde R, Feliu Batlle J, Villalba Yllan A, Jimenez Gordo AM, Redondo Sanchez A, San Jose Valiente B et al (2008) Employment in a cohort of breast cancer patients. Occup Med 58(7):509–511
Murphy BA (2007) Clinical and economic consequences of mucositis induced bychemotherapy and/or radiation therapy. J Support Oncol 5(9 Suppl 4):13–21
Nagarajan R, Neglia JP, Clohisy DR, Yasui Y, Greenberg M, Hudson M et al (2003) Education, employment, insurance, and marital status among 694 survivors of pediatric lower extremity bone tumors: a report from the childhood cancer survivor study. Cancer 97(10):2554–2564
Nonzee NJ, Dandade NA, Markossian T, Agulnik M, Argiris A, Patel JD et al (2008) Evaluating the supportive care costs of severe radiochemotherapy-induced mucositis and pharyngitis: results from a Northwestern University Costs of Cancer Program pilot study with head and neck and nonsmall cell lung cancer patients who received care at a county hospital, a Veterans Administration hospital, or a comprehensive cancer care center. Cancer 113(6):1446–1452
Norredam M, Meara E, Landrum MB et al (2009) Financial status, employment, and insurance among older cancer survivors. J Gen Intern Med 24 Suppl 2:S438-45
Norum J, Moen MA (2008) Practice and costs of red blood cell (RBC) transfusion in an oncological unit. Anticancer Res 28(1B):459–464
Novakovic B, Fears TR, Horowitz ME, Tucker MA, Wexler LH (1997) Late effects of therapy in survivors of Ewing's sarcoma family tumors. J Pediatr Hematol Oncol 19(3):220–225
Park JH, Park EC, Kim SG, Lee SY et al (2008) Job loss and re-employment of cancer patients in Korean employees: a nationwide retrospective cohort study. J Clin Oncol 26(8):1302–1309
Peuckmann V, Ekholm O, Sjøgren P, Rasmussen NK, Christiansen P, Møller S, Groenvold M (2009) Health care utilisation and characteristics of long-term breast cancer survivors: Nationwide survey in Denmark. Eur J Cancer 45(4):625–633. doi: 10.1016/j.ejca.2008.09.027 (Epub 2008 Nov 25)
Short PF, Vasey JJ, Tunceli K (2005) Employment pathways in a large cohort of adult cancer survivors. Cancer 103(6):1292–1301
Skolarus TA, Zhang Y, Miller DC et al (2010) The economic burden of prostate cancer survivorship care. J Urol 184(2):532–538
Smith GL, Smith BD, Buchholz TA, Giordano SH, Garden AS, Woodward WA et al (2008) Cerebrovascular disease risk in older head and neck cancer patients after radiotherapy. J Clin Oncol 26(31):5119–5125
Verdonck-de Leeuw IM, Bleek WJ, Leemans CR, Bree R et al (2010) Employment and return to work in head and neck cancer survivors. Oral Oncol 46(1):56–60
Weaver KE, Rowland JH, Bellizzi KM, Aziz NM et al (2010) Forgoing medical care because of cost: assessing disparities in healthcare access among cancer survivors living in the United States. Cancer 116(14):3493–3504
Weycker D, Malin J, Edelsberg J, Glass A, Gokhale M, Oster G (2008) Cost of neutropenic complications of chemotherapy. Ann Oncol 19(3):454–460
Weycker D et al (2012) Risk and healthcare costs of chemotherapy-induced neutropenic complications in women with metastatic breast cancer. Chemotherapy 58(1):8–18.
Yabroff KR, Kim Y (2009) Time costs associated with informal caregiving for cancer survivors. Cancer 115(18 Suppl):4362–4373.

Radiological and Nuclear Terrorism: Relevance to the Radiation Oncology and Biology Communities

C. Norman Coleman, Nathaniel Hafer, Bert Maidment, Ronald Manning, Pat Prasanna, and Paul Okunieff

Contents

*Katherine Casey-Sawicki from University of Florida provided editorial assistance.Conflicts of interest-none.

C. N. Coleman (✉)
Department of Health and Human Services (HHS), Office of the Assistant Secretary for Preparedness and Response (ASPR), Washington, USA
e-mail: ccoleman@mail.nih.gov

C. N. Coleman · P. Prasanna
Division of Cancer Treatment and Diagnosis (DCTD)/Radiation Research Program (RRP), National Cancer Institute (NCI), Bethesda, USA

N. Hafer · B. Maidment
National Institutes of Health (NIH), National Institute of Allergy and Infectious Diseases (NIAID), Bethesda, USA

N. Hafer
The American Association for the Advancement of Science (AAAS) Science and Technology Policy Fellow, Washington, USA

R. Manning
ASPR, Biomedical Advanced Research and Development Authority (BARDA), Washington, USA

P. Okunieff
Department of Radiation Oncology, University of Florida Shands Cancer Center, Gainesville, USA

Abstract

There are now unique opportunities for research and community service for radiation experts based on a confluence of needs for reducing radiation toxicity for cancer care and preparing a medical response to a potential nuclear or radiological incident. The new opportunities include: (a) the need for agents (e.g., drugs, biologics, and natural products) to prevent and/or mitigate radiation injury; (b) the discovery and validation of biomarkers to predict radiation susceptibility and provide diagnostics for measuring dose (biodosimetry) and guiding clinical care; (c) basic research on mechanisms of radiation injury that are in common with other fields, such as inflammation, regenerative medicine, cancer, and aging; and (d) radiation biology research on mechanisms of radiation injury at the molecular, cellular, and organismal levels. The radiological/nuclear medical preparedness and response field is moving rapidly with a multipronged goal of ever-improving medical preparedness and response. This effort involves basic and translational science, device and medical countermeasure development, deployment of personnel and medical resources, access to up-to-date, just-in-time information for medical management, post-event recovery and resilience, and complex policy issues. The breadth of challenges provides an opportunity for a wide range of experts to participate. This chapter highlights the current state of the radiological/nuclear medical preparedness and response field. Given the rapidity with which research, development, and system solutions are

P. Rubin et al. (eds.), *ALERT – Adverse Late Effects of Cancer Treatment*, Medical Radiology. Radiation Oncology,
DOI: 10.1007/978-3-540-72314-1_20,
 © Springer-Verlag Berlin Heidelberg 2014

evolving, this chapter emphasizes where to find up-to-date information.

Abbreviations and Acronyms

AC	Assembly centers (predetermined site in RTR system)
AFRRI	Armed forces radiobiology research institute
ALC	Absolute lymphocyte count
ARS	Acute radiation syndrome
ASPR	Office of the Assistant Secretary for Preparedness and Response
BAA	Broad Agency announcement (BARDA)
BARDA	Biomedical Advanced Research and Development Authority (ASPR)
CBRN	Chemical, biological, radiological, nuclear
CDC	Centers for Disease Control and Prevention
CMCR	Centers for Medical Countermeasures against Radiation (NIAID)
CTCAE	Common toxicity criteria for adverse events
DARPA	Defense Advanced Research Products Agency
DEARE	Delayed effects of acute radiation exposure
DF	Dangerous fallout zone
DHS	Department of Homeland Security
DHHS	Department of Health and Human Services (also HHS)
DoD	Department of Defense
DOE	Department of Energy
DTPA	Diethylenetriaminepentaacetate
EPR	Electron paramagnetic resonance
FDA	Food and drug administration
FY	Fiscal year
GI	Gastrointestinal
GIS	Geographic information system
GLP	Good laboratory practice (required by FDA)
GMP	Good manufacturing practice (required by FDA)
Gy	Gray
HHS	Department of Health and Human Services
IAEA	International Atomic Energy Agency
IMAAC	Interagency Modeling and Atmospheric Advisory Center
LD	Light damage zone
LINAC	Linear accelerator
MC	Medical care sites (predetermined site in RTR system)
MCM	Medical countermeasures
MD	Moderate damage zone
MTA	Material threat assessment
MTD	Material threat determination
NIA	National Institute on Aging
NCI	National Cancer Institute
NHP	Non-human primate
NIAID	National Institute of Allergy and Infectious Diseases
NIH	National Institutes of Health
NSBRI	National Space Biomedical Research Institute
OPEO	Office of Preparedness and Emergency Operations
PAHPA	Pandemic and all-hazards preparedness act
PDA	Personal digital assistant
PHEMCE	Public Health Emergency Medical Countermeasures Enterprise
PRO-CTCAE	Patient related outcomes-common toxicity criteria for adverse events
R&D	Research and development
RCP	Radiation countermeasures program (NIAID)
RDD	Radiological dispersal device
REMM	Radiation emergency medical management
RERF	Radiation effects research foundation
RFA	Request for application
RFI	Request for information (BARDA)
RFP	Request for proposal (BARDA)
RITN	Radiation injury treatment network
RTR	Radiation triage, treatment and transport system
SALT	Sort, assess, life-saving intervention, treat/triage/transport
SBIR	Small business innovation research (grant)
SD	Severe damage zone
SNS	Strategic national stockpile (CDC)
SSN	Sources sought notice (BARDA)
TRL	Technology readiness level
WHO	World Health Organization

1 Introduction

The spectrum of a terrorist attack includes biological, chemical, and radiological/nuclear events. As the Cold War came to a close, the interest and investment in the consequences of a nuclear attack waned, although there was fortunately ongoing support for long-term epidemiological studies (Mettler et al. 2007; Preston et al. 2007, 2008; Ivanov et al. 2008; Little 2009). However, a National Cancer Institute (NCI) workshop in 2000 stimulated renewed interest in normal tissue injury (Stone et al. 2002) as new information was emerging from other fields, such as inflammatory response and imaging. Although limited, there was some ongoing investment at the Armed Forces Radiobiology Research Institute (AFRRI) in developing radiation protectors (Ledney and Elliott 2010) and biodosimetric assessment. The terrorist attack on September 11, 2001 and the recent growth in the number of actual and potential countries with nuclear weapons have lead to renewed interest and investment in nuclear and radiological terrorism response. The majority of the investment in terrorism response is in biological agents, but there is also solid interest in all-hazards response planning (PHEMC 2010), including natural and man-made disasters since there are response commonalities among all hazards and threats. Over the past 8 years, detailed planning for nuclear and radiological incidents has been undertaken, and there is now investment in the discovery and development of radiological/nuclear medical countermeasures and diagnostics. This work has been supported largely by a funding stream through NIAID (NIAID 2010) that is separate from the National Institutes of Health (NIH) budget. It is specifically dedicated to terrorism response and normal tissue medical countermeasure (called MCM) development.

This chapter highlights the preparedness and response challenges, the spectrum of programs for response to a nuclear detonation, and the relevance of these programs to the radiation oncology, biology, and physics communities. In that these are rapidly moving areas of research and development, this chapter will emphasize key references and websites where opportunities and progress can be followed. The components of the United States' overall response to radiological/nuclear threats include detection, interdiction, render safe, community planning, response, and resilience. Experts from the radiation oncology, biology, physics, hematology, and transplantation fields have the opportunity to be involved in these activities as part of their formal work or through volunteerism. The importance of such involvement is significant (Coleman and Parker 2009) since well-informed expertise must be available to local communities as well as to advisory groups to the federal, state, local, and tribal governments.

2 Preparedness and Planning

The Planning Guidance for Response to a Nuclear Detonation (Homeland Security Council 2010; Buddemeier and Dillion 2010) contains detailed information regarding the physical impact of a nuclear detonation using 10 kT as the example. There are five general damage zones that are considered for response:

- Severe Damage (SD) zone—close to the epicenter with extensive physical damage and radiation with few survivors likely, although people sheltered deep within some modern structures may survive.
- Moderate Damage (MD) zone—physical damage and some radiation, particularly where the dangerous fallout (DF) crosses the zone. Many people in this zone will be injured but salvageable.
- Light Damage (LD) zone—glass damage and car accidents but a limited number of serious injuries. It will have radiation only where the DF crosses this zone. Most victims will be ambulatory and few will have any radiation exposure.
- Dangerous Fallout (DF) zone—the exposure rate will be sufficiently high to potentially cause acute radiation syndrome (Homeland Security Council 2010; Waselenko et al. 2004; Fliedner 2006) in which a person may receive ~2 Gy or more from fallout. Sheltering in place is important for reducing dose. The footprint of the DF zone is determined by about 1–2 h and dose rate declines rapidly thereafter so that it becomes smaller (Homeland Security Council Interagency Policy Coordination Subcommittee for Preparedness and Response to Radiological and Nuclear Threats 2010).
- A Time Limited zone (Fig. 1)—zone above 10 mR/h where responders can work; however, the Incident Commander limits time based on protective action principles (Homeland Security Council 2010).

The medical response is a complex system that has two general components developed by the Office of Preparedness and Emergency Operations (OPEO) in the Office of the Assistant Secretary for Preparedness and Response (ASPR) (ASPR 2010) in the Department of Health and Human Services (HHS). One is the set of spontaneously forming sites at which people will congregate and/or victims may be found; the other is a set of predetermined response sites. This RTR system, which defines functional sites for Radiation TReatment, TRiage, and TRansport (Hrdina et al. 2009; Coleman et al. 2009), is not a medical triage system.

Figure 1 illustrates the five response zones and RTR sites (Homeland Security Council 2010; Buddemeier and Dillion 2010). RTR 1 sites have both physical damage and high radiation (will be near SD and MD zones); RTR 2 has limited or no damage and fallout (will be near DF zone); RTR 3 has limited or no damage, has no radiation, and is where people may spontaneously gather or be sent as the response gets organized (will be near LD zone and beyond). Medical care sites (MC) are predetermined sites that will include alternate care sites. Assembly centers (AC) are predetermined places where people without medical needs will be sent to assemble after the Shelter-in-Place period. Given the initial high exposure rate from fallout, sheltering

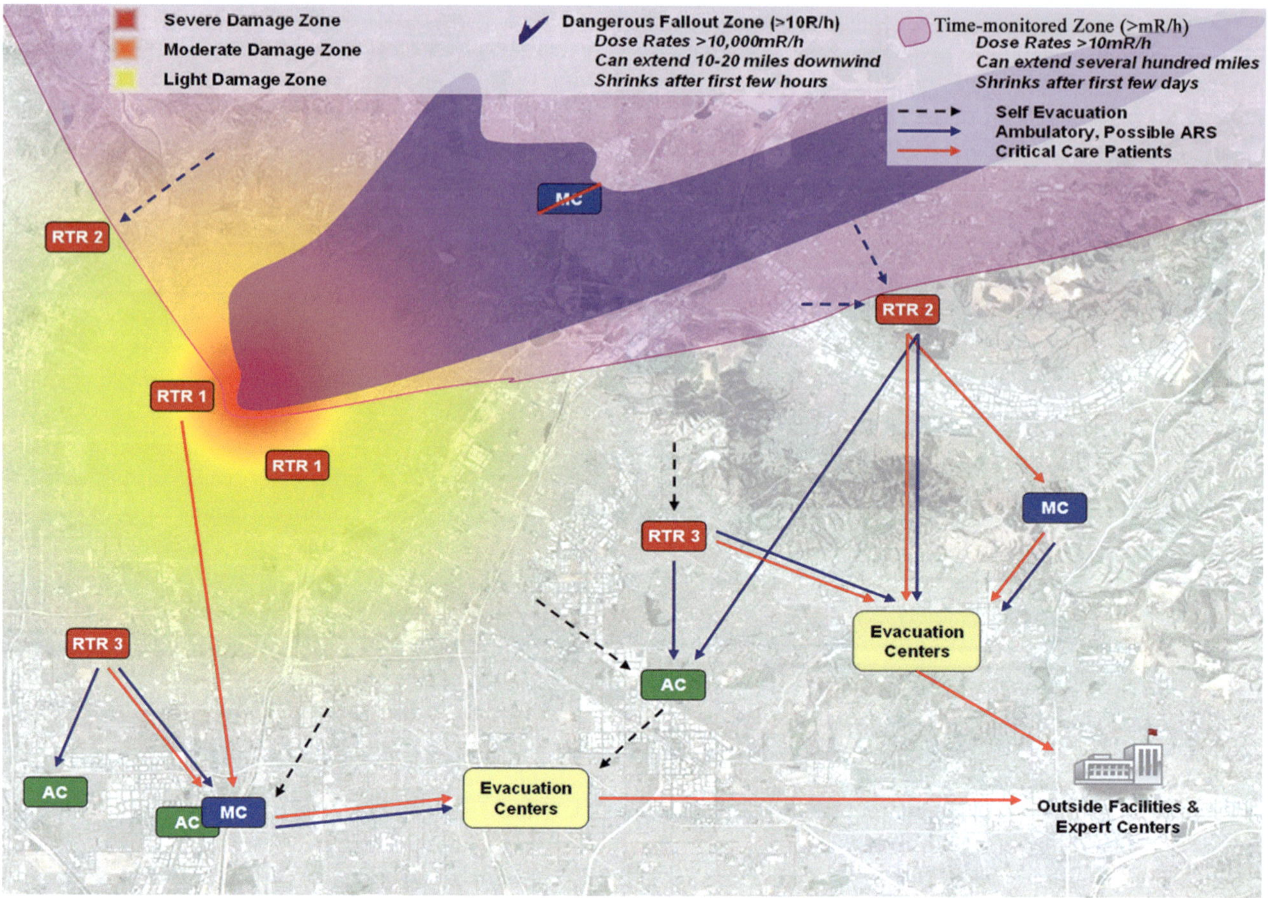

Fig. 1 Response zones and RTR medical system. The five physical damage zones are noted: severe, moderate, and light damage, dangerous fallout, and hot zone. The RTR sites are overlaid, RTR 1–3, medical care sites (MC), assembly centers (AC), evacuation centers, and outside facilities/expert centers (Homeland Security Council 2010; ASPR 2010)

in place is the default recommendation for 12–24 h as responders develop situational awareness. RTR 3 and AC differ in that AC are predetermined; whereas, RTR 3 will form during the event, although they may end up being used as ACs. HHS has advanced geographic information system (GIS) mapping capabilities by which to manage the event in the Med Map system (Homeland Security Council 2010).

Comprehensive medical management and triage are beyond the purpose and scope of this chapter and references are provided below. In addition to the Planning Guidance (Homeland Security Council Interagency Policy Coordination Subcommittee for Preparedness and Response to Radiological and Nuclear Threats 2010), another key reference tool is the Radiation Emergency Medical Management (REMM) website (Coleman et al. 2009), which can be downloaded to a computer or personal digital assistant (PDA). Some key underlying principles and useful references for medical management are presented below.

Radiation injury is often described as consisting of two general types—deterministic, in which the complication severity increases with dose, and stochastic, in which the probability of the complication increases with dose but the severity is not dose dependent. The deterministic injuries are often called Acute Radiation Syndrome (ARS) and include hematological, gastrointestinal, dermatological, and neurovascular effects (Coleman et al. 2009, 2003; Fliedner et al. 2009). The delayed effects of acute radiation exposure (DEARE) occur over time and include lung and kidney injury and soft tissue fibrosis (Homeland Security Council 2010; Coleman et al. 2009; Pellmar and Rockwell 2005) (See Table 1). While radiation injuries are often described as separate organ system injury with differential sensitivity, we now recognize that this is a multiorgan issue, for both diagnostic biomarkers and therapeutic interventions, in which all organs are responding to the radiation (Fliedner et al. 2009, 2009). The stochastic effect of concern is radiation-induced cancer (Suit et al. 2007) for which appropriate biomarker and surveillance studies will be needed. The spectrum of injuries will include one or more of the following: blast, burn, radiation, and secondary trauma (e.g., glass injury and car accidents). Medical management includes appropriate supportive care, specifically hematological growth factors, antibiotics, blood products, and other approaches often used in oncology

Table 1 Basic radiation medicine

Basic radiation medicine
Hematological syndrome (>2 Gy) Occurs after whole-body or substantial partial-body dose Shielding part of the body reduces impact Aggressive treatment can be life saving Death can occur within a few days at high doses but more commonly in 3–8 weeks
Gastrointestinal syndrome (5–10 Gy, although GI dysfunction occurs at lower doses) Occurs after whole-body or if only part of the abdomen is irradiated Can cause immediate symptoms If untreated death occurs in 3–10 days
Dermatological syndrome (5–6 Gy) From the prompt flash to exposed areas Beta-burns can occur from fallout Thermal burns may also occur from secondary fires
Pulmonary syndrome (5–10 Gy) Considered a delayed effect—can be months to years after exposure Occurs if part of the lung is irradiated
Central nervous system syndrome (>10 Gy) Complex brain and cardiovascular collapse Can be fatal immediately and within first few days
Combined injury = radiation plus trauma and/or burns Lowers the threshold for acute radiation syndrome Enhances likelihood of death—prompt intervention needed
Multiorgan dysfunction and failure All organs respond to radiation so that the “syndromes” above describe dominant cause of clinical syndrome Diagnostics such as biomarkers will be impacted by multiple organ changes
Phases Exposure may be followed by latent phase before full syndrome occurs Latent period can be days to weeks for acute radiation syndromes
Radiation medical countermeasures (MCM) Protectors—used before radiation (not likely of major use in nuclear event) Mitigators—used after exposure but before development of major dysfunction to reduce injury Treatment—used as syndrome is developing Internal contamination—issue for a radiological dispersal device but not a nuclear detonation.

(Waselenko et al. 2004; Fliedner 2006; REMM 2010; Fliedner et al. 2009a, 2009b; Dainiak et al. 2003; Koenig et al. 2005; Weinstock et al. 2008; Weisdorf et al. 2006; AFRRI 2009, 2008; REAC/TS 2010). The REMM provides detailed medical management algorithms for radiation injury (Homeland Security Council 2010).

Medical triage will be based on the physical injury and the best possible assessment for radiation dose. Given the size of the event and the limited number of emergency responders, it is expected that the vast majority of those who reach medical care will do so by self-evacuation. The estimation of possible exposure will come from the modeling of the incident by the Interagency Modeling Atmospheric and Advisory Center (IMAAC) (Homeland Security Council 2010), physical dose measurement of the area by responders, and a person’s symptoms. Evaluating the severity of and time to vomiting is helpful but unreliable for definitive triage (Demidenko et al. 2009) due to the possibility other causal factors. After initial sorting of victims, there will be assessment, life-saving intervention, and treatment/transport/triage using a variation of the SALT approach (Lerner et al. 2008). Clearly, a very complex and rapidly changing scarce resources situation will exist (AHRQ 2007). A critical component of medical response is reassessment, especially as conditions change in that someone triaged to receive palliative care only may be changed to aggressive management as resource setting improves. A detailed discussion of triage, medical management in a scarce resources setting, crisis standards of care (IOM 2009), ethical considerations, the importance of serial reassessment (Homeland Security Council 2010), and the need for the Radiation Injury Treatment Network (RITN) (Davids et al. 2010) are in a recent issue of *Disaster Med* (Coleman et al. 2011).

The radiation oncology and biology communities, the National Institutes of Health (NCI and NIAID), AFRRI, and the Radiation Research and Health Physics Societies have responded to the challenge of nuclear terrorism by bringing together the research communities to help determine the preparedness and response and develop research plans (Coleman et al. 2001, 2003; Pellmar and Rockwell 2005; Stone et al. 2004; Augustine et al. 2005; Williams et al. 2010). Aspects of these programs are described below. A recent effort has begun to explore the possibility of using the medical countermeasures developed for normal tissue mitigation for terrorism response for clinical cancer care (Mosvas et al. 2010).

3 Biodosimetry

Using biological methods to assess the dose received by an individual is essential when physical dosimetry is lacking, particularly in a radiation mass casualty setting. Even when there is a physical estimate of exposure, laboratory confirmation is necessary for medical management. Hematological analysis, particularly absolute lymphocyte count (ALC) and the change in ALC over time, are important indicators and this may be sufficient information for managing the higher-radiation dose ranges. In general, the initial goal is to sort or “bin” people with potential exposure to radiation into three bins: (a) <2 Gray (Gy) where no intervention is needed (except in the presence of combined injury); (b) 2–4 Gy where observation and potential treatment for ARS is needed over the next few weeks; and (c) >4 Gy where immediate medical management is needed. A fourth cut off of >8–10 Gy would likely be used to triage a victim into the expectant category (Lerner et al. 2008). The use of hematological growth factors is appropriate only at doses of >2 Gy (and for serious combined injury).

While crude assessment of absorbed dose can be made from the clinical signs and symptoms, such as skin responses (erythema) and peripheral blood cell counts, uncertainties in these dose predictions are quite large because of variability among individuals, potential presence of infection or trauma, and comorbid medical illnesses. Methods are needed to help assess the stochastic risk of radiation-induced cancer to determine who might require long-term follow-up. At present, cytogenetic-based methods are widely used to measure radiation dose and occupy a unique niche in biological dosimetry. Several molecular biomarker and biophysical dosimetric approaches are also rapidly evolving, as noted below.

Radiation induces many types of chromosomal aberrations in an exposed individual's peripheral blood lymphocytes. Due to their radiation specificity, the presence of dicentrics, a common structural aberration, indicates radiation exposure and provides an excellent measure of absorbed dose. It shows a very low background level, low interindividual variation, and good dose-frequency relationship. Exposure of lymphocytes in vitro or in vivo produces similar levels of dicentrics per Gy; therefore, dose can be predicted from observed dicentric yield in an exposed subject's peripheral blood lymphocytes by comparison with a suitable in vitro generated calibration curve. The assay is also useful in determining full- versus partial-body exposures (International Atomic Energy Agency 2001).

Biological dosimetry using dicentrics following an accidental overexposure has been used since the 1962 Recuplex criticality accident at Hanford (Bennder and Gooch 1966), as well as several other radiation accidents involving mass casualties. Estimated doses using cytogenetic methods correlated well with the severity of ARS (Sevankaev 2000). Several countries have established laboratories for chromosome aberration-based biological dosimetry. In addition, harmonized technical manuals (Williams et al. 2010) and laboratory accreditation standards are now available (ISO 2004). Recently, an interlaboratory comparison study further validated the assay by determining variability and accuracy among five laboratories (Wilkins et al. 2008).

Referral guidance for cytogenetic biodosimetry for determining who may need subsequent treatment or surveillance is based on the person's location from knowledge of physical dosimetry, onset of prodromal signs and symptoms, and lymphocyte depletion kinetics. Small volumes of peripheral blood are collected from exposed subjects and sent to a cytogenetic laboratory where the peripheral blood lymphocytes are grown in cultures to harvest cells in metaphase, and the frequency of dicentrics is estimated by analysis of 500–1,000 metaphases for dose prediction by comparison with a calibration curve. However, in order to rapidly diagnosis- or bin- who may be at risk for ARS, rapid and preliminary dose estimation for triage may be needed for scores of 20–50 metaphases per subject. For example, in the Chernobyl accident, an approximate dosimetry was achieved by a preliminary examination of 50 metaphases per person for several individuals (Pyatkin et al. 1989).

Frequency of metaphase spreads without dicentric aberrations and distribution of dicentrics among metaphase spreads can help determine whether exposure is uniform, whole-body, or partial-body and help identify patients' appropriate treatments (Lloyd 1997). Radiation exposures from accidents or terrorist incidents are likely to be partial-body from the prompt radiation (the initial blast) but relatively homogenous for fallout radiation. Recently, a model for triage dose prediction in radiation mass casualties, which is based on determination of equivalent whole-body doses under partial-body exposure conditions, has been proposed (Prasanna et al. 2010). According to the model, an initial screening of metaphases can confirm radiation exposure above 2 Gy and analysis of 50 metaphases will allow risk-based stratification of the exposed cohort.

However, cytogenetic biodosimetry is labor-intensive, time-consuming, and expertise-driven. Therefore, automation of sample preparation analysis is essential to improve throughput for mass casualty events. In addition, laboratory automation improves quality control and assurance. Use of robotic instruments, as well as laboratory information management systems to address data management and sample-tracking, is being established (Martin et al. 2007). National and international cooperative cytogenetic networks are already established to increase throughput in radiation mass casualties (Wilkins et al. 2008; Miller et al. 2007).

Exposure to radiation induces stable radicals in teeth and fingernails. These changes are highly reliable and electron paramagnetic resonance (EPR) analysis can provide useful information for retrospective dose reconstruction (IAEA 2002). The EPR technology may provide rapid capability for dose assessment in mass casualties (Trompier et al. 2007); however, complete mapping of partial-body exposures may not be possible. Currently, bulky instrumentation requires miniaturization.

Alternative biomarkers of DNA damage may be assessed relatively quickly and easily compared to traditional cytogenetic tools providing clinically useful information. Examples of potential alternative methods include: (a) gamma-H2AX assay (Dicky et al. 2009); (b) measurement of micronuclei along with other damage in cytokinesis-blocked binucleated cells (Fenech 2007); and (c) a rapid interphase chromosome assay (RICA), which measures damage to specific chromosomes in interphase cells by fluorescence in situ hybridization after premature chromosomal condensation by mitosis promotion and phosphatase

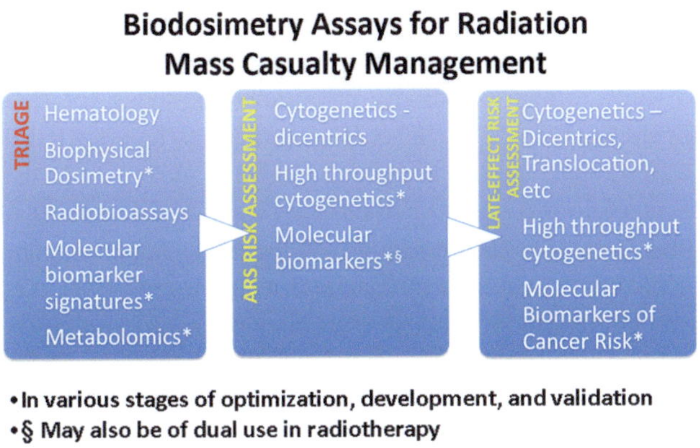

Fig. 2 Biodosimetry and radiobioassay for medical management. The current techniques available include hematology, dicentric-cytogenetic assay, and radio bioassay for some of the radionuclides. There is limited laboratory capacity such that a Radiation Laboratory Network (Rad-LN) has been proposed. Newer approaches include automation of current techniques and novel markers

inhibition (Prasanna et al. 2000). Early gene expression changes, proteomics, metabolomics, and organ-specific biomarkers may also be useful in the near future (Zhang et al. 2009).

Any single assay may not be able to address dose assessment needs in all radiation exposure scenarios, which can be often complex. Therefore, when multiple assays are involved, a multiparameter, comprehensive, and integrated approach for predicting dose is essential (Fig. 2). Some of these approaches to estimate dose are available on REMM (REMM 2010). In a mass casualty event there will be two sets of screens; assays that produce risk assessment for significant radiation exposures (i.e., binning) would be followed by systems that produce a reliable actual physical dose. Because some casualties will have combined injuries, including some degree of trauma, and since combined injuries greatly alter the need for triage for even low-dose whole-body exposures, the first screen should be sensitive to prognosis rather than just radiation dose. Triage will be done based on standard medical triage (trauma, burns, and level of consciousness), radiation-alone triage (dose), and some estimate of the adverse impact of combined injury. When exposure is not homogeneous, the specification of the dose is not possible. For example, individuals with ingestion or inhalation exposures from a Radiological Dispersal Device (RDD), or those partially shielded from prompt radiation by physical structures like cars and walls, will have some marrow protection. The partial-marrow protection will lead to a much greater tolerance to whole-body exposure. Here again, it will be important to have a first screen that determines both medical risk as well as a secondary accurate measure of radiation dose. Medical management will be guided by dose; nevertheless, since the actual patient's clinical progression and organ dysfunction are the most critical issues, physicians with experience in oncology care are necessary.

Additional information is available on multiparameter triage (Blakely et al. 2010; Ossetrova and Blakely 2009; Ossetrova et al. 2010), partial-body exposure (Prasanna et al. 2010), the establishment of laboratory networks (Blakely et al. 2009; Ainsbury et al. 2009), and the criteria for rapid techniques (Grace et al. 2010).

4 Medical Countermeasures Against Radiological and Nuclear Threats- NIAID

Safeguarding people against the threat of nuclear or radiological agents is not only a priority for U.S. national security but also a major public health concern. Should mass exposure to these hazards occur, medical countermeasures that prevent or repair tissue damage will need to be widely available. Because it is unlikely that people will have advanced warning, and it will take time to muster the response, these countermeasures must be effective when given days after radiation exposure. Healthcare providers must be equipped to treat both the acute and long-term effects of radiation damage. However, there are currently no licensed medical products to mitigate or treat the injuries that can result from a nuclear or radiological accident or attack.

The Secretary of the HHS, through the Project BioShield Act of 2004 (Project Bioshield 2010), directed NIAID to develop a strategic plan and research agenda to guide all NIH activities contributing to the development of medical countermeasures against radiological and nuclear threats. The final document, *The National Institutes of Health (NIH) Strategic Plan and Research Agenda for Medical Countermeasures Against Radiological and Nuclear Threats*, was published in June 2005 and describes NIAID's priorities in this area (NIH 2005). Over the past 5 years, the radiation countermeasures program (RCP) has made significant progress toward the goals described within the Strategic Plan, and this section highlights the recent activities supported by the RCP. Current information can be found on RCP's website (NIAID 2010).

The RCP is primarily focused on developing mitigators and treatments for ARS and DEARE, developing biodosimetric tools that can rapidly assess the dose of radiation absorbed by a person post-exposure and also decorporation agents that can speed the removal of internalized radionuclides from the body (Ramakrishnan 2009; Cassatt et al. 2010). Since the type and severity of radiation injury can vary greatly due to the nature of the exposure, ARS/DEARE does not represent a single pathological condition, but rather describes a variety of syndromes affecting the hematopoietic system, gastrointestinal system, lungs, kidneys, skin, and central nervous system (Table 1). Broad classes of compounds that might enhance repair of radiation-induced damage and increase survival include growth factors, cell-signaling molecules, antioxidants, anti-apoptotics, anti-inflammatory agents, and antibiotics. A number of studies in the literature demonstrate that radiation combined with other trauma (such as a burn or wound) significantly alters the course of tissue recovery and survival (Ledney and Elliott 2010; DiCarlo et al. 2008). It is also important to consider that survivors of acute radiation exposure are at risk to develop a variety of late effects, such as cataracts, cardiovascular disease, tissue fibrosis, and cancer. Biodosimetry must accurately assess the amount of radiation received by an individual and must be useful during a mass casualty event. Thus, the signal for a putative biomarker must persist long enough to be measured and must be robust enough to be detected in a population with a great amount of genetic diversity and variability in underlying health status. Decorporation agents, useful for a RDD but not a nuclear detonation, must be developed for a variety of radionuclides that constitute a realistic threat, and each has a unique pharmacokinetic and target organ injury profile (Cassatt et al. 2008; Hafer 2009a, b).

Given that a sizable and diverse group of people may need treatment after a large-scale radiological or nuclear incident, products that address these three scientific needs must also be easily administered to large numbers of people, including special populations (e.g., children, pregnant women, the elderly and immuno-compromised people). It is also likely that Federal Government resources will not be immediately available after a major incident, so medical products and regimens must be effective even when they are administered at least 24 h after radiation exposure. The RCP products must meet all these requirements; consequently, decisions on which candidate product to advance are based on the ability of the product to meet these priority needs.

Research programs. The RCP supports research and product development through a number of funding mechanisms and flexible approaches. Research is supported through grants for basic, translational, and small business research programs. The primary grant program is the Centers for Medical Countermeasures against Radiation (CMCRs). Awarded for the first time in 2005, the eight CMCRs operate under a cooperative agreement and serve as an early stage research and discovery engine for the program. The CMCR accomplishments over the past 5 years, detailed in the next section, include the publication of nearly 200 papers and the submission of over 20 patents. Rodent, canine, non-human primate (NHP), and knockout models of radiation injury have been developed and more than 100 MCMs are currently under various stages of development to mitigate/treat radiation injuries. Several investigators are developing portable and automated biodosimeters with promising results. The CMCRs have reinvigorated the field of normal tissue radiobiology by developing educational tools, recruiting new investigators to study radiation biology, and providing funds for pilot research projects. The CMCR program was recompeted in 2010 and will be supported for another 5 years.

In addition to the CMCRs, the RCP supports a number of grant programs focused on topics including radiation combined injury, immune reconstitution, gastrointestinal (GI) injury, radiation-induced thrombocytopenia, radiation-induced lung injury, cutaneous radiation syndrome, understanding the mechanism of radiation injury, and novel decorporation agents. These programs to date have funded nearly 60 individual projects. To help provide funding opportunities for small businesses, a focused radiation/nuclear medical countermeasures small business innovation research (SBIR) grant program was initiated in 2009 with expanded funding limits and timelines compared to traditional SBIR awards. These are more attractive to small industry and enable companies to achieve more significant progress and results. The success of the CMCR and grant programs sponsored by NIAID is demonstrated by the fact that multiple RCP awardees have gone on to win additional funds from the Biomedical Advanced Research and Development Authority (BARDA) (BARDA 2010) and the Department of Defense (DoD) to support the advanced development of radiation countermeasures.

Early stage product development. In addition to sponsoring research, the RCP is also responsible for the early stage product development of radiation medical countermeasures. In order to operate efficiently and reduce the risk and cost to the Federal Government, the RCP has developed a product development support services contract to perform product development tasks for specific MCM candidates in partnership with industry. To achieve these goals, in 2005 NIAID awarded a contract to the University of Maryland School of Medicine for these services (NIAID 2010; Advanced Radiation Therapeutics- Radiation Injury Mitigation 2010). The contractor, under the direction of NIAID, can perform a number of pre-clinical and early clinical studies with specific MCMs to support licensure by the Food and Drug Administration (FDA). If a product demonstrates efficacy in initial studies, additional evaluations are performed to optimize the dose, schedule, and route of administration. Capabilities also exist in the contract to evaluate toxicology, pharmacology, and safety parameters. Manufacturing facilities capable of compliance with current Good Manufacturing Practice (GMP) are available to provide formulation and stability testing. Finally, the contract can support regulatory services to assist with the preparation of Investigational New Drug and New Drug Application submissions.

Currently, the contract supports five facilities that are capable of performing Good Laboratory Practice (GLP)-compliant pivotal animal efficacy studies and nonclinical safety studies. Animal models for hematological and GI ARS have been developed for the mouse and NHP. Screening facilities have evaluated nearly 20 compounds for efficacy in mitigating the hematological syndrome and almost 10 compounds for the GI syndrome in mice and have identified several promising candidates for further development. Four compounds have been tested for their ability to decorporate Americium-241 from rats. The RCP, through this contract, has assisted with one pre-Investigational New Drug application and two pre-Investigational Device Exemption submissions to the FDA and performed a GLP efficacy study in NHP for the mitigation of hematological ARS.

Collaborations. The RCP actively promotes research and collaborates with other organizations to expand research capacity. Since 2005, RCP has sponsored and participated in almost 30 meetings related to radiation injury and countermeasure development. One recent meeting of particular interest was sponsored by the RCP and the NCI and held in January 2010 (Mosvas et al. 2010). This joint workshop was designed to examine how compounds being developed for a radiation MCM indication might also be developed for a radiation therapy indication (Mosvas et al. 2010). MCM development is often considered a poor business opportunity due to the projected low volume and low margin of product sales and unpredictable need for the product. This problem can be addressed by developing products that could be used for multiple clinical indications. In the case of radiation countermeasures, the radiation oncology market represents an additional clinical opportunity to reduce treatment toxicity for patients treated with radiation therapy or radiation plus chemotherapy.

The RCP has established a number of active collaborations with research groups inside and outside the U.S., including the Radiation Effects Research Foundation (RERF), the National Space Biomedical Research Institute (NSBRI), the Armed Forces Radiobiology Research Institute (AFRRI), the World Health Organization (WHO), and other institutes at NIH, including the NCI, the National Institute on Aging (NIA), and the National Institute of Diabetes and Digestive and Kidney Diseases. Additional information about these programs and collaborations can be found in the reference section (NIAID 2010; Cassatt et al. 2010).

5 Normal Tissue Injury Research Program-Centers for Medical Countermeasures Against Radiation

The CMCRs have reinvigorated translational research for diagnostic technologies and pharmaceuticals to be used for post-exposure mitigation of radiation injury. While these centers have been very successful at increasing understanding of the mechanisms of radiation toxicity, including the reversible components of both acute and late radiation-related and combined modality-mediated toxicity, there are still few agents ready for the strategic national stockpile (SNS) despite efficacy in animal models. The later is largely due to the inability of these agents to overcome the many regulatory hurdles required for approval under the FDA's "Animal Rule" (Williams et al. 2010; Food and Drug Administration, HHS 2009, 2002). More recently, however, it has become clear that many of these agents can also improve wound healing. Other data for some agents indicate that they improve tumor response to radiation and/or chemotherapy, while also reducing radiation and combined modality toxicities (Mosvas et al 2010). Indeed, the approach of the radiation MCM effort has been to emphasize the potential "multi-clinical use" agents that have other indications. This approach might have the benefits of (a) facilitating drug approval, (b) having doctors with experience using the agents, (c) having drugs already available in hospitals and pharmacies, and (d) encouraging investment in drug development by industry as it would have a reasonable market beyond that of government stockpiles.

Biodosimetry technologies are also finding use in oncology clinics. In local radiation treatments, the tumor is the organ largely exposed to the majority of the radiation; thus, damage detection by biodosimetry techniques are under investigation as markers of tumor response. Since the approaches being studied by the CMCR require turnaround within minutes and must be evaluable shortly after exposure, these technologies have the potential for measuring tumor response within hours or days after exposure, instead of the usual long delays currently experienced clinically between staging laboratory or radiographic studies and response evaluation.

The impact of supportive measures has also made important strides over the past 5 years since the CMCR inception. Perhaps more than any other type of mitigation or therapeutic intervention, supportive care to cover the usually short period of highest mortality risk can be very effective (Williams et al. 2010). This includes measures that are easy to implement, such as dietary modification, antibiotics, and hydration, although the surge in the number of patients will stress the healthcare system. As a result, a second category of agents has been identified that prolongs the median survival after otherwise lethal exposure (Williams et al. 2010). Such agents can allow for the time needed to evacuate patients to intensive care units nationally. Indications are that some antibiotic medications also have an independent direct mitigation effect against radiation toxicity allowing them to work on two levels (Epperly et al. 2010; Kim et al. 2009; Xiao et al. 2006).

The CMCRs have put a great deal of thought into animal models that might best identify agents and instruments for and justify agents in the SNS (Augustine et al. 2005;

Williams et al. 2010). While publications developed through these workshops are not necessarily used by the FDA to approve agents, the concepts defined at those meetings provide some guidance to entities trying to develop nuclear or radiological mitigation technologies. The organ of interest must clearly be protected in the identification of appropriate animal models. While a number of radiation toxicities are common to multiple organs, most injury is organ specific; thus, mitigation agents tend to be different for different organs and tend to require different schedules to be most efficacious. Therefore, mitigation and treatment will need cocktails of agents for the multiple organs at risk. Along with these needs, it will be necessary to identify technologies that assess the organ that was most critically damaged by radiation and to be able to follow and measure any organ-specific beneficial effects of the intervention. The multi-clinical use application of these agents and technologies are obvious for the cancer clinic (Mosvas et al. 2010). Figure 3 includes some of the agents currently under development through the CMCRs.

6 Product Development: Biomedical Advanced Research and Development Authority

6.1 BARDA

The Biomedical Advanced Research and Development Authority (BARDA) (BARDA 2010) provides an integrated, systematic approach to the development and purchase of the necessary vaccines, drugs, therapies, and diagnostic tools for public health medical emergencies. BARDA manages Project BioShield (Project Bioshield 2010), which includes the procurement and advanced development of medical countermeasures for chemical, biological, radiological, and nuclear (CBRN) agents, as well as the advanced development and procurement of MCMs for pandemic influenza and other emerging infectious diseases that fall outside the auspices of Project BioShield. In addition, BARDA manages the Public Health Emergency Medical Countermeasures Enterprise (PHEMCE) (PHEMC 2010).

6.2 Project BioShield

The Project BioShield Act of 2004 (Project Bioshield 2010) is part of a broader strategy to defend the United States against weapons of mass destruction. Its purpose is to accelerate the research, development, purchase, and availability of effective MCMs for the adverse health effects of CBRN agents. In addressing radiological and nuclear threats, an interagency group of experts recommended the use of the Special Reserve Fund, described below, authorized under Project BioShield to acquire the following additional countermeasures for the Strategic National Stockpile (SNS):

- A liquid form of potassium iodide (KI) that can be taken more easily than tablets by children. KI is a drug that blocks absorption of radioactive iodide in the thyroid gland.
- Calcium-diethylenetriaminepentaacetate (DTPA) and Zinc-DTPA, 2 forms of a decorporation agent which help remove transuranic radioactive particles from the body.
- Treatments to address the neutropenia associated with ARS.

The Secretaries of HHS and the Department of Homeland Security (DHS) jointly recommended these acquisitions; the Director of the Office of Management and Budget approved the purchases under delegated authority from the President; and, HHS implemented these acquisition programs.

Project BioShield provided unprecedented legislation to facilitate CBRN preparedness. The law authorized HHS to support late-stage procurement programs (8 years to licensure); in addition, it appropriated $5.6 billion in the Special Reserve Fund for fiscal years (FY) 2004–2013, facilitated the NIH mission to develop countermeasures, and permitted use of MCMs not yet FDA approved (under Emergency Use Authorization). However, there were insufficient incentives to entice large pharmaceutical companies due to the risk being placed primarily on developers. Advance payments refundable upon contract failure and insufficient support for advanced product development caused products to languish in the so-called "Valley of Death".

6.3 Pandemic and All-Hazards Preparedness Act

In 2006, the Pandemic and All-Hazards Preparedness Act (PAHPA) (PAHPA 2010) established BARDA as the focal point within HHS for the advanced development and acquisition of MCMs to protect the American civilian population against CBRN and naturally occurring threats to public health. Using its advanced research and development authority, BARDA strengthens HHS efforts to bridge the "Valley of Death" funding gap that exists between the early stages of product development and the acquisition of approved or approvable MCMs for the SNS. The PAHPA provided for the establishment of the Biodefense MCM Development Fund ($1.07 billion of funding were authorized but funds were not provided, i.e. appropriated,), and PAHPA authorized milestone-payments under Project BioShield (up to 50 % nonrefundable).

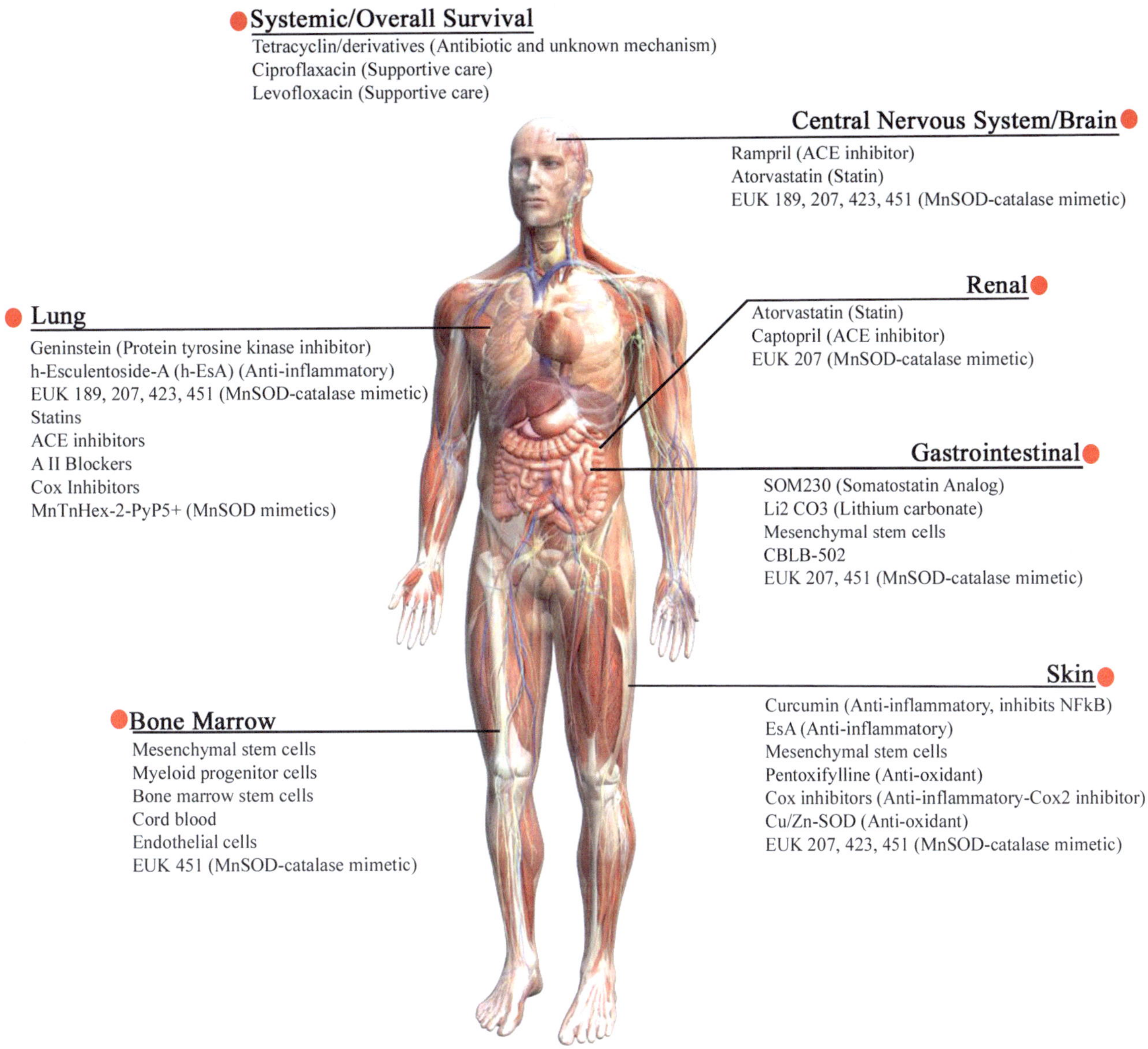

**Each drug's mechanism of action is listed in parentheses.*
***Image used courtesy of ZYGOTE.*

Fig. 3 Radiation mitigators under development through the CMCRs. This is a partial list of agents that have been studied by various CMCR as potential protection, mitigation, or therapeutic agents against radiation. These agents generally come in classes including anti-inflammatory, antioxidant, antiapoptotic, and growth factors. Those agents in the first two categories have commonly shown a doubly beneficial effect wherein tumor response to radiation is improved as is the normal tissue toxicity. Regarding the anti-inflammatory agents, the mechanism of this apparently contradictory effect appears to be a reduction in inflammatory cytokines. In tumors, these cytokines augment tumor aggressiveness and in normal tissue they promote deleterious normal tissue reactions. Thus, inhibition of these signaling molecules after radiation benefits both processes

6.4 Integrated National Biodefense Medical Countermeasures Portfolio: Promoting a One-Portfolio Approach

Under the Integrated National Biodefense Medical Countermeasure Portfolio "One-Portfolio Approach", the DoD and HHS each identify MCM requirements to address their different missions and foci. DoD's focus is on protecting the armed forces prior to exposure; whereas, HHS's focus is on response to threats to the civilian population after exposure in a CBRN event. However, there are areas of common requirements or interest where MCM candidates, resources, and information can be appropriately shared to maximize opportunities for success in the development of MCMs for the highest priority threats. BARDA, in partnership with other HHS and DoD partners, is leading an Integrated National Biodefense Medical Countermeasure Portfolio to leverage resources and programs across the agencies that develop and acquire CBRN MCMs to more effectively address the broad range of common threats and requirements. Members of this Integrated Portfolio include BARDA, NIAID and other Institutes of NIH, and multiple elements of the DoD Chemical and Biological Defense Program.

Integrated Portfolio objectives include:

- Collect information and report on the overall state of the Integrated Portfolio CBRN MCM programs.
- Evaluate portfolio probability of success and articulate required investment.
- Identify portfolio gaps and overlaps.
- Develop recommendations for portfolio ("Implementation Planning").
- Implement joint portfolio oversight.
- Enhance intradepartmental and interdepartmental collaboration.
- Build portfolio plan into budget planning.

Accomplishments to date:

- DoD and HHS harmonization of a common set of Technology Readiness Levels (TRLs - discussed below, Table 2) (Project BioShield 2006) to define the research pipeline and candidate maturity.
- An improved understanding of the expected impact of the FDA "Animal Rule" on MCM product development.
- Mapping of pipelines for several biological threat MCMs.
- Establishment by program officers of focused networks with colleagues in other agencies.
- MCM development of "projects in common" between DoD and HHS and across HHS.
- Approaches to portfolio integration: cost-sharing, knowledge sharing, and program sharing.
- Establishment of memorandums of understanding (MOUs) between agencies to facilitate cooperation.

6.5 The MCM Requirements Process

MCMs are developed and acquired in a requirements process. This consists of four pillars:

1. Pillar 1 is to identify and assess threats. This includes development of Material Threat Assessments (MTAs) and Material Threat Determinations (MTDs). In the former, DHS and HHS collaborate to identify and model plausible, high consequence scenarios, and the number of individuals likely to be exposed to each threat agent under those scenarios. The latter are issued by the Secretary of Homeland Security for threat agents deemed to pose a material threat to national security; these are necessary for Project BioShield acquisitions.
2. Under Pillar 2, HHS evaluates medical and public health consequences based on DHS scenarios. Questions to be answered include: How many people will require diagnostics and MCMs? What is the potential public health impact (i.e., reductions in morbidity/mortality) of existing or future medical countermeasures? How do response times at the federal, state, and local levels affect MCM effectiveness?
3. Pillar 3 is the establishment of MCM requirements. Deliverables are based on a scientific background assessment in which the biochemical, epidemiological, and pathogenic characteristics of threat agents are examined. A follow-on deliverable is then a scenario-based requirement in which medical-consequence modeling defines classes and quantities of necessary MCMs. Product-specific requirements are determined next. Minimum and desired features for individual MCM products (e.g., characteristics and quantity) for development and acquisition are identified. Next, a utilization policy is developed. This policy consists of a framework of operational policies and procedures for MCM utilization and deployment.
4. Pillar 4 involves determination of near-, mid-, and long-term development and acquisition strategies. In stage 1 (strategy), overarching guiding principles and framework for priority-setting are determined. In stage 2 (implementation planning), near- (FY07 – 08), mid- (FY09 – 13), and long-term (FY14 – 23) goals for research, development, and acquisition of MCMs were developed.

6.6 BARDA Radiological and Nuclear Activities

6.6.1 Biodosimetry

A request for information (RFI) was issued in May 2008 in Federal Business Opportunities for *Physical and Biological Dosimetry Techniques and Devices Useful in Initial Triage after Radiologic and Nuclear Events* (https://www.fbo.gov/index?s=opportunity&mode=form&id=3e7743eb3535970 91efeb4194cb685b4&tab=core&_cview=1). In February 2009, a Broad Agency Announcement (BAA) was issued for *Point of Care or High-Throughput Biological Assays for Determining Absorbed Ionizing Radiation Dose (Biodosimetry) After Radiologic and Nuclear Events* (https://www.fbo.gov/index?id=9079d4e9d8f113c4b79b8785051d69f4). Subsequently, BARDA awarded contracts for tests and devices to help the nation respond to a radiological emergency. Nine contracts for the advanced research and development of more effective tests and devices to determine the level of radiation a person has absorbed after a nuclear or radiological incident were awarded. The

Table 2 Technology Readiness Levels (TRLs) For Medical Countermeasure Products (Drugs And Biologics)[a,b]. Based on October 2004 DOD Medical TRLs and May 2008 HHS PHEMCE TRLs

TRL 1	*Review of scientific knowledge Base* Active monitoring of scientific knowledge base. Scientific findings are reviewed and assessed as a foundation for characterizing new technologies
TRL 2	*Development of hypotheses and experimental designs* Scientific "paper studies" to generate research ideas, hypotheses, and experimental designs for addressing related scientific issues. Focus on practical applications based on basic principles observed. Use of computer simulation or other virtual platforms to test hypotheses
TRL 3	*Target/Candidate identification and characterization of preliminary candidate(s)* Begin research, data collection, and analysis in order to test hypothesis. Explore alternative concepts, identify and evaluate critical technologies and components, and begin characterization of candidate(s). Preliminary efficacy demonstrated in vivo *3A* Identify target and/or candidate *3B* Demonstrate in vitro activity of candidate(s) to counteract the effects of the threat agent *3C* Generate preliminary in vivo proof-of-concept efficacy data (non-Good Laboratory Practice (GLP))
TRL 4	*Candidate optimization and non-GLP in vivo demonstration of activity and efficacy* Integration of critical technologies for candidate development. Initiation of animal model development. Non-GLP in vivo toxicity and efficacy demonstration in accordance with the product's intended use. Initiation of experiments to identify markers, correlates of protection, assays, and endpoints for further nonclinical and clinical studies *Animal models.* Initiate development of appropriate and relevant animal model(s) for the desired indications *Assays.* Initiate development of appropriate and relevant assays and associated reagents for the desired indications *Manufacturing.* Manufacture laboratory-scale (i.e., non-GMP (Good Manufacturing Practice)) quantities of bulk product and proposed formulated product *4A* Demonstrate non-GLP in vivo activity and potential for efficacy consistent with the product's intended use (i.e., dose, schedule, duration, route of administration, and route of threat agent challenge) *4B* Conduct initial non-GLP toxicity studies and determine pharmacodynamics and pharmacokinetics and/or immune response in appropriate animal models (as applicable) *4C* Initiate experiments to determine assays, parameters, surrogate markers, correlates of protection, and endpoints to be used during nonclinical and clinical studies to further evaluate and characterize candidate(s)
TRL 5	*Advanced characterization of candidate and initiation of GMP process development* Continue non-GLP in vivo studies and animal model and assay development. Establish draft Target Product Profiles. Develop a scalable and reproducible manufacturing process amenable to GMP *Animal models.* Continue development of animal models for efficacy and dose-ranging studies *Assays.* Initiate development of in-process assays and analytical methods for product characterization and release, including assessments of potency, purity, identity, strength, sterility, and quality as appropriate *Manufacturing.* Initiate process development for small-scale manufacturing amenable to GMP *Target product profile.* Draft preliminary Target Product Profile. Questions of shelf life, storage conditions, and packaging should be considered to ensure that anticipated use of the product is consistent with the intended use for which approval will be sought from FDA *5A* Demonstrate acceptable *A*bsorption, *D*istribution, *M*etabolism and *E*limination characteristics and/or immune responses in non-GLP animal studies as necessary for IND filing *5B* Continue establishing correlates of protection, endpoints, and/or surrogate markers for efficacy for use in future GLP studies in animal models. Identify minimally effective dose to facilitate determination of "humanized" dose once clinical data are obtained
TRL 6	*GMP pilot lot production, IND submission, and phase 1 clinical trial(s)* Manufacture GMP-compliant pilot lots. Prepare and submit Investigational New Drug (IND) package to FDA and conduct Phase 1 clinical trial(s) to determine the safety and pharmacokinetics of the clinical test article *Animal models.* Continue animal model development via toxicology, pharmacology, and immunogenicity studies *Assays.* Qualify assays for manufacturing quality control and immunogenicity, if applicable *Manufacturing.* Manufacture, release, and conduct stability testing of GMP-compliant bulk and formulated product in support of the IND and clinical trial(s) *Target Product Profile.* Update target product profile as appropriate. *6A* Conduct GLP nonclinical studies for toxicology, pharmacology, and immunogenicity as appropriate *6B* Prepare and submit full IND package to FDA to support initial clinical trial(s) *6C* Complete phase 1 clinical trial(s) that establish an initial safety, pharmacokinetics, and immunogenicity assessment as appropriate
TRL 7	*Scale-up, initiation of GMP process validation, and phase 2 clinical* 3 *Trial(s)* Scale-up and initiate validation of GMP manufacturing process Conduct animal efficacy studies as appropriate.[d] Conduct Phase 2 clinical trial(s)[c] *Animal models.* Refine animal model development in preparation for pivotal GLP animal efficacy *Assays.* Validate assays for manufacturing quality control and immunogenicity if applicable *Manufacturing.* Scale-up and validate GMP manufacturing process at a scale compatible with USG requirements. Begin stability studies of the GMP product in a formulation, dosage form, and container consistent with Target Product Profile. Initiate manufacturing process validation and consistency lot production *Product profile.* Update target product profile as appropriate *7A* Conduct GLP animal efficacy studies as appropriate for the product at this stage[d] *7B* Complete expanded clinical safety trials as appropriate for the product (e.g., Phase 2)[c]

(continued)

Table 2 (continued)

TRL 8	*Completion of GMP validation and consistency lot manufacturing, pivotal animal efficacy studies or clinical trials 3, and FDA approval or licensure* Finalize GMP manufacturing process. Complete pivotal animal efficacy studies or clinical trials (e.g., Phase 3), and/or expanded clinical safety trials as appropriate. Prepare and submit NDA/BLA *Manufacturing.* Complete validation and manufacturing of consistency lots at a scale compatible with USG requirements. Complete stability studies in support of label expiry dating *Target product profile.* Finalize target product profile in preparation for FDA approval *8A* Complete pivotal GLP animal efficacy studies or pivotal clinical trials (e.g., Phase 3) and any additional expanded clinical safety trials as appropriate for the product[c] *8B* Prepare and submit New Drug Application (NDA) or Biologics Licensing Application (BLA) to the FDA. *8C* Obtain FDA approval or licensure
TRL 9	*Post-Licensure and post-approval activities* *9A* Commence post-licensure/post-approval and phase 4 studies (post-marketing commitments), such as safety surveillance, studies to support use in special populations, and clinical trials to confirm safety and efficacy as feasible and appropriate[e] *9B* Maintain manufacturing capability as appropriate

Note When using these criteria, a medical countermeasure product should be rated at a particular level only after the sponsor has completed all activities listed in that level (e.g., a product is rated at TRL 4 once it completes all of the activities listed in TRL 4)

[a] This document is designed for evaluating the maturity of medical countermeasure development programs. For a detailed description of development processes for assays and animal models, please consult the Technology Readiness Levels for Product Development Tools (PDTs), developed by the PDT Working Group of the HHS Public Health Emergency Medical Countermeasures Enterprise (PHEMCE) and available at http://www.medicalcountermeasures.gov

[b] This document does not serve as official FDA Guidance nor does it represent FDA's current thinking on this topic. For the purposes of a regulatory application seeking licensure or approval for a specific medical product, additional data may be required by FDA

[c] Identification of later regulatory stages of clinical development in this document (e.g., Phase 2, Phase 3) may not apply to some products being developed under the "Animal Rule." Other than human safety studies, no additional clinical data may be feasible or ethical to obtain. For additional information on the "Animal Rule," please see http://www.fda.gov/OHRMS/DOCKETS/98fr/053102a.htm

[d] These could include GLP animal efficacy studies required by the FDA at this stage in support of an Emergency Use Authorization (EUA). The scientific evidence required for issuance of an EUA will be handled on a case-by-case basis and will depend on, among other things, the nature and extent of the threat at any point during the product development timeline, from the initiation of Phase 1 studies through licensure or approval. GLP animal efficacy study requirements may also vary by product type (e.g., vaccine, therapeutic, prophylactic) and U.S. government agency program office

[e] For products approved under the "Animal Rule," confirmatory efficacy data are required, if such studies are feasible and ethical, and may be obtained from use during an event

contracts total $35 million for the initial phase and up to $400 million over 5 years (names of awardees available on BARDA website) (BARDA 2010).

Each contract awardee identified particular physical or biological characteristics, known as biomarkers, of radiation dose to help health care responders determine the most appropriate treatment. In the first year of the contract, the contractors conduct tests of the accuracy of the biomarkers as an indicator for the level of absorbed radiation and determine if their proposed devices measure these biomarkers effectively. If successful, the contractors develop prototypes of portable devices that can be used in the field by responders. These are developed under the U.S. Food and Drug Administration (FDA) Investigational Device Exemption process that allows the devices to be used in a clinical study to collect safety and effectiveness data required to support a premarket approval application or a premarket notification submission to FDA. If the products are approved by the FDA in future years, the products may become eligible for consideration and procurement by the U.S. government.

6.6.2 Acute Radiation Syndrome

In October 2004 and May 2005, Requests for Information (RFIs) were issued for *Therapeutics to Treat Neutropenia and Thrombocytopenia Associated with the Acute Radiation Syndrome (ARS)* (http://grants.nih.gov/grants/guide/notice-files/not-ai-05-007.html). A sources sought notice (SSN) for *Therapeutics Applicable for the Treatment of Neutropenia Resulting from Exposure to Ionizing Radiation* (https://www.fbo.gov/index?s=opportunity&mode=form&tab=core&id=13c9de1649a4a12754124bd0e5cf02ee&_cview=1) was issued in May 2007. A Request for Application (RFA) for *BARDA/NIAID Medical Countermeasures to Mitigate and/or Treat Ionizing Radiation-Induced Pulmonary Injury: Project Bioshield* (http://grants.nih.gov/grants/guide/rfa-files/rfa-ai-07-040.html) was issued in December 2007 and a Request for Proposal (RFP) for *Advanced Therapeutics for Treating Neutropenia Resulting from Acute Exposure to Ionizing Radiation* (https://www.fbo.gov/index?id=7d5aae491592d213faf9489aaceab5eb) was posted in March 2009. One or more contract awards are pending.

A BAA was posted in 2008 for *Therapies for Hematopoietic Syndrome, Bone Marrow Stromal Cell Loss, And Vascular Injury Resulting From Acute Exposure to Ionizing Radiation* (https://www.fbo.gov/index?s=opportunity&mode=form&id=a8f8740158d15c32d4f9f4a8defdfcb2&tab=core&_cview=1). Over $20 Million was awarded to seven respondents in September 2008. The BAA targeted the following 3 R & D areas:

1. Area 1 was for the development of MCMs that can replenish the normal hematopoietic profile, in whole or in part (i.e., treat neutropenia, lymphopenia, and thrombocytopenia), following acute radiation exposure that induces lethal hematopoietic dysfunction.
2. Area 2 targeted the development of MCMs to replenish bone marrow niche and progenitor cells that normally populate the bone marrow stroma and niche environments and that can restore normal functioning hematopoietic cell lineages following acute exposure to ionizing radiation that induces lethal hematopoietic dysfunction.
3. Area 3 aimed at the development of MCMs that address injury to the vascular system induced following acute exposure to ionizing radiation, including changes in intimal integrity and clotting propensity, macrophage repair mechanisms and trafficking, vascular leak, endothelial repair, endovascular surface chemistry, alteration of angiogenesis, and other changes in anatomical or molecular pathology.

6.6.3 Chronic Effects of Radiation Exposure

BARDA awarded a contract for a Pediatric Formulation (Liquid) Potassium Iodide (KI) in March 2005 and a contract for acquisition of Calcium and Zinc Diethylenetriamine-pentaacetate (Ca DTPA and Zn DTPA) in December 2005.

6.6.4 Rolling BAA

BARDA has reissued a long-range BAA: (BARDA-CBRN-BAA-10-100-SOL-00012) (https://www.fbo.gov/index?id=c1d5b56d7a9026456191e372b856f469) to identify innovative and promising MCM technologies for advanced development across several CBRN Research Areas. The focus is on TRLs 5–7 (pre-IND to Phase 2) (https://www.fbo.gov/index?s=opportunity&mode=form&id=3e7743eb353597091efeb4194cb685b4&tab=core&_cview=1) in the following areas:

- Vaccines
- Antitoxins and Therapeutics
- Antimicrobial Drugs
- Radiological/Nuclear Threat Countermeasures
- Chemical Threat Countermeasures
- Diagnostics.

The BAA application is a two stage process. The initial stage involves submission of a 5–15 page white paper/quad chart that is reviewed for BARDA program relevance, technical merit, and capabilities. Within 90 days, BARDA provides specific technical feedback to the offeror if the white paper/quad chart is deemed acceptable. If acceptable, the offeror will receive an invitation letter to submit a full proposal based on technical guidance provided by BARDA. The second stage of the BAA process involves submission of a full proposal (technical and cost) based on guidance provided by BARDA.

6.6.5 BARDA Animal Model Development RFI-BARDA-2010-Animal Models-001

Under this RFI, the USG is seeking appropriate facilities that are adequate and available to develop new animal tests or models and also update existing animal tests or models that are accepted by FDA (https://www.fbo.gov/index?s=opportunity&mode=form&id=399f56eafb7b181ff66327e2134e34fe&tab=core&_cview=0). Laboratories that can conduct pilot studies to establish the natural history of selected CBRN agents in appropriate animal species are included. Also of interest are laboratories that can perform efficacy evaluations in various species on candidate compounds. BARDA is seeking laboratories that can provide analytical support to monitor the progression of the disease in animal models and demonstrate prospective correlates of protection. Finally, BARDA seeks laboratories with the capability to perform radiation exposure studies using Cs-137, Co-60, Linear Accelerator (LINAC), X-ray, or other accepted instrumentation for controlled exposures of animals to lethal radiation within the constraint of acceptable dose rates and with uniform field flux and field sizes for both large and small animals.

6.6.6 Continuum between BARDA and NIAID

The experience with the initial efforts in Project Bioshield (Project Bioshield 2010) demonstrated that translational science, typically interpreted as bench to bedside and back, required a component of technology transfer to be successful. There are few if any customers or demand for radiological and nuclear terrorism products other than the government; thus, there is little incentive for major pharmaceutical companies to enter the business of creating expensive and hard-to-test terrorism products. The CMCR and related grantees funded by NIAID were found to be fertile breeding places for the identification of mechanisms and example products but were not sufficiently large or focused enough for commercialization. Since BARDA funds advanced research required to reach a commercialization stage, it was able to fill the gap between the research funded by NIAID and that required for regulatory approval and commercialization.

The rigorous distinction between NIAID- and BARDA-funded efforts are usually based on TRLs that range from the most basic level 1 to a final level of FDA approval in level 9 (Table 2) (Project BioShield 2006). BARDA funds TRLs that are typically higher than those supported by the CMCRs and NIAID. The focus of BARDA is to oversee the steps and help guide the studies needed to create a product of interest to the government with FDA approval.

Figure 4 illustrates the continuum of effort among the federal agencies ranging from basic science to translational work to product development and implementation.

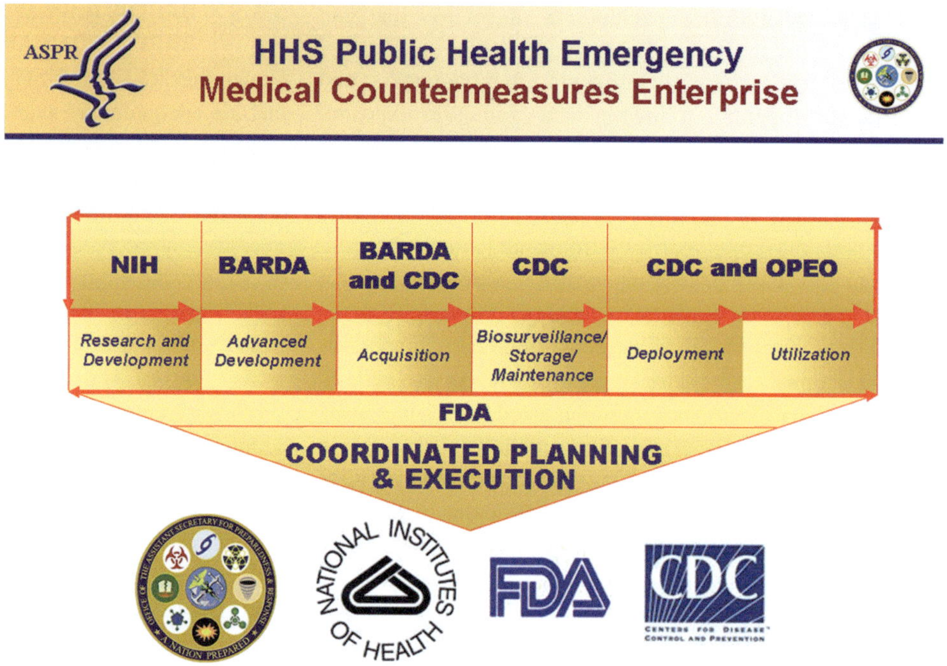

Fig. 4 Continuum of product development by the Federal agencies. The funding for MCM and biodosimetric development comes from several different funding streams. It builds on the research and development of NIH and other agencies, such as the Department of Energy (DOE), the Department of Defense (DoD), and the Defense Advanced Research Products Agency (DARPA)

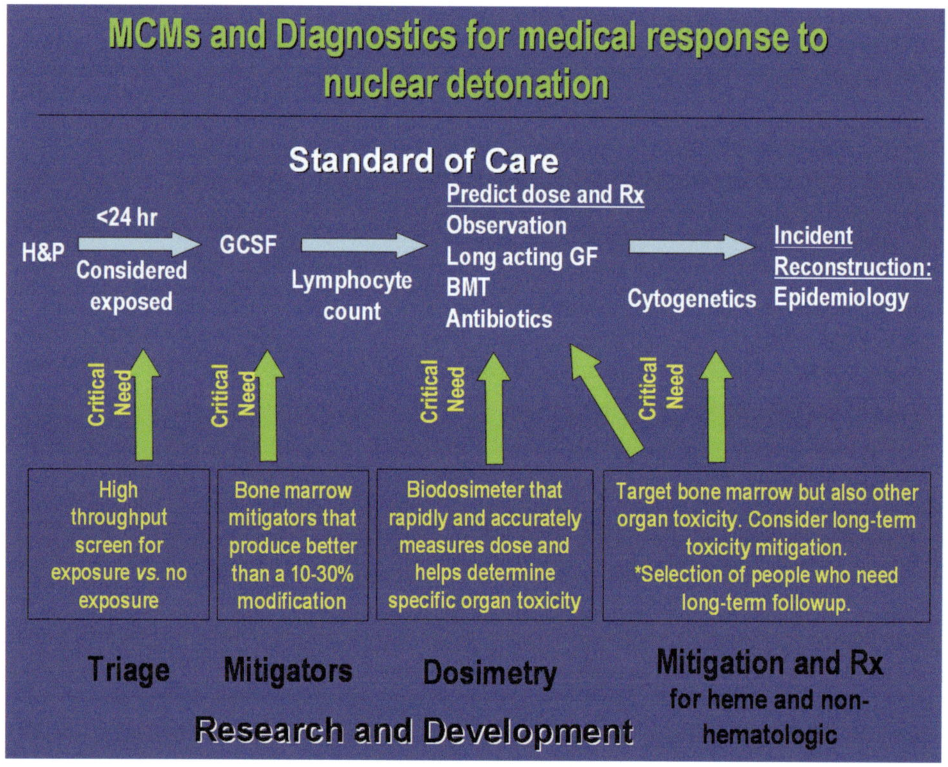

Fig. 5 Medical countermeasures and diagnostics for medical response to a nuclear detonation. A typical scenario after a radiation event will include a triage stage (best if within 1–2 days), wherein identification of individuals who might have had significant radiation exposure are identified. These individuals will likely be offered a dose of the appropriate growth factor until validation of their exposure is obtained. They will be followed with more detailed biodosimetry and supportive and mitigative care. At present, the gold standard biodosimetry remains cytogenetics, which will be available later for epidemiological study

7 Conclusions

Over the last 6–7 years, there has been substantial progress in the organization of the medical response to a nuclear/radiological incident built on (a) a resurgence in the interest in normal tissue radiation biology; (b) the description of new mechanisms of injury, including inflammation; (c) the inclusion of late toxicity into clinical toxicity criteria for cancer care (Common Toxicity Criteria for Adverse Events, or CTCAE and now Patient Related Outcomes- PRO-CTCAE) (https://www.fbo.gov/index?s=opportunity&mode

=form&id=3e7743eb353597091efeb4194cb685b4&tab=core&_cview=1); (d) programs developed through NIAID, BARDA, AFRRI, NCI, and others; and (e) the "multi-clinical use" concept whereby technologies and medicines that are used to treat injuries caused by terrorism are also used in day-to-day medical care. Figure 5 illustrates how the ongoing research and development can impact the current state of the art.

There are tools available for those involved in medical response preparedness and planning, including REMM (REMM 2010), the Planning Guidance (Homeland Security Council 2010), and the Scare Resources project soon to be published (Coleman, personal communication). Those interested in these areas of research can find information on the websites noted in this chapter. There are substantial opportunities for research and development, community participation, public communication and education, and recruitment/retention of talented people to assist in the science, policy, and clinical application of these advances for both terrorism preparedness and spin-off benefits to cancer care.

References

AFRRI (2008) AFRRI emergency radiation medicine pocket guide. http://www.afrri.usuhs.mil/outreach/pdf/AFRRI-Pocket-Guide.pdf. Accessed 07 May 2010

Advanced Radiation Therapeutics- Radiation Injury Mitigation (2010). National Cancer Institute and the National Institute of Allergy and Infectious Disease. http://www3.cancer.gov/rrp/workshop_2010/rrp_workshop.pdf. Accessed 07 May 2010

Ainsbury EA, Livingston GK, Abbott MG, Moquet JE, Hone PA, Jenkins MS, Christensen DM, Lloyd DC, Rothkamm K (2009) Interlaboratory variation in scoring dicentric chromosomes in a case of partial-body X-ray exposure: implications for biodosimetry networking and cytogenetic "triage mode" scoring. Radiat Res 172(6):746–752

Armed Forces Radiobiology Research Institute (AFRRI), US Department of Defense AFRRI (2009) Medical Management of Radiological Casualties, 3rd edn. http://www.afrri.usuhs.mil/outreach/pdf/2edmmrchandbook.pdf. Accessed 07 May 2010

Augustine AD, Gondre-Lewis T, McBride W, Miller L, Pellmar TC, Rockwell S (2005) Animal models for radiation injury, protection and therapy. Radiat Res 164(1):100–109

Bennder MA, Gooch PC (1966) Somatic chromosome aberrations induced by human whole-body irradiation: The "Recuplex" criticality accident. Radiat Res 18:389–396

Biomedical Advanced Research and Development Authority (BARDA). Available at: http://www.hhs.gov/aspr/barda/index.html. Accessed 14 May 2010

Blakely WF, Carr Z, Chu MC, Dayal-Drager R, Fujimoto K, Hopmeir M et al (2009) WHO 1st consultation on the development of a global biodosimetry laboratories network for radiation emergencies (BioDoseNet). Radiat Res 171(1):127–139

Blakely WF, Ossetrova NI, Whitnall MH, Sandgren DJ, Krivokrysenko VI, Shakhov A et al (2010) Multiple parameter radiation injury assessment using a nonhuman primate radiation model-biodosimetry applications. Health Phys 98(2):153–159

Buddemeier BR, Dillion MB (2010) Key response planning factors for the aftermath of a nuclear detonation. LLNL-TR-410067. http://www.remm.nlm.gov/IND_ResponsePlanning_LLNL-TR-410067.pdf. Accessed 07 May 2010

Cassatt DR, Kaminski JM, Hatchett RJ, DiCarlo AL, Benjamin JM, Maidment BW (2008) Medical countermeasures against nuclear threats: radionuclide decorporation agents. Radiat Res 170: 540–548

Coleman CN, Parker GW (2009) Radiation terrorism: what society needs from the radiobiology-radiation protection and radiation oncology communities. J Radiol Prot 29(2A):A159-69

Coleman CN, Blakely WF, Fike JR, MacVittie TJ, Metting NF, Mitchell JB et al (2003) Molecular and cellular biology of moderate-dose (1–10 Gy) radiation and potential mechanisms of radiation protection: report of a workshop at Bethesda, Maryland, December 17–18. Radiat Res 159(6):812–834

Coleman CN, Stone HB, Alexander GA, Barcellos-Hoff MH, Bedford JS, Bristow RG et al (2003) Education and training for radiation scientists: radiation research program and American Society of Therapeutic Radiology and Oncology Workshop, Bethesda, Maryland, May 12–14. Radiat Res 160(6):729–737

Coleman CN, Hrdina C, Bader JL, Norwood A, Hayhurst R, Forsha J et al (2009) Medical response to a radiologic/nuclear event: integrated plan from the office of the assistant secretary for preparedness and response, Department of Health and Human Services. Ann Emerg Med 53(2):213–222

Coleman CN, Knebel AR, Hick JL, Weinstock DM, Casagrande R, Jaime Caro J, DeRenzo EG, Dodgen D, Norwood AE, Sherman SE, Cliffer KD, McNally R, Bader JL, Murrain-Hill P (2011) Scarce resources for nuclear detonation: project overview and challenges. Disaster Med Public Health Preparedness (Suppl 1):13–19

Dainiak N, Waselenko JK, Armitage JO, MacVittie TJ, Farese AM (2003) The hematologist and radiation casualties. Hematology/the Education Program of the American Society of Hematology, pp 473–496

Davids MS, Case C Jr, Hornung R 3rd, Chao NJ, Chute JP, Coleman CN, Weisdorf D, Confer DL, Weinstock DM (2010) Assessing surge capacity for radiation victims with marrow toxicity. Biol Blood Marrow Transplant. [Epub ahead of print]

Demidenko E, Williams BB, Swartz HM (2009) Radiation dose prediction using data on time to emesis in the case of nuclear terrorism. Radiat Res 171(3):310–319

DiCarlo AL, Hatchett RJ, Kaminski JM, Ledney GD, Pellmar TC, Okunieff P, Ramakrishnan N (2008) Medical countermeasures for radiation combined injury: radiation with burn, blast, trauma and/or sepsis. Report of an NIAID Workshop, 26–27 March 2007. Radiat Res 169:712–721

Dicky JS, Redon CE, Nakumara AJ, Baird BJ, Sedelnikova OA, Bonner WM (2009) H2AX: Functional roles and potential applications. Chromosoma 118:683–692

Epperly MW, Franicola D, Shields D, Rwigema JC, Stone B, Zhang X, McBride W, Georges G, Wipf P, Greenberger JS (2010) Screening of antimicrobial agents for in vitro radiation protection and mitigation capacity, including those used in supportive care regimens for bone marrow transplant recipients. In Vivo 24(1):9–19

Fenech M (2007) Cytokinesis-block micronucleus cytome assay. Nat Protoc 2:1084–1104

Fliedner TM (2006) Nuclear terrorism: the role of hematology in coping with its health consequences. Curr Opin Hematol 13(6):436–444

Fliedner TM, Friesecke I, Beyrer K. Medical management of radiation accidents: manual on the acute radiation syndrome. (METREPOL) http://vts.uni-ulm.de/docs/2009/6891/vts_6891_9572.pdf Compendium to the main METREPOL document http://vts.uni-ulm.de/docs/2009/6891/vts_6891_9573.pdf Accessed 07 May 2010

Fliedner TM, Chao NJ, Bader JL, Boettger A, Case C Jr, Chute J, Confer DL, Ganser A, Gorin NC, Gourmelon P, Graessle DH, Krawisz R, Meineke V, Niederwieser D, Port M, Powles R, Sirohi B, Weinstock DM, Wiley A, Coleman CN (2009) Stem cells, multiorgan failure in radiation emergency medical preparedness: a U.S./European Consultation Workshop. Stem Cells 27(5):1205–1211

Food and Drug Administration, HHS (2002) New drug and biological drug products; evidence needed to demonstrate effectiveness of new drugs when human efficacy studies are not ethical or feasible. http://www.fda.gov/OHRMS/DOCKETS/98fr/053102a.htm. Accessed 10 May 2010

Food and Drug Administration, HHS (2009, January) Guidance for industry: animal models—essential elements to address efficacy under the animal rule. http://www.fda.gov/downloads/Drugs/GuidanceComplianceRegulatoryInformation/Guidances/UCM078923.pdf. Accessed 10 May 2010

Grace MB, Moyer BR, Prasher J, Cliffer KD, Ramakrishnan N, Kaminski J, Coleman CN, Manning RG, Maidment BW, Hatchett R (2010) Rapid radiation dose assessment for radiological public health emergencies: roles of NIAID and BARDA. Health Phys 98(2):172–178

Hafer, N. Cassatt, D, DiCarlo, A, Ramakrishnan, N, Kaminski, J, Norman,M-K, Maidment, B and Hatchett, R. (2010) NIAID/NIH radiation/nuclear medical countermeasures product research and development program. Health Phys J 98(6):903–905

Hafer N (2009a) Radionuclide medical countermeasures development programs. Paper presented at tenth international meeting on the conference on the health effects of incorporated radionuclides. May 10–14, 2009. http://www.lrri.org/heir/Program/HEIR/Presentations/Tuesday/11%20-%20Tue%20-%201340%20-%20HaferNathaniel24421.pdf. Accessed 07 May 2010

Hafer N (2009b) NIH/NIAID radionuclide decorporation agent development program. Nov 5, 2009. Paper presented at: GHSI public health emergency medical countermeasures workshop. http://www.blsmeetings.net/2009GHSImeetingsmcm/presentations/RadNuc/Hafer-GHSIpresentationFINAL.pdf. Accessed 07 May 2010

Homeland Security Council Interagency Policy Coordination Subcommittee for Preparedness and Response to Radiological and Nuclear Threats (2010). Planning guidance for response to a nuclear detonation. http://www.whitehouse.gov/files/documents/ostp/press_release_files/Planning%20Guidance%20for%20Nuclear%20Detonation%20Response.pdf. Accessed 07 May 2010

Hrdina CM, Coleman CN, Bogucki S, Bader JL, Hayhurst RE, Forsha JD et al (2009) The "RTR" medical response system for nuclear and radiological mass-casualty incidents: a functional TRiage-TReatment-TRansport medical response model. Prehosp Disaster Med 24(3):167–178

https://www.fbo.gov/index?id=7d5aae491592d213faf9489aaceab5eb

https://www.fbo.gov/index?id=c1d5b56d7a9026456191e372b856f469

https://www.fbo.gov/index?s=opportunity&mode=form&id=399f56eafb7b181ff66327e2134e34fe&tab=core&_cview=0

https://www.fbo.gov/index?s=opportunity&mode=form&tab=core&id=13c9de1649a4a12754124bd0e5cf02ee&_cview=1

https://www.fbo.gov/index?s=opportunity&mode=form&id=3e7743eb353597091efeb4194cb685b4&tab=core&_cview=1

https://www.fbo.gov/index?id=9079d4e9d8f113c4b79b8785051d69f4

http://grants.nih.gov/grants/guide/notice-files/not-ai-05-007.html

http://grants.nih.gov/grants/guide/rfa-files/rfa-ai-07-040.html

https://www.fbo.gov/index?s=opportunity&mode=form&id=a8f8740158d15c32d4f9f4a8defdfcb2&tab=core&_cview=1

IAEA (2002) Use of electron paramagnetic resonance dosimetry with tooth enamel for retrospective dose assessment. TECDOC-1331, IAEA, Vienna, Austria

International Atomic Energy Agency (2001) Cytogenetic analysis for radiation dose assessment: a manual. Technical Report Series No 405, IAEA, Vienna, Austria

Institute of Medicine (IOM) (2009) Guidance for establishing crisis standards of care for use in disaster situations http://www.iom.edu/Reports/2009/DisasterCareStandards.aspx. Accessed 07 May 2010

ISO (2004) Radiation protection—performance criteria for service laboratories performing biological dosimetry by cytogenetics, ISO 19238. International Standardization Organization, Geneva

Ivanov VK, Chekin SY, Kashcheev VV, Maksioutov MA, Tumanov KA (2008) Risk of thyroid cancer among chernobyl emergency workers of Russia. Radiat Environ Biophys 47(4):463–467

Kim K, Pollard JM, Norris AJ, McDonald JT, Sun Y, Micewicz E, Pettijohn K, Damoiseaux R, Iwamoto KS, Sayre JW, Price BD, Gatti RA, McBride WH (2009) High-throughput screening identifies two classes of antibiotics as radioprotectors: tetracyclines and fluoroquinolones. Clin Cancer Res 15(23):7238–7245

Koenig KL, Goans RE, Hatchett RJ, Mettler FA Jr, Schumacher TA, Noji EK et al (2005) Medical treatment of radiological casualties: current concepts. Ann Emerg Med 45(6):643–652

Ledney GD, Elliott TB (2010) Combined injury: factors with potential to impact radiation dose assessments. Health Phys 98:145–152

Lerner EB, Schwartz RB, Coule PL, Weinstein ES, Cone DC, Hunt RC, Sasser SM, Liu JM, Nudell NG, Wedmore IS, Hammond J, Bulger EM, Salomone JP, Sanddal TL, Markenson D, O'Connor RE (2008) Mass casualty triage: an evaluation of the data and development of a proposed national guideline. Disaster Medicine and Public Health Preparedness 2:S25–S34

Little MP (2009) Cancer and non-cancer effects in Japanese atomic bomb survivors. J Radiol Prot 29(2A):A43–59

Lloyd DC (1997) Chromosomal analysis to assess radiation dose. Stem Cells 15(Suppl. 2):195–201

Martin PR, Berdechevsky RE, Subramanian U, Blakely WF, Prasanna PGS (2007) Sample tracking in an automated cytogenetic biodosimetry laboratory for radiation mass casualties. Radiat Meas 42:1119–1124

Mettler FA Jr, Gus'kova AK, Gusev I (2007) Health effects in those with acute radiation sickness from the chernobyl accident. Health Phys 93(5):462–469

Miller SM, Ferrarotto CL, Vlahovich S, Wilkins RC, Boreham DR, Dolling JA (2007) Canadian cytogenetic emergency network (CEN) for biological dosimetry following radiological/nuclear accidents. Int J Radiat Biol 83:353–361

Mosvas B et al. (2010) Decreasing the adverse effects of cancer therapy: National Cancer Institute Guidance for the Clinical Development of Radiation Injury Mitigators (submitted). Advanced radiation therapeutics-radiation injury mitigation. http://www3.cancer.gov/rrp/workshop_2010/rrp_workshop.pdf. Accessed 07 May 2010

NIAID-National Institute of Allergy and Infectious Diseases, (2010) Medical countermeasures against radiological and nuclear threats. Available at: http://www.niaid.nih.gov/topics/radnuc/Pages/default.aspx. Accessed 07 May 2010

National Institutes of Health (2005). NIH Strategic Plan and Research Agenda for medical countermeasures against radiological and nuclear threats (online). Washington, DC: U.S. Department of Health and Human Services; NIH Publication No. 05-5608; 2005. Available at: http://www.niaid.nih.gov/about/whoWeAre/Documents/radnucstrategicplan.pdf. Accessed 14 May 2010

Ossetrova NI, Blakely WF (2009) Multiple blood-proteins approach for early-response exposure assessment using an in vivo murine radiation model. Int J Radiat Biol 85(10):837–850

Ossetrova NI, Sandgren DJ, Gallego S, Blakely WF (2010) Combined approach of hematological biomarkers and plasma protein SAA for improvement of radiation dose assessment triage in biodosimetry applications. Health Phys 98(2):204–208

Office of the Assistant Secretary for Preparedness and Response (ASPR) (2010). http://www.hhs.gov/aspr/. Accessed 07 May 2010

Pandemic and All-Hazards Preparedness Act (PAHPA). http://www.hhs.gov/aspr/opsp/pahpa/index.html. Accessed 07 May 2010

Patient-Reported Outcomes Version of the Common Terminology Criteria for Adverse Events (PRO-CTCAE). http://outcomes.cancer.gov/tools/pro-ctcae.html. Accessed 07 May 2010

Pellmar TC, Rockwell S (2005) Priority list of research areas for radiological nuclear threat countermeasures. Radiat Res 163(1):115–123

PHEMC,(2010) Public health emergency medical countermeasures (PHEMC) enterprise. http://www.hhs.gov/aspr/barda/phemce/index.html. Accessed 07 May 2010

Prasanna PGS, Escalada ND, Blakely WF (2000) Induction of premature chromosome condensation by a phosphatase inhibitor and a protein kinase in unstimulated human peripheral blood lymphocytes: a simple and rapid technique to study chromosome aberrations using specific DNA hybridization probes for biological dosimetry. Mutat Res 466:131–141

Prasanna PGS, Moroni M, Pellmar TC (2010a) Triage dose assessment for partial-body exposure: dicentric analysis. Health Phys 98:244–251

Prasanna PG, Blakely WF, Bertho JM, Chute JP, Cohen EP, Goans RE, Grace MB, Lillis-Hearne PK, Lloyd DC, Lutgens LC, Meineke V, Ossetrova NI, Romanyukha A, Saba JD, Weisdorf DJ, Wojcik A, Yukihara EG, Pellmar TC (2010b) Synopsis of partial-body radiation diagnostic biomarkers and medical management of radiation injury workshop. Radiat Res 173(2):245–253

Preston DL, Ron E, Tokuoka S, Funamoto S, Nishi N, Soda M et al (2007) Solid cancer incidence in atomic bomb survivors: 1958–1998. Radiat Res 168(1):1–64

Preston DL, Cullings H, Suyama A, Funamoto S, Nishi N, Soda M et al (2008) Solid cancer incidence in atomic bomb survivors exposed in utero or as young children. J Natl Cancer Inst 100(6):428–436

Project Bioshield. http://www.hhs.gov/aspr/barda/bioshield/index.html. Accessed 07 May 2010

Project BioShield: Annual Report to Congress (2006–2007) http://www.hhs.gov/aspr/barda/documents/bioshieldannualreport2006.pdf. Accessed 07 May 2010

Pyatkin EK, Nugis VY, Chrikov AA (1989) Absorbed dose estimation according to the results of cytogenetic investigation of lymphocyte cultures of persons who suffered in the accident at Chernobyl atomic power station. Radiat Med 4:52–58

Radiation Emergency Medical Management (REMM). http://www.remm.nlm.gov/. Accessed 07 May 2010

Radiation Emergency Assistance Center/Training Site (REAC/TS). http://orise.orau.gov/reacts/. Accessed 07 May 2010

Ramakrishnan, N (2009) NIAID/NIH radiation/nuclear medical countermeasures development program. GHSI public health emergency medical countermeasures workshop, Nov 4 2009. http://www.blsmeetings.net/2009GHSImeetingsmcm/presentations/RadNuc/Ramakrishnan-GHSIRamakrishnanNov4.pdf. Accessed 07 May 2010

Sevankaev AV (2000) Results of cytogenetic studies of the consequences of the chernobyl accident. Radiat Biol Radioecol 40:589–595

Stone HB, McBride WH, Coleman CN (2002) Modifying normal tissue damage postirradiation. Report of a workshop sponsored by the radiation research program, National Cancer Institute, Bethesda, Maryland, Sept 6–8 2000. Radiat Res 157(2):204–223

Stone HB, Moulder JE, Coleman CN, Ang KK, Anscher MS, Barcellos-Hoff MH et al (2004) Models for evaluating agents intended for the prophylaxis, mitigation and treatment of radiation injuries. Report of an NCI Workshop, Dec 3–4 2003. Radiat Res 162(6):711–728

Suit H, Goldberg S, Niemierko A, Ancukiewicz M, Hall E, Goitein M et al (2007) Secondary carcinogenesis in patients treated with radiation: a review of data on radiation-induced cancers in human, non-human primate, canine and rodent subjects. Radiat Res 167(1):12–42

Trompier F, Kornak L, Calas C, Romanyuka A, Leblanc B, Mitchell CA, Swartz HM, Clairand I (2007) Protocol for emergency EPR dosimetry in fingernails. Radiat Meas 42:1085–1088

US DHHS. Agency for Healthcare Research and Quality (AHRQ) (2007) Mass medical care with scarce resources: a community guide. http://www.ahrq.gov/research/mce/mceguide.pdf. Accessed 07 May 2010

Waselenko JK, MacVittie TJ, Blakely WF, Pesik N, Wiley AL, Dickerson WE et al (2004) Medical management of the acute radiation syndrome: recommendations of the strategic national stockpile radiation working Group. Ann Intern Med 140(12):1037–1051

Weinstock DM, Case C Jr, Bader JL, Chao NJ, Coleman CN, Hatchett RJ et al (2008) Radiologic and nuclear events: contingency planning for hematologists/oncologists. Blood 111(12):5440–5445

Weisdorf D, Chao N, Waselenko JK, Dainiak N, Armitage JO, McNiece I et al (2006) Acute radiation injury: contingency planning for triage, supportive care, and transplantation. Biol Blood Marrow Transplant 12(6):672–682

Williams JP, Brown SL, Georges GE, Hauer-Jensen M, Hill RP, Huser AK, Kirsch DG, Macvittie TJ, Mason KA, Medhora MM, Moulder JE, Okunieff P, Otterson MF, Robbins ME, Smathers JB, McBride WH (2010) Animal models for medical countermeasures to radiation exposure. Radiat Res 173(4):557–578

Wilkins RC, Romm H, Kao TC, Awa AA, Yoshida MA, Livingston GK, Jenkins MS, Oestereicher U, Pellmar TC, Prasanna PGS (2008) Inter-laboratory comparison of the dicentric chromosome assay for radiation biodosimetry in mass casualty events. Radiat Res 169:551–560

Xiao Z, Su Y, Yang S, Yin L, Wang W, Yi Y, Fenton BM, Zhang L, Okunieff P (2006) Protective effect of esculentoside A on radiation-induced dermatitis and fibrosis. Int J Radiat Oncol Biol Phys 65(3):882–889

Zhang H, Zhang SB, Sun W, Yang S, Zhang M, Wang W, Liu C, Zhang K, Swarts S, Fenton BM, Keng P, Maguire D, Okunieff P, Zhang L (2009) B1 sequence-based real-time quantitative PCR: a sensitive method for direct measurement of mouse plasma DNA levels after gamma irradiation. Int J Radiat Oncol Biol Phys 74(5):1592–1599

MIX
Papier aus verantwortungsvollen Quellen
Paper from responsible sources
FSC® C105338

If you have any concerns about our products,
you can contact us on
ProductSafety@springernature.com

In case Publisher is established outside the EU,
the EU authorized representative is:
Springer Nature Customer Service Center GmbH
Europaplatz 3, 69115 Heidelberg, Germany

Printed by Libri Plureos GmbH
in Hamburg, Germany